Encyclopedia of
Nursing Education

Mary Jane Smith, PhD, RN, earned bachelor's and master's degrees from the University of Pittsburgh and a doctorate from New York University. She has held faculty positions at the following nursing schools: University of Pittsburgh, Duquesne University, Cornell University-New York Hospital, and the Ohio State University; and she is currently professor of nursing at West Virginia University School of Nursing. She has been teaching theory to nursing students at the master's and doctoral levels for over three decades.

Roger D. Carpenter, PhD, RN, CNE, earned a bachelor's degree from Kent State University, a master's degree from Case Western Reserve University, and a doctorate from West Virginia University. He has held staff development positions at University Hospitals of Cleveland, and faculty positions at Wheeling Jesuit University and at West Virginia University School of Nursing. He is currently assistant professor and teaches courses in adult health and leadership at the undergraduate and graduate levels.

Joyce J. Fitzpatrick, PhD, MBA, RN, FAAN, is Elizabeth Brooks Ford Professor of Nursing, Frances Payne Bolton School of Nursing, Case Western Reserve University where she was dean for 15 years. She has been involved in nursing education for over four decades, teaching nursing at the undergraduate, master's, and doctoral levels, and developing a range of innovative nursing education programs. She has published several books with Springer Publishing Company, including three editions of the *Encyclopedia of Nursing Research*.

Encyclopedia of Nursing Education

Mary Jane Smith, PhD, RN

Roger D. Carpenter, PhD, RN, CNE

Joyce J. Fitzpatrick, PhD, MBA, RN, FAAN

SPRINGER PUBLISHING COMPANY

NEW YORK

Springer Publishing Company, LLC
11 West 42nd Street
New York, NY 10036
www.springerpub.com

Acquisitions Editor: Margaret Zuccarini
Composition: Newgen Knowledge Works

ISBN: 978-0-8261-2031-1
e-book ISBN: 978-0-8261-2032-8

Instructor's materials are available by contacting textbook@springerpub.com

15 16 17 18 / 5 4 3 2 1

The author and the publisher of this Work have made every effort to use sources believed to be reliable to provide information that is accurate and compatible with the standards generally accepted at the time of publication. Because medical science is continually advancing, our knowledge base continues to expand. Therefore, as new information becomes available, changes in procedures become necessary. We recommend that the reader always consult current research and specific institutional policies before performing any clinical procedure. The author and publisher shall not be liable for any special, consequential, or exemplary damages resulting, in whole or in part, from the readers' use of, or reliance on, the information contained in this book. The publisher has no responsibility for the persistence or accuracy of URLs for external or third-party Internet websites referred to in this publication and does not guarantee that any content on such websites is, or will remain, accurate or appropriate.

Library of Congress Cataloging-in-Publication Data

Encyclopedia of nursing education / [edited by] Mary Jane Smith, Roger Carpenter, Joyce Fitzpatrick.
   p. ; cm.
Includes bibliographical references and index.
ISBN 978-0-8261-2031-1 — ISBN 978-0-8261-2032-8
I. Smith, Mary Jane, editor. II. Carpenter, Roger (Roger D.), editor. III. Fitzpatrick, Joyce J., editor.
[DNLM: 1. Education, Nursing—Encyclopedias—English. WY 13]
RT21
610.7303—dc23   2014044297

Printed in the United States of America by Bradford & Bigelow.

To Ursula Springer, president of Springer Publishing Company from 1970 to 2004, for her unfailing support of nursing education, research, and professional practice. And for her continued investment in new and experienced nurse authors.

Dr. Springer has left a legacy for nurse educators throughout the world, in her commitment to advancing the profession through dissemination of the best work available, and for her risk-taking and cutting-edge ideas about what nursing could be and what nurses might provide to their patients and communities.

Dr. Springer was the exemplary educator, striving for excellence, and pushing the boundaries open for nurses, nurse scientists, and especially nurse educators.

With gratitude . . .

CONTENTS

PREFACE

The growing demand for well-prepared nurse educators was a key factor in our decision to launch this first edition of the *Encyclopedia of Nursing Education*. Furthermore, we were aware of the success of the *Encyclopedia of Nursing Research* (now in its third edition) and the use of encyclopedias in other academic disciplines. We believe that this compilation of the key content will provide a valuable reference and source of important information for nurse educators. To prepare this work, we reviewed all six volumes of the *Annual Review of Nursing Education (ARNE*; published by Springer, 2003–2008) and the three most recent years of the two leading nursing education journals: *Journal of Nursing Education JNE* and *Nursing Education Perspectives NEP*. These reviews were used to compile a list of topics and potential authors. Then, colleague recommendations were solicited for additional topics and potential authors.

The book will be most useful to new nurse educators and to students in graduate programs in nursing education, either at the master's or doctoral level. In addition, the encyclopedia will serve as a resource for all levels of faculty in schools of nursing. For each entry, the reader will have a beginning introduction to a topic along with both the most recent and the classic references relevant to nursing education. The alphabetical ordering of entries offers the reader ease in locating a topic. For consistency and comparison, each topic is organized using the following headings: Definition, Application, Synopsis, and Recommendations. This consistent format for all entries gives the reader focused information on the topic and facilitates understandings across topics, particularly when there are related topics in large content areas such as simulation and mentoring.

The Editors

ACKNOWLEDGMENTS

This work would not have been possible without the support and contributions of a number of persons. First, we would like to acknowledge the work of Tracy Hudgins who assisted in the review of the previous publications, identifying potential topics and authors through the *ARNE, NEP,* and *JNE.* This was a significant part of Tracy's doctoral practicum in nursing education. Importantly, we would like to acknowledge the nurse educators who wrote the entries. Their dedication to scholarship in nursing education is evident in their work. We thank all of them for their contributions to the book. We thank Margaret Zuccarini and Joanne Jay at Springer Publishing Company for their guidance and thoughtful review of this work. This work was indeed a team effort and we are immensely proud of each person who made a difference to our work.

Contributors

Roxanne Amerson, PhD, RN, CNE, CTN-A
Assistant Professor
School of Nursing
Clemson University
Greenville, SC

Daniella Arieli, PhD
Senior Lecturer
Department of Nursing/Sociology and
    Anthropology
Max Stern Yezreel Valley College
Emek Yezreel, Israel

Yolanda Babenko-Mould, PhD, RN
Assistant Professor
Arthur Labatt Family School of Nursing
Western University
London, Ontario, Canada

Barbara H. Baker, PhD, RN
Assistant Professor
Department of Nursing
University of Central Missouri
Warrensburg, MO

Janet M. Banks, MSN, RN
Instructor
School of Nursing
University of Portland
Portland, OR

Diane M. Billings, EdD, RN, FAAN, ANEF
Chancellor's Professor Emeritus
Indiana University School of Nursing
Indianapolis, IN

Pamela L. Bonnett, MSN, RN
Instructor
School of Nursing
College of Health Professions
The University of Akron
Akron, OH

Carol Boswell, EdD, RN, CNE, ANEF
Professor
James A. "Buddy" Davidson Charitable
    Foundation Endowed Chair for
    Evidence-Based Practice
Codirector of the Center of Excellence in
    Evidence-Based Practice
School of Nursing
Texas Tech University Health Sciences Center
Odessa, TX

Diane M. Breckenridge, PhD, RN, ANEF
Professor and Director Nursing Workforce
    Strategies for Success Program
School of Nursing and Health Science
La Salle University
Philadelphia, PA

Remylin S. Bruder, DNP, RN
Dean of Nursing
Rochester College
Rochester Hills, MI

Carrie Buch, PhD, RN
Associate Professor
School of Nursing
Oakland University
Rochester, MI

Ellen B. Buckner, PhD, RN, CNE
Professor
College of Nursing
University of South Alabama
Mobile, AL

Corazon B. Cajulis, DNP, RN, ANP-BC, NEA-BC
Nurse Practitioner
The Tisch Cancer Institute
The Mount Sinai Hospital
New York, NY

Theresa M. Campo, DNP, APRN, FNP-C, ENP-BC
Assistant Professor Graduate Nursing
Coordinator Family Nurse Practitioner Program
School of Nursing
Felician College
Lodi, NJ

Carli A. Carnish, MSN, RN, AGNP-C
Clinical Faculty
Frances Payne Bolton School of Nursing
Case Western Reserve University
Cleveland, OH

Roger D. Carpenter, PhD, RN, CNE
Assistant Professor
School of Nursing
West Virgnia University
Morgantown, WV

Freida Chavez, DNP, MHSc, RN
Director, Global Affairs Office
Senior Lecturer
Lawrence Bloomberg Faculty of Nursing and
    Dalla Lana School of Public Health
University of Toronto
Toronto, Ontario, Canada

Laura H. Clayton, PhD, RN, CNE
Professor of Nursing Education
Department of Nursing Education
Shepherd University
Shepherdstown, WV

Elizabeth R. Click, ND, RN, CWP
Medical Director
Case Western Reserve University
Assistant Professor
Frances Payne Bolton School of Nursing
Case Western Reserve University
Cleveland, OH

Jaclyn Conelius, PhD, FNP-BC
Assistant Professor
Fairfield University
School of Nursing
Fairfield, CT

Frances H. Cornelius, PhD, RN-BC, CNE
Clinical Professor of Nursing
College of Nursing and Health Professions
Drexel University
Philadelphia, PA

Marie Cox, DNP, RN, NP-BC
Clinical Assistant Professor of Nursing
Adelphi University
Garden City, NY
Assistant Director of Nursing Administration
North Shore—LIJ Medical Center
New Hyde Park, NY

Susan B. Coyle, PhD, RN
Teaching Assistant Professor
Coordinator, Rural Health Education
WVU School of Nursing
West Virginia University
Morgantown, WV

Sandra Davidson, PhD, RN
Assistant Professor
Faculty of Nursing
University of Alberta
Edmonton, Alberta, Canada

Kathleen de Leon, BSN, RN
Masters Student—Health Policy Nursing
University of California, San Francisco
San Francisco, CA
Registered Nurse
Santa Clara Valley Medical Center
San Jose, CA

Barbara DeVoe, DNP, FNP-BC
Vice President for Interprofessional Education
and Learning
Director of The Patient Safety Institute
North Shore—LIJ Health System
Center for Learning and Innovation
Assistant Professor of Science Education
Hofstra North Shore—LIJ School of Medicine
Lake Success, NY

John Distler, DPA, MBA, MS, FNP-C, FAANP
Dean
Nurse Practitioner Tracks
Chamberlain College of Nursing
Westminster, MD

Mary A. Dolansky, PhD, RN
Associate Professor
Case Western Reserve University
Frances Payne Bolton School of Nursing
Cleveland, OH

Ruby K. Dunlap, EdD, APRN-BC
Professor of Nursing
School of Nursing
Belmont University
Nashville, TN

Karen S. Dunn, PhD, RN, FGSA
Associate Professor
School of Nursing
Oakland University
Rochester, MI

Emerson E. Ea, DNP, APRN, CNE
Clinical Assistant Professor
College of Nursing
New York University
New York, NY

Ruth A. Eby, MSN, RNC
Chair
Associate Dean
School of Nursing
Indiana Wesleyan University
Marion, IN

Debbie Faulk, PhD, RN
Professor of Nursing
RN to BSN (EARN) Coordinator
Auburn University Montgomery School of
Nursing
Auburn University Montgomery
Montgomery, AL

Joyce J. Fitzpatrick, PhD, MBA, RN, FAAN
Elizabeth Brooks Ford Professor of Nursing
Frances Payne Bolton School of Nursing
Case Western Reserve University
Cleveland, OH

Lisa Sue Flood, DNP, RN, CNE
Professor
School of Nursing
Northern Michigan University
Marquette, MI

**M. Isabel Friedman, DNP, MPA, RN, BC,
CCRN, CNN, CHSE**
Program Director Nurse Fellowship Programs
North Shore—LIJ Health System
The Center for Learning and Innovation
Lake Success, NY
Assistant Professor of Science Education
Hofstra North Shore—LIJ School of Medicine
Hempstead, NY

Kari Gali, DNP, RN, CPNP
Pediatric Nurse Practitioner
Be Well Kids
Cleveland Clinic Children's Hospital
Cleveland, OH

Kelly A. Gallagher, MSN, RN
Program Director
Professional Nursing Practice Innovations
Center for Professional Nursing Practice
New York Presbyterian Hospital
New York, NY

Mary Joy Garcia-Dia, MA, RN
Director, Clinical Applications, Information
Technology
Mount Sinai Health System
New York, NY
Adjunct Faculty
New York University College of Nursing
New York, NY

Faye Gary, EdD, MS, RN, FAAN
The Medical Mutual of Ohio Kent W. Clapp Chair
Professor of Nursing
Frances Payne Bolton School of Nursing
Case Western Reserve University
Cleveland, OH

Sally O. Gerard, DNP, RN
Associate Professor
School of Nursing
Fairfield University
Trumbull, CT

Sarah E. Givens, BSN, RN
Doctoral Student
Frances Payne Bolton School of Nursing
Case Western Reserve University
Painesville, OH

Robin S. Goodrich, EdD, RN
Dean
Chamberlain College of Nursing
North Brunswick, NJ

Mary Grady, MSN, RN, CNE, CHSE
Assistant Professor
Lorain County Community College
Elyria, OH

Mary T. Quinn Griffin, PhD, RN, FAAN, ANEF
Associate Professor
Frances Payne Bolton School of Nursing
Case Western Reserve University
Cleveland, OH

Claudia Grobbel, DNP, RN, CNL
Assistant Professor
School of Nursing
Oakland University
Rochester Hills, MI

Cynthia Hadenfeldt, EdD, RN
Assistant Professor
College of Nursing
Creighton University
Omaha, NE

Lourance Abdul Razzaq Enad Alzyarah Al Hadid, PhD, RN, CCN
Assistant Professor
Al-Ghad International College for Applied Medical Sciences
Nursing Department
Tabouk Campus- Male
Tabouk, Saudi Arabia

Ann Hallyburton, MSLS, MPH, AHIP
Research and Instruction Librarian, Liaison to the Health and Human Sciences
Hunter Library
Western Carolina University
Cullowhee, NC

Vicki Sullivan Hannah, MSN, APRN, FNP-BC
Nursing Faculty
Department of Nursing
Shelton State Community College
Tuscaloosa, AL

Gerardina Harnett, M Comm, MSc, LLB, RN, RM, RPHN, RNT, RNP
Head of Department of Nursing and Health Care Sciences
Department of Nursing and Health Care Sciences
Institute of Technology
Tralee, County Kerry, Ireland

Margaret A. Harris PhD, RN
Associate Professor
School of Nursing
Oakland University
Rochester, MI

Barbara E. Harrison, PhD, APRN, FNP-BC
Associate Professor of Nursing
College of Health Sciences
West Chester University of Pennsylvania
West Chester, PA

Susan D. Hart, PhD, RN
Chair and Assistant Professor
Department of Collaborative Nursing Care
College of Nursing
The University of Southern Mississippi
Hattiesburg, MS

Patricia Hartley, MSN, RN
Assistant Professor
School of Nursing
Indiana Wesleyan University
Marion, IN

April Richardson Hatcher, PhD
Associate Professor
Anatomy and Neurobiology Department
College of Medicine
Chandler Medical Center
University of Kentucky
Lexington, KY

Barbara Head, PhD, CHPN, ACSW, FPCN
Associate Professor
University of Louisville School of Medicine
Louisville, KY

Catrina Heffernan, MSc, RNT, RN
Doctoral Student
Department of Nursing and Health Care Studies
Institute of Technology Tralee
Tralee, Co. Kerry, Ireland

Josephine Hegarty, PhD, RNT, RGN
Professor of Nursing
Director of Graduate Studies
Catherine McAuley School of Nursing and
    Midwifery
University College Cork
Cork, Ireland

Judith W. Herrman, PhD, RN, ANEF, FAAN
Professor
School of Nursing
University of Delaware
Newark, DE

Ronald L. Hickman, Jr., PhD, RN, ACNP-BC
Assistant Professor
School of Nursing
Case Western Reserve University
Acute Care Nurse Practitioner
Department of Anesthesiology and Perioperative
    Medicine
University Hospitals Case Medical Center
Cleveland, OH

Josiane Hickson, EdD, RN, NE-BC
Director of Nursing, Emergency Services
St. John's Riverside Hospital
Adjunct Associate Professor
Teachers College, Columbia University
New York, NY

Patricia Hodges, MSN, RN
Assistant Professor
School of Nursing
Indiana Wesleyan University
Marion, IN

Catherine Houghton, PhD, MHSc, RGN, RCN
Lecturer
School of Nursing and Midwifery
Áras Moyola
National University of Ireland
Galway, Ireland

Therese Hulme, ARNP, FNP-BC
Doctoral Student
Case Western Reserve University
Cleveland, OH

Immaculata N. Igbo, PhD
Associate Professor
College of Nursing
Prairie View A&M University
Houston, TX

Sonya L. Jakubec, MN, RN
Associate Professor
School of Nursing and Midwifery
Faculty of Health and Community Studies
Mount Royal University
Calgary, Alberta, Canada

Marianne R. Jeffreys, EdD, RN
Professor, Nursing
Graduate College and College of Staten Island
The City University of New York (CUNY)
Staten Island, NY

Janet H. Johnson, MA, ANP-BC, ACNP, FAANP
Acute Care Nurse Practitioner
The Mount Sinai Hospital
Saugerties, NY

Elsie A. Jolade, DNP, RN, FNP-BC, CCRN
Clinical Nurse Specialist
Cardiac Service Line
New York Presbyterian Hospital
The University Hospital of Columbia and Cornell
Adjunct Assistant Professor of Nursing
Hunter-Bellevue School of Nursing
The City University of New York
New York, NY

Amy Jones, MSN, RN
Assistant Professor
Director for Associate Degree of Nursing
    Program
Mercy College of Nursing and Health Sciences
    Southwest Baptist University
Springfield, MO

Janice M. Jones, PhD, RN, CNS
Clinical Professor
Coordinator
MS Nursing Leadership and Health Care Systems
University at Buffalo, School of Nursing
Buffalo, NY

Karen D. Joris, MSN, RN
Assistant Professor
Associate Degree Nursing Program
Lorain County Community College
Elyria, OH

Rachel Joseph, PhD, CCRN
Assistant Professor
College of Health Sciences
West Chester University of Pennsylvania
West Chester, PA

Debbie Kane, PhD, RN
Associate Professor
Faculty of Nursing
University of Windsor
Windsor, Ontario, Canada

Karen A. Karlowicz, EdD, RN
Associate Professor and Chairperson
School of Nursing
Old Dominion University
Norfolk, VA

Irena L. Kenneley, PhD, APHRN-BC, CIC
Associate Professor
Faculty Development Director
Frances Payne Bolton School of Nursing
Case Western Reserve University
Cleveland, OH

Monica Metrick Kennison, EdD, RN
Professor
Wheeling Jesuit University
Wheeling, WV

Laura Killam, MScN, RN
Professor
School of Health Sciences and Emergency
  Services
Cambrian College
Sudbury, Ontario, Canada

Sheryl Kirk, MSN, APRN-C
Doctoral Student
Frances Payne Bolton School of Nursing
Case Western University
Cleveland, OH

**Robin Kirschner, EdD, RN, NEA-BC,
  CNE, CRA**
Dean, MSN Specialty Tracks
Associate Professor
Graduate Division
Chamberlain College of Nursing
Gilbert, AZ

Robin S. Krinsky, MSN, RN-BC, CCRN
Adjunct Instructor
Lehman College—Department of Nursing
The City University of New York
Bronx, New York

Aoife Lane, MSc, BNS, RNT, RGN
Doctoral Candidate
School of Nursing and Midwifery
University College Cork
Cork, Ireland

William T. Lecher, MS, MBA, RN, NE-BC
Senior Clinical Director
Patient Services
Cincinnati Children's Hospital Medical Center
Cincinnati, OH
Immediate Past President
American Assembly for Men in Nursing
Philadelphia, PA

**Seatbyul Diane Lee, DNP, ANP-BC, CCRN,
  OCN**
Assistant Professor
Molloy College
Rockville Centre, NY

Shirleatha T. Lee, PhD, RN, CNE
Associate Professor
Loewenberg School of Nursing
The University of Memphis
Memphis, TN

Julie C. Lehrer, MSN, APRN-BC, RN
Family Nurse Practitioner
Northern Ohio Medical Specialists
Sandusky, OH

Mary C. Lemp, DNP, ANP-BC
Senior Administrative Director of Cardiac
  Services
North Shore—LIJ Health System
Huntington Hospital
Huntington, NY
Adjunct Faculty
Adelphi University
School of Nursing
Garden City, NY
Assistant Clinical Faculty
Columbia University
School of Nursing
New York, NY

Lynne P. Lewallen, PhD, RN, ANEF, CNE
Professor and Assistant Dean for Academic
  Affairs
UNCG School of Nursing
The University of North Carolina at Greensboro
Greensboro, NC

Kezia Lilly, DNP, MBA, RN, HC
Nursing Administrator
Assistant Professor
Nursing Informatics Specialist Consultant
Department of Nursing and Health Sciences
Mercy College of Nursing and Health Sciences
Southwest Baptist University
Springfield, MO

Fidelindo A. Lim, DNP, CCRN
Clinical Faculty
New York University College of Nursing
New York, NY

Marilyn J. Lotas, PhD, RN, FAAN
Associate Professor
Frances Payne Bolton School of Nursing
Case Western Reserve University
Cleveland, OH

Kari L. Luoma, PhD, RN
Faculty Development Specialist
Chamberlain College of Nursing
Downers Grove, IL

Gina Maiocco, PhD, RN, CCNS
Clinical Associate Professor
School of Nursing
West Virginia University
Morgantown, WV

Deborah Mandel, PhD, RNC-OB
Assistant Professor
Department of Nursing
West Chester University of Pennsylvania
Ephrata, PA

Linda Mayne, PhD, RN
Associate Professor
College of Nursing
East Carolina University
Greenville, NC

Sarah McCloskey, MSc, RGN, BA (Hons),
  Doctoral Student, University College Cork
Director of Nursing and Allied Health Services
Marymount University Hospital and Hospice
Curraheen, Cork, Ireland

Deborah McElligott, DNP, ANP-BC, HWNC-BC
Voluntary Nurse Practitioner
Katz Institute of Women's Health
NSLIJ Health System
Lake Success, NY
Assistant Professor
Department of Science Education
Hofstra-North Shore--LIJ School of Medicine
Hempstead, NY

Dee McGonigle, PhD, RN, CNE, FAAN, ANEF
Chair, Virtual Learning Environments
Professor, Graduate Programs
Chamberlain College of Nursing
Dillon, SC

Tamara Hertenstein McKinnon, RN, DNP
Lecturer and Global Programs Chair
School of Nursing at San Jose State University
The Valley Foundation
San Jose, CA

Dawn McMeekin, DNP, RN
Assistant Professor
Department of Nursing
South University
Tampa, Fl

Maria A. Mendoza, EdD, RN, ANP,
  GNP-BC, CDE, CNE
Clinical Assistant Professor
Program Coordinator, Nursing Education
  Master's and Advanced Certificates
College of Nursing
New York University
New York, NY

Sharon Elizabeth Metcalfe, EdD, RN
Program Director—Nursing Network: Careers
  and Technology Program
Associate Professor
School of Nursing
Western Carolina University
Cullowhee, NC

Anne Marie Mitchell, PhD, RN, CNM, WHNP
Associate Professor
School of Nursing
Oakland University
Rochester, MI

Margory A. Molloy, MSN, RN, CNE, CHSE
Director
Center for Nursing Discovery
School of Nursing
Duke University
Durham, NC

Phyllis Montgomery, PhD, RN
Full Professor
School of Nursing
Laurentian University
Sudbury, Ontario, Canada

Cheryl Ann Monturo, PhD, RN, MBE, ACNP-BC
Associate Professor of Nursing
John A. Hartford Claire M. Fagin Fellow
Department of Nursing
West Chester University of Pennsylvania
West Chester, PA

Hope M. Moon, MSN, RN, CNS
Dean and Professor
Allied Health and Nursing
Lorain County Community College
Elyria, OH

Martha S. Morrow, MSN, RN, CNE
Associate Professor
Mercy College of Nursing
Southwest Baptist University
Springfield, MO

Nancy R. Mosser, EdD, RN
Chairperson/Professor
Department of Nursing
Waynesburg University
Waynesburg, PA

Sharolyn Mossey, MScN, RN
Assistant Professor
School of Nursing
Laurentian University
Sudbury, Ontario, Canada

Florence Myrick, PhD, RN
Professor Emerita
Faculty of Nursing
University of Alberta
Edmonton, Alberta, Canada

Jan M. Nick, PhD, RNC-OB, CNE, ANEF
Professor of Nursing
Director, Pipeline Program for a Diverse Nursing
  Workforce
School of Nursing
Loma Linda University
Loma Linda, CA

Kathleen M. Nokes, PhD, RN, FAAN
Professor Emerita
Hunter College and Graduate Center
City University of New York (CUNY)
New York, NY

Rachel Nye, MS, RN-C, CNE
Associate Professor
School of Nursing
Northern Michigan University
Marquette, MI

Marilyn H. Oermann, PhD, RN, ANEF, FAAN
Thelma M. Ingles Professor of Nursing and
  Director of Evaluation and Educational
  Research
School of Nursing
Duke University
Durham, NC

JoAnn S. Oliver, PhD, RN, ANP-BC, CNE
Associate Professor
Capstone College of Nursing
The University of Alabama
Tuscaloosa, AL

Debra O'Shaughnessy, MSN, RN
Faculty
Associate Degree Nursing Program
Lorain County Community College
Elyria, OH

Brian Parker, PhD, RN, RPN
Faculty
Psychiatric Nursing Program
Faculty of Health and Community Studies
MacEwan University
Edmonton, Alberta, Canada

Susan Pauly-O'Neill, DNP, RN, PPCNP
Assistant Professor of Nursing
School of Nursing and Health Professions
University of San Francisco
San Francisco, CA

Barbara Penprase, PhD, RN, CNE, ANEF
Professor
School of Nursing
OUSON/Crittenton Endowed Professor
Oakland University
Rochester, MI

Kathryn E. Phillips, PhD, RN, APRN
Assistant Professor
School of Nursing
Fairfield University
Fairfield, CT

Grant A. Pignatiello, BSN, RN
Doctoral Student
Frances Payne Bolton School of Nursing
Case Western Reserve University
Cleveland, OH

Letty R. Piper, EdD, RN
Adjunct Faculty
University of Pennsylvania
Assistant Professor
LaSalle University
Philadelphia, PA

Ellen Pokorny, MA, RN NEA-BC
Director—Nursing Education
North Shore—LIJ Plainview and Syosset
  Hospitals
Plainview, NY

Carole A. Pomarico, MSN, MA, RN
Adult Program Director
School of Nursing
Fairfield University
Fairfield, CT

**Cathlin Buckingham Poronsky, PhD, RN,
  APRN, FNP-BC**
Assistant Professor and Director—Family Nurse
  Practitioner Program
Marcella Niehoff School of Nursing
Loyola University Chicago
Chicago, IL

Patricia Prufeta, MS, RN, NEA-BC
Director of Surgical Nursing
New York-Presbyterian Hospital
New York, NY

Theresa Tavella Quell, PhD, RN
Assistant Dean for Academic Programs
School of Nursing
Fairfield University
Fairfield, CT

Deborah A. Raines, PhD, EdS, RN, ANEF
Associate Professor
School of Nursing
University at Buffalo (SUNY)
Buffalo, NY

Anthony R. Ramsey, PhD, RN, FNP
Assistant Professor and Director
Waldron College of Health and Human Services
School of Nursing
Radford University
Radford, VA

Janet Resop Reilly, DNP, RN, APRN-BC
Associate Professor and Director
MSN Leadership and Management in Health
  Systems
Professional Programs in Nursing
University of Wisconsin
Green Bay, WI

Anita C. Reinhardt, PhD, RN
Associate Director of Undergraduate Programs
Associate Professor
College of Health and Social Services
School of Nursing
New Mexico State University
Las Cruces, NM

Deanna L. Reising, PhD, RN, ACNS-BC, ANEF
Associate Professor
School of Nursing
Indiana University
Bloomington, IN

Amy Reiterman, MSN, RN
Clinical Informaticist, Information Technology
Mount Sinai Health System
New York, NY

Cheryl Riley-Doucet, PhD, RN, FGSA
Associate Professor
School of Nursing
Oakland University
Rochester, MI

Teresa D. Ritchie, DNP, RN, APRN, FNP-BC
Senior Lecturer
School of Nursing, West Virginia University
Morgantown, WV

Reynaldo R. Rivera, DNP, RN, NEA-BC, FAAN
Director of Nursing Research and Innovations
Center for Professional Nursing Practice
Department of Nursing
New York-Presbyterian Hospital
New York, NY

Tonya Rutherford-Hemming, EdD, RN, ANP-BC, CHSE
Senior Nurse Researcher
Office of Nursing Research and Innovation
Cleveland Clinic
Cleveland, OH

Darlene M. Salas, MSN, RN, ANP
DNP Student
Frances Payne Bolton School of Nursing
Case Western Reserve University
Cleveland, OH

Medel Salvador-Paguirigan, EdD, RN, CNE, CNN
Senior Manager
Nursing Research and Education
The Mount Sinai Hospital
New York, NY

Susan Sanner, PhD, RN, APRN, FNP-BC, CNE
Senior Manager of Graduate Practicum Operations
Family Nurse Practitioner Program
Chamberlain College of Nursing
Morrow, GA

Judith M. Scanlan, PhD, RN
Associate Professor
Faculty of Health Sciences
College of Nursing
University of Manitoba
Winnipeg, Manitoba, Canada

Maura C. Schlairet, EdD, MA, MSN, RN, CNL
Associate Professor of Nursing and Bioethicist
College of Nursing and Health Sciences
Valdosta State University
Valdosta, GA

Cheryl D. Schlamb, DNP, RN, CRNP
Assistant Professor
Graduate Coordinator
Department of Nursing
West Chester University of PA
West Chester, PA

Cheryl K. Schmidt, PhD, RN, CNE, ANEF, FAAN
Associate Professor
College of Nursing
University of Arkansas for Medical Sciences
Little Rock, AR

Terri L. Schmitt, PhD, RN, ARNP, FNP-BC, CDE
Assistant Professor
Family Nurse Practitioner Track
Chamberlain College of Nursing
Boynton Beach, FL

Patricia L. Schrull, MSN, MBA, MEd, RN, CNE
Professor and Nursing Programs Administrator
Lorain County Community College
Elyria, OH

Patricia A. Sharpnack, DNP, RN, CNE, NEA-BC, ANEF
Dean and Strawbridge Professor
Ursuline College
The Breen School of Nursing
Pepper Pike, OH

Teresa Shellenbarger, PhD, RN, CNE, ANEF
Professor
Department of Nursing and Allied Health Professions
Indiana University of Pennsylvania
Indiana, PA

Rebecca J. Sisk, PhD, RN, CNE
Associate Professor
Online MSN Program
Chamberlain College of Nursing
Downers Grove, IL

Larry Z. Slater, PhD, RN-BC, CCRN
Clinical Assistance Professor
College of Nursing
New York University
New York, NY

Suzanne C. Smeltzer, EdD, RN, FAAN
Professor and Director
Center for Nursing Research
College of Nursing
Villanova University
Villanova, PA

Jackie A. Smith, PhD
Professor (Clinical)
College of Nursing
University of Utah
Salt Lake City, UT

Mary Jane Smith, PhD, RN
Professor of Nursing
School of Nursing, West Virginia University
Morgantown, WV

Angel Smothers, DNP, RN, FNP-BC, RN
Senior Lecturer, School of Nursing
School of Nursing, West Virginia University
Morgantown, WV

Azizeh Sowan, PhD
Faculty of Nursing
Department of Adult Health Nursing
The Hashemite University
Zarqua, Jordan

Lauraine Spano-Szekely, MBA, RN
Senior Vice President Patient Care Services and
    Chief Nursing Officer
Northern Westchester Hospital Center
Mount Kisco, NY

Pam Springer, PhD, RN, CEN, ANEF
Director
Clinical Learning Services
St. Luke's Health System
Boise, ID

Lori Stier, EdD, RN
Assistant Vice President
Institute for Clinical Excellence and Quality
North Shore—LIJ Health System
Lake Success, NY

Sharon L. Strang, DNP, RN, APRN, FNP-BC
Associate Professor
School of Nursing
James Madison University
Harrisonburg, VA

Martha Summers, DNP, RN, FNP-BC
MSN/DNP Program Director
School of Nursing, West Virginia University
Morgantown, WV

Siobhan Sundel, DNP, RN, GNP-BC, ANP
Geriatric Nurse Practitioner
Coffey Geriatric Associates at the Martha Stewart
    Center for Living
Mount Sinai Hospital
Lab Coordinator
Physical Assessment Lab for Nurse Practitioner
    Students
New York University
New York, NY

Karen Gahan Tarnow, PhD, RN
Clinical Associate Professor
School of Nursing
University of Kansas
Kansas City, KS

George E. Thibault, MD
President
Josiah Macy Jr. Foundation
New York, NY

Christine M. Thomas, PhD, RN
Associate Professor
Department of Nursing
West Chester University of Pennsylvania
West Chester, PA

Brent W. Thompson, PhD, RN
Associate Professor
Department of Nursing
West Chester University of Pennsylvania
West Chester, PA

Carolyn Kollar Tieppo, DNP, RN, CPNP-PC
Special Instructor
School of Nursing
Oakland University
Rochester, MI

Susan Peck Tipperman, MSN, RN, CCM
Adjunct Faculty
Department of Nursing
West Chester University of Pennsylvania
West Chester, PA

Jacqueline Vaughn, BSN, RN, CHSE
Clinical Lab Instructor
Duke University School of Nursing
Center for Nursing Discovery
Durham, NC

Maria L. Vezina, EdD, RN, NEA-BC
Vice President, Nursing/Chief Nursing Officer
Mount Sinai St. Luke's
New York, NY

Suzy Mascaro Walter, PhD, RN, FNP-BC, CNRN
Assistant Professor
School of Nursing, West Virginia University
Health Sciences South
Morgantown, WV

Kathryn S. Whitcomb, DNP, RN, CHSE
Simulation Center Coordinator and Assistant
   Professor
School of Nursing and School of Pharmacy
Texas Tech University Health Sciences Center
Abilene, TX

Mary A. White, PhD, RN
Lecturer
Wellstar School of Nursing
Kennesaw State University
Kennesaw, GA

**Barbara L. Morrison Wilford, MSN, MBA/
   HCA, RN**
Associate Professor
Allied Health and Nursing
Lorain County Community College
Elyria, OH

Tami H. Wyatt, PhD, RN, CNE, ANEF, FAAN
Associate Professor and Director of Graduate
   Studies
Chair of Master's Program
Chair of Educational Technology and Simulation
Codirector
Health Information Technology and
   Simulation Lab
University of Tennessee, Knoxville
Knoxville, TN

**Patricia S. Yoder-Wise, EdD, RN, NEA-BC,
   ANEF, FAAN**
President
The Wise Group
Faculty
Texas Tech University Health Sciences Center
   School of Nursing
Lubbock, TX

Olive Yonge, PhD, RN
Professor
Faculty of Nursing
University of Alberta
Edmonton, Alberta, Canada

Margarete L. Zalon, PhD, RN, ACNS-BC, FAAN
Professor
Director, Health Informatics Program
Department of Nursing
University of Scranton
Scranton, PA

Jean Ellen Zavertnik, DNP, RN, ACNS-BC, CNE
Simulation Director and Lecturer
School of Nursing
Clemson University
Clemson, SC

Brenda K. Zierler, PhD, RN, FAAN
Professor, Biobehavioral Nursing
   and Health Systems
University of Washington School of Nursing
Codirector, Center for Health Sciences
Interprofessional Education, Practice, and Research
Director of Faculty Development, Institute for
   Simulation and Interprofessional Studies
University of Washington
Seattle, WA

List of Entries

A

ACADEMIC ADVISING

DEFINITION

Academic advising is a dynamic process that is executed in order to facilitate student development and assist in the formulation of long-term professional goals. The primary purpose of academic advising is to guide students in developing educational goals that will further enable them to achieve life aspirations (Harrison, 2009a). Academic advising is an important faculty role that is an integral part of the student experience where choices are made about personal and career goals (Schultz, 1998). Students are navigated through the experience of developing a meaningful program of study, becoming informed of administrative procedures of the institution, promoting the development of long-term personal and professional aspirations, and providing students with referrals when deemed necessary (Harrison, 2009a).

APPLICATION

Effective academic advising is central to the success of the nursing student in order to gain foundational knowledge of the degree program and other general education requirements of the institution. The roles and duties of the academic adviser have often been viewed as bureaucratic, involving tedious record keeping and ensuring that students have fulfilled major requirements for graduation (Harrison, 2009b). In contrast, advisers play a significant role in student development and academic success, which makes effective advising a well-paying investment for the student and the institution (Harrison, 2009b).

There are several models used as frameworks to guide the advising of practice and research. One model is the prescriptive model in which the adviser relationship is used as a means of control for dispensing information on technical matters. Another model is customer service where students' needs are met by providing responsive services and support (Schultz, 1998). Advising has also been used as a model of teaching where all of the characteristics that make an exemplary teacher are put into practice for effective advising. Developmental advising, based on developmental principles, is a goal-directed and continuous process (Schultz, 1998). Schultz (1998), in the theory of modeling and role modeling, offers an effective framework to practice academic advising. In modeling, the adviser seeks understanding of the student's view of the world and then frames advising issues from the student's perspective.

Harrison (2009a) notes that advising interventions should be aimed at building trust, encouraging positive orientation, promoting control, acknowledging strengths, and setting mutual goals for success. In addition, the adviser needs to be: accessible, knowledgeable, focused on academic requirements, reliable, and one who shows respect for the learner (Kearney, 1994). Advising of a nursing student presents challenges based on: course sequence for the major, designation of course sections, and frequency of visits by the student to the adviser. The role of the academic adviser is a complex one, requiring a certain degree of clinical and academic competence, as well as personal qualities of creativity, flexibility, and good communication skills (Sobralske & Naegele, 2001).

SYNOPSIS

Literature shows that advising needs of students who hold a degree and are advancing toward a higher degree differ from those of traditional students entering a college/university for a first professional degree (Wendler, Fyans, & Kirkbride, 2013). Trent (1997) recommends that academic advising for adult students should follow constructs of adult learning encompassing a caring attitude, problem-solving strategies, attentiveness to student issues, and realistic expectations. Few studies in the nursing literature have addressed the unique needs of career-oriented nurses who are seeking a higher degree.

RECOMMENDATIONS

Research on the nature of the adviser–advisee relationship is at an early stage (Harrison, 2009b). There is a definite need to revitalize and redefine academic advisement. Ongoing research studies are needed to increase knowledge and awareness of the issues and needs of nursing students at all phases of their educational and career development. Harrison (2009a) recommends that undergraduate academic advising responsibilities can be shared with teaching assistants. This incorporation of peer advising could be a course requirement for graduate students and may assist in preparing nurse educators for an essential component of the role. However, there are privacy and confidentiality issues with peer advising. Academic advisers should continue to develop knowledge and self-awareness about the advising process in relation to the adviser–student relationship (Harrison, 2009a).

Harrison, E. (2009a). (Re)Visiting academic advising. *Nurse Educator, 34*(2), 64–68.

Harrison, E. (2009b). Faculty perceptions of academic advising: "I don't get no respect." *Nursing Education Perspectives, 30*(1), 229–233.

Kearney, R. T. (1994). Academic advisement and the RN-to-BSN student. *The Journal of Continuing Education in Nursing, 25*(1), 11–16.

Schultz, E. (1998). Academic advising from a nursing theory perspective. *Nurse Educator, 23*(2), 22–25.

Sobralske, M., & Naegele, L. M. (2001). Worth their weight in gold: The role of clinical coordinator in a family nurse practitioner program. *Journal of the American Academy of Nurse Practitioners, 13*(12), 537–544.

Trent, B. A. (1997). Student perceptions of academic advising in an RN-to-BSN program. *The Journal of Continuing Education in Nursing, 28*(6), 276–283.

Wendler, M. C., Fyans, P. M., & Kirkbride, G. (2013). No more "fumbling alone": Effect of a nurse-led academic advising service in a magnet hospital. *The Journal of Continuing Education in Nursing, 44*(5), 218–224.

Julie C. Lehrer
Mary T. Quinn Griffin

ACADEMIC DISHONESTY

DEFINITION

Academic dishonesty (AD) refers to "students giving or receiving unauthorized assistance in an academic exercise (all forms or work submitted for credit hours) or receiving credit for work that is not their own" (Kibler, Nuss, Patterson, & Pavela, 1988, p. 1). In contrast, academic integrity (AI) is "a commitment, even in the face of adversity, to five fundamental values; honor, trust, fairness, respect and responsibility" (Centre for Academic Integrity, 2014).

Common forms of AD that can occur together or alone include plagiarism (using another's words or ideas without appropriate recognition of the source); fabrication (making up data or information); falsification (falsely manipulating and reporting data or results); misrepresentation (falsifying personal identity, paying for someone to complete assignments, and/or purchasing papers or projects); and cheating (using or attempting to use unauthorized methods or information). Common forms of "e-cheating" (Rogers, 2006) include collusion (the most common form of online cheating) and technology manipulation (citing untrue technology problems).

APPLICATION

All forms of AD are universally recognized and common across all levels of education worldwide. While online courses have increased in popularity and have become a valid means of formal education, research indicates that online courses do not yield higher rates of AD (Spaulding, 2009). Faculty and students both admit that AD occurs and agree that some types are more serious than others. Each form of AD represents a serious breach in ethical behavior that many faculty members are reluctant to deal with; however, many students believe that it is acceptable. Damaged school reputations, unfair advantage for dishonest students, repeat cheating, and backlash to honest students are immediate and delayed concerns (Josien & Broderick, 2013).

The rate at which AD occurs across all levels of nursing education (70%–95%) is disheartening (Kolanko et al., 2006; LaDuke, 2013). McCabe (2009) reported higher rates among nursing undergraduates than those in other disciplines, with highest rates among accelerated bachelor of science in nursing (BSN) students—77% versus 58% for all nursing undergraduates. A major concern for nursing is that dishonesty will transcend into unethical clinical practice (LaDuke, 2013) where dishonest behaviors can have "potentially dire consequences" (DiBartolo, 2010, p. 543). Jeffreys and Stier (1995) developed a conceptual model to assist nurse educators define, prevent, and confront AD. An updated version illustrates the interaction among predisposing factors, student and educator behaviors, and potential outcomes

impacting the profession (Jeffreys & Stier, 2004). Whatever the cause, circumstance, rate, or setting, it is incumbent to develop proactive approaches to AD.

SYNOPSIS

The following main assumptions about student AD (SAD) provide a framework for understanding complexities, issues, and guidance for faculty action (Jeffreys & Stier, 1995, 2004). SAD is a widespread problem affecting all disciplines including nursing; it can be damaging to future professional development; it may adversely affect client care; AI, professionalism, and quality health care are important values to the nursing profession and society; and PROACTIVE communication is the key strategy to prevent and confront dishonest behavior.

PROACTIVE communication focuses on *Policy*, *Responsibility*, *Ongoing* action, *Accountability*, *Commitment*, *Trust*, *Initiative*, *Values*, and *Expectations*, and is aimed at creating a culture of AI. This is the core of the solution. Clearly communicating what constitutes AD and ways to avoid it include clearcut and accessible definitions and policies in syllabi and handbooks, required tutorials and orientations, self-assessment quizzes, case examples of workplace dishonesty, AI peer educators, posters and slogans, hyperlinks to AI websites and resources, honor codes, anti-plagiarism software, online passwords, and just-in-time reminders (beginning of test or online submission of an assignment; Gallant, 2011; Griffith, 2013; McGee, 2013). Incorporating learner-centered education and varying methods of student evaluation also discourage AD. Institutionalizing AI through centralized organizational structures and processes that support a culture of AI and address AD incidents is essential (Gallant, 2011).

RECOMMENDATIONS

Administrators need to take the lead by recognizing that AD is a serious problem and make a commitment to foster a culture of AI.

Schools should aim to infuse the values of AI into the structures, processes, and culture of the organization so that ethical behavior is supported (Gallant, 2011). Faculty members must acknowledge their role in promoting AI and be supported by their administrators and peers. Resources such as an Office for Academic Integrity and a designated administrator send a message that AI is a priority (Griffith, 2013).

Administrators, faculty, and students share the responsibility of fostering AI and must work together to achieve it. Students need to be inducted into the larger academic and professional community that expects integrity and appeal to peer disapproval of AD (McGee, 2013). This necessitates a proactive, publicized pedagogical approach that values AI over a punitive (after-the fact) approach.

If AD occurs, faculty needs to act swiftly and consistently, match the response to the violation within the institutional policies and guidelines, and gather data to determine what may have led to the AD incident. Resources such as the International Centre for Academic Integrity, Plagiarismadvice.org, Impact of Policies for Plagiarism in Higher Education across Europe (IPPHAE) project (Glendenning, 2012), outside experts and consultants, and scholarly multidisciplinary literature can be used to design, implement, and evaluate evidence-based strategies that fit within the organizational culture. Additional research is required to inform the broader academic community about strategies that work best.

Centre for Academic Integrity. (2014). *Definition*. Retrieved from http://www.academicintegrity.org/icai/resources-2.php

DiBartolo, M. C. (2010). Desperate times call for desperate measures: Where are we in addressing academic dishonesty? *Journal of Nursing Education, 49*(10), 543–544.

Gallant, T. (2011). Building a culture of academic integrity. In J. Garrett (Ed.), *Helping students learn from ethical failures (and changing organizational responses to cheating). White Paper* (pp. 1–44). Madison, WI: Magna Publications.

Glendenning, I. (2012). *European responses to student plagiarism in higher education.* Retrieved from http://archive.plagiarismadvice.org/document/conference2012/finalpapers/Glendenning_fullpaper.pdf

Griffith, J. (2013). Pedagogical over punitive: The academic integrity websites of Ontario universities. *Canadian Journal of Higher Education, 43*(1), 1–22.

Jeffreys, M. R., & Stier, L. A. (1995). SPEAKING against student academic dishonesty: A communication model for nurse educators. *Journal of Nursing Education, 34,* 297–304.

Jeffreys, M. R., & Stier, L. A. (2004). Student academic dishonesty. In M. Oermann & K. Heinrich (Eds.), *Annual review of nursing education, Volume II.* New York, NY: Springer.

Josien, L., & Broderick, B. (2013). Cheating in higher education: The case of multimethod cheaters. *Academy of Educational Leadership Journal, 17*(3), 93–105.

Kibler, W. L., Nuss, E. M., Patterson, B. G., & Pavela, G. (1988). *Academic integrity and student development: Legal issues and policy perspectives.* Asheville, NC: College Administration Publications.

Kolanko, K. M., Clark, C., Heinrich, K. T., Olive, D., Farley Serembus, J., & Sifford, K. S. (2006). Academic dishonesty, bullying, incivility, and violence: Difficult challenges facing nurse educators. *Nursing Education Perspectives, 27*(1), 34–43.

LaDuke, R. D. (2013). Academic dishonesty today, unethical practices tomorrow? *Journal of Professional Nursing, 29*(6), 402–406.

McCabe, D. L. (2009). Academic dishonesty in nursing schools: An empirical investigation. *Journal of Nursing Education, 48*(11), 614–623.

McGee, P. (2013). Supporting academic honesty in online courses. *Journal of Educators Online, 10*(1), 1–31.

Rogers, C. F. (2006). Faculty perceptions about e-cheating during online testing. *Journal of Computing Sciences in Colleges*, 22(2), 206–212.

Spaulding, M. (2009). Perceptions of academic honesty in online vs. face-to-face classrooms. *Journal of Interactive Online Learning*, 8(3), 183–198.

Marianne R. Jeffreys
Lori Stier

ACADEMIC FAILURE

DEFINITION

Academic failure in nursing education occurs when there is involuntary attrition of a student due to academic reasons such as course failure, resulting in withdrawal or dismissal from the program (Jeffreys, 2012). This is closely tied with failure to meet the institutional academic progression outcomes as measured by nursing course grade, cumulative grade point average (GPA) in nursing courses, and overall GPA. It is a result of the interplay of many factors: inadequate knowledge base from prerequisites; inappropriate perception of the rigors of nursing upper-division curricula; and personal issues concerning financial needs, family demands, and health.

APPLICATION

Academic failure in nursing education impacts the student's psychological and financial well-being with lifelong effects. It is costly to the academic institutions given the current limited financial resources and nursing faculty shortage. Furthermore, it perpetuates the national nursing shortage.

The literature reveals many factors that contribute to academic failure. These factors have been classified under personal, academic, and environmental categories (Igbo et al., 2011; Jeffreys, 2012; Kuh, Kinzie, Buckley, Bridges, & Hayek, 2006; Williams, 2010). Personal factors identified include financial and family commitments, failure to assume responsibility for the outcome, and inadequate language skills. Academic factors include unrealistic perception of academic rigor, transitional shock (Igbo, Landson, & Straker, in press), and inadequate pre-nursing academic preparation. The environmental factors include fit with nursing major, inclusive of institutional learning environment, mentoring, student engagement, supportive institutional resources, and appropriate interventions.

While there are issues that affect all nursing students, the nontraditional student has certain characteristics that put him or her at higher risk of academic failure (Igbo et al., 2011). These factors include being older, nursing as a second degree, increased family responsibilities, English as a second language, and first generation attending college. The Nursing Undergraduate Retention and Success (NURS) model (Jeffreys, 2012) proposes that decisions preventing academic failure should be based on the following multidimensional factors: student affect, the environment, professional integration, academic outcomes, and psychological outcomes. These factors must be considered when addressing the matter of student academic failure (Igbo et al., 2011).

SYNOPSIS

Academic failure has personal, institutional, and larger societal implications. Academic failure can slow the rate at which graduates enter the workforce. A literature review has revealed models addressing nursing student success, thus preventing academic failure. These models have been tested in different student populations and are focused on decreasing barriers to academic success (Dapremont, 2013). The results of this review indicate that successful models included various combinations of academic support, mentoring, student financial support, and community partnerships that were

A

effective in recruiting, retaining, and graduating minority students in nursing education (Dapremont, 2013). Student engagement (McCarthy & Kuh, 2006) has also been identified as an important strategy in preventing academic failure and increasing retention.

RECOMMENDATIONS

Increased nursing student retention and prevention of academic failure are key to addressing the national nursing shortage. It is important to target students from minority backgrounds who are at higher risk of academic failure.

To address the problem of academic failure and increase nursing student retention, it is recommended that every nursing program should create a model that best fits the student population characteristics; embark on training faculty to empower students and embrace cultural diversity; and provide a supportive campus climate and available resources to increase student engagement.

Dapremont, J. A. (2013). A review of minority recruitment and retention models implemented in undergraduate nursing programs. *Journal of Nursing Education and Practice, 3*(2), 112.

Igbo, I. N., Landson, M. J., & Straker, K. C. (in press). Nursing student retention: An integrated study skills elective. *Journal of Nursing Education Perspectives.*

Igbo, I. N., Straker, K. C., Landson, M. J., Symes, L., Bernard, L. F., Hughes, L. A., & Carroll, T. L. (2011). Multidisciplinary approach: An innovative strategy to improve retention of students from disadvantaged backgrounds. *Journal of Nursing Education Perspectives, 32*(6), 375–379.

Jeffreys, M. R. (2012). *Nursing student retention: Understanding the process and making a difference* (2nd ed.). New York, NY: Springer Publishing Company.

Kuh, G. D., Kinzie, J., Buckley, J. A., Bridges, B. K., & Hayek, J. C. (2006). *What matters to student success: A review of the literature.* Commissioned Report for the National Symposium on Postsecondary Student Success: Spearheading a Dialog on Student Success. Retrieved from https://www.ue.ucsc.edu/sites/default/files/WhatMattersStudentSuccess(Kuh,July2006.pdf

McCarthy, M. M., & Kuh, G. D. (2006). Are students ready for college? What student engagement data say. *Phi Delta Kappa, 87*(9), 664–669.

Williams, M. (2010). Attrition and retention in the nursing major: Understanding persistence in beginning nursing students. *Journal of Nursing Education Perspectives, 31*(6), 362–367.

Immaculata N. Igbo

ACADEMIC INTEGRITY

DEFINITION

Academic integrity is defined as a commitment to six fundamental values: honesty, trust, fairness, respect, responsibility, and courage in scholarship and research (International Center for Academic Integrity, 2013). Without these fundamental values, teaching and research lose credibility, leading to a questioning of personal and professional integrity.

APPLICATION

Academic integrity rests on the foundations of personal accountability. Upholding academic integrity is reflective of a person's personal integrity, ethical principles, and moral character. Accountability also extends to the academic institution to address academic infractions and take action when necessary (International Center for Academic Integrity, 2013).

Nursing has a long history of being regarded by the public as a profession that is ethical and trustworthy (Fontana, 2009; Tippitt et al., 2009). Hence, personal integrity and ethical principles are essential for all nurses and student nurses to embrace. Research shows that students who do not possess academic integrity will likely engage in unethical or even illegal activities, both as students and as professional nurses (Balik, Sharon, Kelishek, & Tabak, 2010; Fontana, 2009; LaDuke, 2013; Tippitt et al., 2009).

Nursing educators serve as the gatekeepers of the nursing profession (Fontana, 2009). They are given the task of preparing students intellectually and developmentally with personal and academic integrity (Tsokris & Struminger, 2013). Throughout the curriculum nurse educators model these behaviors through their own actions. Furthermore, the importance of professional standards can be taught by guiding students to practice following the American Nurses Association (ANA) Code of Ethics (ANA, 2001; Tippitt et al., 2009). Nurse educators must also address academic integrity infractions to assure that the students who progress through the program are ethical in practice and well versed in the course material.

SYNOPSIS

Greater access to online resources may put academic and personal integrity at risk of being compromised. The Internet offers an abundance of information on numerous scholarly topics and therefore may pose a temptation for students to plagiarize. With a simple click of a mouse, sections of an author's work can be copied and pasted into a student's paper without giving proper citation of the source (Mohr, Ingram, Fell, & Mabey, 2011). Furthermore, the perception of academic transgressions by students differs from that of faculty. Students may believe that cheating in an examination, buying papers, and plagiarizing are acceptable (Mohr et al., 2011; Tsokris & Struminger, 2013).

Technology is a welcome addition to most classrooms but poses a serious threat to maintaining academic integrity. Handheld devices and laptops accepted in classrooms can be misused to photograph and transmit examinations. Mobile phones, never far from students' hands, can be used to send text-messaged answers (Mohr et al., 2011). Strict technological policies must be developed to govern proper use to maintain academic integrity.

Maintaining academic integrity in an online environment has also been called into question. Researchers examined the levels of academic integrity violations in both online and face-to-face classes, and reported higher rates of academic dishonesty in face-to-face classes than in online counterparts (Miller & Young-Jones, 2012; Watson & Sottile, 2010). Having student and faculty conversations about academic integrity as well as formal instruction has been noted to improve students' understanding of what constitutes academic integrity violations. Therefore, discussions about academic integrity should be incorporated in all courses (Piascik & Brazeau, 2010). Morgan and Hart (2013) in their quasi-experimental study examined ways to promote academic integrity in an online RN-BSN program. The standard academic integrity policy and student handbook was given to the control group, and the treatment group received a faculty-designed program including discussion and instruction. The students in both groups reported low levels of academic dishonesty. However, the treatment group reported higher levels of faculty and student support for academic integrity policies and perceived these policies to be more effective.

RECOMMENDATIONS

It is essential that institutional standards, policies, and procedures are aligned with the fundamental values of honesty, trust, fairness, respect, responsibility, and courage for academic integrity to be supported and upheld (International Center for Academic Integrity, 2013). The principles of professional behavior and academic integrity must start from day 1 (Piascik & Brazeau, 2010; Tippitt et al., 2009). It is essential that

A

students be provided with a formal orientation. The orientation should include approved resources, student handbook, and information on academic integrity (Tippitt et al., 2009). Policies regarding the misuse of technology in classrooms should also be reviewed at the beginning of each course outlining expectations and defining violation consequences.

Nurse educators must model professionalism and academic integrity and uphold the standards of academic integrity in their practice and teaching (Eby et al., 2013). Modeling these behaviors has been found to be the most successful method to promote academic honesty and integrity among students. Finally, nurse educators need to be supported in their efforts to promote in-class and online environments that maintain academic integrity, as well as address issues related to breaches in academic integrity. As gatekeepers of the profession, educators assure that those entering into practice demonstrate not only exceptional knowledge and skill, but also personal and academic integrity.

American Nurses Association (ANA). (2001). *Code of ethics for nurses with interpretive statements.* Retrieved from http://www.nursingworld.org/MainMenuCategories/EthicsStandards/CodeofEthicsforNurses.aspx

Balik, C., Sharon, D., Kelishek, S., & Tabak, N. (2010). Attitudes towards academic cheating during nursing studies. *Medicine and Law, 29*(4), 547–563.

Eby, R. A., Hartley, P. L., Hodges, P. J., Hoffpauir, R., Newbanks, S., & Kelley, J. H. (2013). Moral integrity and moral courage: Can you teach it? *Journal of Nursing Education, 52*(4), 229–233.

Fontana, J. S. (2009). Nursing faculty experiences of students' academic dishonesty. *Journal of Nursing Education, 48*(4), 181–185.

International Center for Academic Integrity. (2013). *The fundamental values of academic integrity.* Retrieved from http://www.academicintegrity.org/icai/resources-2.php

LaDuke, R. D. (2013). Academic dishonesty today, unethical practices tomorrow? *Journal of Professional Nursing, 29*(6), 402–406.

Miller, A., & Young-Jones, A. (2012). Academic integrity: Online classes compared to face-to-face classes. *Journal of Instructional Psychology, 39*(3), 138–145.

Mohr, T., Ingram, D., Fell, N., & Mabey, R. (2011). The case for academic integrity in physical therapy education. *Journal of Physical Therapy Education, 25*(2), 51–56.

Morgan, L., & Hart, L. (2013). Promoting academic integrity in an online RN-BSN program. *Nursing Education Perspectives, 34*(4), 240–243.

Piascik, P., & Brazeau, G. A. (2010). Promoting a culture of academic integrity. *American Journal of Pharmaceutical Education, 74*(6), 113.

Tippitt, M. P., Ard, N., Kline, J. R., Tilghman, J., Chamberlain, B., & Meagher, P. G. (2009). Creating environments that foster academic integrity. *Nursing Education Perspectives, 30*(4), 239–244.

Tsokris, M., & Struminger, S. (2013). Does academic misconduct influence professional integrity? *Access, 27*(4), 22.

Watson, G., & Sottile, J. (2010). Cheating in the digital age: Do students cheat more in online courses? *Online Journal of Distance Learning Administration, 13*(1). Retrieved from http://www.westga.edu/~distance/ojdla/spring131/watson131.html

Deborah Mandel

ACADEMIC LEADERSHIP

DEFINITION

The National Academy for Academic Leadership (2014) defines leadership as helping people identify, confront, and solve problems that require adaptation to new realities for which there are no routine solutions. Leadership involves a willingness to modify or change values, beliefs, and behaviors in the academic environment. Academic leadership is the practical and everyday process of supporting, managing, developing, and inspiring academic colleagues (Ramsden, 1998). Furthermore, academic leadership positions include managers of personnel and managers of programs (Ramsden, 1998).

APPLICATION

In 1965, the American Nurses Association (ANA) issued its *First Position on Education for Nursing*. The central tenet of the position statement was that the education for all those who are licensed to practice nursing should take place in institutions of higher education (ANA, 1965). Today, the nursing profession has arrived at a place in history where the expectation of faculty and leaders are in alignment with expectations of the academy. Academic leaders in nursing are those who provide leadership of baccalaureate and higher nursing programs in the academic setting. Although terminology differs across institutions, common titles that embody the role of academic leadership in nursing education include dean, director, department chair, and coordinator.

Formal leadership development programs in nursing share the common mission of developing, supporting, and reenergizing nurse leaders across all settings. Robert Wood Johnson Foundation (RWJF) Executive Nurse Fellows program is a 3-year advanced leadership program for nurses who aspire to lead and shape health care locally and nationally. Fellows strengthen leadership capacity and improve abilities to lead teams and organizations in improving health and health care (RWJF, 2014). The National League for Nursing (NLN) Leadership Institute is comprised of three full-year programs that help nurse faculty develop strong leadership skills. Programs within the Nursing Leadership Institute are designed for nurse educators who have experienced a rapid transition to leadership, those who wish to assume a leadership role in simulation, and senior deans and directors (NLN, 2013). The American Association of Colleges of Nursing (AACN) sponsors an executive leadership fellowship specifically for those aspiring for leadership positions in nursing. This professional development experience includes assessment and evaluation of leadership skills, opportunities for networking, and consultation to achieve long-term goals (AACN, 2014).

SYNOPSIS

Multiple responsibilities (Minnick, Norman, Donaghey, Fisher, & McKirgan, 2010); leadership development (Broome, 2013; Minnick et al., 2010); and lack of succession planning (Broome, 2013; McNamara, 2009; Minnick et al., 2010) have been identified as challenges to the role of academic leadership in nursing. Minnick, Norman, Donaghey, Fisher, and McKirgan (2010) found that directors of doctoral nursing programs carried multiple responsibilities in addition to the role of director. Effort allocation, multiple responsibilities, lack of stability, rotating directorships, workload, and tenure contribute to academic planning.

Over the past decade there has been a lack of attention paid to developing strong academic leaders (Broome, 2013). The academic work environment is extremely challenging and requires a comprehensive skill set that allows leaders to recognize new opportunities, mobilize and motivate faculty, and secure opportunities. It is equally important that leaders stay focused on priorities and initiatives (Broome, 2013). Although formal leadership development programs in nursing exist (RWJF, NLN, and Commission on Collegiate Nursing Education [CCNE]), these programs tend to be selective. The most common mechanism for leadership training may be informal mentorship followed by internal leadership development (Minnick et al., 2010).

Many deans of schools of nursing are approaching an age at which retirement may be expected (Minnick et al., 2010). Given the demographics of deans in nursing, there is a critical need for succession planning and for the development of emerging academic leaders (Broome, 2013). Minnick et al. found that the majority of schools in their survey of doctoral nursing programs reported no succession plan. Academic leaders can ensure succession planning through recruitment and development programs for the next generation of leaders.

RECOMMENDATIONS

Since the time of the Crimean War, nursing has gone through many stages in search for a professional identity and devoted time to defining its domain of knowledge and practice (Meleis, 2012). In the early stage of practice, the mission of nursing was defined as providing care and comfort to enhance healing and a sense of well-being (Meleis, 2012). Amid the complexity of academic systems, there is a need for leadership that appreciates and supports the basic values that have historically sustained the profession (Moody, Horton-Deutsch, & Pesut, 2007). Academic leaders in nursing need to be mindful that whatever the landscape and architecture of health care will be in the future, the mission and values of nursing should remain clear and constant (Graham, 2010).

Leaders need to pay close attention to reaching out to younger academic nurses who have potential to become academic leaders in the future (Broome, 2013). The significance of leadership development and succession planning cannot be underestimated. Goodrich (2014) found that nurse educators with greater than 5 years in the role demonstrated high levels of personal control and intended to stay in the role of an academic nurse educator. Therefore, existing processes that support academic nurse educators need to be reexamined and enhanced.

Academic nursing leadership in the context of the complex academic setting requires a discussion on leadership styles, priorities, activities, and the future of the profession. Leadership in academic settings is not a solo activity. Transformative behaviors on the part of a leader require reciprocity between the leader and other members of the organization (Broome, 2013). Knowledge related to finances, resource acquisition, interprofessional collaboration, development, and advancement is critical (Broome, 2013).

American Association of Colleges of Nursing (AACN). (2014). *Leadership for academic nursing.* Washington, DC: Author.

American Nurses Association (ANA). (1965). American Nurses' Association first position on education for nursing. *American Journal of Nursing, 65*(12), 106–111.

Broome, M. (2013). Self-reported leadership styles of deans of baccalaureate and higher degree nursing programs in the United States. *Journal of Professional Nursing, 29*(6), 323–329.

Goodrich, R. S. (2014). Transition to academic nurse educator: A survey exploring readiness, confidence, and locus of control. *Journal of Professional Nursing, 30*(3), 203–212.

Graham, I. (2010). The search for the discipline of nursing. *Journal of Nursing Management, 18*, 355–362.

McNamara, M. (2009). Academic leadership in nursing: Legitimating the discipline in contested spaces. *Journal of Nursing Management, 17*, 484–493.

Meleis, A. (2012). *Theoretical nursing: Development and progress* (5th ed.). Philadelphia, PA: Lippincott.

Minnick, A., Norman, L., Donaghey, B., Fisher, L., & McKirgan, I. (2010). Leadership in doctoral nursing research programs. *Journal of Nursing Education, 49*(9), 504–510.

Moody, R., Horton-Deutsch, S., & Pesut, D. (2007). Appreciative inquiry for leading in complex systems: Supporting the transformation of academic nursing culture. *Journal of Nursing Education, 46*(7), 319–324.

The National Academy for Academic Leadership. (2014). *Mission of the national academy.* Syracuse, NY: Author.

National League for Nursing (NLN). (2013). *The NLN leadership institute.* Washington, DC: Author.

Ramsden, P. (1998). *Learning to lead in higher education.* London: Routledge.

Robert Wood Johnson Foundation (RWJF). (2014). *Executive nurse fellows.* Chapel Hill, NC: Center for Creative Leadership and University of North Carolina at Chapel Hill School of Nursing.

Robin S. Goodrich

ACADEMIC MISCONDUCT

DEFINITION

Academic misconduct is "intentional participation in deceptive practices regarding one's academic work" that can occur in the classroom and clinical setting (Gaberson, 1997, p. 14). Students frequently define academic misconduct as things that they should not do, such as "do not cheat on exams" (Woith, Jenkins, & Kerber, 2012).

APPLICATION

The incidence of academic dishonesty among undergraduate nursing students has ranged from 58% to 94% (McCabe, 2009; Roberson, 2009). Academic dishonesty has been reported by 77% of students in accelerated programs, 57% of master's candidates with a non-nursing baccalaureate degree, 48% of all graduate nursing students, 37% of RN to BSN students, and 25% of doctoral students (McCabe, 2009).

Similar forms of academic misconduct occur in both graduate and undergraduate nursing students (McCabe, 2009). The six most frequently self-reported examples of academic misconduct in undergraduate students include: collaborating with others on individual assignments (38%), copying sentences from the Internet (28%) or published text (24%) without citing the reference, receiving assistance on an assignment that is not permitted (19%), getting answers to an examination from someone who took it previously (18%), and using a false or forged excuse to delay an examination or assignment (10%; McCabe, 2009). Other less commonly self-reported instances of academic misconduct are copying from someone else in an examination with or without his or her knowledge, assisting someone to cheat in an examination, turning a paper in copied from another student, copying most or part of a paper from a written or Web source, using cheat notes in an examination, turning in an assignment completed by someone else, or purchasing papers from online services (McCabe, 2009).

Unfortunately, students do not view academic misconduct as unethical. Undergraduate nursing students believe that working with another student on an assignment (22%), getting answers to examination questions from another student (19%), and paraphrasing or copying material from a reference without an appropriate citation (17%) are not unethical behaviors (McCrink, 2010). "Students rationalize their behavior by denying wrongdoing, pleading time constraints, citing unfair course requirements forcing them to cheat or shifting the blame for their behaviors onto nurse educators" (McCrink, 2010, p. 654). Students cite competition to achieve high grades (Gaberson, 1997; Kolanko et al., 2006; Roberson, 2009; Woith et al., 2012); perfectionism; impaired morals; and inadequate role models (Gaberson, 1997) as reasons for academic misconduct.

The use of high-tech cheating is rapidly increasing. High-tech academic misconduct occurs when copies of examinations or test banks are purchased online, handheld devices are used to text answers or access the Internet for answers during the examination, or by taking photos of examination pages to share with others (Arhin, 2009; Kolanko et al., 2006). Additionally, high-tech cheating can occur with use of micro-recorders; still cameras that are concealed in wristwatches, cigarette lighters, or campaign buttons; audio or video transmitters that are no larger than the size of a quarter; and ultraviolet pens (Kolanko et al., 2006).

SYNOPSIS

Research has shown that students who engage in academic misconduct are more likely to become professionals who engage in unethical behaviors in the clinical setting (Baxter & Boblin, 2007; Roberson, 2009; Tippitt et al., 2009).

Clinical misconduct may negatively impact patient outcomes and violate national practice standards (McCrink, 2010). Thirty-five percent of nursing students reported discussing patients in public places or with nonmedical personnel, thus breeching patient confidentiality (McCrink, 2010). Nursing students self-reporting clinical misconduct acknowledged that they reported or recorded vital signs that were either not taken or accurately recalled (13%), treatments that were not performed or observed (9%), patient responses to treatments or medications that were not assessed (7%), or recorded medications that were not administered (2%; McCrink, 2010). Less frequently reported unethical clinical behaviors included failing to report errors and failing to question incorrect provider orders (Baxter & Boblin, 2007).

RECOMMENDATIONS

"Faculty need to create an ethical community that clearly communicates expectations of academic integrity and penalties for cheating" (Morgan & Hart, 2013, p. 240). It is imperative that nursing faculty model ethical behavior, show accountability, and confront students in a discrete manner when episodes of academic misconduct occur. The nursing program should clearly define academic misconduct and post the statements in every syllabus and on the online course management system (Bristol, 2011). The statement should be reviewed at the beginning of every course and periodically throughout the semester.

Nursing faculty is more likely to use different versions of the examination, more closely monitor students during examination, and remind students of the university's policy regarding academic misconduct more frequently than non-nursing faculty (McCabe, 2009). Strategies to minimize academic dishonesty include using honor codes, assigning seats or moving seats farther apart during examinations, requiring students to leave all personal belongings at the front of the room, using at least two proctors who walk around the room during examinations, and placing time limits on examinations (Arhin, 2009; Kolanko et al., 2006; McCabe, 2009; Roberson, 2009; Tippitt et al., 2009). Students should not be allowed to leave the classroom during the examination and should provide proof prior to making up a missed examination (Kolanko et al., 2006). The use of plagiarism detection software (Bristol, 2011) and computerized examination programs that allows for password protection and requires the proctor to start the examination for every student is an additional strategy that can minimize academic misconduct (Woith et al., 2012).

Faculty should discuss the importance of integrity, personal accountability, and time management skills with students (Dibartolo & Walsh, 2010; Tippitt et al., 2009). Only meaningful assignments that include a rationale for the assignment with written objectives should be given to students. The dates for examinations and assignments should be provided to students at the beginning of the semester and coordinated with other courses.

Arhin, A. O. (2009). A pilot study of nursing student's perceptions of academic dishonesty: A generation Y perspective. *The ABNF Journal, 20*(1), 17–21.

Baxter, P. E., & Boblin, S. L. (2007). The moral development of baccalaureate nursing students: Understanding unethical behavior in classroom and clinical settings. *Journal of Nursing Education, 46*(1), 20–27.

Bristol, T. J. (2011). Plagiarism prevention with technology. *Teaching and Learning in Nursing, 6,* 146–149. doi:10.1016/j.teln.2011.05.002

Dibartolo, M. C., & Walsh, C. M. (2010). Desperate times call for desperate measures: Where are we in addressing academic dishonesty? *Journal of Nursing Education, 49*(10), 543–544.

Gaberson, K. B. (1997). Academic dishonesty among nursing students. *Nursing Forum, 32*(3), 14–20.

Kolanko, K. M., Clark, C., Heinrich, K. T., Olive, D., Serembus, J. F., & Sifford, K. S. (2006). Academic dishonesty, bullying, incivility, and violence: Difficult challenges facing nurse educators. *Nursing Education Perspectives, 27*(1), 34–43.

McCabe, D. L. (2009). Academic dishonesty in nursing schools: An empirical investigation. *Journal of Nursing Education, 48*(11), 614–623.

McCrink, A. (2010). Academic misconduct in nursing students: Behaviors, attitudes, rationalizations, and cultural identity. *Journal of Nursing Education, 29*(11), 653–659. doi: 10.3928/01484834–20100831-03

Morgan, L., & Hart, L. (2013). Promoting academic integrity in an online RN-BSN program. *Nursing Education Perspectives, 34*(4), 240–243.

Roberson, D. W. (2009). Using a student response system to reduce academic cheating. *Nurse Educator, 34*(2), 60–63.

Tippitt, M. P., Ard, N., Kline, J. R., Tilghman, J., Chamberlain, B., & Meagher, P. G. (2009). Creating environments that foster academic integrity. *Nursing Education Perspectives, 30*(4), 239–244.

Woith, W., Jenkins, S. D., & Kerber, C. (2012). Perceptions of academic integrity among nursing students. *Nursing Forum, 47*(4), 253–259.

Laura H. Clayton

ACADEMIC PARTNERSHIPS

A

DEFINITION

Academic partnerships are formalized relationships between an academic nursing program and a care setting, which may include other professionals, corporations, government entities, and foundations (AACN, 2010). Academic partnerships provide an organizational association between academia and service that propose to share a common vision and collaboration to advance nursing practice and health of the public.

APPLICATION

Academic practice partnerships exist in all types of care settings and academic programs. Based on recommendations of the Institute of Medicine (IOM), greater emphasis has been placed on the development of sustained partnerships between academia and nursing service to improve student transition to practice, clinical environments, and patient outcomes. Crucial principles guiding an intentional relationship between academia and practice include mutual trust, respect, shared vision and goals, commitment to the partnership, and transparent, sustained communication (Beal, 2012).

One exemplar of an academic partnership is a collaborative clinical model called dedicated education unit (DEU), an innovative approach to clinical teaching/learning with an intentional emphasis on systems-thinking, clinical reasoning, accountability, and collaboration. Nurses selected to work on a DEU take on the role of a clinical teacher, establishing a one-to-one relationship with the student while in clinical practice. These nurses are prepared for this role by faculty who serve as coach to facilitate teaching strategies, enable the transfer of classroom learning to practice, assure achievement of expected learning outcomes, and assist with the resolution of problems that may arise.

The faculty member establishes a collaborative working relationship with the nurse manager, charge nurses, and DEU nurses to facilitate an optimal clinical environment for student learning.

Other academic partnerships involve dual enrollment affiliation agreements between universities and community colleges to provide a seamless transition between programs. Opportunities for students to enroll in classes at a 4-year university, while enrolled at a community college, offer students the opportunity to become familiar with academic expectations while creating an effective educational pathway for academic advancement.

Additional types of academic partnerships include statewide workforce coalitions, nurse residency programs, clinical nurse leader initiatives, interprofessional educational opportunities, graduate nurse education, clinical faculty boot camps, partnerships with free clinics, school-based health center partnerships, and collaborations and exchange of faculty between nursing programs.

SYNOPSIS

Academic partnerships are essential to nursing practice for positioning leaders to advance health care outcomes; however, the challenges to establish effective and sustained relationships are many. In an effort to promote effective partnerships, the American Association of Colleges of Nursing (AACN) and American Organization of Nurse Executives (AONE) collaborated to create the Task Force of Academic Practice Partnerships. This task force identified barriers and developed guidelines to cultivate and sustain effective academic partnerships (AACN, 2010). Barriers to successful partnerships include reduction in funding for education and health care; lack of financial support from universities; and increased faculty workloads. Successful partnerships between academia and practice are sustained through formal affiliations established at the senior leadership level and replicated at all levels of the management team. A common vision with clear expectations and mutually established goals with a systematic plan for evaluation are essential to the partnership. The foundation of a partnership includes respect, trust, transparent communication, shared commitment, and persistence in achieving established goals (AACN, 2010).

Research on academic partnerships has shown that these models can be effective in reducing health care costs, improving patient outcomes, improving quality and safety, and providing opportunities for staff development. For the academy, these partnerships have increased enrollment capacity within schools of nursing, enhanced research and evidence-based practice opportunities, improved transition to the clinical setting, and increased opportunities for employment (Lindahl, Dagborn, & Nilsson, 2009; Lovecchio, DiMattio, & Hudacek, 2012; Moore & Nahigian, 2013; Springer et al., 2012).

Springer et al. (2012) found that a DEU model resulted in significantly lower expenses incurred by the health care agency and school than traditional clinical models, while reaping higher student satisfaction and outcomes. Lovecchio et al. (2012) used clinical liaison faculty to facilitate student learning in a community hospital. This partnership improved students' perceptions of the clinical learning environment. A collaboration between a school of nursing and hospital system resulted in student-initiated quality improvement (QI) projects being implemented on nursing units with positive quality outcomes (Flores, Hickenlooper, & Saxton, 2013). Finally, a cooperative partnership between schools of nursing and hospitals documented the use and advancement of clinical nursing research (Boland, Kamikawa, Inouye, Latimer, & Marshall, 2010).

Academic practice partnerships provide an opportunity for academia and practice to share a common vision in a framework that optimizes health system performance. Initiating and sustaining effectively focused partnerships improve patient outcomes and reduce costs, while facilitating student transition to practice. Providing better care at lower cost requires application of the best evidence available. Academic partnerships that facilitate the generation of new evidence for practice will foster goal attainment for the academy and the health care agency.

RECOMMENDATIONS

It is essential that nursing leaders in practice and education continue to design and develop new approaches to solve the challenges of clinical education. These challenges include problems related to the lack of clinical faculty and clinical placements; costs associated with orientation, quality, and safety initiatives; and transition to practice issues. Nurse educators need to become attentive to establishing partnerships that facilitate transfer of relevant knowledge, improve student outcomes, and maximize enrollment capacity. Academic partnerships must be sensitive to transition issues and the need for health systems to improve quality while reducing costs. Effective partnerships can provide for outcomes that support both agendas.

There are numerous studies and explanations of academic partnerships that provide anecdotal evidence of success. However, because there is insufficient objective evidence to provide support for the positive patient and student outcomes of these relationships, the ability to generalize the research published to date is limited. Academic partnerships are a promising area for rigorous inquiry that distinguishes quantifiable and achievable outcomes.

American Association of Colleges of Nursing (AACN). (2010). *AACN-AONE task force on academic-practice partnerships. Guiding principles.* Retrieved from www.aacn.nche.edu/leading-initiatives/academic-practice-partnerships/GuidingPrinciples.pdf

Beal, J. A. (2012). Academic-service partnerships in nursing: An integrative review. *Nursing Research and Practice, 2012*(1), 1–9. doi:10.1155/2012/501564

Boland, M., Kamikawa, C., Inouye, J., Latimer, R., & Marshall, S. (2010). Partnership to build research capacity. *Nursing Economics, 28*(5), 314–321, 336.

Flores, D., Hickenlooper, G., & Saxton, R. (2013). An academic practice partnership: Helping new registered nurses to advance quality and patient safety. *The Online Journal of Issues in Nursing, 18*(3), Manuscript 3.

Lindahl, B., Dagborn, K., & Nilsson, M. (2009). A student-centered clinical educational unit—description of a reflective learning model. *Nursing Education in Practice, 9*(1), 5–12. doi:10.1016/j.nepr.2008.03.008

Lovecchio, C., DiMattio, M. J. K., & Hudacek, S. (2012). Clinical liaison nurse model in a community hospital: A unique academic–practice partnership that strengthens clinical nursing education. *Journal of Nursing Education, 51*(11), 609–615.

Moore, J., & Nahigian, E. (2013). Nursing student perceptions of nurse-nurse collaboration in dedicated education units and traditional learning units. *Journal of Nursing Education, 52*(6), 346–350. doi:10.3928/01484834-20130509-01.

Springer, P., Johnson, P., Lind, B., Walker, E., Clavelle, J., & Jensen, N. (2012). The Idaho dedicated education unit model: Cost-effective, high-quality education. *Nurse Educator, 37*(6), 262–267.

Patricia A. Sharpnack
Mary T. Quinn Griffin

ACADEMIC PROGRESSION: ARTICULATION

DEFINITION

Academic progression refers to articulation models that promote lifelong learning through the addition of academic credentials (National League for Nursing [NLN], 2011).

A

APPLICATION

In 2010, the Institute of Medicine (IOM) in the Future of Nursing Report advocated for changes in nursing education (IOM, 2010). In addition, the IOM (2010) recommended that educational programs should be structured to enable the learner to progress from basic to advanced education with minimal disruption. Nursing continues to have multiple entry options (Raines & Taglaireni, 2008). These entry options include bachelor of science in nursing (BSN) completion programs for registered nurses (RNs), baccalaureate to master's programs, and BSN to research or clinical doctorate programs. Some individuals first enter nursing through associate degree programs and then advance with the achievement of higher degrees (Raines & Taglaireni, 2008). In order to implement the IOM recommendation, nurse education programs need to develop and implement innovative approaches to prepare nurses needed for the future. The report emphasized that flexibility will be needed in both delivery and scheduling of courses on the part of academic institutions. Examples of flexibility include online distance programs, hybrid courses, virtual learning, and nontraditional hours for course offerings such as weekends and late evenings.

SYNOPSIS

In 2010, the United States Health Resources and Services Administration (HRSA) published the results of the 2008 national sample of RN survey and reported that 32% of RNs with a baccalaureate or higher degree entered the profession with a diploma or associate degree. However, in this report, it was stated that many nurses continue to pursue advanced degrees after attaining initial licensure (HRSA, 2010). Munkvold, Tanner, and Herinckx (2012) studied the graduates from an associate degree program who were eligible to obtain a bachelor's degree with 1 year additional study and chose not to advance. The top three factors that influenced these associate degree graduates to

not pursue further nursing education were financial concerns, work, and family issues. Jeffreys (2007) identified several important trends that may influence nursing student progress and graduation. Students entering nursing exhibit diversity in age, ethnicity, and prior academic experience (Jeffreys, 2007). Students at highest risk of either dropping out or taking breaks in their program were older, female, and belonged to a minority group (Jeffreys, 2007). Awareness of these diverse student characteristics highlights the need for and implementation of culturally diverse academic advisement and mentoring. Nurse administrators need to provide additional resources so that nurse educators may develop and implement innovative teaching strategies and evaluation measures that are culturally congruent (Jeffreys, 2007). These students also took longer to complete their degrees.

RECOMMENDATIONS

The Tri-Council for Nursing (2010), a coalition of American Association of Colleges of Nursing (AACN), American Nurses Association (ANA), NLN, and American Organization of Nurse Executives (AONE), issued a consensus statement calling for all RNs to advance their education in the interest of offering patients the best possible care. The Tri-Council ends its statement with a twofold call to action for nurses to understand the importance of academic progression and embrace lifelong learning; and for policy makers at all levels to provide funding and to develop and implement collaborative initiatives that facilitate nurses obtaining advanced education (Tri-Council for Nursing, 2010). They emphasized that not only should graduates of associates degree in nursing (ADN) programs advance to the BSN, but also that the BSN and master of science in nursing (MSN) graduates should advance to the doctoral level in order to meet the need for educators and leaders (Tri-Council for Nursing, 2010).

The NLN, AACN, American Association of Community Colleges, Associations of Community College Trustees, and the

National Organization for Associate Degree Nursing are the authors of a position statement endorsing the academic progression of nursing students and graduates through partnership and collaboration with the goal of a "well educated diverse workforce to advance the nation's health" (NLN, 2011, p. 1). This group has developed the NLN Education Competencies Model, a model that embraces all types of nursing and identifies the graduate competencies for each program along with articulation of each program to the other (NLN, 2011). This model ensures that the core competencies are present in basic programs and that all graduates are educated to care for increasingly complex patients in a safe and competent manner.

There is a need for research in the area of academic progression to identify the best approaches to achieve the IOM recommendation of a seamless transition for nurses seeking to advance education. Pittman, Kurtzman, and Johnson (2014) examined the design and implementation of alternative pathways for academic progression. They conducted interviews with 31 educational leaders in the United States and developed four case studies representing different design approaches, such as sharing faculty, provision of online courses, and recognition of previous work experience as part of the admission criteria. There is a need for additional research, including evaluation of outcomes of models in current use. Academic progression is a multifaceted topic that needs to be carefully addressed to create a diverse well-educated nursing workforce ready to meet the nursing needs of an increasingly complex patient population.

Health Resources and Services Administration (HRSA). (2010). *The registered nurse population: Initial findings from the March 2008 National Sample Survey of Registered Nurses.* Washington, DC: U.S. Department of Health and Human Services.

Institute of Medicine (IOM). (2010). *The future of nursing: Leading change, advancing health.* Retrieved from http://books.nap.edu/openbook.php?record_id=12956&page=R1

Jeffreys, M. R. (2007). Tracking students through program entry, progression, graduation, and licensure: Assessing undergraduate nursing student retention and success. *Nursing Education Today, 27,* 406–419.

Munkvold, J., Tanner, C. A., & Herinckx, H. (2012). Factors affecting the academic progression of associate degree graduates. *Journal of Nursing Education, 51*(4), 232–235. doi: 10.3928/01484834–20120224-04

National League for Nursing (NLN). (2011). *Academic progression in nursing a living document from the NLN board of governors.* New York, NY: Author.

Pittman, P. M., Kurtzman, E. T., & Johnson, J. E. (2014). Academic progression models in nursing: Design decisions faced by administrators in four case studies. *Journal of Nursing Education, 53*(6), 329–335. doi: 10.3928/01484834–20140520-03

Raines, C. F., & Taglaireni, M. E. (2008). Career pathways in nursing: Entry points and academic progression. 2008. *OJIN: The Online Journal of Issues in Nursing, 13*(3) Manuscript 1.

Tri-Council for Nursing. (2010). *Consensus policy statement on the educational advancement of nurses.* Retrieved from http://www.nln.org/newsreleases/tri-council.pdf

Mary T. Quinn Griffin
Ellen Pokorny

ACADEMIC RETENTION

DEFINITION

Academic retention is defined as the number of nursing students enrolled in a specific program who are tracked to graduation (Baker, 2010). On the other hand, attrition is defined as the number of students who enter a program without progressing to graduation.

A

APPLICATION

The impact of academic retention is far reaching for the student, faculty, college or university, and community. Students have mounting costs in loans and tuition fees as well as possible lost wages from lack of progression to graduation. Student retention is essential for an institution in carrying out its purpose and mission. Retention is associated with students of traditional age, full-time status, and residing in campus. Retention rates in nursing programs may be as low as 50% (McLaughlin, 2008). Therefore, retention of nursing students is a key factor in nursing education.

The retention rate for U.S. higher education is 50% to 70% (O'Keeffe, 2013). Risk factors for noncompletion are related to mental health issues, disability, socioeconomic status, and ethnicity. Furthermore, a disconnection of students with the college, lack of a caring and supportive environment, and poor student–faculty relationships can also affect college retention.

In nursing, retention of students is often hard to predict due to students attending part time, withdrawing for personal or financial reasons, and changing majors. Dropout, withdrawal, and loss of students within the first year of nursing are issues affecting academic retention. Students may drop out due to poor academic performance, motivation, and stress. Self-perception and past academic performance have been listed as the two most important predictors of success (Peterson, 2009). Selecting qualified applicants, identifying at-risk students, and implementing strategies to promote student success are efforts to increase student retention. Faculty are encouraged to identify program characteristics that describe a clear picture of what constitutes academic success as well as what contributes to risk of academic failure (Jeffreys, 2006).

Low academic retention rates have been associated with minority students, and are linked to poor academic preparation, financial need, ineffective study habits, and poor English-language skills. Faculty team support has been effective in providing study skills, test-taking and critical thinking seminars, career coaching, and social interaction activities (Igbo et al., 2011). Baker (2010) sampled faculty at various nursing programs across 16 states to investigate the types of retention strategies used for retaining minority students. Retention strategies ranged over seminars, tutors, mentoring, study groups, financial aid, timely feedback, and faculty availability. Direct interaction between nursing faculty and students and timely feedback were rated by faculty as the most effective strategies.

Persistence is an emerging theme in retention climates with many key players. The institution plays a significant role in setting the tone for retention possibilities. The student's academic preparation as well as the student's peers can influence persistence. A student's persistence is also influenced by socioeconomic status and financial concerns (Oseguera & Rhee, 2009).

SYNOPSIS

Research has been conducted to identify factors impacting student academic performance and retention. Pitt, Powis, Levett-Jones, and Hunter (2012) conducted an integrative literature review and found that multiple factors can have an impact on student's academic performance. These factors are English as a second language, employment status, preadmission and in-school performance, social engagement, and support systems.

Research studies suggest that academic retention can be improved through assisting students with persistence and understanding of the importance of prerequisites required for entering nursing education. In addition, early identification of at-risk students should include setting specific goals and providing opportunities for socialization (McLaughlin, 2008). Other retention strategies that have been found to influence persistence include four themes as researched by Williams (2010). The themes are "keeping up" with the rigor of nursing, "not giving up" by having a clear vision and self-determination, "doing it" with a positive mind-set, and "connecting" in order to make use of all available resources for success.

The research continues to support prenursing experiences, advisement, peer tutoring, mentoring, financial assistance, and connection to the educational environment in providing positive strategies for success in nursing programs. These strategies can be applied with traditional and nontraditional undergraduate nursing students in a culturally diverse population (Jeffreys, 2012; Valencia-Go, 2005).

RECOMMENDATIONS

Successful retention programs must focus on providing stipends, scholarships, and seminars to increase academic retention. Key components of a strong retention plan for success should focus on developing and maintaining partnerships, counseling, tutoring, and social networking (Melillo, Dowling, Abdallah, Findeisen, & Knight, 2013).

Efforts should be centered on recruitment, retention, and graduation of minority nursing students. Reaching out to these students through pre-nursing activities in middle and high school offers potential for preparing them for success in an academic nursing program. Further research is needed to validate successful strategies for recruiting students early so that they can relate to the rigor of nursing education and the preparation required for program completion.

Faculty support to students has been described as a cornerstone of academic retention (Ramsburg, 2007). Faculty support includes creating a sense of community, ongoing advisement, conducting success seminars, and providing opportunities for social interaction.

Baker, B. H. (2010). Faculty ratings of retention strategies for minority nursing students. *Nursing Education Perspectives, 31*(4), 216–220.

Igbo, I. N., Straker, K. C., Landson, M. J., Symes, L., Bernard, L. F., Hughes, L. A., & Carroll, T. L. (2011). An innovative, multidisciplinary strategy to improve retention of nursing students from disadvantaged backgrounds. *Nursing Education Perspectives, 32*(6), 375–379.

Jeffreys, M. R. (2006). Tracking students through program entry, progression, graduation, and licensure: Assessing undergraduate nursing student retention and success. *Nurse Education Today, 27*, 406–419.

Jeffreys, M. R. (2012). *Nursing student retention: Understanding the process and making a difference.* New York, NY: Springer Publishing Company.

McLaughlin, B. N. (2008). Retention issues: What can we do? *Teaching and Learning in Nursing, 3*, 83–84.

Melillo, K. O., Dowling, J., Abdallah, L., Findeisen, M., & Knight, M. (2013). Bring diversity to nursing: Recruitment, retention, and graduation of nursing students. *Journal of Cultural Diversity, 20*(2), 100–104.

O'Keeffe, P. (2013). A sense of belonging: Improving student retention. *College Student Journal, 47*(4), 605–613.

Oseguera, L., & Rhee, B. S. (2009). The influence of institutional retention climates on student persistence to degree completion: A multilevel approach. *Research in Higher Education Journal, 50*, 546–569.

Peterson, V. (2009). Predictors of academic success in first semester baccalaureate nursing students. *Social Behavior and Personality, 37*(3), 411–418.

Pitt, V., Powis, D., Levett-Jones, T., & Hunter, S. (2012). Factors influencing nursing students' academic and clinical performance and attrition: An integrative literature review. *Nursing Education Today, 32*, 903–913.

Ramsburg, L. (2007). Strive for success: A successful retention program for associate of science in nursing students. *Teaching and Learning in Nursing, 2*, 12–16.

Valencia-Go, G. (2005). Growth and access increase for nursing students: A retention and progression project. *Journal of Cultural Diversity, 12*(1), 18–25.

Williams, M. (2010). Attrition and retention in the nursing major: Understanding persistence in beginning nursing students. *Nursing Education Perspectives, 31*(6), 362–367.

Susan D. Hart

ACADEMIC STRESSORS

DEFINITION

Academic stress includes actual and perceived stressors within the occupational environment. Compensation, role expectations, and job satisfaction have been found to be stress inducers (Whalen, 2009). Time constraints are a significant academic stressor (Hendel & Horn, 2008). Sources of stress for nurse educators include workload, lack of student achievement, and clinical supervision. Female gender and working in a public institution (Hendel & Horn, 2008), as well as technology are related to increased stress in academia (Burke, 2009).

APPLICATION

Finding balance among teaching, clinical assignments, and research obligations is challenging, yet may lead to lower levels of stress in nursing faculty. Clinical workload has been identified as the most significant issue for some nurse educator groups (Kaufman, 2007). Stressors experienced by clinical faculty may include challenges in meeting job expectations, energy depletion from work, imbalance between work and other responsibilities, and handling the needs of students who may not be well prepared (Oermann, 1998). Personnel shortages and continual change, which can be outcomes of dysfunctional and unhealthy work environments, may also contribute to stress in academia (Rudy, 2001).

Nursing faculty may be a vulnerable population (DalPezzo & Jett, 2010). Issues such as incivility, horizontal violence, and administrative power as potential sources of harm and stress for nursing faculty have been described (Clark, 2008; Clark & Springer, 2010; DalPezzo & Jett, 2010). Additional stressors for nurse educators include burnout related to demands within the work environment, clinical responsibilities, turnover, and role stress.

SYNOPSIS

Academic stress is experienced by nursing faculty. Workload, clinical supervision, role expectations, personnel shortages, lack of student preparation, technology, and poor coping skills have been identified as stressors for nurse educators.

RECOMMENDATIONS

Incorporating new support mechanisms within academic nursing environments may reduce stress for faculty and students. Chung and Kowalski (2012) studied mentor relationships, salary, tenure status, psychological empowerment, and job stress and found that all influenced job satisfaction. Nurses in mentoring relationships had higher job satisfaction. Mentoring would be particularly helpful for new faculty and may help establish a base, which could strengthen the ability to cope with stress.

Exploration of the working lives of part-time clinical faculty was advised by Whalen (2009) to encourage retention of those valuable clinicians. Whalen suggested development of an orientation program for faculty with inclusion of a mentoring program, maintenance of competitive salaries, open lines of communication, and keeping up-to-date on best practices.

Creation of positive academic environments for faculty includes structures that facilitate faculty choice and support faculty independence. Leadership influences work environment by utilization of excellent communication, celebration of success, and support of faculty decisions. Nursing faculty must realize the responsibility that all bear to create healthy work environments (Rudy, 2001).

Healthy work environments facilitate the provision of quality nursing education (National League for Nursing [NLN], 2006). Brady (2010) identified the NLN's toolkit as the guiding framework for healthy work environments. The NLN Healthful Work Environment Tool Kit (NLN, 2006) presents a structured method for academic administrators to evaluate the current environment of a school.

Fostering civility among faculty in nursing is a method to enhance collegial relationships and decrease stress in the working environment (Clark & Springer, 2010). The impact of leaders in forming the culture and climate of an organization is critical. Stress can be decreased and performance among academicians enhanced when civil work environments are established. Additional suggestions include stress management sessions for faculty, counseling, and integration of civility training.

Brady, M. S. (2010). Healthy nursing academic work environments. *The Online Journal of Issues in Nursing, 15*(1), 9.

Burke, M. S. (2009). The incidence of technological stress among baccalaureate nurse educators using technology during course preparation and delivery. *Nurse Education Today, 29*(1), 57–64.

Chung, C. E., & Kowalski, S. (2012). Job stress, mentoring, psychological empowerment, and job satisfaction among nursing faculty. *Journal of Nursing Education, 51*(7), 381–388.

Clark, C. M. (2008). Faculty and student assessment and experience with incivility in nursing education: A national perspective. *Journal of Nursing Education, 47,* 458–465.

Clark, C. M., & Springer, P. J. (2010). Academic nurse leaders' role in fostering a culture of civility in nursing education. *Journal of Nursing Education, 49*(6), 319–325.

DalPezzo, N., & Jett, K. T. (2010). Nursing faculty: A vulnerable population. *Journal of Nursing Education, 49*(3), 132–136.

Hendel, D. D., & Horn, A. S. (2008). The relationship between academic life conditions and perceived sources of faculty stress over time. *Journal of Human Behavior in the Social Environment, 17*(1–2), 61–88.

Kaufman, K. (2007). Headlines from the NLN. Introducing the NLN Carnegie national survey of nurse educators: Compensation, workload, and teaching practice. *Nursing Education Perspectives, 28,* 164–167.

National League for Nursing (NLN). (2006). *The healthful work environment tool kit.* Retrieved from http://www.nln.org/facultyprograms/HealthfulWorkEnvironment/toolkit.pdf

Oermann, M. H. (1998). Work-related stress of clinical nursing faculty. *Journal of Nursing Education, 37*(7), 302–304.

Rudy, E. B. (2001). Supportive work environments for nursing faculty. *AACN Clinical Issues: Advanced Practice in Acute & Critical Care, 12*(3), 401–410.

Whalen, K. S. (2009). Work-related stressors experienced by part-time clinical affiliate nursing faculty in baccalaureate education. *International Journal of Nursing Education Scholarship, 6*(1), Art. 30.

Elizabeth R. Click

ACADEMIC SUCCESS

DEFINITION

Success is the achievement of desired results. Therefore, academic success is defined as the ability of a student to achieve a desired academic outcome.

A

APPLICATION

Within the scope of nursing education and nursing practice, success in the National Council Licensure Examination-Registered Nurse (NCLEX-RN) is directly related to success in the nursing program. One hundred percent success by students in the NCLEX-RN is a benchmark that nursing programs strive to meet. However, more than 20% of nursing students from 4-year institutions and more than 30% of students from 2-year institutions withdraw from the program within 1 year (National League for Nursing, 2008). In addition, students who are unsuccessful in nursing programs drain institutional resources, costing more than $750,000 per year, per institution. Because personal success in an academic program is related to a program's student retention rate, efforts to understand factors and create programs that evoke academic success have turned out to be of paramount importance to nursing institutions.

SYNOPSIS

Evidence supports the notion that higher grade point average (GPA), excelling in nursing courses, and above-average scores on standardized tests provide a reliable predictor of the likelihood of success in the NCLEX-RN. Sayles, Shelton, and Powell (2003) evaluated the relationship between scores in the Nurse Entrance Test (NET) and the Comprehensive Achievement Profiles, Exit/Mobility Test. While success in the NET and Pre-RN Examinations was positively correlated with success in the NCLEX-RN, Sayles et al. (2003) emphasized the need to understand the significance of a student's learning style in his or her success. Such learning styles include visual, oral dependent, writing dependent, tactile, and kinesthetic (Sayles & Shelton, 2005; Sayles et al., 2003). Further understanding of these learning styles allows for implementation of various academic instruction methods that are compatible with a student's unique learning style.

In addition to learning style, subsequent studies have evaluated the effect of cognitive disposition on academic success. Wood, Saylor, and Cohen (2009) recognized that locus of control (LOC), an internal and external continuum of recognized factors that contribute to a particular outcome, influences nursing student academic success. Moreover, nursing students with a stronger external LOC orientation, which is a belief that outcomes are related to circumstances outside one's control, had a lower propensity for academic success. Furthermore, Peterson (2009) identified that although self-esteem and self-efficacy are positively correlated, neither variable was significantly related to academic success.

Another way to support students is to develop intrainstitutional programming to perpetuate success. Findings from Robinson and Niemer (2010) align with findings from previous studies that identify the merit of a peer tutor program for students who are at risk of nonsuccess in a nursing major. Mentees in this program were shown to score higher in examinations and earn a higher GPA than students who were not a part of the mentoring program. Also, a review of the literature by Weaver (2011) revealed that the use of high-fidelity patient simulation (HFPS) increased the overall knowledge of nursing students. However, the impact on knowledge transfer and confidence was inconclusive. Furthermore, Sportsman, Schumacker, and Hamilton (2011) emphasized the need for further evaluation of the relationship between HFPS and indicators of academic success and success in the NCLEX-RN.

RECOMMENDATIONS

Promoting academic success in nursing programs serves the dual purposes of promoting the efficient use of administrative expenditures and perpetuating the likelihood for success on the NCLEX-RN. Further research should be devoted to understanding and implementing educational programs that facilitate learning for students of various learning styles. Furthermore, research is needed to assess the relationship between HFPS and academic success. In addition, evidence supports the benefits of implementing a peer-tutoring program with conclusions that such programming will promote academic success and contribute to higher student retention rates. Further research is needed to evaluate the impact of psychosocial factors, such as self-confidence and self-efficacy, on academic success. Finally, it is important to consider the rapidly evolving demographics of the college student. These students are characterized by technological competence, propensity for multitasking, inability to communicate through traditional channels, distaste for reading and writing, and expression of self-doubt regarding academic abilities and readiness for college (Pardue & Morgan, 2008). Therefore, it is imperative to include interventions and programs designed to promote academic success for this unique and diverse cohort.

National League for Nursing. (2008). *One-year retention status of full time nursing students and full time U.S. undergraduates by program/institution type.* Retrieved from http://www.nln.org/researchgrants/slides/pdf/AS0607_23.pdf

Pardue, K. T., & Morgan, P. (2008). Millennials considered: A new generation, new approaches, and implications for nursing education. *Nursing Education Perspectives, 29*(2), 74–79.

Peterson, V. (2009). Predictors of academic success in first semester baccalaureate nursing students. *Social Behavior & Personality: An International Journal, 37*(3), 411–417.

Robinson, E., & Niemer, L. (2010). A peer mentor tutor program for academic success in nursing. *Nursing Education Perspectives, 31*(5), 286–289.

Sayles, S., & Shelton, D. (2005). Student success strategies. *ABNF Journal, 16*(5), 98–101.

Sayles, S., Shelton, D., & Powell, H. (2003). Predictors of success in nursing education. *ABNF Journal, 14*(6), 116–120.

Sportsman, S., Schumacker, R. E., & Hamilton, P. (2011). Evaluating the impact of scenario-based high-fidelity patient simulation on academic metrics of student success. *Nursing Education Perspectives, 32*(4), 259–265. doi: 10.5480/1536-5026- 32.4.259

Weaver, A. (2011). High-fidelity patient simulation in nursing education: An integrative review. *Nursing Education Perspectives, 32*(1), 37–40.

Wood, A., Saylor, C., & Cohen, J. (2009). Locus of control and academic success among ethnically diverse baccalaureate nursing students. *Nursing Education Perspectives, 30*(5), 290–294.

Grant A. Pignatiello
Ronald L. Hickman

ACCELERATED NURSING PROGRAMS

DEFINITION

Accelerated nursing (fast-track) programs have evolved to hasten the time in which nursing students can complete the bachelor of science nursing degree (BSN). The goal of an accelerated nursing program is to develop baccalaureate (BSN)-prepared graduates who are qualified to take the National Council Licensure Examination for Registered Nurses (NCLEX-RN) licensing examination in a shorter period of time than the typical 4-year nursing program (Penprase & Koczara, 2009).

APPLICATION

Accelerated nursing programs offer an innovative solution to the nursing shortage that is expected to grow from 2.74 million in 2010 to 3.45 million in 2020, an increase of 712,000 or 26% (American Association of Colleges of Nursing [AACN], 2014b). These programs focus on attracting potential adult candidates who have already completed a bachelor degree in another discipline. Accelerated degree nursing programs afford non-nursing

A

college graduates the opportunity to earn a BSN with a rapid transition into nursing practice. These programs hold that accelerated nursing students are adult learners, have already proven that they can complete the rigor of upper-level education through the first degree, and can transition through the accelerated program because of experience in education and previous employment.

Adults who have science degrees tend to be better prepared to enter the accelerated programs because they need fewer prerequisites in science-related courses such as pathophysiology, biology, and chemistry. Students generally can earn a BSN in 12 to 18 months. The time frame of the program completion varies related to what courses are considered prerequisites. Thus, the 12-month accelerated program may have more prerequisites, whereas the 18-month program integrates several prerequisites into the nursing curriculum.

Accelerated nursing programs have grown rapidly over the past three decades to more than 232 accelerated baccalaureate programs (AACN, 2014a). Associate of science degree in nursing (ASDN) programs attract new, previously untapped students to nursing, including professionals and mature individuals from a variety of educational fields seeking a second career (Cangelosi, 2008). Because ASDN programs are rigorous and intense, admission standards are high, typically requiring a minimum 3.0 grade point average (GPA) from the bachelor degree.

SYNOPSIS

Reasons for adults being attracted to accelerated nursing programs as a second degree include shifts in the U.S. economy, secure employment, steady income, recognition of the prior degree(s), and the desire to make a difference in other people's lives. Accelerated nursing students perform better than traditional students, as measured between NCLEX-RN first-time pass rates and other pass rates in the nursing program. Generally, attrition rates of accelerated

nursing studies are much lower than those of traditional nursing students (Penprase & Harris, 2013). Highest attrition is noted in the first semester either for academic reason or a mismatch with nursing practice. Accelerated nursing students are at academic risk related to personal background preparation, pre-entrance examinations, GPA in nursing programs, and NCLEX-RN preparation examinations (Bentley, 2006; Penprase, Harris, & Qu, 2013).

Accelerated nursing students are successful in the fast-past curriculum because they are college graduates who have already completed many of the science and liberal arts requirements (Rico, Beal, & Davies, 2010). These students tend to be highly motivated and excel academically (Seldomridge & DiBartolo, 2005). They are mature and understand the commitment required to succeed based on past experiences. Accelerated nursing students are older than traditional nursing students, predominately female and Caucasian, and more diverse than traditional students (Penprase et al., 2013). The proportion of men in the programs is notably higher than the national average of traditional nursing programs (AACN, 2014c; Penprase et al., 2013).

RECOMMENDATIONS

Accelerated nursing program curricula must cover the same content as a traditional nursing program; however, the content may be altered in delivery. Because the pace of information is accelerated, creative ways are used to deliver content in an accelerated format. In addition, an accelerated student is an adult learner who needs to be motivated differently from the traditional nursing student. Acknowledgment of the diverse knowledge and experience these unique students bring to the nursing classes is necessary. A variety of teaching modalities offers engagement of the student with less emphasis on passive-learning and more focus on active-learning methods.

Accelerated nursing programs are for mature, highly motivated students who have already demonstrated success in earning an undergraduate degree. The program is intensive during the 12 to 18 months in which it is offered. It is best that students do not work and plan for the lack of income during this period. Some students report being highly stressed during the program; thus, accelerated nursing programs are not for all adults. Consideration of other life commitments, time pressures, and financial security must be assessed before entering an accelerated nursing program.

American Association of Colleges of Nursing (AACN). (2014a). *Accelerated nursing programs.* Retrieved from http://www.aacn.nche.edu/students/accelerated-nursingprograms

American Association of Colleges of Nursing (AACN). (2014b). *Fact sheet: Accelerated nursing programs.* Retrieved from http://www.aacn.nche.edu/media/factsheets/acceleratedprog.htm

American Association of Colleges of Nursing (AACN). (2014c). *Nursing shortage.* Retrieved from http://www.aacn.nche.edu/media-relations/fact-sheets/nursing-shortage

Bentley, R. (2006). Comparison of traditional and accelerated baccalaureate nursing graduates. *Nurse Educator, 31*(2), 79–83.

Cangelosi, P. R. (2008). Accelerated nursing students and theater students: Creating a safe environment by acting the part. *Nursing Education Perspectives, 29*(6), 342–346.

Penprase, B. B., & Harris, M. A. (2013). Accelerated second-degree nursing students: Predictors of graduation and NCLEX-RN first-time pass rates. *Nurse Educator, 38*(1), 26–29.

Penprase, B., Harris, M., & Qu, H. (2013). Academic success: Which factors contribute significantly to NCLEX success for students? *Journal of Nursing Education and Practice, 3*(7), 1.

Penprase, B., & Koczara, S. (2009). Understanding the experiences of accelerated second-degree nursing students and graduates: A review of the literature. *Journal of Continuing Education in Nursing, 40*(2), 74–78.

Rico, S., Beal, J., & Davies, T. (2010). Promising practices for faculty in accelerated nursing programs. *Journal of Nursing Education, 49*(3), 150–155. Retrieved from http://dx.doi.org/10.3928/01484834-20100115-01

Seldomridge, L. A., & DiBartolo, M. C. (2005). A profile of accelerated second bachelor's degree nursing students. *Nurse Educator, 30*(2), 65–68.

Barbara Penprase

ACTIVE LEARNING

DEFINITION

Active learning includes several models of instruction that put the responsibility of learning on the learner. This approach to instruction was popularized in the 1990s and a key report was published by the Association for the Study of Higher Education (ASHE; Bonwell & Eison, 1991). This report detailed various methods used to promote active learning. The report indicated that to learn, students must do more than just listen. They must read, write, discuss, and be engaged in solving problems. This type of instruction relates to the domains of learning referred to as knowledge, skills, and attitudes. In order to learn, students must engage in higher-order thinking tasks such as analysis, synthesis, and evaluation. Active learning engages students in two crucial aspects. These are doing things, and thinking about the things they are doing (Bonwell & Eison, 1991).

APPLICATION

Active learning involves the learner engaging in activities and reflecting. Some activities include learner engagement in debates, simulations, guided design, small group

A

problem solving, and case studies. The classic example of passive learning is seen when a learner is listening to a lecture. To make learning more active, experiential learning and opportunities for reflective dialogue need to be included.

When educators prepare a teaching session, they need to design learning activities that involve reading, writing, discussion, and active engagement in solving problems. In order to create substantial learning, tools and innovative methods of teaching and learning are needed. It is necessary to understand how to incorporate more active learning in the teaching session.

Learning is not a passive spectator sport, and the more actively engaged learners are, the more learning and retention take place. Evidence shows that different instructional methods have greater rates of retention (Kolb, Boyatzis, & Mainemelis, 1999). Most people learn best when actively involved in the learning process.

There are several strategies to consider depending on the level of the audience and the purpose of the educational offering. Some strategies are particularly relevant for diverse audiences. For example, role-playing could be incorporated by having participants practice talking to a clinical preceptor, patient, or family about noncompliance with hand washing. Other active learning strategies include quizzes, games, brainstorming, problem solving, case studies, and simulation.

SYNOPSIS

Active learning is an influential model that emerged in the literature on teaching and learning in the 1990s. Research supports the concept of active learning. Many studies show that learners retain learning longer when instructional methods used were active rather than passive (Anderson, Mitchell, & Osgood, 2005; Armbruster, Patel, Johnson, & Weiss, 2009; Freeman et al., 2007; Smith, Wood, Krauter, & Knight, 2011).

Research has also shown that the use of a wide assortment of active-learning strategies

to reach nursing students in a holistic manner promotes learning (Ulrich & Glendon, 2005). As adult learners, nursing students learn through all senses, including vision, hearing, smell, touch, taste, and emotional connections.

RECOMMENDATIONS

Students learn more effectively if they are active rather than passive during the learning process. Learning by doing is generally more effective than learning by listening or reading. Experiential learning is more effective. When students engage in active participation in the learning process, they are more likely to remember what they have learned and to process the learning in a meaningful way. Providing incentives for learning is important.

Numerous studies have pointed to the success of active-learning strategies in nursing education. Additional research including systematic studies is needed to augment and broaden the knowledge base of active learning in nursing education. Studies of specific teaching methods that fully maximize student competencies in the clinical setting are needed.

Anderson, W. L., Mitchell, S. M., & Osgood, M. P. (2005). Comparison of student performance in cooperative learning and traditional lecture-based biochemistry classes. Biochemistry and molecular biology education: A bimonthly publication of the *International Union of Biochemistry and Molecular Biology, 33*(6), 387–393.

Armbruster, P., Patel, M., Johnson, E., & Weiss, M. (2009). Active learning and student-centered pedagogy improve student attitudes and performance in introductory biology. *Education, 8*, 203–213.

Bonwell, C., & Eison, J. (1991). *Active learning: Creating excitement in the classroom AEHE-ERIC higher education report No. 1.* Washington, DC: Jossey-Bass. ISBN 1–878380-08–7.

Freeman, S., Connor, E. O., Parks, J. W., Cunningham, M., Hurley, D., Haak, D.,...Wenderoth, M. P. (2007). Prescribed active learning increases performance in introductory biology. *Education, 6*, 132–139.

Kolb, D., Boyatzis, R. E., & Mainemelis, C. (1999). *Experiential learning: Experience as the source of learning and development.* Department of Organizational Behavior Weatherhead School of Management, Case Western Reserve University. Retrieved from http://www.d.umn,edu/~kgilbert/educ5165–731/Readings/experiential-learningtheory.pdf

Smith, M. K., Wood, W. B., Krauter, K., & Knight, J. K. (2011). Combining peer discussion with instructor explanation increases student learning from in-class concept questions. *CBE—Life Sciences Education, 10*, 55–63.

Ulrich, D. L., & Glendon, K. J. (2005). *Interactive group learning: Strategies for nurse educators* (2nd ed., pp. 73–126). New York, NY: Springer Publishing Company.

Irena L. Kenneley

ADULT LEARNING

DEFINITION

Adult learning is also known as *andragogy*. Andragogy emphasizes the process of learning through approaches that are problem oriented and collaborative. It is defined as principles and processes that help adults learn (Utley, 2011). Knowles identified six principles of adult learning. Adults are internally motivated and self-directed, bring life experiences and knowledge to learning experiences, are goal oriented, are relevancy oriented, are practical, and want to be respected (Knowles, 1984).

APPLICATION

The use of adult learning principles is recommended in the nursing classroom, lab, and simulation and clinical settings. Nurse educators who teach nursing students should utilize the principles of andragogy. Nursing students who are adults and have practice experience can build their nursing skills either in a lab or a clinical setting.

SYNOPSIS

Nursing research linked to adult learning principles has been implemented in a variety of nursing classroom and clinical settings, which include facilitating graduate students' knowledge and development in science and theory; application of a new graduate transition model to clinical practice (Schoessler & Waldo, 2006); breastfeeding workshops (Noel-Weiss, Rupp, Cragg, Bassett, & Woodend, 2006); development of professionalism in registered nurse-bachelor of science in nursing (RN-BSN) students (Morris & Faulk, 2007); and growing leaders in an organization (Shekleton, Preston, & Good, 2010).

RECOMMENDATIONS

Nurse educators should liberate students from the traditional process of nursing education through lecture. Innovative and effective educators create conditions where students can test new knowledge to gain clinical competence, which will foster life-long learning. Themes emerging from the literature include problem-solving methodology and student-centered and self-directed learning to foster professional knowledge and growth. Adult learning principles should be applied across the nursing curriculum. Principles of adult learning should be used to teach both students and adult patients. Teaching practices should migrate from a parochial methodology to a collaborative learner-centered teaching style.

A

Knowles, M. (1984). *Andragogy in action*. San Francisco, CA: Jossey-Bass.

Morris, A., & Faulk, D. (2007). Perspective transformation: Enhancing the development of professionalism in RN-to-BSN students. *Journal of Nursing Education, 46*(10), 445–451.

Noel-Weiss, J., Rupp, A., Cragg, B., Bassett, V., & Woodend, A. (2006). Randomized controlled trial to determine effects of prenatal breastfeeding workshop on maternal breastfeeding self-efficacy and breastfeeding duration. *JOGNN: Journal of Obstetric, Gynecologic & Neonatal Nursing, 35*(5), 616–624. doi:10.1111/j.1552–6909.2006.00077.x

Schoessler, M., & Waldo, M. (2006). The first 18 months in practice: A developmental transition model for the newly graduated nurse. *Journal for Nurses in Staff Development, 22*(2), 47–54.

Shekleton, M., Preston, J., & Good, L. (2010). Growing leaders in a professional membership organization. *Journal of Nursing Management, 18*(6), 662–668. doi: 10.1111/j.1365–2834.2010.01152.x

Utley, R. (2011). *Theory and research for academic nurse educators*. Boston, MA: Jones and Bartlett Publishers.

Cheryl D. Schlamb

Art and Reflection

DEFINITION

Art has various definitions including: the expression or application of human creative skill and imagination used in the creation of aesthetic objects, environments, or experiences that can be shared with others. Art is further described in the field of aesthetics as a branch of philosophy that includes the critical reflection on art, nature, and culture.

Reflection is giving something serious thought. Self-reflection is an inner awareness of thoughts, feelings, beliefs, judgments, and perceptions. Both the creation of art and the experience of viewing art enhance the reflective process and support both knowing and healing. In viewing art one recreates a vision, similar to the creator of the piece, as the details are gathered into an expression of the whole.

APPLICATION

The practice of art and reflection, initially used by art therapists, is increasingly being used in the education of students. Art media, the creative process, and the resulting artwork can be used to facilitate student learning on interventions to promote client well-being. Reflecting on art can assist clients explore feelings, resolve emotional conflicts, increase self-awareness and self-esteem, manage behavior and addictions, reduce anxiety, and develop social skills (American Art Therapy Association [AATA], 2014). The benefit of art in the patient care setting occurs through the professional relationship, artistic self-expression, communication, and reflection for individuals who experience illness, trauma, and developmental, social, or psychological impairment.

Reflecting on art may also be used to improve interpersonal skills, manage problematic behaviors, reduce negative stress, and achieve personal insight (AATA, 2014). Initiatives such as the inclusion of art and reflection in curriculum, workshops, and training programs (O'Donnell, Rabow, & Remen, 2007) are providing experiences for nurses and physicians with various forms of art, including reflection, imagery, ritual, poetry, writing, and journaling. When programs are conducted with a spirit of discovery and recognition of the collective wisdom of the group, outcomes include increased group cohesiveness, increased meaning in work, tools to maintain personal and professional satisfaction, validation of self-care and self-reflection, increased empathy, and the exploration of difficult concepts such as suffering and healing (Kearsley & Lobb, 2014).

Students viewing art in a gallery, often with a prompt, followed by group debriefing have cultivated emotional self-awareness and empathetic responses to particular health care situations. Works of art may communicate a broad range of human experience and thoughts, and thus are useful in studying interpersonal and social situations (Wikstrom, 2000). Drama performances and visual arts seminars also allow students to increase visual observation and develop empathetic understanding. The use of drama skills in patient communication courses, as opposed to role-play, allows students to portray the role of patient, physician, and nurse, for the purpose of enhancing empathy. Other forms of art such as drawing, storytelling, poetry, collages, and photographic imagery have increased understanding and uncovered students' emotions with agonizing and traumatic clinical encounters. Drawing, in many forms, focused on images, nature, abstract thoughts, or mandala have also been used to increase self-awareness through both self- and critical reflection.

SYNOPSIS

Creative and expressive art is used in various patient populations and different environments by health care professionals ranging from art therapists to physicians and nurses. The use in nursing education is increasing with the goal of assisting student development in various areas such as self-awareness, empathy, critical thinking, and socialization. In addition, peer-to-peer, interprofessional team, and student–faculty relationships may benefit from expressive art. Through these approaches, understanding is enhanced, thus transcending the limits of language and capturing what cannot be articulated (Barone & Eisner, 2012).

RECOMMENDATIONS

The value of art and reflection in education and practice is grounded in the expression of personal philosophy, spirituality, self-awareness,

and nonverbal communication. The process aids in the development of a holistic perspective of health and healing, patient-centered care, and increased interprofessional collaboration. In addition, personal reflections and experiences are shared in a safe setting.

Teaching and learning strategies are needed to support learner-centered curricula and prepare nurses and physicians for today's challenging health care environments. Innovative approaches are needed to support discussion, debate, critical reflection, and lifelong learning. Involving the arts in learning is one strategy with a potential to engage learners while fostering understanding of multiple perspectives (Rieger & Chernomas, 2013). An increased use of these modalities as well as research supporting these efforts is needed. Research studies may be designed around art that represents specific medical conditions, patient or social issues, cultural diversity, and population health, and involve both quantitative and qualitative designs as new rubrics are established.

American Art Therapy Association (AATA). (2014). *Art therapy*. Retrieved from http://www.arttherapy.org/upload/whatisart-therapy.pdf

Barone, T., & Eisner, E. W. (2012). *Arts based research*. Washington, DC: Sage.

Kearsley, J. H., & Lobb, E. A. (2014). Workshops in healing for senior medical students: A 5-year overview and appraisal. *Medical Humanities*. doi:10.1136/medhum-2013–010438. (Epub ahead of print.)

O'Donnell, J., Rabow, M., & Remen, R. (2007). The healer's art: Awakening the heart of medicine. *Medical Encounter, 21*(1), 7–11.

Rieger, K. L., & Chernomas, W. M. (2013). Arts-based learning: Analysis of the concept for nursing education. *International Journal of Nursing Education Scholarship, 10*. doi:10.1515/ijnes-2012–0034.

Wikstrom, B. M. (2000). Nursing education at an art gallery. *Journal of Nursing Scholarship, 32*(2), 197–199.

Deborah McElligott

A

ART OF NURSING

DEFINITION

The art of nursing verbally and/or non-verbally conveys caring, an interpersonal connection, human touch, a presence that calms the fears and soothes the soul of a hurting person. "(T)he art of nursing is the intentional creative use of oneself, based upon skill and expertise, to transmit emotion and meaning to another" (Jenner, 1997, p. 5). "The art of nursing is the expert use and adaptation of empirical and metaphysical knowledge and values. It involves sensitively adapting care to meet the needs of individual patients, and in the face of uncertainty, the discretionary use of creativity" (Finfgeld-Connett, 2008a, p. 387).

APPLICATION

The art of nursing is more complex and difficult to teach than psychomotor skills or scientific facts. It involves knowledge, skills, attitudes, and values. Role modeling allows faculty to teach by example through interactions with patients and their families, and also students, other faculty, nursing staff, and other health care providers. Role modeling should occur in all interactions both in and out of the classroom or clinical arena. Students can use other nurses as role models with reading assignments from the *Journal of Holistic Nursing* or *American Journal of Nursing*'s feature called Reflections.

Most students have laboratory experiences teaching them psychomotor skills. Often they are so focused on the skill that they say nothing. Faculty can help them talk to the simulated patient and learn the process of building a nurse–patient relationship. Some techniques that can be used include: giving each mannequin a name and using narrative pedagogy to tell a story about who he or she is, providing a context for why the skill needs to be performed.

Recording the interaction can help students see themselves as others see them. Many are uncomfortable watching and hearing themselves, but it is a valuable teaching/learning modality. Also asking the student how it might feel to be the patient in each situation is helpful. For example, ask: "Is that the way you would want it done for you or a family member?"

Use case studies to add the person to the medication or procedure scenario. The National League for Nursing has several unfolding case studies in its Advancing Care Excellence for Seniors (ACES) Program (www.nln.org/facultyprograms/faculty resources/ACES/index.htm). The Julia Morales/Lucy Grey case has been used as the narrative pedagogical background for a simulated patient encounter.

The fine arts, both visual and written, convey powerful emotions. Students could be asked to reflect on a painting or poem. Freda Kahlo is one artist who might be used. Blogs are used by some patients and families to share their lived experiences and some can be accessed.

Reflection helps nursing artistry grow. It puts an experience into context for a greater understanding of what occurred by reflecting on both the patient and self. Ask students to write their thoughts and feelings about illness and nursing. For self-evaluation, ask: "What did I do well?' and "What could I have done better?" More detailed questions might be: Did I do everything I could to make the patient comfortable? Was my teaching understood? Did I prepare the patient adequately for the procedure? How did the patient feel before, during, and after the procedure? How did I feel? It can include an examination of values, beliefs, and assumptions that came into play during the encounter. This can occur individually or in groups, verbally or written. Journaling may help the student grow in nursing artistry. Warn students about digital blogs as they could violate patient confidentiality. Reflection can move a nurse toward a humanistic, holistic nursing practice that actualizes the art of nursing.

SYNOPSIS

Florence Nightingale (1868) said that nursing is an art that requires devotion and preparation. Both Nightingale (1868) and Donahue (1985) consider nursing the finest art. For decades, students have been told that nursing is both an art and a science (Potter & Perry, 2009; Stewart, 1929). The science provides the knowledge base, but the art is the core of how that knowledge is applied and truly what nursing is (Tarnow & Butcher, 2005). Jacobs-Kramer and Chinn (1988) indicated that "empirical, ethical, and personal knowledge to bring about a harmonious and pleasing whole—an artful nursing act" (p. 137). The art of nursing is not merely the knowing, but the act, the intervention, the application of nursing care in an artful manner.

There is concern about technology becoming too prominent in nursing. "The real essence of nursing, as of any fine art, lies not in the mechanical details of execution, nor yet in the dexterity of the performer, but in the creative imagination, the sensitive spirit, and the intelligent understanding lying back of these techniques and skills" (Smith, 1930). Technology can provide valuable information, but cannot replace listening to the patient and being with the patient, which is the art of nursing.

RECOMMENDATIONS

Nursing has advanced the profession through research. Yet, there is limited research centered on the art of nursing. Finfgeld-Connett's (2008a) review of the literature from 1982 to 2006 revealed varying interpretations and implementation of the art of nursing. They found that not only the patients but also the nurses benefited from implementing the art of nursing; nurses had more professional and personal satisfaction and growth. Her qualitative study examining the concepts of art of nursing, caring, and presence in the literature concluded that there is a need to "substantiate core elements of nursing practice and to provide a better understanding of the discipline" (Finfgeld-Connett, 2008b, p. 534).

Gramling's (2004) qualitative study from conversations with patients identified these elements of artful care: perpetual presence, knowing the other, intimacy in agony, deep detail, and honoring the body (p. 387). These patients/subjects said, "... the presence or absence of nursing art...becomes a healing force or a cause of further suffering" (p. 394).

In summary, the study, education, and practice of the art of nursing is important for both patient and nurse satisfaction with nursing.

Donahue, M. P. (1985). *Nursing, the finest art: An illustrated history.* St. Louis, MO: Mosby.

Finfgeld-Connett, D. (2008a). Concept synthesis of the art of nursing. *Journal of Advanced Nursing, 62*(3), 381–388. doi: 10.1111/j.1365–2648.2008.04601.x

Finfgeld-Connett, D. (2008b). Qualitative convergence of three nursing concepts: Art of nursing, presence and caring. *Journal of Advanced Nursing, 63*(5), 527–534. doi: 10.1111/j.1365–2648.2008.04622.x.

Gramling, K. L. (2004). A narrative study of nursing art in critical care. *Journal of Holistic Nursing, 22,* 379–398.

Jacobs-Kramer, M. K., & Chinn, P. L. (1988). Perspectives on knowing: A model of nursing knowledge. *Scholarly Inquiry for Nursing Practice: An International Journal, 2*(2), 129–143.

Jenner, C. A. (1997). The art of nursing. A concept analysis. *Nursing Forum, 32*(4), 5–11.

Nightingale, F. (1868). Una and the lion. *Good Works.* London: Strahan & Co.

Potter, P. A., & Perry, A. G. (2009). *Fundamentals of nursing, 7th edition.* St. Louis, MO: Mosby.

Smith, M. R. (1930). How to evaluate existing nursing procedures. *American Journal of Nursing, 30*(4), 391–398.

Stewart, I. (1929). The science and art of nursing (Editorial). *Nursing Education Review, 2,* 1.

Tarnow, K. G., & Butcher, H. K. (2005). Teaching the art of professional nursing in a learning laboratory. In M. Oermann & K. Heinrich (Eds.), *Annual review of nursing education. Vol. 3* (pp. 375–392). New York, NY: Springer Publishing Company.

Karen Gahan Tarnow

ATTRITION

DEFINITION

The California Postsecondary Education Commission (2003) defines attrition as "departure from a nursing program without successful completion of the program; but can also be defined to include students who are delayed in their progress toward program completion" (p. 12).

APPLICATION

Attrition is a serious concern in nursing education. As the profession struggles to remedy the current and projected nursing shortage, there is a strong and urgent need to understand factors that influence attrition. In addition, the problem of attrition in nursing education hampers efforts to efficiently manage education-related resources.

SYNOPSIS

There have been many nursing education studies that explore factors that contribute to attrition among nursing students. These factors can be divided into two major factors: intrinsic and extrinsic. Intrinsic factors influencing attrition include demographic variables such as age, gender, and ethnicity. Results of several studies show that younger students and those with English as a second language are more likely to leave a nursing program (Higgins, 2005; Jeffreys, 2007; Pitt, Powis, Levett-Jones, & Hunter, 2012). Various personal, academic, and psychosocial attributes have also been found to significantly influence attrition. These attributes are: critical-thinking ability, self-efficacy, level of acculturation, self-determination, prerequisite and preexamination performance, anxiety, support-seeking behaviors, financial burden, and health-related issues (Higgins, 2005; Jeffreys, 2007; McLaughlin, Moutray, & Muldoon, 2007; Pitt et al., 2012; Rouse & Rooda, 2010; Williams, 2010). In addition, perception of burn out and dissonance between theory and practice has been found to impact the decision to leave a nursing school (O'Donnell, 2010; Williams, 2010).

External factors that influence the decision to leave a nursing program include: support from family, significant others, peers, friends, and other social systems such as faith-based organizations. Other external factors are academic assistance, orientation program, motivational and morale-boosting workshops, time management, test-taking, stress relief, anxiety management, tutoring, library and laboratory services, support from faculty and counselors, and remediation and mentoring programs (Higgins, 2005; Jeffreys, 2007; Pitt et al., 2012; Rudel, 2006). These intrinsic and extrinsic factors have universal relevance for baccalaureate, associate degree, and traditional, nontraditional, and accelerated programs.

RECOMMENDATION

Studies that explore nursing student attrition have recommended several strategies to address this serious nursing education issue that include: (a) the need to closely examine the variables that predict attrition, (b) establishing a set of criteria and methods to identify students at risk early in the program, (c) offering programs and workshops shown to increase student retention, (d) constantly evaluating the curriculum and program outcomes to ensure that they produce nurses who have the competency and skills needed to practice in a complex health care environment, (e) developing a culture of openness and support, (f) establishing a structured advisement program to specifically address the needs of those students who are struggling in the program, (g) offering assistance to students how to access possible sources of financial aid and scholarships, and (h) creating a system to support faculty to address issues that relate to attrition and retention.

Addressing attrition in nursing education has a significant relevance to our future as a profession. A review of the literature on student attrition and retention reveals that although there are many extenuating circumstances that could influence attrition, schools of nursing have a primary responsibility to ensure that students accepted into a nursing program are provided with support and resource in order to succeed.

The literature search also reveals that there is limited information on this topic especially among nontraditional or accelerated-degree students. There is a need to explore the pattern and nature of attrition among this growing cohort of nursing students.

California Postsecondary Education Commission. (2003). *Admission policies and attrition rates in California community college nursing programs. Commission report 03–2.* Retrieved March 19, 2014, from http://www.cpec.ca.gov./completereports/2003reports/03–02.pdf

Higgins, B. (2005). Strategies for lowering attrition rates and raising NCLEX-RN pass rates. *Journal of Nursing Education, 44*(12), 541–547.

Jeffreys, M. (2007). Nontraditional students: Perceptions of variables influencing retention: A multisite study. *Nurse Educator, 32*(4), 161–167.

McLaughlin, K., Moutray, M., & Muldoon, O. (2007). The role of personality and self-efficacy in the selection and retention of successful nursing students: A longitudinal study. *Journal of Advanced Nursing, 61*(2), 211–221.

O'Donnell, H. (2010). Expectations and voluntary attrition in nursing students. *Nursing Education in Practice, 11,* 54–63.

Pitt, V., Powis, D., Levett-Jones, T., & Hunter, S. (2012). Factors influencing nursing students' academic and clinical performance and attrition: An integrative literature review. *Nursing Education Today, 32,* 903–913.

Rouse, S., & Rooda, L. (2010). Factors for attrition in an accelerated baccalaureate nursing program. *Journal of Nursing Education, 49*(6), 359–362.

Rudel, R. (2006). Nontraditional nursing students: The social influences on retention. *Teaching and Learning in Nursing, 1,* 47–54.

Williams, M. (2010). Attrition and retention in the nursing major: Understanding persistence in beginning nursing students. *Nursing Education Perspectives, 31*(6), 362–367.

Emerson E. Ea

AUDIENCE RESPONSE SYSTEM

DEFINITION

The Audience Response System (ARS) is an active learning and teaching strategy that utilizes computer software and a handheld remote control device also termed a clicker to wirelessly communicate with a receiver connected to a universal serial bus (USB) port on the computer (Vana, Silva, Muzyka, & Hirani, 2011). The ARS transmits question responses for display using graphics and frequency distributions to provide instant feedback for both the lecturer and students (Vana et al., 2011).

APPLICATION

Traditional lecture is widely used in nursing education, although it has been identified as passive, with student learning often disconnected from knowledge application (Johnson & Mighten, 2005). Nursing lectures often include a great deal of information covering new and often complex topics. The ARS allows the instructor to present a question to students. Then students use their handheld device clickers to select the correct answers and the instructor can display the aggregate student responses anonymously in real time (Clauson, Alkhateeb, & Singh-Franco, 2012). The utilization of the ARS in the nursing classroom can transform a traditional passive lecture into a multidimensional active learning environment.

ARS questions can be embedded into PowerPoint presentations to assess student learning. When used in this format, the educator must prepare ARS questions prior to class; however, preconstructed questions may be readily available from the textbook publisher. It is beneficial to space the questions in the lecture, about 1 question every 15 to 20 minutes or 3 to 4 questions per hour to prevent overloading. When the question appears on the slide students are given a specified time to provide an answer. One minute is usually sufficient for the length of the question. During this time, students read the question and provide an answer using their clicker devices. At the conclusion of the specified time, polling is closed. The instructor can then view results, which are instantly tabulated and displayed. Next, students are queried to share which answer they chose, the rationale, and how other choices were eliminated. This usually leads to a discussion among students who either respectfully agree or disagree with peers. During this time, students discover and learn from peers. After discussion of the question, the educator can: display the correct answer, identify correct decisions by students, clarify any misconceptions, and reteach any content that was not fully understood. Therefore, when ARS responses are polled the educator must be flexible, prepared, and feel comfortable engaging in open discussion with students. The discussion that follows an ARS question can help students think like a nurse (Russell, McWilliams, Chasen, & Farley, 2011) and to improve test-taking skills (Stein, Challman, & Brueckner, 2006). The educator can serve as the moderator during discussions and support, correct, and clarify misconceptions. At the conclusion of each lecture the educator can save all student responses for further review and analysis.

SYNOPSIS

The practice of nursing education requires students to bring together content learned in the classroom for application in clinical practice. The ability to think critically and make accurate and appropriate decisions aimed at providing safe patient care is imperative. When using the ARS in the classroom setting the lecturer can present questions and case studies to students using the ARS to bridge the gap between classroom and clinical practice. This teaching strategy has been found to be effective in both small and large classes (Stein et al., 2006; Thomas, Monturo, & Conroy, 2011; Vana et al., 2011).

There are several benefits to utilizing the ARS in nursing education, which includes the ability to reinforce student learning, increase student participation, improve student engagement and active learning, and identify misconceptions for clarification (Efstathiou & Bailey, 2012; Stein et al., 2006). These benefits are increasingly valuable as nursing-class sizes steadily increase making it difficult to discern whether students understand information taught (Russell et al., 2011). In addition to the increased benefit of active student learning, research finding demonstrates that student satisfaction with the ARS system combined with lecture is higher than that with lecture alone (Lee & Dapremont, 2012; Stein et al., 2006).

RECOMMENDATIONS

Nurse educators are challenged to teach students how to provide patient care in an increasingly complex health care system. Although, the impact of ARS usage on examination scores is inconclusive (Vana et al., 2011), overall student satisfaction is high. The ARS system provides prompt feedback for both students and faculty to improve student learning.

The educator must be prepared to integrate ARS questions into lecture and plan ahead accordingly. Time must be allowed to present and discuss the question and reteach content if necessary (Vana et al., 2011). Although, time must be allotted to prepare the ARS questions (Stein et al., 2006; Vana et al., 2011), many textbook publishers have begun to provide preconstructed ARS questions with resources that are readily available for faculty use.

The ARS system increases student participation, interaction, and engagement in the classroom (Stein et al., 2006). The anonymity of ARS responses also decreases student apprehension about answering questions in class. Although, preparation time for educators can be a slight drawback, the technology is easy to use, and requires minimal training (Efstathiou & Bailey, 2012). The pedagogical benefits support the use of this active learning technology (Thomas et al., 2011).

Clauson, K. A., Alkhateeb, F. M., & Singh-Franco, D. (2012). Concurrent use of an audience response system at a multi-campus college of pharmacy. *American Journal of Pharmaceutical Education, 76*(1), 6. doi: 10.5688/ajpe7616; 10.5688/ajpe7616

Efstathiou, N., & Bailey, C. (2012). Promoting active learning using audience response system in large bioscience classes. *Nurse Education Today, 32*(1), 91–95. doi: 10.1016/j.nedt.2011.01.017; 10.1016/j.nedt.2011.01.017

Johnson, J. P., & Mighten, A. (2005). A comparison of teaching strategies: Lecture notes combined with structured group discussion versus lecture only. *Journal of Nursing Education, 44*(7), 319–322.

Lee, S. T., & Dapremont, J. A. (2012). Engaging nursing students through integration of the audience response system. *Nursing Education Perspectives, 33*(1), 55–57.

Russell, J. S., McWilliams, M., Chasen, L., & Farley, J. (2011). Using clickers for clinical reasoning and problem solving. *Nurse Educator, 36*(1), 13–15. doi: 10.1097/NNE.0b013e3182001e18; 10.1097/NNE.0b013e3182001e18

Stein, P. S., Challman, S. D., & Brueckner, J. K. (2006). Using audience response technology for pretest reviews in an undergraduate nursing course. *Journal of Nursing Education, 45*(11), 469–473.

Thomas, C. M., Monturo, C., & Conroy, K. (2011). Experiences of faculty and students using an audience response system in the classroom. *Computers, Informatics, Nursing: CIN, 29*(7), 396–400. doi: 10.1097/NCN.0b013e3181fc405b; 10.1097/NCN.0b013e3181fc405b

Vana, K. D., Silva, G. E., Muzyka, D., & Hirani, L. M. (2011). Effectiveness of an audience response system in teaching pharmacology to baccalaureate nursing students. *Computers, Informatics, Nursing: CIN, 29*(6 Suppl), TC105–113. doi: 10.1097/NCN.0b013e3182285d71; 10.1097/NCN.0b013e3182285d71.

Shirleatha T. Lee

Best Practice Guidelines

DEFINITION

Evidence-based practice (EBP) is the conscientious use of current best evidence for clinical decisions about patient care. Best practice guidelines or evidence-based guidelines are defined as outcomes from systematic reviews that are synthesized and appraised to determine the current best knowledge in an area of specific interest. These outcomes provide nurses and/or other clinicians with up-to-date information to formulate guidelines for practice such as clinical guidelines, protocols, policies, and procedures. Evidence-based guidelines support optimal clinical decisions and standardized best practice to enhance efficiency and better patient outcomes (Cajulis, Beam, & Davis, 2010). These guidelines uphold the American Nurses Association (ANA) practice standard for professional nurses to integrate evidence and research findings into practice (ANA, 2010). Utilization of these guidelines can reduce inappropriate variations in patient care, provide optimal timely clinical intervention, and promote autonomy in clinical practice. Understanding the impact of EBP on patient outcomes and cost of services is essential for every nurse.

APPLICATION

Education of nurses at all levels from theoretical and/or practical experiences is requisite for best practice. The need to be educated and updated about practice begins as a nursing student moves forward with the career as a graduate nurse. Every nurse has the professional responsibility to attain knowledge and skills to improve practice (Fitzpatrick, 2013). Likewise, every nurse has a responsibility to use best evidence in the delivery of patient care.

Creating a work environment of EBP for nurses is a fundamental component in the education of nurses. A paradigm shift is occurring from traditional practice to EBP.

Undergraduate- and graduate-level students are educated in formal courses on research and EBP in the curriculum. Students review, discuss, and critique research articles, and report on evidence-based interventions for a specific clinical population. Students in clinical practice experience real-time patient care delivery. Most clinical sites provide students with access to evidence-based clinical guidelines, policies, and procedures. Clinical instructors and nurse mentors are expected to be knowledgeable about evidence-based guidelines, as well as be readily available to guide students to solve clinical issues using best practice guidelines.

Education is a continuous process of knowledge and skill acquisition obtained from formal education programs, continuing education, or self-learning (Fitzpatrick, 2013). Continuing education is essential for the delivery of the current best available evidence for patient care interventions. With a considerable body of information and advanced technology, many evidence-based guidelines are available for nurses at all levels to guide clinical decisions for best possible patient care.

SYNOPSIS

Understanding the concept of EBP is essential for staff nurses and advanced practice nurses (APN) in order to deliver high-quality and cost-effective care. Improving knowledge about EBP improves implementation of best practice guidelines. Several steps in implementing EBP include assessing the need for EBP, reviewing the current literature, implementing EBP at all organizational levels, and evaluating the implementation. Increased understanding of EBP facilitates implementation of EBP in clinical settings. Cullen and Adams (2012) presented an EBP model consisting of four phases: organizational interest, education, implementation, and evaluation.

Shulman (2008) emphasized the importance of organizational leadership in promoting an environment of clinical inquiry and constant learning. Access to clinical information, education of staff members on how to evaluate the literature, strategies to ensure implementation of practice changes, and promotion of EBP projects are factors that support EBP. Cable-Williams et al. (2014) described a program using best practice guidelines for curricula development in a baccalaureate nursing program. They emphasized several key points for project management and sustainability including shared governance, ongoing communication among members, identifying outcomes, promoting new opportunities for students and faculty, and disseminating project information.

Mahanes, Quatrara, and Shaw (2013) described implementation of APN rounds in which identification of evidence-based patient issues are discussed by staff nurses. They found that a proactive approach improves implementation of evidence-based guidelines. In addition, evidence-based guidelines are frequently not implemented because they are not disseminated to the staff nurses.

RECOMMENDATIONS

APNs are at the forefront in developing and implementing EBP guidelines in the clinical setting. Their clinical expertise and ability to interpret research findings can help staff nurses translate research into practice guidelines. Nursing rounds can promote education and practice improvement strategies by helping staff nurses apply evidence-based knowledge to clinical situations (Mahanes et al., 2013).

Shulman (2008) suggested that staff nurses should have access to EBP databases 24 hours/day. Promoting use of databases by providing support to nurses on how to access the databases through continuing education programs and mentorship can increase access and use of the guidelines.

Promotion of EBP skills by staff nurses and APN can translate into improved patient care and professional satisfaction. These best practices can facilitate the use of practice guidelines in patient care. Research on implementation of these guidelines is needed in order to promote nurses' understanding and utilization of EBP.

American Nurses Association (ANA). (2010). *Nursing: Scope and standards of practice* (2nd ed.). Silver Spring, MD: Author.

Cable-Williams, B., Rush, J., Mowry, A., MacLeod, A., Gilmer, C., Graham, C., & White, S. (2014). An educational innovation to foster evidence-informed practice. *Journal of Nursing Education, 53*(X), 1–4. doi:10.3928/0148434–20140217-06

Cajulis, C. B., Beam, P. S., & Davis, S. B. (2010). Making evidence-based decisions in nursing. In F. Chiappelli, M. H. Ramchandani, N. Neagos, O. O. Oluwadara, & X. M. Caldeira Brant (Eds.), *Evidence-based practice: Toward optimizing clinical outcomes*. New York, NY: Springer. Science and Media

Cullen, L., & Adams, S. L. (2012). Planning for implementation of evidence-based practice. *The Journal of Nursing Administration, 42*(4), 222–230. doi:10.1097/NNA.0b013e31824ccd0a

Fitzpatrick, J. J. (2013). Professional standards for nurses. In M. M. Glembocki & J. J. Fitzpatrick (Eds.), *Advancing professional nursing practice* (pp. 51–74). Minneapolis, MN: Creative Health Care Management.

Mahanes, D., Quatrara, B. D., & Shaw, K. D. (2013). APN-led nursing grand rounds:

An emphasis on evidence-based nursing care. *Intensive and Critical Care Nursing, 29,* 256–260.

Shulman, C. S. (2008). Strategies for starting a successful evidence-based practice program. *AACN Advanced Critical Care, 19*(3), 301–311.

Corazon B. Cajulis
Siobhan Sundel

BLOGGING

DEFINITION

A weblog or a blog is a web-based collection of thoughts or information, similar to a diary or a log. Blogs are arranged chronologically and may be hosted by one or more people (Curry, 2012). Blogs are also described by Bonk and Zhang (2008) as websites that provide a personal opinion or viewpoint on a topic of interest and is open for comments. Blog entries are posted sequentially, with the most recent post appearing first on the list. Blogs cannot be edited or rearranged; they can be created for internal use and be password protected; and media files can be linked to blogs (Billings, 2009).

APPLICATION

There is increasing need for nurse educators to incorporate technology in nursing education. More than 80% of nursing students are Millennials, or the Net Generation. These students are considered to be digital natives and view new technologies as a normal part of everyday life (Peck, 2014). In addition, Schmitt, Sims-Giddens, and Booth (2012) noted that it is expected that many nurses will return to school for further education. The demographics of current undergraduate and graduate nursing students varies from millennials to baby boomers.

SYNOPSIS

Blogs can be an empowering tool for personally publishing ideas and communicating with a worldwide audience. However, blogs in online courses and academic settings typically relate to course readings, course tasks and activities, field experiences, and extra course-related work (Bonk & Zhang, 2008).

Results of the pilot study conducted by Roland, Johnson, and Swain (2011) suggest that blogs help students become more adept in written communication. A blog can be used for reflection to enable the student to express thoughts and feelings about a learning situation. Carozza (2012) noted that blogging promotes reflection and greater understanding needed for writing. She further identified blogging as a tool that can help those students with some fear of technology.

Peck (2014) identified how social media is changing the communication paradigm from a traditional face-to-face model to the one that uses a variety of web-based applications. She further noted that online interactive and social media platforms are changing the way nursing students communicate and that one third of faculty in academic institutions report using social media to communicate with students. The major privacy concerns related to the use of social media include the potential to violate the Health Insurance Portability and Accountability Act (HIPAA) of 1996, and the Family Educational Rights and Privacy Act (FERPA) that protects students' privacy in the school environment. However, the overall benefits of social media in the classroom far outweigh the challenges. Blogging can help students develop problem-solving skills, and enhance networking, collaboration, and student engagement in the course.

RECOMMENDATIONS

Blogs are another way to facilitate internal and external communication and dialogue among nurses and nurse educators. When used in clinical agencies, they have been shown to promote interprofessional collaboration, simplify project development, provide peer support, and link users to information provided by national health care organizations (Billings, 2009). It is therefore recommended that blogs be incorporated into nursing curricula for faculty's and students' use.

It is also recommended that educators are provided with technical support and necessary training on how to use blogs. Due to the ethical and legal issues associated with the use of social media, it is essential that educators be familiar with the policy for the responsible use of social media in their institution before adopting the use of blogging or any other social media in the courses.

According to the National Council of State Boards of Nursing (NCSBN, 2011), improper use of social media by nurses may violate state and federal laws established to protect patient privacy and confidentiality. Such violations may result in both civil and criminal penalties, including fines and possible jail time. Therefore, there is the need for further research into the use of blogging in nursing education. More nursing faculty should also be trained and encouraged to incorporate blogging as a form of social media in their courses.

Billings, D. M. (2009). Wikis and blogs: Consider the possibilities for continuing nursing education. *Journal of Continuing Education in Nursing, 40*(12), 534–535.

Bonk, C. J., & Zhang, K. (2008). *Empowering online learning: 100+ activities for reading, reflecting, displaying and doing.* San Francisco, CA: Jossey-Bass.

Carozza, B. (2012). *5 Reasons educators should blog.* Retrieved from http://connected-principals.com/archives/5835

Curry, K. (2012). Increasing communications in the intensive care unit. Is blogging the answer? *Critical Care Nursing Quarterly, 35*(4), 328–334.

The National Council of State Boards of Nursing (NCSBN). (2011). *White paper: A nurses guide to the use of social media.* Retrieved from https://www.ncsbn.org/Social_Media.pdf

Peck, J. L. (2014). Social media in nursing education: Responsible integration for meaningful use. *Journal of Nursing Education, 53*(3), 164–169.

Roland, E. J., Johnson, C., & Swain D. (2011). Blogging as an educational enhancement tool for improved student performance: A pilot study in undergraduate nursing education. *New Review of Information Networking, 16,* 151–166.

Schmitt, T., Sims-Giddens, S., & Booth, R. (2012). Social media use in nursing education. *The Online Journal of Issues in Nursing, 17*(3), 2.

Elsie A. Jolade

BULLYING

DEFINITION

Bullying is defined as repeated, unreasonable actions intended to intimidate, degrade, humiliate, or undermine. It generally occurs when there is a power differential and can result in harm to one's physical and mental health (Canadian Centre for Occupational Health and Safety, 2005). Bullying behaviors may be overt, such as yelling or using profanity, threatening abuse, publicly belittling or humiliating, or spreading malicious rumors or gossip; the more covert behaviors, such as isolating an individual; changing expectations, guidelines, and deadlines; or providing incorrect information to sabotage one's work, are equally destructive but less obvious to prove.

APPLICATION

The phrase "Nurses eat their young" has been around for generations and refers to the aggressive and unsupportive behavior senior nurses exhibit toward newer and younger student nurses. This often-quoted phrase suggests that bullying is unique to nursing; however, in contrast, bullying occurs in all occupational sectors (Namie, 2014) and across the age span (Longo, 2013). It is vital that nursing recognizes the existence of bullying, across all domains (clinical practice, administration, education, and research) in order to develop prevention strategies, establish reporting protocols, and implement education and awareness programs to promote quality workplaces, free of bullying behaviors.

Within the academic domain, bullying has been reported as occurring from educator to student, student to student, student to educator, and educator to educator. In all instances, the bullying behaviors negatively impact student recruitment, retention, satisfaction, and the overall quality of the educational setting (Beckman, Cannella, & Wantland, 2013) and ultimately the quality of patient care. Within the educational domain, students must be prepared to recognize and manage bullying behaviors and be aware of the dynamics so that they themselves do not develop behaviors consistent with bullying interactions.

SYNOPSIS

Bullying in nursing education is a double-edged sword as health care and education are the occupational sectors reporting the largest proportion of bullying experiences (Namie, 2014). It is suggested that individuals attracted to both nursing and education possess caring and nurturing qualities that make them susceptible targets to bullying. It has also been theorized that nursing, as an oppressed group, experiences horizontal violence (bullying staff to staff) as a result of being a predominantly female group that is devalued within a hierarchical health care system (Purpora, Blegen, & Stotts, 2012; Roberts, 1983). Nurse educators have a responsibility to empower nursing students so that they do not adopt the oppressive group behaviors associated with bullying and lateral violence.

Nurse educators also have a responsibility to ensure that they are not perpetuating bullying behavior. As a practice-based discipline, the education of future nursing practitioners requires that students gain knowledge and competency through clinical experience. While nursing educators are valued for their nursing expertise, they may not necessarily be equipped with theories of teaching and learning that prepare them to effectively provide feedback while recognizing the students' efforts and building on the students' strengths. Anecdotally, clinical instructors and staff nurses routinely define their feedback to students as constructive criticism; students define it as bullying. In a recent study of Canadian undergraduate baccalaureate nursing students, 88% reported having experienced at least one act of bullying, with the clinical instructor identified as the greatest source of the bullying behavior, followed by staff nurses (Clarke, Kane, Rajacich, & Lafreniere, 2012). The most frequently reported bullying behavior was the perception from students that their efforts were undervalued, followed by reports of being unjustly criticized. Nursing students who self-labeled as being bullied were significantly more likely to consider leaving nursing and believed that the bullying behavior had a negative impact on their learning experience (Clarke et al., 2012).

The academic setting is a perfect opportunity to provide role-playing or simulated scenarios for students and educators to act out aggressive interactions and problem-solve a nonaggressive resolution. Students may share experiences they perceive as negative and demeaning and identify effective communication strategies to discuss with the instructor. Because bullies often do not identify their behavior as bullying (Thompson, 2012) role-playing provides educators the opportunity to reflect on behaviors and determine if they are contributing, directly or indirectly, to a bullying culture.

RECOMMENDATIONS

There is a need to ensure that nursing students are equipped with effective communication and conflict-resolution skills. Nursing students will not only benefit by being prepared to address bullying behavior when it occurs they will also be able to support their colleagues should they experience it. Equally important is the need to ensure that all nurses who interact with nursing students are able to do so in a constructive and empowering manner. Promoting reflective nursing practice will encourage nurses to reflect on their own behavior and identify if they are guilty of bullying behaviors. Since nursing education does not exist in a vacuum, every member of the health care team must play an active role in eliminating bullying from the health care sector.

Research into the phenomenon of bullying needs to begin with the development of a unified definition of bullying and valid and reliable standardized tools for measuring bullying. Studies that evaluate the implementation of policies and legislation that address the existence and management of workplace violence, including bullying, are needed to create and sustain quality learning environments for nursing students.

Beckman, C., Cannella, B., & Wantland, D. (2013). Faculty perception of bullying in schools of nursing. *Journal of Professional Nursing, 29*(5), 287–294.

Canadian Centre for Occupational Health and Safety. (2005). *Bullying in the workplace.* Retrieved from www.ccohs.ca/oshanswers/

Clarke, C., Kane, D., Rajacich, D., & Lafreniere, K. (2012). Bullying in undergraduate clinical nursing education. *Journal of Nursing Education, 51*(5), 269–276.

Longo, J. (2013). Bullying and the older nurse. *Journal of Nursing Management, 21,* 950–955.

Namie, G. (2014). *US workplace bullying survey.* Workplace Bullying Institute. Retrieved April 15 from www.workplacebullying.org/multi/pdf/WBI-2014-US-Survey.pdf

Purpora, C., Blegen, M., & Stotts, N. (2012). Horizontal violence among hospital staff nurses related to oppresses self or oppressed group. *Journal of Professional Nursing, 28,* 306–314.

Roberts, S. (1983). Oppressed group behavior: Implications for nursing. *Advances in Nursing Science, 5,* 21–30.

Thompson, R. (2012). *"Do No Harm" applies to nurses too!* Pittsburgh, PA: inCredible Messages Press.

Debbie Kane

CAPSTONE PROJECT

DEFINITION

Capstone projects are identified by many different names such as capstone experiences, senior exhibition, or senior project. In a capstone project, the individual is expected to identify a contemporary challenge or issue with a clinical focus that can be evaluated using "evidence-based search strategies and critical appraisal of the literature" (Newland, 2013, p. 6). The Great Schools Partnership (n.d.) defines a capstone project as a complex and intricate assignment that is a concluding academic experience demonstrating a body of knowledge about a topic of interest. A capstone project is characterized by incorporating a strong decision-making process to guide the inquiry.

APPLICATION

While capstone projects can be found in any educational setting, they tend to be used primarily in master and/or doctoral programs in nursing education. The fundamental and central target of a capstone project is to investigate problems and issues identified in health care. Through the investigation, evidence related to the identified focus can be confirmed to build on the topic being analyzed. The ultimate outcome for each project embraces the idea of improving the quality of care delivered to individuals. A key point in the development and management of a capstone project is mentoring to ensure that each step of the project is carefully and efficiently carried out.

Each project is specific to the setting and individual choice. The projects embrace all of the steps of critical thinking. A capstone endeavor can take the direction of a research venture, quality improvement undertaking, or an evidence-based practice venture. It is expected that the entire process results in careful consideration of how to improve an aspect of health care.

Capstone projects tend to be directed toward a clinical situation. According to Clarke (2013), the linkages between academia and practice need to be directed toward patient/family-centered care, including finance and policy. Attention is directed on merging clinical and best practices to improve health care.

SYNOPSIS

In the DNP Essentials developed by the American Association of Colleges of Nursing (AACN, 2006), it is suggested that the final DNP project delivers conclusions that ensued from practice engagement experiences. The entire process should be carefully reviewed and evaluated by experts in the program. While discussion continues on the need for research to be incorporated in the projects, the main focus is that the project demonstrates sound decision making and analytical management. Rutledge and Renaud (2013) list examples of doctor of nursing practice (DNP) capstone projects that include pilot studies, program development and evaluation efforts, quality improvement projects, incorporation of interprofessional collaborative models, evaluation of cost-effectiveness, and provider outcome efficiency.

Overcash (2013) believes that there is a need for small projects to validate nursing research. The outcome of a capstone project is to "cultivate perceptions of empowerment and confidence that pave the way for a career of nursing inquiry" (Overcash, 2013, p. 22). Through a mentor, the capstone project student is moved forward to provide evidence and best practices related to the topic addressed. Active engagement by individuals to manage challenges identified in innovative and creative ways allows new solutions for problems to be studied. The research and/or quality improvement projects can create the essential and crucial evidence imperative for health care.

The Great Schools Partnership (n.d.) asserts that a capstone project develops the following skills: critical thinking, precise oral communication, problem solving, media literacy, and self-sufficiency. Each capstone experience is envisioned to result in some form of dissemination. The individual is expected to provide a final product such as a manuscript for publication, oral presentation, and/or poster presentation. For some projects, the dissemination of results must be provided in more than one venue. Some educational goals for the capstone projects are increasing the rigor of the educational aspects of the final year of the program; engaging students to be more motivated and engaged in discovery of solutions; escalating the educational and career aspirations of students; advancing confidence, maturity, and self-perception of students; and documenting learning and proficiency resulting from the project.

RECOMMENDATIONS

Capstone experiences are opportunities for expanding the evidence available for use in advancing health care. Scholars have the responsibility for seeking the best evidence and knowledge for enhancing and improving methods used for provision of health care. Capstone projects are guided by mentors through successful completion of the project. The mentor is frequently called the capstone adviser. These individuals are strategically placed to provide ongoing support and guidance to effectively develop the skills and expertise needed. Mentors are purposefully

selected and used in the process to aid the scholar to thoroughly investigate problems. In addition, experts are identified and used as the project is planned and implemented. These experts provide the scholar with additional insight into the project topic. These networking connections are deliberately selected to augment information provided in conjunction with the mentor.

Capstone projects provide support and engagement with students to develop an in-depth evidence-based learning outcome. An expectation of the capstone project is the commitment to lifelong learning through the use of decision making and evidence-based practice.

American Association of Colleges of Nursing (AACN). (2006). *The essentials for doctoral nursing for advanced nursing practice.* Washington, DC: Author.

Clarke, S. P. (2013). Practice-academia collaboration in nursing: Contexts and future directions. *Nursing Administration Quarterly, 37*(3), 184–193.

Great Schools Partnership. (n.d.). *Capstone project.* Retrieved from http://edglossary. org/capstone-project/

Newland, J. A. (2013). DNP scholarly projects change practice. *The Nurse Practitioner, 38*(4), 6.

Overcash, J. (2013, August). Nursing research: Speaking up for the value of small projects. *Oncology Nurse Advisor,* 21–23.

Rutledge, C. M., & Renaud, M. (2013). Back to school! Selecting a DNP program. *Nursing Management, 44*(11), 30–36; quiz 36. doi: 10–1097/01.NUMA.0000436363.14645.15

Carol Boswell

CARING

DEFINITION

Caring is a moral ideal demonstrated through caritas processes. Caritas processes described by Watson (1985) are practicing loving kindness, honoring others, nurturing individual beliefs, developing helping/trusting relationships, listening, creative decision making, respecting human dignity, and being open to mystery. Caring is a value, an attitude, a will, an intention, and a commitment (Watson, 1985). Thus, caring is a moral imperative focusing on maintaining dignity and respect of patients. Caring is an intersubjective process involving humanistic aspects initialized through the demonstration of the caritas processes.

APPLICATION

The teaching of caring is central to nurse education. According to Watson and Smith (2002), knowledge about caring is the key to understanding human health, healing, and quality of life. Caring is being present with the patient in the here and now. The use of a theory to guide the teaching of caring is crucial for nursing and knowledge development. Caring theories fall into the category of middle-range theories and are best suited to teach caring because these theories can directly be applied to practice. There are several teaching strategies available to assist the teaching of caring. Such strategies include the use of case studies, reflection, caring scenarios, objective structured clinical examinations, and role-play.

SYNOPSIS

The teaching of caring is fundamental to nursing. Caring is the essence of nursing, a core professional value, and a paradigm unique to nursing (Cohen, 1991; Kitson, 1987; Leininger, 1977; Roach, 1998; Schwerin, 2004; Swanson, 1993; Watson, 1979). Caring is defined and conceptualized in various ways. Teachers who have a solid grasp on the meaning of caring and practice a caring way of being, make a unique contribution to nursing education. Caring is defined according to the theoretical perspective

that is proposed or presented. Therefore, in teaching the concept of caring, it is key to understand the assumptions and worldview of the caring theory (Smith, 1999).

The findings from research studies exploring student nurses' and nurses' perceptions of caring show that the clinical aspects of caring are rated highly. In addition, knowing what to do and technical competency were rated high (Omari, AbuAlRub, & Ayasreh, 2013; Papastavrou et al., 2012; Zamanzadeh, Azimzadeh, Rahmani, & Valizadeh, 2010). However, practicing a caring approach goes beyond clinical competence, and includes creating a healing environment. Therefore, teaching from a theoretical framework that includes caring is a moral imperative.

RECOMMENDATIONS

It is recommended that a caring philosophy should be integrated throughout the curriculum of a nursing program. Integration can be accomplished through a theoretical framework on caring that makes explicit the caritas processes of practicing loving kindness, honoring others, nurturing individual beliefs, developing helping/trusting relationships, listening, creative decision making, respecting human dignity, and being open to mystery.

Cohen, J. A. (1991). Two portraits of caring: A comparison of the artists, Leininger and Watson. *Journal of Advanced Nursing, 16*(8), 899–909.

Kitson, A. L. (1987). A comparative analysis of lay-caring and professional (nursing) caring relationships. *International Journal of Nursing Studies, 24*(2), 155–165.

Leininger, M. (1977). The phenomenon of caring. Part V. Caring: The essence and central focus of nursing. *Nursing Research Report, 12*(1), 2, 14.

Omari, F. H., AbuAlRub, R., & Ayasreh, I. R. (2013). Perceptions of patients and nurses towards nurse caring behaviors in coronary care units in Jordan. *Journal of Clinical Nursing, 22*(21–22), 3183–3191.

Papastavrou, E., Efstathiou, G., Tsangari, H., Suhonen, R., Leino-Kilpi, H., Patiraki, E.,...Merkouris, A. (2012). A cross-cultural study of the concept of caring through behaviours: Patients' and nurses' perspectives in six different EU countries. *Journal of Advanced Nursing, 68*(5), 1026–1037.

Roach, M. S. (1998). Caring ontology: Ethics and the call of suffering. *International Journal for Human Caring, 2*(2), 30–34.

Schwerin, J. I. (2004). The timeless caring connection. *Nursing Administration Quarterly, 28*(4), 265–270.

Smith, M. C. (1999). Caring and the science of unitary human beings. *Advances in Nursing Science, 21*(4), 14–28.

Swanson, K. M. (1993). Nursing as informed caring for the well-being of others. *Image—The Journal of Nursing Scholarship, 25*(4), 352–357.

Watson, J. (1979). *Nursing: The philosophy and science of caring.* Boston, MA: Little Brown. Reprinted/republished 1985. Boulder: Colorado Associated University Press.

Watson, J. (1985). *Nursing: Human science and human care—A theory of nursing.* New York, NY: National League for Nursing.

Watson, J., & Smith, M. C. (2002). Caring science and the science of unitary human beings: A trans-theoretical discourse for nursing knowledge development. *Journal of Advanced Nursing, 37*(5), 452–461.

Zamanzadeh, V., Azimzadeh, R., Rahmani, A., & Valizadeh, L. (2010). Oncology patients' and professional nurses' perceptions of important nurse caring behaviors. *BMC Nursing, 9,* 10.

Catrina Heffernan

CASE SCENARIOS

DEFINITION

A case scenario is a comprehensive analysis of a real-life situation used to promote active learning during instruction of course material (Rowles, 2012). Case scenarios encourage critical thinking through application of theory and didactic content to real or simulated life situations. The term *case scenario* is used interchangeably with *case study, case problem, case report,* and *research case.* Attributes of case scenarios may be exemplified through sociodrama and role-play methodologies that incorporate theatrical presentation of classroom theory.

APPLICATION

Development of critical thinking and clinical reasoning is essential to the education of nurses. Clinical reasoning encompasses reflection (Benner, Sutphen, Leonard, & Day, 2010) and ability to use critical thinking skills to accommodate the ever-changing nature of clinical environments (Rowles, 2012). Throughout history, nurse educators have relied on clinical rotations to provide experiential learning for students; however, clinical learning opportunities vary depending on care needs of patients and available clinical sites. Considering the impact of multiple variables on clinical learning, there is a call for nursing education to be transformed through the use of active teaching and learning strategies, one of which is the case scenario. Many students learn through inductive rather than deductive reasoning; they learn better from examples, and benefit from applying what they have learned in the classroom to real world situations. Case scenarios, written from rich clinical experiences, may be used as an adjunct to a minilecture or customized to assist students with applying course-specific theory to real life in an active learning environment. Multiple case scenarios incorporated in a classroom setting allow smaller groups of students to identify similarities and differences among cases. Well-designed cases should illustrate critical concepts in a nonthreatening environment to ensure active student participation. Engagement in case study discussion promotes development of analytical and problem-solving skills and improves students' decision-making abilities in complex situations. Comprehension of concepts may be reinforced by pairing the case with a reading assignment and/or through utilization of concept maps, chalkboards, and electronic resources.

Use of a framework to foster development of clinical reasoning promotes integration and application of theory to practice in the clinical setting. The concept of case-based reasoning (CBR), born of research in the 1980s, suggested that individuals not only organize different types of knowledge through identifying schema-like knowledge structures, they also simultaneously make inferences determined by those knowledge structures (Kolodner, 2006). Researchers' observations further indicated that there are processes that allow a reasoner to reason on the basis of previous experiences. Considering these findings, the use of a framework based on principles of CBR has potential for designing learning environments, including adult education, K–12 classrooms, and undergraduate education.

In CBR, a case includes a setting, actors and actors' goals, sequence of events, expected results, and explanations that link outcomes to goals and means; intelligent behavior is determined by a person's ability to identify significant features of a new situation and apply previous experiences to solve problems (Kolodner, 2006). Although reflection on learning has been linked to more complex thinking, particularly in the practice dimension of clinical reasoning, students must actively engage with the theoretical, psychomotor, and affective content inherent in nursing to transform information into their own knowledge (Rowles, 2012). Students use focused reflection to reason on the basis of previous experiences and critical thinking to find answers they will not find in a book. Use of a holistic nursing knowledge base allows nurses to think through patient situations and provide individualized evidence-based care as opposed to following a routine procedure. Nurses engage in metacognition (reflective thinking), a self-communication process, before, during, and after performance of a task or skill (Rowles, 2012). Metacognition

and critical thinking, when combined, have been described as the thinking required in nursing (Kuiper & Pesut, 2004). Participation in a case study discussion promotes formulation of varied and unique ideas at both the individual and collaborative levels, thus broadening the knowledge integration perspective (Linn, 2006).

SYNOPSIS

Learning involves a relatively permanent change in cognition that results from experience and directly influences behavior. Active learning strategies such as case scenarios that prepare students for challenges of the health care environment are supported by the American Association of Colleges of Nursing (AACN, 2009). Benner et al. (2010) support radical transformation in learning, whereby educators promote clinic-like experiences that inspire students to apply knowledge and practice thinking to changing situations to improve patient health outcomes. According to Benner's theory, students' perceptual awareness of emerging clinical problems closely parallels their level of clinical competency (Larew, Lessans, Spunt, Foster, & Covington, 2006). Case scenarios can be written for simulated learning opportunities, designed to emphasize various nursing concepts, and utilized in collaborative education environments at multiple levels of learning (Hannah & Oliver, 2011). This evidence-based teaching methodology promotes exchange of ideas between information and practice, and assists students with identifying "practice evidence" on which they can base care of clients in the future.

RECOMMENDATIONS

Nurse educators have a professional responsibility to incorporate established standards and clearly articulated student learning and program outcomes consistent with contemporary practice in the educational preparation of students (Accreditation Commission for Education of Nurses [ACEN], 2013). Benner et al. (2010) and the National League for

C

Nursing (2005) recognize the need to transform knowledge by designing nursing curricula that mirror contemporary health care trends, thus preparing graduates to perform effectively in the health care arena. The nurse educator facilitates learning by modeling critical and reflective thinking. Use of case-based scenarios promotes the cognitive, psychomotor, and affective development of nursing students. Case scenarios stimulate critical thinking, may be presented in more practical context, can be utilized in a safe environment without threat to a patient (Rowles, 2012), and have potential to simulate real-life situations, particularly among an aging population with multiple-organ disease and disabilities.

Accreditation Commission for Education of Nurses (ACEN). (2013). *ACEN accreditation manual.* Retrieved from http://www.acenursing.net/manuals/SC2013_ASSOCIATE.pdf

American Association of Colleges of Nursing (AACN). (2009). *Faculty tool kit for the essentials of baccalaureate education for professional nursing practice.* Retrieved from http://www.aacn.nche.edu/Education/pdf/BacEssToolkit.pdf

Benner, P. B., Sutphen, M., Leonard, V., & Day, L. (2010). *Educating nurses: A call for radical transformation.* San Francisco, CA: Jossey-Bass.

Hannah, V., & Oliver, J. S. (2011). Teaching principles of assessment, data collection, and prioritization: Using a case scenario. *Journal of Nursing Education, 50*(4), 235–236.

Kolodner, J. L. (2006). Case-based reasoning. In R. Keith Sawyer (Ed.), *The Cambridge handbook of the learning sciences* (pp. 225–242). New York, NY: Cambridge University Press.

Kuiper, R. A., & Pesut, D. J. (2004). Promoting cognitive and metacognitive reflective reasoning skills in nursing practice: Self-regulated learning theory. *Journal of Advanced Nursing, 45*(4), 381–391.

Larew, C., Lessans, S., Spunt, D., Foster, D., & Covington, B. G. (2006). Innovations in clinical simulation: Application of Benner's theory in an interactive patient care simulation. *Nursing Education Perspectives, 27*(1), 16–21.

Linn, M. C. (2006). The knowledge integration perspective on learning and instruction. In R. Keith Sawyer (Ed.), *The Cambridge handbook of the learning sciences* (pp. 243–264). New York, NY: Cambridge University Press.

National League for Nursing. (2005). *Core competencies of nurse educators.* Retrieved from http://www.nln.org/profdev/pdf/corecompetencies.pdf

Rowles, C. J. (2012). Strategies to promote critical thinking and active learning. In D. M. Billings & J. A. Halstead (Eds.), *Teaching in nursing: A guide for faculty* (4th ed., pp. 258–284). St. Louis, MO: Elsevier Saunders.

Vicki Sullivan Hannah

CIVILITY

DEFINITION

Civility is a type of behavior demonstrated in an encounter between two individuals who are not in agreement. The dictionary defines civility as "polite, reasonable, and respectful behavior" toward another person (Civility, n.d.). The concept of civility includes having respect for another's viewpoint, being willing to communicate openly and honestly about the conflict, and having the mutual purpose of seeking some form of agreement (Clark & Carnosso, 2008).

APPLICATION

To illustrate the importance of civility in nursing education, incivility must be first understood. Incivility that occurs in academic settings has been defined as "rude or disruptive behavior often resulting in psychological or physiological distress for the people involved" (Clark, 2013, p. 98). Incivility in interactions between nurse educators and students is damaging to both parties' sense of self-worth and can create lasting effects. It has been cited as a barrier to education and can lead to violent behaviors (Clark, 2009; Clark & Springer, 2010).

Incivility can occur during interactions between students and faculty, students and peers, or between students and staff nurses in the clinical setting. Examples of student incivility in the academic setting include tardiness or leaving class early, rude comments, participating in side conversations during class, and misusing technology during class (Clark & Springer, 2010). Researchers studied faculty incivility toward students in online nursing courses (Rieck & Crouch, 2007). Students have cited incivility from faculty in the forms of "unfairness, rigidity, insistence on conformity, and overt discrimination" (Clark & Springer, 2010, p. 319). Incivility can occur in the form of vertical violence toward nursing students in the clinical setting by staff nurses (Thomas & Burk, 2009).

Civility is the practice of being fully present in an encounter with another whose views are not the same, being willing to listen to an opposite viewpoint, having respect for the other individual, and finding some form of mutual agreement. In nursing education, civility between faculty and students is essential for student learning in both the classroom and clinical setting. The topic of civility can be found in the American Nurses Association Code of Ethics as well as in recommendations from the Joint Commission and the Institute of Medicine (IOM) as an adjunct to increasing patient safety (ANA, 2001; IOM, 2003; Woods, 2010). Nursing faculty can demonstrate civility during encounters with students as a way of role modeling effective communication for students' future patient interactions and as a way of fostering a culture of civility in the academic environment to facilitate learning.

SYNOPSIS

Recent developments have included research studies on the impact of civility and incivility in nursing education. In 2001, a survey was conducted asking program directors of 611 nursing schools to describe problematic student behaviors. Three behaviors that were cited in all responses were inattentiveness in class, attendance problems, and lateness. Objectionable physical contact and verbal abuse toward faculty were also mentioned frequently (Lashley & DeMeneses, 2001). The investigators recommended strategy development to decrease these behaviors, now seen as examples of incivility, as well as directing further attention to the topic of problematic behavior in nursing education.

Luparell (2004) further explored uncivil student behaviors noted by faculty that were similar in nature and caused negative physical and psychological results to occur in educators. She questioned the effect that student incivility may have on faculty recruitment and retention in the face of a nursing shortage. In 2007, Luparell interviewed 21 faculty members to investigate the effects uncivil encounters with nursing students had on them. These uncivil encounters were on a continuum of relatively mild to highly aggressive. The faculty members reported short- and long-term effects, both physical and psychological. In addition, they included effects on their teaching abilities and an overall negative effect on the teaching/learning process. A small number of faculty resigned from teaching and cited student behavior as a factor in their decision.

Incivility can be reciprocal between nursing students and faculty. Clark (2008) interviewed both faculty and nursing students to find that civility was lacking on the part of both faculty and students in many interactions. She found that the occurrence of incivility on the part of one of the members of the dyad led to an uncivil response from the other and the cycle continued. Clark and Carnosso (2008) developed a concept analysis of civility concluding that civility is necessary to maintain safe and respectful teaching–learning experiences.

Civility in interactions between students and faculty in nursing education is inversely related to stress. In a conceptual model

C

developed by Clark, both faculty stresses related to arduous workloads and student stressors such as multiple role obligations contributed to uncivil exchanges (2008). As stress increased for either faculty or student, civil behaviors decreased. This atmosphere is not conducive to learning and may even prove dangerous if allowed to continue or escalate.

RECOMMENDATIONS

Civility is an essential component in effective communication. There is much information that nurse educators must communicate to students during their progression to becoming safe and effective professional nurses. Providing instruction about civility in interactions and modeling civility in communication allows both faculty and students to communicate needs and expectations openly and without fear or anxiety. Using civility in educational encounters by both faculty and students will improve the students' understanding of content and allow application of knowledge in an environment that promotes acceptance and understanding. Incorporating civility into nursing education will allow students to practice communication skills that will serve them in their future encounters with patients. Strategies to promote civility awareness and usage among students and faculty include policy development for dealing with incivility, creation of classroom and communication expectation using both faculty and student input, and incorporation of opportunities for better communication between students and faculty (Clark, 2008). Civility awareness and training for both faculty and nursing students may be an important component in the development of safe patient care and should be included during student and faculty orientation, faculty meetings, and at regular intervals throughout the curriculum.

American Nurses Association (ANA). (2001). *Code of ethics for nurses with interpretive statements*. Washington, DC: American Nurses Association.

Civility. (n.d.). *Merriam-Webster*. Retrieved from http://www.merriam-webster.com/dictionary/civility

Clark, C. (2008). The dance of incivility in nursing education as described by nursing faculty and students. *Advances in Nursing Science, 31*(4), E37–E54. doi:10.1097/01.ANS.0000341419.96338.a3

Clark, C. M. (2009). Faculty field guide for promoting student civility in the classroom. *Nurse Educator, 34*(5), 194–197. doi:10.1097/NNE.0b013e3181b2b589

Clark, C. M. (2013). National study on faculty-to-faculty incivility: Strategies to foster collegiality and civility. *Nurse Educator, 38*(3), 98–102. doi:10.1097/NNE.0b013e31828dc1b2

Clark, C. M., & Carnosso, J. (2008). Civility: A concept analysis. *The Journal of Theory Construction & Testing, 12*(11), 11–15.

Clark, C. M., & Springer, P. J. (2010). Academic nurse leaders' role in fostering a culture of civility in nursing education. *Journal of Nursing Education, 49*(6), 319–325. doi:10.3928/01484834–20100224-01

Institute of Medicine (IOM). (2003). *Health professions education: A bridge to quality*. Washington, DC: National Academy Press.

Lashley, F.R.., & DeMeneses, M. (2001). Student civility in nursing programs: A national survey. *Journal of Professional Nursing, 17*, 81–86.

Luparell, S. (2004). Faculty encounters with uncivil nursing students: An overview. *Journal of Professional Nursing, 20*(1), 59–67. doi:10.1016/j.profnurs.2003.12.007

Rieck, S., & Crouch, L. (2007). Connectiveness and civility in online learning. *Nurse Education in Practice, 7*(6), 425–432. doi:10.1016/j.nepr.2007.06.006

Thomas, S. P., & Burk, R. (2009). Junior nursing students' experiences of vertical violence during clinical rotations. *Nursing Outlook, 57*(4), 226–231. doi:10.1016/j.outlook.2008.08.004

Woods, M. S. (2010). *Civil leadership: The final step to achieving safety, quality, innovation, and profitability in health care.* Oakbrook Terrace, IL: Joint Commission Resources.

Karen D. Joris
Mary T. Quinn Griffin

CLICKER TECHNOLOGY

DEFINITION

Clicker technology is a teaching strategy that promotes active learning in the classroom setting. It is an interaction between presenter and participants that uses electronic polling to elicit immediate response and feedback that are tallied automatically, usually in the form of a bar graph (Caldwell, 2007; Skiba, 2006; Woolforde & Lopez-Zhang, 2012). Clickers are also synonymous with audience response system (ARS), personal response system (PRS), student response system (SRS), and classroom response system (CRS). The ARS has three components: wireless-technology or browser-based software such as Turning Technologies® ARS system, a compatible receiver, and the remote-control clicker. The software can be downloaded free from the software company. The receiver and ARS are sold separately. The financial implication for implementing this program is minimal.

APPLICATION

The ARS is widely used in the academic setting but is slowly gaining ground in the hospital setting (Paguirigan & Vezina, 2013; Woolforde & Lopez-Zhang, 2012). For example, the utility of the ARS technology in the hospital setting is used as an approach to improve an orientation program.

At the beginning of each session, the participants receive their individual remote-control ARS that is used to answer questions by pressing a keypad to make a selection. Although the ARS has the capability to identify responders, it is usually used anonymously to create a nonthreatening atmosphere. The clicker technology works by asking participants to respond to multiple choice, true/false, priority ranking, Likert, and even essay questions embedded in the electronic slide (e.g., PowerPoint®) lecture presentation. After a choice is made, responses are transmitted and are tallied automatically usually in the form of a bar graph (Caldwell, 2007; Skiba, 2006; Woolforde & Lopez-Zhang, 2012).

SYNOPSIS

Adopting innovative technologies to stimulate active engagement in nursing education continues to be a challenge for nursing educators. The literature is replete with information making the claim that promoting active learning improves learning outcomes. The use of innovative teaching and learning strategies is grounded in Chickering and Gamson's (1991) seminal article on principles for optimal practice in education that includes "encouraging contact between learners and faculty; developing reciprocity and cooperation among learners; encouraging active learning; giving prompt feedback; emphasizing time on task; communicating high expectations; and respecting diverse talents and ways of learning."

This technology encourages contact between learners and faculty through immediate response and feedback. It also raises the "level of participation and effectiveness of interaction" (DeBourgh, 2008; Lymn & Mostyn, 2010; Russell, McWilliams, Chasen, & Farley, 2011; Woolforde & Lopez-Zhang, 2012). Although responses are anonymous, shy learners are encouraged to participate, creating a nonthreatening atmosphere. Learning outcomes are improved through peer learning and evaluation (Caldwell, 2007; Skiba, 2006).

One of the most important benefits of this technology is to encourage active learning (Efstathiou & Bailey, 2012; Thomas, Monturo, & Conroy, 2011). The interactive environment keeps learners involved (Skiba, 2006), enhances their participation (Caldwell, 2007;

C

Jones, Henderson, & Sealover, 2009; Russell et al., 2011), and reinforces concepts using the "learning-by-doing" format (Efstathiou & Bailey, 2012).

Because responses are immediately compiled, analyzed, and displayed, giving prompt feedback is another benefit of this system (Menon et al., 2004). The faculty can assess the learner's level of comprehension of the concepts or mastery of material to monitor individual and class progress (Skiba, 2006). The pace of the lecture can be adjusted by slowing down or focusing on a specific subject with more depth. The faculty receives valuable input about teaching effectiveness, as well as student interest and comprehension (Caldwell, 2007; Menon et al., 2004). The immediate feedback also fosters communication to clarify incorrect thinking (DeBourgh, 2008) and identify gaps in knowledge (Collins, 2007). By rapidly quizzing learners in an open, yet welcoming format, the clicker method communicates high expectations.

ARS fosters learning that includes analyzing difficult concepts at the synthesis level, thereby promoting advanced reasoning (Caldwell, 2007; Collins, 2007; DeBourgh, 2008; Skiba, 2006). The traditional classroom is bound to quizzes that telegraph rote repetition of basic knowledge, while clicking pushes the learners to think critically. Time on task is greatly facilitated by the swift question-and-answer format of clicking, which can be much quicker than the traditional pen-and-paper format of quizzing or by "show of hands." ARS increases satisfaction and enthusiasm (Caldwell, 2007; DeBourgh, 2008; Jones et al., 2009; Lee & Dapremont, 2012; Woolforde & Lopez-Zhang, 2012); decreases attrition rate (Caldwell, 2007); and increases attendance (Jones et al., 2009).

RECOMMENDATIONS

The use of clicker technology has several implications in education in the academic and hospital-based setting. The challenge lies in engaging educators to embrace new technology in integrating the ARS in their respective educational programs (Woolforde & Lopez-Zhang, 2012). The use of clickers can be an effective teaching strategy that provides a balanced approach between active and passive learning. It is still the responsibility of the nurse educator to be creative in developing other teaching strategies to provide a learning environment that promotes critical thinking and clinical decision making. This technology also has a significant implication to nursing research in terms of evaluating outcomes in nursing education both from a qualitative and quantitative perspective.

Caldwell, J. E. (2007). Clickers in the large classroom: Current research and best-practice tips. *CBE Life Sciences Education, 6*(1), 9–20.

Chickering, A. W., & Gamson, Z. F. (1991). Applying the seven principles for good practice in undergraduate education. *New Directions for Teaching and Learning.* San Francisco, CA: Jossey-Bass Inc.

Collins, L. J. (2007). Livening up the classroom: Using audience response systems to promote active learning. *Medical Reference Services Quarterly, 26*(1), 81–88.

DeBourgh, G. A. (2008). Use of classroom "clickers" to promote acquisition of advanced reasoning skills. *Nurse Education in Practice, 8*(2), 76–87.

Efstathiou, N., & Bailey, C. (2012). Promoting active learning using audience response system in large bioscience classes. *Nurse Education Today, 32*(1), 91–95.

Jones, S., Henderson, D., & Sealover, P. (2009). "Clickers" in the classroom. *Teaching and Learning in Nursing, 4,* 2–5.

Lee, S. T., & Dapremont, J. A. (2012). Engaging nursing students through integration of the audience response system. *Nursing Education Perspectives, 33*(1), 55–57.

Lymn, J. S., & Mostyn, A. (2010). Audience response technology: Engaging and empowering non-medical prescribing students in pharmacology learning. *BMC Medical Education, 10,* 73.

Menon, A. S., Moffett, S., Enriquez, M., Martinez, M. M., Dev, P., & Grappone,

T. (2004). Audience response made easy: Using personal digital assistants as a classroom polling tool. *Journal of the American Medical Informatics Association, 11*(3), 217–220.

Paguirigan, M., & Vezina, M. (2013). *Use of clicker technology in nursing education at The Mount Sinai Hospital.* Poster Presentation at the ANCC National Magnet Conference, Orlando, FL.

Russell, J. S., McWilliams, M., Chasen, L., & Farley, J. (2011). Using clickers for clinical reasoning and problem solving. *Nurse Educator, 36*(1), 13–15.

Skiba, D. J. (2006). Got large lecture hall classes? Use clickers. *Nursing Education Perspectives, 27*(5), 278–280.

Thomas, C. M., Monturo, C., & Conroy, K. (2011). Experiences of faculty and students using an audience response system in the classroom. *Computers, Informatics, Nursing, 29*(7), 396–400.

Woolforde, L., & Lopez-Zang, D. (2012). Transforming engagement in learning through innovative technologies: Using an audience response system in nursing orientation. *Journal of Continuing Education in Nursing, 43*(3), 102–103.

Maria L. Vezina
Medel Salvador-Paguirigan

CLINICAL COMPETENCY

DEFINITION

Benner (1982) defined nursing competency as the ability to perform a task with desirable outcomes under the varied circumstances of the real world. Benner (1984) famously placed competence in the middle of a continuum, ranging from novice to advanced beginner, to competent, to proficient, to expert. Competent practitioners are understood to be able to consciously plan their activities, but can lack flexibility and speed (Benner, 1984). Chapman (1999) defined competence as being more concerned with what people can do rather than with what they know. Similarly, competency-based training and education are believed to have concentrated on what people can do as opposed to what they know and not on the learning process itself, with emphasis on observable and measurable outcomes, requiring a consistent standard of practice (Winskill, 2000).

APPLICATION

Competence is much more than an array of skills attained by the clinician. The interface of professional skills with knowledge, attitudes, and values works in tandem with the cognitive and emotional intellect in nursing practice. Other critical qualities involved in competent practice include motivation, personal insight, explanatory capacity, maturity, and self-assessment ability (Axley, 2008).

The importance of clinical competence must not be underestimated. One study explored competency levels of nurses working in accident and emergency departments in Ireland. Findings demonstrated a positive correlation between level of perceived competence and frequency of practice, and a positive relationship between competence and frequency of activities, as well as competence and years of experience (McCarthy, Cornally, O'Mahoney, White, & Weathers, 2013).

SYNOPSIS

There is a wealth of literature on clinical competence, particularly on the advantages and disadvantages as a measure of practice ability. Nurse managers and educators have been increasingly required to demonstrate that a process is in place to assess, validate, audit, and maintain or improve the competence of staff on an annual basis. Recommended competencies have included the following: provision of patient-centered care; collaboration as a member of an interdisciplinary team; understanding of how to access, interpret,

C

and synthesize information; and use of evidence to guide nursing practice and clinical decision making (Billings, 2008).

Lejonqvist, Eriksson, and Meretoja (2012) conducted a study by exploring the views of clinical staff, students, and nurse educators. They found clinical competence was evident in practice as encountering, knowing, performing, maturing, and improving. These authors discuss the core of nursing as the ethical foundation of clinical competence. The ethical foundation includes nurse–patient relationships, the aim of doing good, and maintaining the dignity of the patient. Clinical competence becomes evident in thought, words, and actions, thus constituting the culture of nursing. Competence is believed to be the essence of nursing expertise and is grounded in meaning that is transferable between contexts (Lejonqvist et al., 2012). Another view on competence considers the relationship with accountability to self. There is evidence that competence is related to continuous learning, professional career advancement, actively adopting self-care strategies, and taking control of work and life (Meretoja & Koponen, 2012).

While some discuss the complexities of competence development, others argue competence-based nursing is reductionist. There is consensus that the perception of nurse competence as a task-based activity is redundant, and a holistic framework is more appropriate (Cowan, Norman, & Coopamah, 2005). One study found that an individual nurse's education level and years of experience influence level of expertise, thus enhancing the probability of becoming a competent expert (McHugh & Lake, 2010).

The importance of competence should not be underestimated. It is most evident in terms of quality of care and patient safety. Ensuring patient safety is considered a major principle of clinical competence together with problem-solving competence, critical thinking ability, and the capacity to anticipate factors, which may impact on patient care outcomes (Axley, 2008). The absence of competence may lead to clinical errors resulting in serious consequences or harm for patients (Axley, 2008). Nurses are fundamental in the systematic identification, assessment, and implementation of good care for patients, as well as recognizing potential adverse events. It is, therefore, essential that the acquisition and maintenance of competence for nurses is mandatory, particularly given the fast-evolving health care settings (Ponte, Kruger, DeMarco, Hanley, & Conlin, 2004). Educators and clinical managers should therefore safeguard patients by leading nurses in a culture of lifelong learning, which is critical in the maintenance of competence and safe practice.

RECOMMENDATIONS

Nursing requires a combination of knowledge, performance, skills, and attitudes; hence, a holistic definition of competence is a requisite. This holistic approach could then underpin the development of competency standards and associated tools required for assessment (Cowan et al., 2005).

Nurse educators and managers must be challenged to promote learning that builds competence, capability, and resilience. The ever-changing health care environment requires competent frontline clinical staff; thus, nurse educators need to prepare nurses to manage practice improvement and change. Collaboration between educators and clinicians is key to positively influencing current competent, safe practice. Competence planning and monitoring of programs needs to consider a broad view of nursing, encompassing factors such as ethos, ethics, peer review, self-assessment, and the cultural context.

Axley, L. (2008). Competency: A concept analysis. *Nursing Forum, 43*(4), 214–222.

Benner, P. (1982). Issues in competency-based testing. *Nursing Outlook, 30*(5), 303–309.

Benner, P. (1984). *From novice to expert: Excellence and power in clinical nursing practice*. California: Addison-Wesley.

Billings, D. M. (2008). Quality care, patient safety and the focus on technology. *Journal of Nursing Education, 47*(2), 51–52.

Chapman, H. (1999). Some important limitations of competency-based education with respect to nurse education: An Australian perspective. *Nurse Education Today, 19*(2), 129–135.

Cowan, D. T., Norman, I., & Coopamah, V. P. (2005). Competence in nursing practice: A controversial concept—a focused review of literature. *Nurse Education Today, 25*(5), 355–362.

Lejonqvist, G. B., Eriksson, K., & Meretoja, R. (2012). Evidence of clinical competence. *Scandinavian Journal of Caring Sciences, 26*(2), 340–348.

McCarthy, G., Cornally, N., O' Mahoney, C., White, G., & Weathers, E. (2013). Emergency nurses: Procedures performed and competence in practice. *International Emergency Nursing, 21*(1), 50–57.

McHugh, M. D., & Lake, E. T. (2010). Understanding clinical expertise: Nurse education, experience, and the hospital context. *Research in Nursing & Health, 33*(4), 276–287.

Meretoja, R., & Koponen, L. (2012). A systematic model to compare nurses' optimal and actual competencies in the clinical setting. *Journal of Advanced Nursing, 68*(2), 414–422.

Ponte, P. R., Kruger, N., DeMarco, R., Hanley, D., & Conlin, G. (2004). Reshaping the practice environment. *Journal of Nursing Administration, 34*(4), 173–179.

Winskill, R. (2000). Is competency based training/education useful for workplace training. *Contemporary Nurse, 9*(2), 115–119.

Sarah McCloskey

CLINICAL DECISION MAKING

DEFINITION

Clinical decision making is a process that involves the interaction among the knowledge of preexisting pathological conditions, patient data, clinical experience, and judgment (Banning, 2008). Clinical decision making is defined as the ability by which a clinician identifies, prioritizes, establishes plans, and evaluates data.

APPLICATION

Clinical decision making is central to the education of nurses. A critical issue in clinical decision making is the educational level, preparation, and experience of the nurses who are formulating decisions. The use of a decision-making framework to guide clinical decision making by students and practicing nurses fosters the integration of knowledge, skills, and confidence. Students are prepared to engage in clinical decision making using a variety of teaching strategies, including the use of technology. Also, students are encouraged to engage patients/clients in the decision-making process regarding their care. Above all, clinical decision making is about the welfare of the patient, doing what is best in his or her interest.

There are several models that can be used to teach clinical decision making. One approach that has been used often in nursing education is the case study method. A patient scenario is presented to students and they are engaged in decision making based on the key dimensions of the patient's experience, including pathophysiology, social, cultural, and ethical aspects as related to the patient's presenting symptoms. Another teaching methodology is the gathering of a patient's story, a theory-based approach built on story theory (Smith & Liehr, 2013). The story is focused on what matters most to the patient about his or her complicating health challenge. The student is taught to engage in intentional dialogue and invite the telling of the story. Gathering the story from the patient's perspective facilitates a comprehensive approach to clinical decision making.

SYNOPSIS

There are three key points in understanding clinical decision making. (a) Educating

C

students in clinical decision making requires different approaches at various levels of education. (b) Clinical decision making is a complex process that includes high levels of knowledge and skills (Standing, 2008). (c) Clinical decision making has been studied across a number of clinical settings and among students at all levels (Gillespie & Peterson, 2009; Hoffman, Aitken, & Duffield, 2009). Banning (2008) found that nurses gained a sense of saliency in clinical decision making with increased experience. When investigating the decision-making process, researchers have utilized simulations, together with interviews regarding the thought processes individuals use to reach decisions. Decision-support technology serves as an adjunct to, not as a replacement for, actual clinical decision making. Advanced practice nurses integrate clinical decision systems into their practices to provide more objective, scientifically derived, technology-based data for their patient care decisions (Traynor, Boland, & Buus, 2010). There are some inherent difficulties with technology-based decision support systems. Nurses who are unfamiliar or uncomfortable with the technology are less likely to value the utilization of the systems (Weber, Crago, Sherwood, & Smith, 2009). Also, nurses' decision making has been shown to be affected by the sociodemographics of the patient. Age, sex, race, religion, and socioeconomic status can impact on decision making. Disparities in health care may be due to biases when formulating clinical decisions. In a study of more than 400 patients, it was shown that females, those with a high school or college education and those with previous hospital experience, are significantly more likely to prefer an active role in clinical decision making (Florin, Ehrenberg, & Ehnfors, 2008). Competent clinical decision making by nurses requires being cognizant of potential biases.

Clinical decision making is critical to nursing practice and held in high regard by nurses as it is viewed to be essential in the provision of safe effective care and the promotion of desired outcomes. Gathering, organizing, and prioritizing data are major components of the nursing process. Continued research in this area can foster the development of decision-making skills in novice nurses and cultivate high clinical decision-making ability in expert nurses.

RECOMMENDATIONS

Nurses have a professional responsibility to provide patients with opportunities to participate in clinical decision making. However, patients' preferences to participate vary greatly. Patient participation in clinical decision making has been studied from a variety of perspectives. Guiding students to understand the unique cultural values and beliefs that patients bring to the decision-making process will influence their judgments, and their participation rates.

As advances in technology are implemented in nursing education it is important for nurse faculty to understand that the technology is not a substitute for the nurse–patient relationship that is the core of nursing professional practice. Nursing educators must be cognizant of the need to integrate all learning modalities and assist the student in synthesizing the content and applying it to their nursing interventions.

There is a need for current research on clinical decision making, particularly in relation to new knowledge regarding cognitive processes and applications of technology to student nurse learning. As nursing education research expands, this is a promising area for scholarly inquiry.

Banning, M. (2008). A review of clinical decision making: Models and current research. *Journal of Clinical Nursing, 17*(2), 187–195.

Florin, J., Ehrenberg, A., & Ehnfors, M. (2008). Clinical decision-making: Predictors of patient participation in nursing care. *Journal of Clinical Nursing, 17*(21), 2935–2944.

Gillespie, M., & Peterson, B. L. (2009). Helping novice nurses make effective clinical decisions: The situated clinical decision-making framework. *Nursing Education Perspectives, 30*(3), 164–170.

Hoffman, K. A., Aitken, L. M., & Duffield, C. (2009). A comparison of novice and expert nurses' cue collection during clinical decision-making: Verbal protocol analysis. *International Journal of Nursing Studies, 46*(10), 1335–1344.

Smith, M. J., & Liehr, P. R. (2013). Story theory. In M. J. Smith & P. R. Liehr (Eds.), *Middle range theory for nursing* (pp. 225–251). New York, NY: Springer Publishing.

Standing, M. (2008). Clinical judgement and decision-making in nursing—nine modes of practice in a revised cognitive continuum. *Journal of Advanced Nursing, 62*(1), 124–134.

Traynor, M., Boland, M., & Buus, N. (2010). Professional autonomy in 21st century healthcare: Nurses' accounts of clinical decision-making. *Social Science & Medicine, 71*(8), 1506–1512.

Weber, S., Crago, E. A., Sherwood, P. R., & Smith, T. (2009). Practitioner approaches to the integration of clinical decision support system technology in critical care. *The Journal of Nursing Administration, 39*(11), 465–469.

Joyce J. Fitzpatrick
Mary Jane Smith

CLINICAL FAILURE

DEFINITION

Clinical failure occurs when evidence-based assessment and evaluation processes implemented by faculty identify unsafe student behavior (Larocque & Luhanga, 2013; Luhanga, Yonge, & Myrick, 2008; Tanicala, Scheffer, & Roberts, 2011).

APPLICATION

Determination of clinical failure arises through the use of evidence-based tools and evaluation processes created through the use of public, professional, and academic standards (Killam, Montgomery, Luhanga, Adamic, & Carter, 2010; Larocque & Luhanga, 2013). Tools and processes need to be appropriate at the program level and timing of the clinical experience (Tanicala et al., 2011). The use of checklists with clearly defined behaviors and practices that align with each objective ensures accurate assessment, clear documentation, objectivity, and transparency (Larocque & Luhanga, 2013; Luhanga et al., 2008). Students are evaluated and advised of their performance at each clinical experience, followed by identified remediation needs with required completion in a designated time frame (Larocque & Luhanga, 2013; Luhanga et al., 2008). Examples of behavior and practices that indicate clinical failure include clear knowledge deficits, psychomotor skills below expectations, lack of motivation, inappropriate interpersonal skills, actions that place others at risk for harm, poor attitude, lack of preparation, unethical or unprofessional conduct, failure to identify and seek help for deficits, lack of calculation competency, violation of policies, inability to apply theory to practice, and cheating or falsification of documentation (Killam et al., 2010; Larocque & Luhanga, 2013; Luhanga et al., 2008; Tanicala et al., 2011).

SYNOPSIS

Clinical failure may be determined to be due to professional, academic, and personal reasons. The National League for Nursing (NLN, 2005) identified the core competencies for nurse educators related to assessment and evaluation strategies. Based on these core competencies, the challenge for clinical faculty is recognition of students who are unsafe. If students are unable to remediate to a level of competence by the end of the clinical experience, then failing the student is the only option. However, clinical faculty are hesitant to fail a student based on lack of preparation, risk of an appeals process, required time to complete

C

adequate documentation, concern about being thought of negatively by others, institutional expectations that all students will pass, concern that teaching ability will be considered the reason for a student's lack of success, financial implications for the student, and concern that a second failure means dismissal from the nursing program (Killam et al., 2010; Larocque & Luhanga, 2013; Luhanga et al., 2008; Tanicala et al., 2011). Supporting clinical faculty with thorough orientation to the clinical evaluation tools and organizational policies promotes faculty–student assessments that are objective, reliable, and valid. Clinical faculty who have administrative support understand the importance of being the gatekeeper for the profession, demonstrating responsibility and accountability to the profession and society, as well as ethical and legal obligations to determine clinical failure when established criteria are not met.

RECOMMENDATIONS

The literature supports the fact that challenges when determining clinical failure originate from lack of clear and concise evaluation tools and sustained organizational policies (Larocque & Luhanga, 2013). Evidence-based evaluation tools and processes must be established that clearly and concisely define behaviors and practices at each level of clinical practice within the program of study. Furthermore, problems associated with observing each student over a sufficient period of time may interfere with identification of unsafe students. When the unsafe student is not identified, then students who are marginal or borderline may pass the clinical experience because the faculty member gives the student the benefit of the doubt (Killam et al., 2010; Larocque & Luhanga, 2013; Tanicala et al., 2011).

Organizational policies must be in place to support clinical faculty decision making based on policies and documentation that will make the case for failure during an academic appeals process. In addition, selection

of clinical faculty must not only ensure expert practitioners, evaluators, and supervisors, but also ensure that they are fully immersed in translation of theory into practice and skilled in assisting students to close the theory–practice gap. Orientation and ongoing education should be implemented to address specific clinical faculty issues based on identified needs. Clinical faculty must be effective in engaging students where open and transparent communication of performance is presented with each clinical experience (Tanicala et al., 2011).

Establishment of policy, tools, and guidelines as well as further research into these areas, offer the evidence required to ensure that safe students pass the clinical experience, that unsafe students have the opportunity to remediate to safety, and those that remain unsafe will be assigned a clinical failure.

Killam, L. A., Montgomery, P., Luhanga, F. L., Adamic, P., & Carter, L. M. (2010). Views on unsafe nursing students in clinical learning. *International Journal of Nursing Education Scholarship, 7,* Article 36.

Larocque, S., & Luhanga, F. L. (2013). Exploring the issue of failure to fail in a nursing program. *International Journal of Nursing Education Scholarship, 10*(1).

Luhanga, F., Yonge, O. J., & Myrick, F. (2008). "Failure to assign failing grades": Issues with grading the unsafe student. *International Journal of Nursing Education Scholarship, 5,* Article 8.

National League for Nursing. (NLN). (2005). *Core competencies of nurse educators with task statements*. Retrieved from http://www.nln.org/profdev/corecompetencies.pdf

Tanicala, M. L., Scheffer, B. K., & Roberts, M. S. (2011). Defining pass/fail nursing student clinical behaviors phase I: Moving toward a culture of safety. *Nursing Education Perspectives, 32*(3), 155–161.

Robin Kirschner

CLINICAL PRECEPTOR

DEFINITION

The clinical preceptor is a nurse who works one-on-one with a nursing student during a time-limited experience in the clinical area. This activity is accomplished with the support of nursing faculty for guidance and evaluation of objectives. The triad relationship among the preceptor, student, and faculty member assists in bridging the gap between theory and practice in the education of the student. Clinical preceptors perform complex, multifaceted roles: functioning as a role model, teaching clinical skills, and modeling critical thinking for the student while delivering optimal patient care (Billings & Halstead, 2012; McClure & Black, 2013; Omansky, 2010; Udlis, 2008).

APPLICATION

Preceptorship models developed in the 1970s were used for new nursing graduates in the orientation process. The 1970s model was quickly adapted into undergraduate education, with administrators in the 1980s and 1990s recognizing the value of the registered nurse (RN) preceptor (McClure & Black, 2013). The use of the clinical preceptor has been widely accepted and used in a variety of countries, such as Australia, Canada, United States, United Kingdom, and the Scandinavian countries (Luhanga, Billay, Grundy, Myrick, & Yonge, 2010). Clinical preceptors are used in both undergraduate and advanced practice nursing programs. For both levels, preceptors create an opportunity for students to synthesize theoretical knowledge and incorporate evidence into practice (Billings & Halstead, 2012). The American Association of Colleges of Nursing (AACN, 2012) provides specific criterion for advanced practice clinical preceptors. Requirements of the preceptor include appropriate educational experience, 1 year of clinical experience, orientation to the educational program requirements, and ongoing contact with the advanced practice faculty. In the undergraduate programs, preceptors are used with senior students during a clinical immersion experience throughout the semester (Omansky, 2010). AACN (2009) suggests that preceptors have formal mentoring in the academic and practice partnership. The literature suggests that when preceptors function fully in their role, they know the expectations of the role, the best methods to role model practice, and how to socialize the student in the profession of nursing (Martin, Brewer, & Barr, 2011).

SYNOPSIS

The one-to-one relationship with a consistent preceptor is a critical attribute for developing an effective preceptor relationship. This relationship allows the preceptor to provide immediate feedback on actions and questions in a safe learning environment (Luhanga et al., 2010). In multiple studies, an overwhelming number of students report a positive professional and learning relationship with preceptors. It was found that student knowledge, integration, autonomy, confidence, authority, and advocacy all increase (Kim, 2007; Rebeschi & Aronson, 2009; Wieland, Altmiller, Dorr, & Wolf, 2007). In a review of 16 studies from the late 1980s and 1990s, the preceptor model was equal and, in some cases, better than traditional clinical experience in preparing students for the nursing role (Udlis, 2008). Common views from preceptors are their enjoyment of working with students and assisting with the development of nursing (Raines, 2012). The preceptor model is beneficial to educational institutions in addressing the faculty shortage, decreasing the high cost of clinical education, and providing clinical expertise (Sedgwick & Harris, 2012). One overall benefit of the preceptor model is the development of an academic–service relationship or partnership. In the past, the relationship between academia and health care institutions was primarily faculty practice models and centers for research. Today, the majority of academic–service relationships is focused on increasing the nursing workforce, with safe, competent nurses (Beal, 2010).

RECOMMENDATIONS

Clinical preceptors are integral to the success of graduate and undergraduate nursing students. Adequate preparation and orientation are imperative for the preceptor role (McClure & Black, 2013). Role ambiguity, conflict, and role overload may cause stress for the preceptor. Sedgwick and Harris (2012) identify necessary supports for the clinical preceptor to include financial and educational support. Clinical preceptors deserve recognition and support from leadership, faculty, and peers (Luhanga et al., 2010; Omansky, 2010). Future empirical research should focus on preceptor characteristics, orientation methods, and other educational needs to identify how these relate to successful preceptor programs (Martin et al., 2011; Udlis, 2008).

American Association of Colleges of Nursing (AACN). (2009). *Faculty tool kit: The essentials of baccalaureate education for professional nursing practice*. Retrieved from http://www.aacn.nche.edu/education-resources/BacEssToolkit.pdf

American Association of Colleges of Nursing. (2012). *Criteria for evaluation of nurse practitioner programs*. Retrieved from http://www.aacn.nche.edu/education-resources/evalcriteria2012.pdf

Beal, J. A. (2010). Academic-service partnerships in nursing: An integrative review. *Nursing Research and Practice, 7*(1), 1–15. Retrieved from http://dx.doi.org/10.1155/2012/501564

Billings, D. M., & Halstead, J. A. (2012). *Teaching in nursing: A guide for faculty* (4th ed.). St. Louis, MO: Elsevier Saunders.

Kim, K. H. (2007). Clinical competence among senior nursing students after their preceptorship experiences. *Journal of Professional Nursing, 23*(6), 369–375.

Luhanga, F. L., Billay, D., Grundy, Q., Myrick, F., & Yonge, O. (2010). The one-to-one relationship: Is it really key to an effective preceptorship experience? A review of the literature. *International Journal of Nursing Education Scholarship, 7*(1), 1–15. Retrieved from http://dx.doi.org/10.2202/1548–923X.2012

Martin, D. L., Brewer, D., & Barr, N. (2011). Gradually guiding nursing students through their capstone course: Registered nurse preceptors share their experiences. *Nursing Research and Practice*. Retrieved from http://dx.doi.org/10.1155/2011/645125

McClure, E., & Black, L. (2013). The role of the clinical preceptor: An integrative literature review. *Journal of Nursing Education, 52*(6), 335–341.

Omansky, G. L. (2010). Staff nurses' experiences as preceptors and mentors: An integrative review. *Journal of Nursing Management, 18*, 697–703. Retrieved from http://dx.doi.org/10.1111/j.1365–2834.2010.01145.x

Raines, D. A. (2012). Nurse preceptors' views of precepting undergraduate nursing students. *Nursing Education Perspectives, 33*(2), 76–79.

Rebeschi, L., & Aronson, B. (2009). Assessment of nursing students learning outcomes and employment choice after the implementation of a senior capstone course. *International Journal of Nursing Education Scholarship, 6*(1), 1–15. Retrieved from http://dx.doi.org/10.2202/1548–923X.1775

Sedgwick, M., & Harris, S. (2012). Review article: A critique of the undergraduate nursing preceptorship model. *Nursing Research and Practice*. Retrieved from http://dx.doi.org/10.1155/2012/248356

Udlis, K. A. (2008). Preceptorship in undergraduate nursing education: An integrative review. *Journal of Nursing Education, 47*(1), 20–29.

Wieland, D. M., Altmiller, G. M., Dorr, M. T., & Wolf, Z. R. (2007). Clinical transition of baccalaureate nursing students during preceptored, pregraduation practicums.

Nursing Education Perspectives, 28(6), 315–321.

Martha S. Morrow
Mary T. Quinn Griffin

CLINICAL REMEDIATION

DEFINITION

Clinical remediation is the act or process of correcting deficiencies in nursing practice and promoting safe patient care through the implementation of learning strategies to improve critical thinking and clinical performance (Evans & Harder, 2013; *Merriam-Webster Dictionary Online*). Clinical remediation may result from academic, clinical practice, and regulatory deficiencies identified through examination, observation, peer review, or failure to successfully complete the minimum standard of care (Evans & Harder, 2013; Walker-Cillo & Harding, 2013).

APPLICATION

The application of clinical remediation is multifaceted in nursing education. Nursing education does not end with the conferring a degree or giving a diploma. Continuing education is a journey that all nurses, regardless of field of practice, travel for successful and safe clinical practice. Remediation plans can be used in academia and clinical practice, as well as for regulatory policies to maintain minimum practice standards.

Remediation begins with identification of deficiencies that can lead to unsafe practice. Clinical remediation is an organized process comprising objectivity, openness, and transparency. It is essential that the process respects the right to due process when engaging in clinical remediation. Remediation can be achieved through student-centered remediation that is adaptable to learning needs and deficiencies. Plans should be individualized using supportive strategies, including tutoring, advising, counseling, and skill building. Activities supporting remediation are simulation, case presentation, and incorporation of theoretical and scholarly resources (Evans & Harder, 2013; Gallant, MacDonald, & Smith Higuchi, 2006; Walker-Cillo & Harding, 2013).

Remediation is useful to assist a struggling student to learn and achieve the minimum standards for practice and to successfully complete the academic program. Nurse educators can identify individuals who have performed poorly on actual and simulated clinical encounters and examinations. Once the individual is identified, a structured plan can be developed. This plan is structured to facilitate a positive and supportive learning environment. It should include clearly stated learning objectives, utilize multiple sources of evidence, and give timely feedback (Evans & Harder, 2013; Gallant et al., 2006).

SYNOPSIS

Remediation methods used include close observation, repetition, self-directed learning, structured classes, scenarios, and case studies. Mechanical simulators and standardized patients can be used to bring particular clinical populations to the remediation experience. Regardless of the method, it is important to keep the remediation focused on the individual (Audétat, Laurin, & Dory, 2013; Evans & Harder, 2013; Klamen & Williams, 2011; Lynn & Twigg, 2011).

The use of mechanical simulators is an effective method of remediation. Case scenarios allow for repetitious learning with immediate feedback and debriefing. This method allows for identification of weaknesses and strengths of the individual. Case scenarios can also be used with standardized patients who are trained to portray a real patient encounter to simulate a set of symptoms with realistic interaction with the nurse (Klamen & Williams, 2011).

Challenges to remediation include underutilization or no utilization of theoretical and conceptual frameworks in the development of the intervention(s), delay in remediation, as well as stress and anxiety. These challenges can be overcome with the use of a well-developed plan and intervention. Early identification of a problem followed by early intervention is the key to remediation success. Mutual respect between the educator and the individual is the foundation for the initiation of any plan, as well as guiding the individual to reflect and discuss progress (Audétat et al., 2013; Evans & Harder, 2013).

RECOMMENDATIONS

Clinical remediation has been a mainstay of nursing education and will remain an integral part of a student's education. Technological advancements, computerization, and simulation will continue to be an important component of the remediation process. Integrating case scenarios with mechanical simulation and the use of standardized patients can lead to proficient actual patient encounters and care. The use of virtual simulation can also be integrated in the remediation plan.

The cost of the faculty, technology, and resources may have an impact on the future of nursing education and remediation. Sharing of resources by various schools can help overall financial viability through the sharing of simulation labs, faculty, and computer resources. Collaboration among health care professionals is integral to safe patient care. Patient safety, standards of care, and professional development are the ultimate goal of remediation.

Audétat, M. C., Laurin, S., & Dory, V. (2013). Remediation for struggling learners: Putting an end to "more of the same." *Medical Education, 47*(3), 230–231.

Evans, C. J., & Harder, N. (2013). A formative approach to student remediation. *Nurse Educator, 38*(4), 147–151.

Gallant, M., MacDonald, J. A., & Smith Higuchi, K. A. (2006). A remediation process for nursing students at risk for clinical failure. *Nurse Educator, 31*(5), 223–227.

Google.com. Retrieved from https://www .google.com/#q=remediation+definition and https://www.google.com/#q= clinical+definition

Klamen, D. L., & Williams, R. G. (2011). The efficacy of a targeted remediation process for students who fail standardized patient examinations. *Teaching and Learning in Medicine, 23*(1), 3–11.

Lynn, M. C., & Twigg, R. D. (2011). A new approach to clinical remediation. *Journal of Nursing Education, 50*(3), 172–175.

Merriam-Webster Dictionary Online. Retrieved from http://www.merriam-webster.com/ dictionary/remediation.

Walker-Cillo, G. A., & Harding, A. (2013). The art of remediation in professional emergency nursing practice. *Advanced Emergency Nursing Journal, 35*(2), 129–142.

Theresa M. Campo

CLINICAL SCENARIOS

DEFINITION

The term *scenario* is derived from the Latin word *scaenarium*, indicating a place for building a stage; *scaena* is the term for the stage itself. A scenario is a collage of events or series of actions that unfold during a performance. Clinical scenarios in nursing address relevant events that occur in the actual execution of health care. During the last decade, a theoretical model and guidelines have emerged to steer the advancement of interactive student learning scenarios in nursing education and clinical practice.

APPLICATION

Clinical scenario applications have been used by the aeronautic, automotive, military, and other industries to develop the best defensive tactics for the prevention of error and promotion of safety. Scenarios are a component of the broader category of simulation education that incorporates low- and high-fidelity manikins, skill and task trainers, virtual reality trainers, and computer-based simulators. The scenario requires a model or laboratory that represents the real-world clinical process. Simulation characterizes the operation of the model or activities that mimic the clinical reality (Jefferies, 2005). A scenario is the enacted performance creating opportunity for a high level of realistic inter-activity for students to learn and develop confidence. A specification of the details of the enactment and the order of the activities is required. Written materials are prepared for the faculty and a separate script is designed for the student. An important aspect of the clinical scenarios is the debriefing segment, which includes reflection on the experience, the student's performance, and what was learned (Schneider Sarver, Senczakowicz, & Slovensky, 2010).

SYNOPSIS

Scenarios have been written to address essential domains of nursing practice including technical and functional training, problem solving, decision making, and team-based competencies (Schneider Sarver et al., 2010). They are increasingly used in nursing education throughout the United States and internationally. Both prelicensure and advanced clinical skills require active listening, effective communication, knowledge, and competence appropriate to the individual's education and experience. The scenario must match the specific level of the undergraduate student while advancing in various degrees of complexity. Both simple vignettes and complex scenarios were rated by students as beneficial in helping them to set priorities, develop critical thinking, acquire assessment skills, and gain an awareness of the nurse's role (Guhde, 2011). Scenarios used in graduate programs, particularly the post-scenario reflection, have been identified as an effective teaching method for graduate faculty and a positive learning experience for graduate students (Einion, 2013; Velok & Smedley, 2014).

Simulation scenarios have been incorporated into the employment setting for licensed providers to learn new techniques and maintain and strengthen skills that are necessary for events that rarely occur. Clinical scenarios are a mechanism for integrating individual skills into complex operational capabilities. Clinical scenarios are designed to develop and enhance team interaction, giving students the opportunity to improve communication, decision making, and team discipline (Liaw et al., 2014).

Although simulation scenarios can be traced back to several decades, current designs are more realistic and congruent with the complexity nurses encounter in the workplace. Clinical scenarios provide students with a means to safely understand the potential for failure while gathering the necessary data to make critical decisions in real-time replication. Jefferies (2005) identified six critical areas as essential components for clinical scenarios: objectives, planning, fidelity, complexity, cues, and debriefing. Continued efforts in simulation scenario education produced theoretical frameworks for generating scenarios (Jeffries & Rogers, 2009). Sixteen studies from the United States and the United Kingdom have used frameworks in undergraduate and graduate curricula to design and evaluate respective simulation scenarios. Students reported that participation in clinical scenarios provided more opportunity for problem solving and that the experience positively affected critical thinking. Analysis of the student outcomes demonstrated improvement in patient safety competencies, higher levels of student satisfaction with the learning method, and increased confidence regarding clinical skills (LaFond & Van Hulle Vincent, 2013).

Waxman (2010) introduced an evidence-based practice (EBP) template for constructing clinical scenarios as a means to promote effective learning. The template was derived from EBP data to advance clinical reasoning skills. Key elements of the template include techniques to measure learning and validation criteria for written scenarios. Data from the SIMulated Professional Learning Environment (SIMPLE) provided further evidence of the value of clinical scenarios for baccalaureate students. The students believed that they were better prepared for transitioning to the workplace as a result of the clinical scenario experience (Liaw et al., 2014). The health care environment is continuously changing, thus challenging educators to provide a safe platform for learning while preparing graduates to apply clinical reasoning skills in the actual setting. Clinical scenarios prepare the learner to quickly organize data derived from multiple sources, process the data, and identify priority needs. Evaluation, reflection, and feedback provide the learner with the opportunity to safely advance in proficiency.

RECOMMENDATIONS

Multisite trials with large sample sizes have been called for to thoroughly evaluate the effect of simulation scenarios on prelicensure students (Shinnick, Woo, & Mentes, 2011). Jeffries et al. (2011) reported on the effectiveness of a highly complex simulation-based cardiovascular assessment curriculum for advanced practice nurses (APN). There was participation from four university-based nursing programs distributed across the United States, with a small number of participants from each institution. Logistic challenges, human resources, and cost have posed obstacles to conducting more multisite trials. Complex and well-constructed clinical scenarios have emerged primarily in the medical surgical practice areas. Future effort should include the development of maternal infant and child scenarios that address childbearing and parenting. Substantial validation of the efficacy and cost-effective improvement of student learning and patient outcomes will provide valuable information for broadening the use of clinical scenarios in nursing education.

Einion, A. (2013). OSCE assessment for emergency scenarios in midwifery education: A reflection and evaluation. *British Journal of Midwifery, 21*(12), 893–897.

Guhde, J. (2011). Nursing students' perceptions of the effect on critical thinking, assessment, and learner satisfaction in simple versus complex high-fidelity simulation scenarios. *Journal of Nursing Education, 50*(2), 73–78.

Jeffries, P. R. (2005). A framework for designing, implementing and evaluating simulations used as teaching strategies in nursing. *Nursing Education Perspective, 26*(2), 96–103.

Jeffries, P. R., & Rogers, K. (2009). Theoretical framework for simulation design. In P. R. Jeffries (Ed.), *Simulation in nursing education: From conceptualization to evaluation* (pp. 21–34). New York, NY: National League for Nursing.

Jeffries, P. R., Beach, M., Decker, S. I., Dlugasch, L., Groom, J., Settles, J., & O'Donnell, J. M. (2011). Multi-center development and testing of a simulation-based cardiovascular assessment curriculum for advanced practice nurses. *Nursing Education Perspectives, 32*(5), 316–322.

LaFond, C. M., & Van Hulle Vincent, C. (2013). A critique of the National League for Nursing/Jeffries simulation framework. *Journal of Advanced Nursing, 69*(2), 465–480.

Liaw, S. Y., Koh, Y., Dawood, R., Kowitlawakul, Y., Zhou, W., & Lau, S. T. (2014). Easing student transition to graduate nurse: A SIMulated Professional Learning Environment (SIMPLE) for final year student nurses. *Nurse Education Today, 34*(3), 349–355.

Schneider Sarver, P. A., Senczakowicz, E. A., & Slovensky, B. M. (2010). Development of simulation scenarios for an adolescent patient with diabetic ketoacidosis. *Journal of Nursing Education, 49*(10), 578–586.

Shinnick, M. A., Woo, M. A., & Mentes, J. C. (2011). Human patient simulation: State of the science in prelicensure nursing education. *Journal of Nursing Education, 50*(2), 65–72.

Velok, K., & Smedley, A. (2014). Using reflection to enhance the teaching and learning of midwifery students. *British Journal of Midwifery, 2*(22), 129–133.

Waxman, K. T. (2010). The development of evidence-based clinical simulation scenarios: Guidelines for nurse educators. *Journal of Nursing Education, 49*(1), 29–35.

Anne Marie Mitchell

CLINICAL TEACHING

DEFINITION

The definition of clinical teaching has evolved over the years. Clinical teaching is a time-limited process, whereby the teacher and student develop a partnership within a shared environment in such a way that the teacher's primary, operational frame of reference is maintained as the legitimate means for affecting the student's behavior toward intended purposes (White & Ewan, 2002). While many of these core aspects remain active today, progress in the area of clinical teaching in nursing has led to expansion of this definition to include aspects such as clinical preceptorship, peer-learning dyads, and simulation (Sims-Giddens, Helton, & Hope, 2010).

APPLICATION

When considering the application of clinical teaching in the education of nurses and their future nursing practice, several themes emerge as being important. Clinical teaching can occur in any setting where a nurse is actively providing care for a patient. The primary settings utilized in the clinical education of nurses include acute care settings, community-based settings, clinic settings, and simulation settings. In each of these settings, an environment-specific approach to clinical education can be provided. The methods of clinical education that are provided across these settings include preceptorship, education-based units, peer education teams, and simulation support.

Clinical nursing education in the acute care setting often encompasses a faculty member taking a group of 8 to 10 nursing students into the acute care setting after a patient has been assigned to the student the day before. Clinical preplanning often occurs in the setting where the student gains insight and knowledge the day before the clinical experience and develops a plan of care for the patient in advance. Preceptorship is also utilized in the acute care setting. Student nurses can be assigned to a preceptor, and the student and the preceptor develop a schedule for clinical experiences for the student. Education-based units are emerging in the acute care setting where a unit is identified as an education unit and the nurses in this unit receive training in their role as a preceptor or a clinical support nurse. These units have a strong focus on clinical education for nursing students, and the environment is often a student-friendly setting that research supports as a method to enhance learning (Balakas & Sparks, 2010).

In the community-based setting, nursing students most often gain their clinical experience through the use of preceptors who agree to develop a relationship with the educational institution where they will precept students during their care of patients in the community. Most often, these agencies are home care or hospice affiliated. The clinic setting is considered a unique environment within the community experience in general but with many overlapping experiences found in the traditional community setting. Many clinic settings are located near acute care facilities and provide care to patients who mainly remain in the community after the clinic visit but may be admitted to the acute care setting (Balakas & Sparks, 2010).

By definition, the simulation experience could occur in any of the available clinical settings if the appropriate simulation equipment were available. Most often, this is accomplished through the use of a trained faculty member who maintains the simulation equipment in a central location. The simulation experiences can be tailored to address multiple care situations that could occur in any of the settings, promoting critical thinking skills (Goodstone et al., 2013).

SYNOPSIS

The literature, as it relates to clinical nursing education, is considered weaker when compared to clinical nursing research (Schneider, Nicholas, & Kurrus, 2013). The literature supports the use of clinical preceptors as an effective means for supporting clinical nursing education (Hendricks, Wallace, Narwold, Guy, & Wallace, 2013). The use of clinical peer dyads, where students work in peer groups with senior-level students mentoring lower-level students, is also supported as an effective method for clinical instruction (Austria, Baraki, & Doig, 2012; Christiansen & Bell, 2010). Clinical peer dyad data show positive results from both the student and patient perspectives. Simulation experiences for nursing students, including standardized patient encounters, are supported in the literature as a supplementary experience for students and can help improve patient safety and enhance the students' critical thinking skills (Kaplan & Ura, 2010; Pacsi, 2008). Ongoing concerns documented in the literature that have had an impact on clinical teaching include nursing shortage, lack of clinical space, restrictions on the number of students per faculty or per unit, and competition with other schools of nursing (Benner, Stuphen, Leonard, & Day, 2010). Also supported in the literature would be the utilization of clinical staff nurses who have joint appointments with schools of nursing to improve access to clinical specialists. The utilization of staff nurses who are not jointly hired is also supported, with the majority of these nurses receiving additional training on clinical teaching (Kowalski et al., 2007; Seldomridge & Walsh, 2006). The literature supports the development of clinical partnerships between schools of nursing and units in acute care settings that are designated as educational units (Moscato, Nishioka, & Coe, 2013). Overall, the literature supports the need for development and utilization of unique clinical learning opportunities to meet the growing demands for nurses.

RECOMMENDATIONS

In nursing education, while classroom and simulation experiences make essential contributions to students' knowledge and skill development, the clinical experience remains the cornerstone of nursing education (Luhanga, Billay, Grundy, Myrick, & Yonge, 2010). The culture of evidence-based practice should start in the clinical teaching setting and continue on in clinical nursing practice (Balakas & Sparks, 2010). Continued growth in the quantity and quality of nursing research focused on nursing education will help to continue to address the clinical teaching needs of future nursing students.

Austria, M., Baraki, K., & Doig, A. (2012). Collaborative learning using nursing student dyads in the clinical setting. *International Journal of Nursing Education Scholarship, 10*(1), 1–8.

Balakas, K., & Sparks, L. (2010). Teaching research and evidence-based practice using a service-learning approach. *Journal of Nursing Education, 49*(12), 691–695.

Benner, P., Stuphen, M., Leonard, V., & Day, L. (2010). *Education nurses: A call for radical transformation.* San Francisco, CA: Jossey Bass.

Christiansen, A., & Bell, A. (2010). Peer learning partnerships: Exploring the experience of pre-registration nursing students. *Journal of Clinical Nursing, 19*(5–6), 803–810.

Goodstone, L., Goodstone, M. S., Cino, K., Glaser, C. A., Kupferman, K., & Dember-Neal, T. (2013). Effect of simulation on the development of critical thinking in associate degree nursing students. *Nursing Education Perspectives, 34*(3), 159–162.

Hendricks, S. M., Wallace, L. S., Narwold, L., Guy, G., & Wallace, D. (2013). Comparing the effectiveness, practice opportunities, and satisfaction of the preceptored clinical and the traditional clinical for nursing students. *Nursing Education Perspectives, 34*(5), 310–314.

Kaplan, B., & Ura, D. (2010). Use of multiple patient simulators to enhance prioritizing and delegating skills for senior nursing students. *Journal of Nursing Education, 49*(7), 371–377.

Kowalski, K., Homer, M., Carroll, K., Center, D., Foss, K., Jarrett, S., & Kane, L. A. (2007). Nursing clinical faculty revisited: The benefits of developing staff nurses as clinical scholars. *Journal of Continuing Education in Nursing, 38*(2), 69–75.

Luhanga, F., Billay, D., Grundy, Q., Myrick, F., & Yonge, O. (2010). The one-to-one relationship: Is it really key to an effective preceptorship experience? A review of the literature. *International Journal of Nursing Education Scholarship, 7*(1), 1–15.

Moscato, S. R., Nishioka, V. M., & Coe, M. T. (2013). Dedicated education unit: Implementing an innovation in replication sites. *Journal of Nursing Education, 52*(5), 259–267.

Pacsi, A. L. (2008). Human simulators in nursing education. *The Journal of the New York State Nurses' Association, 39*(2), 8–11.

Schneider, B. S., Nicholas, J., & Kurrus, J. E. (2013). Comparison of methodologic quality and study/report characteristics between quantitative clinical nursing and nursing education research articles. *Nursing Education Perspectives, 34*(5), 292–297.

Sims-Giddens, S., Helton, C., & Hope, K. L. (2010). Student peer mentoring in a community-based nursing clinical experience. *Nursing Education Perspectives, 31*(1), 23–27.

Seldomridge, L. A., & Walsh, C. M. (2006). Evaluating student performance in undergraduate preceptorships. *Journal of Nursing Education, 45*(5), 169–176.

White, R., & Ewan, C. (2002). *Teaching in nursing.* Gloucester, UK: Nelson Thornes Ltd.

Angel Smothers

COACHING

DEFINITION

Coaching is an art where a coach uses conversation to create an environment that facilitates moving toward goals in a fulfilling manner (Timothy, 2000). The coaching process is supported and guided by nursing theories (Dossey, Luck, & Schaub, 2014) and theories from social sciences including the transtheoretical model of behavioral change, motivational interviewing, and appreciative inquiry (Moore & Tschannen-Moran, 2010). These theories create a foundation for development of the collaborative coaching relationship such as reflection, therapeutic presence, powerful questions, enhanced listening, formative feedback, and summarization. The client is defined as the expert in the coaching process that is time limited, and involves creating awareness and moving to action (O'Grady, 2011, p. 85).

APPLICATION

Coaching in nursing education applies to both the specialty of nurse coach and a practice skill. A nurse coach is defined as a registered nurse who integrates coaching competencies into any setting or specialty area of practice to facilitate a process of change that assists individuals or groups to realize potential (Hess et al., 2013). The nurse coaching practice aligns with the nursing process including: assessment—establishing the relationship and identifying readiness for change; diagnosis—identifying opportunities and concerns; outcome—establishing client-centered goals; plan—creating the structure of the coaching sessions; implementation—empowering clients to reach goals; and evaluation—assisting clients to determine how well goals were achieved (Hess et al., 2013). Coaching skills include open-ended questions, effective listening, and providing feedback to promote learning, self-awareness, and action (Glasgow,

C

C

Weinstock, Lachman, Suplee, & Dreher, 2009). Rather than telling students what to do, the educator as coach uses conversation skills and therapeutic presence to empower students to formulate and move toward goals. The role of a coach is more evocative than didactic, as the educator facilitates the student's empowerment by assisting him or her to discover strengths, identify values, set goals, and decide on action (Hess et al., 2013). Coaching has also been introduced as an innovative leadership strategy for new nursing academic administrators (Glasgow et al., 2009) and for nursing leaders seeking to improve practice and build skills (O'Grady, 2011). Effectiveness of the educator's coaching skills relies on continuous self-development through self-reflection, self-assessment, self-evaluation, and self-care (Dossey et al., 2014). Tobin (2004) identifies coaching as one of the seven roles related to mentoring. Both coaching and mentoring can be used simultaneously with nursing students, but there are distinct differences. As opposed to the time-limited structure of coaching, mentoring often spans several years. It includes a teaching–learning process, encouragement to grow professionally and personally, and formal evaluation (Donner & Wheeler, 2009).

SYNOPSIS

Formerly popular in sports, coaching moved into organizations in the 1960s. During the 1990s, coaching models began to appear in nursing administration, clinical practice, and education. In 2013, the coach role was endorsed by the American Nurses Association and 20 other professional nursing organizations with defined scope and competencies, standardized preparation/supervision process, and a recognized board certification examination (Hess et al., 2013). Educators are in a pivotal role to apply coaching strategies to the self-development of students in the classroom, nursing leaders in academia and clinical practice, or clients in the clinical setting. Coaching goals may include the acquisition of new skills in the clinical setting, leadership development, lifestyle modifications, or chronic disease management. Applications are only limited by the nurse educator's imagination and skill. The principles and acts of coaching, present in nursing education for years, are reflected in the words of exemplary teachers (Smith & Fitzpatrick, 2006) who were asked to give advice to new educators. Their recommendations on teaching as changing behavior included engaging in reflection, facilitating growth, developing self-awareness and understanding, and inviting feedback. Thus, each of those recognized educators highlighted the importance of foundational coaching skills and indirectly alluded to the coaching process for behavior change.

RECOMMENDATIONS

The Institute of Medicine (IOM, 2010) has recommended that nurses practice at the full extent of their education and training, and that education be a seamless progression partnering with health care professionals to redesign the country's health care. Coaching, both the art and specialty, aligns with these national goals. Educators can benefit from the development and refinement of coaching skills, and students can benefit from educators who model coaching skills.

Donner, G., & Wheeler, M. (2009). *Coaching in nursing.* International Council of Nurses and The Honor Society of Nursing Sigma Theta Tau. Indianapolis, IN: Printing Partners.

Dossey, B. M., Luck, S., & Schaub, B. G. (2014). *Nurse coaching: Integrative approaches for health and wellbeing.* North Miami, FL: International Nurse Coach Association.

Glasgow, M. E., Weinstock, B., Lachman, V., Suplee, P., & Dreher, M. (2009). The benefits of a leadership program and executive coaching for new nursing academic administrators: One college's experience. *Journal of Professional Nursing, 25*(4), 204–210.

Hess, D. R., Dossey, B. M., Southard, M. E., Luck, S., Schaub, B. G., & Bark, L. (2013). *The art and science of nurse coaching: The provider's guide to coaching scope and competencies.* Silver Spring, MD: Nursesbooks.org.

Institute of Medicine (IOM). (2010). *Future of nursing: Leading change, advancing health.* Washington, DC: The National Academies Press. Retrieved from http://www.iom.edu/Reports/2010/The-Future-of-Nursing-Leading-Change-Advancing-Health.aspx

Moore, M., & Tschannen-Moran, B. (2010). *Coaching psychology manual.* New York, NY: Wolters Kluwer/Lippincott Williams & Wilkins.

O'Grady, E. (2011). Coaching. In H. R. Feldman, G. R. Alexander, M. J. Greenberg, and M. Jaffe-Ruiz (Eds.), *Nursing leadership: A concise encyclopedia* (2nd ed., pp. 84–86). New York, NY: Springer Publishing Company.

Smith, M. J., & Fitzpatrick, J. (2006). *Stories of exemplary teachers.* New York, NY: Springer Publishing Co.

Timothy, G. W. (2000). *The inner game of work.* New York, NY: Random House.

Tobin, M. J. (2004). Mentoring: Seven roles and some specifics. *American Journal of Respiratory and Critical Care Medicine, 170,* 114–117.

Deborah McElligott

COMMUNICATION

DEFINITION

Communication is the act or process of using words, sounds, signs, or behaviors to express ideas, thoughts, feelings, or exchange information (Merriam-Webster, 2014).

Teaching communication skills requires imparting relevant knowledge, guiding learners to develop and enhance their skills, and coaching effective communication behaviors.

APPLICATION

Communication is an essential component of nursing care. Nurses communicate with patients and families in order to build relationships, to provide comfort and caring, to treat and heal, and to educate. Nurses communicate with other professionals to exchange patient information and ensure safe practices. The Institute of Medicine, The Joint Commission, the Agency for Healthcare Research and Quality's Patient Safety Initiative, and the Quality and Safety in Nursing Education (QSEN) Initiative all support the importance of communication to improve patient care (Cronenwett et al., 2007). While effective communication is clearly essential to nursing practice, the best practices in teaching this skill are still being debated (Aebersold, Tschannen, & Sculli, 2013).

Teaching communication skills, both oral and written, requires didactic and experiential pedagogies. Examining theories of communication, foundational aspects of the nurse–patient relationship, therapeutic communication, and active listening, along with application of these basic skills in clinical settings, are foci in many nursing curricula. Behavioral improvement requires a combination of written information and clinical interactions. Students bring distinctive sets of interpersonal skills, cultural influences, learning styles, and life experiences that directly affect their ability to engage in effective communication. Nursing faculty must build on students' personal strengths and experiences to enhance their communication skills.

Educators must utilize an organized instructional plan that articulates all curricular communication components and emphasizes active learning (Boschma et al., 2010). Communication modules or courses should be aligned with clinical learning throughout the curriculum. Important concepts in a communication skill-training course can include the significance of communication in nursing and common barriers and challenges to effective communication, the

C

development of a therapeutic relationship, empathy, patient-centered communication, breaking bad news, conflict management, and communication with various patient populations such as children, older adults, or cognitively or mentally impaired individuals (Lau & Wang, 2013). Skill development should focus on topics such as self-awareness styles, observation and active listening skills, and communication to assess needs (Lau & Wang, 2013). Other vital components include both knowledge and skill development in interprofessional team communication (Interprofessional Education Collaborative Expert Panel, 2011).

Teaching strategies for communication involve provision of feedback on communication skills and performance utilizing simulation, role-play, modeling, oral presentations, written information, and group discussion (Berkhof, van Rijssen, Schellart, Anema, & van der Beek, 2011). Practicing communication skills through simulation allows students to develop communication skills and faculty to evaluate and provide feedback in a safe, nonthreatening environment (Zavertnik, Huff, & Munro, 2010). The use of human simulators and standardized patients can be effective in enhancing students' interpersonal and communication skills (Lin, Chen, Chao, & Chen, 2013; Reising, Carr, Shea, & King, 2011). Standardized assessment and evaluation tools for measuring outcomes from these various teaching strategies are needed (O'Shea, Pagano, Campbell, & Caso, 2013; Zavertnik et al., 2010), particularly in simulation.

SYNOPSIS

Development of skilled communication is an integral element of nursing education and a core competency of nursing practice. Methods for teaching and assessing this competency are important to nursing practice. While teaching communication skills in the classroom provides students with basic knowledge and improves performance on objective testing, didactic education does not allow for practice of patient–nurse interactions. Experiential and innovative approaches to teaching communication are necessary.

RECOMMENDATIONS

While recent studies show promise in improving the quality of communication education in nursing, evaluation of teaching strategies and student outcomes is not well researched. Nurse educators need to continue to develop and test innovative teaching strategies such as role-playing in clinical conferences; peer-to-peer teaching (Cooper, Martin, Fisher, Marks, & Harrington, 2013); forum theater (Middlewick, Kettle, & Wilson, 2012); and standardized patient scenarios to teach communication skills to diverse groups of learners (Spinner-Gelfars, 2013). Communication skills should be routinely emphasized in simulation and clinical practice experiences throughout the nursing program. Managing information technology and the increasing demands for high-tech communication will be important in nursing education as a more complex health care system emerges. Research on the effectiveness of structured, objective tools to evaluate communication skills will build an evidence-based nursing curriculum.

Aebersold, M., Tschannen, D., & Sculli, G. (2013). Improving nursing students' communication skills using crew resource management strategies. *Journal of Nursing Education, 52*(3), 125–130.

Berkhof, M., van Rijssen, H. J., Schellart, A. J., Anema, J. R., & van der Beek, A. J. (2011). Effective training strategies for teaching communication skills to physicians: An overview of systematic reviews. *Patient Education and Counseling, 84*(2), 152–162.

Boschma, G., Einboden, R., Groening, M., Jackson, C., MacPhee, M., Marshall, H.,...Roberts, E. (2010). Strengthening communication education in an undergraduate nursing curriculum. *International Journal of Nursing Education Scholarship, 7*, Article 28.

Cooper, J. R., Martin, T., Fisher, W., Marks, J., & Harrington, M. (2013). Peer-to-peer teaching: Improving communication techniques for students in an accelerated nursing program. *Nursing Education Perspectives, 34*(5), 349–350.

Cronenwett, L., Sherwood, G., Barnsteiner, J., Disch, J., Johnson, J., Mitchell, P., ... Warren, J. (2007). Quality and safety education for nurses. *Nursing Outlook, 55*(3), 122–131.

Interprofessional Education Collaborative Expert Panel. (2011). *Core competencies for interprofessional collaborative practice. Report of an expert panel.* Washington, DC: Interprofessional Education Collaborative.

Lau, Y., & Wang, W. (2013). Development and evaluation of a learner-centered training course on communication skills for baccalaureate nursing students. *Nurse Education Today, 33*(12), 1617–1623.

Lin, E. C., Chen, S. L., Chao, S. Y., & Chen, Y. C. (2013). Using standardized patient with immediate feedback and group discussion to teach interpersonal and communication skills to advanced practice nursing students. *Nurse Education Today, 33*(6), 677–683.

Merriam-Webster Online Dictionary. (2014). Retrieved from www.merriam-webster/dictionary/communication.

Middlewick, Y., Kettle, T. J., & Wilson, J. J. (2012). Curtains up! Using forum theatre to rehearse the art of communication in healthcare education. *Nurse Education in Practice, 12*(3), 139–142.

O'Shea, E., Pagano, M., Campbell, S., & Caso, G. (2013). A descriptive analysis of nursing student communication behavior. *Clinical Simulation in Nursing, 9*(1), e5–12.

Reising, D. L., Carr, D. E., Shea, R. A., & King, J. M. (2011). Comparison of communication outcomes in traditional versus simulation strategies in nursing and medical students. *Nursing Education Perspectives, 32*(5), 323–327.

Spinner-Gelfars, A. (2013). Using simulation to promote effective communication with a diverse student population. *Teaching and Learning in Nursing, 8,* 96–101.

Zavertnik, J. E., Huff, T. A., & Munro, C. L. (2010). Innovative approach to teaching communication skills to nursing students. *Journal of Nursing Education, 49*(2), 65–71.

Jean Ellen Zavertnik

COMMUNITY-BASED NURSING

DEFINITION

Community-based nursing (CBN) is defined as a setting-specific nursing practice in which the care for illnesses (both acute and chronic) is provided for individuals and families where they live, work, or go to school. The goal of CBN is to provide as many health care services as possible in the community (not in hospital settings) and is based on the philosophy that patients and families maintain health and dignity in their own environment. The practice of CBN is comprehensive, coordinated, and continuous (Stanhope & Lancaster, 2014).

APPLICATION

Community-based (CB) nursing principles are the required content for baccalaureate-prepared professional nurses. Students are prepared to deliver both direct and indirect care to individuals and populations with an emphasis on health promotion and disease prevention. Teaching strategies for community competencies have been identified that focus on integration of didactic and clinical education, thus providing opportunities for learning (Callen et al., 2013). Students learn CB nursing skills through direct and indirect practice with individuals in the community. For example, students collect health history, assess environmental and genetic factors, determine health and illness beliefs, and use evidence-based information to guide health teaching. Students learning CBN also evaluate individuals in relation to literacy,

C

self-care abilities, and resources to maintain health and prevent crisis of chronic diseases. Health promotion, education, and management, as well as coordination and continuity of care, are parts of a holistic approach with individuals in a community setting. CB settings include homes, schools, workplaces, faith-based clinics, prisons, and retail locations. Thus, CB nurses apply autonomous practice skills in assessment, communication, collaboration, analysis, planning, and evaluation.

There are several models used to teach CBN. Some nursing programs form community partnerships (Visiting Nurses Association, hospice programs) in which students practice CB skills with homebound individuals. Community may also be defined by geographic (city or county) or demographic factors (age, ethnicity, or common issue). Thus, students may develop CB skills with individuals at senior centers, a faith-based clinic, school health centers, or within a breast cancer survivors' community group.

There are also several faculty practice models used for teaching CBN. An increasing number of nursing programs are establishing CB nurse centers or clinics. A community nursing center can be staffed by faculty who provide a geographic community with varied services and activities related to health improvement. Another CBN model is a primary care center, where nursing faculty and students provide primary care in a clinic setting. Services may range from screening and education to primary health care. A third model is a CBN service in which services are provided in the home and community with faculty as mentors (Yeh et al., 2009). CBN practice models often engage diverse groups of people with common social and/or geographic ties in which they practice collaborative skills to achieve active involvement of all stakeholders.

SYNOPSIS

CBN is a synthesis of nursing practice with individuals, public health principles, and transcultural nursing applied to promoting and preserving the health of individuals. A common theoretical framework for CBN is the transcultural nursing model by Leininger and McFarland (2002). They describe the importance of understanding cultural universalities and diversities when providing culturally competent CBN care. When CB nurses understand an individual's cultural factors, they can then negotiate and try to accommodate cultural beliefs and needs into holistic care (Leininger & McFarland, 2002). Negotiation and accommodation skills require that CB nurses establish mutual relationships with individuals and other health care professionals that respect the needs of everyone involved. This approach often differs from traditional acute care relationships.

Teaching strategies for CBN practice have been identified (Callen et al., 2013) and focus on comprehensive approaches that include individuals across the life span and care that is continuing, not episodic. Content on health promotion, health maintenance, and health education and management, as well as coordination and continuity of care, are taught in a holistic approach to the management of the health care of individuals in a community.

CBN focuses on individuals and is different from public health nursing (PHN), where the focus is on populations with emphasis on preventing illness and improving quality of life (Stanhope & Lancaster, 2014). CBN differs from acute/hospital-based nursing where the focus is on stabilizing illness and reducing length of stay, whereas CBN focuses on holistic care for chronic illnesses, identifying social determinants of health, preventing exacerbations, and reducing complications that require use of acute/hospital-based care for individuals and families in the community (Stanhope & Lancaster, 2014). Common CBN roles include home health, occupational health, environmental health, forensic/prison nursing, school nursing, and faith-based nursing. Nursing faculty teaching CBN need to be prepared to address competencies in these specific CB specialties, and explain the clinical application of concepts of public health concepts such as epidemiology (Levin, Swider, Breakwell, Cowell, & Reising, 2013). Other programs have utilized the technology of high-fidelity simulated clinical experiences to meet CBN competencies by observing students completing simulated home health visits (Gotwals & Yeager, 2014; Smith & Barry, 2013). One study suggests that some nursing programs still face barriers in establishing CB partnerships that serve the community and needs of students learning CBN (Shannon, 2014).

RECOMMENDATIONS

Nursing education for CBN has moved to teaching in a competency-based curriculum, thus requiring direct and indirect practice experiences that validate student achievement of CBN competencies. Approaches developed by some nursing faculty to increase CBN content include expanding the use of case studies and seminars (Levin et al., 2013). Clinical community preceptors and clinical activities supplement classroom activities to guide students toward meeting specific CB specialty competencies. Nursing programs are also including CBN elective courses offered within the university or from other universities via cooperative arrangements (Levin et al., 2013). However, some nursing programs still report barriers to establishing CBN partnership for education, and these barriers potentially limit student experience with real-world CBN (Shannon, 2014).

Callen, B., Smith, C. M., Joyce, B., Lutz, J., Brown-Schott, N., & Block, D. (2013). Teaching/learning strategies for the essentials of baccalaureate nursing education for entry-level community/public health nursing. *Public Health Nursing, 30*(6), 537–547.

Gotwals, B., & Yeager, S. T. (2014). Improving the process of community-based student nurse practice through a high-fidelity simulated clinical experience. *Nurse Educator, 39*(1), 26–30.

Leininger, M., & McFarland, M. R. (2002). *Transcultural nursing: Concepts, theories, research & practice* (3rd ed.). New York, NY: McGraw-Hill Companies, Inc.

Levin, P. F., Swider, S. M., Breakwell, S., Cowell, J. M., & Reising, V. (2013). Embracing a competency-based specialty curriculum for community-based nursing roles. *Public Health Nursing, 30*(6), 557–565.

Shannon, C. (2014). Community-based health and schools of nursing: Supporting health promotion and research. *Public Health Nursing, 31*(1), 69–78.

Smith, S. J., & Barry, D. G. (2013). An innovative approach to preparing nursing students for care of the elderly in the home. *Geriatric Nursing, 34*(1), 30–34.

Stanhope, M., & Lancaster, J. (2014). *Foundations of nursing in the community: Community-oriented practice* (4th ed.). St. Louis, MO: Elsevier.

Yeh, M. L., Rong, J. R., Chen, M. L., Chang, S. F., & Chung, U. L. (2009). Development of a new prototype for an educational partnership in nursing. *Journal of Nursing Education, 48*(1), 5–10.

Barbara E. Harrison

COMPUTER-BASED TESTING

DEFINITION

Computer-based testing (CBT) is defined as any assessment or examination that utilizes a computer to measure one's knowledge level, competency, or other abilities related to a specific field. CBT was initially introduced in 1985 as college placement tests, aiming to evaluate the domains of reading comprehension, writing, arithmetic, and elementary algebra (Luecht & Sireci, 2011). CBT has since evolved with numerous models administered via a variety of delivery formats to serve various purposes.

APPLICATION

The National Council of State Boards of Nursing (NCSBN) transitioned the National Council Licensure Examination (NCLEX) from the traditional method of paper–pencil testing to CBT in 1994 (NCSBN: NCLEX Examinations, 2014). Since then, advance practice nursing organizations have similarly adopted CBT for certification examinations.

Many nursing schools have begun to implement CBT throughout their programs to better prepare students for licensure or certification examinations. CBT practice during graduate nurse programs of study has demonstrated that students with a lower grade point average (GPA; less than or equal to 3.50) improved on national certification examination scores (Dosch, 2012). In addition, in an attempt to improve or maintain NCLEX pass rates, a number of nursing schools implemented CBT in progression policies. CBT, designed to mimic the NCLEX, provides students the opportunity to practice and demonstrate knowledge prior to taking the licensure examinations.

SYNOPSIS

CBT has appeal for both educators and students. Academic institutions realize the economic benefits of CBT due to decreased use of resources (paper, print ink, etc.) in addition to reduced faculty time spent in grading examinations (Dosch, 2012). Faculty members enjoy test-scoring accuracy and the ability to review and compare group scores through the rapid generation of test and item analysis reports (Zwirn & Muehlenkord, 2009). As a result, students appreciate a faster turnaround in receiving test scores. In relation to standardized exit examinations, faculty members and students are provided with a detailed summary regarding specific areas of weakness. This provides a unique opportunity to develop an appropriate and individualized remediation strategy. When faculty members identify trends in weak areas, they can make curriculum changes (Oermann & Gaberson, 2014).

The use of CBT has expanded dramatically since 1985 from its initial use in college placement examinations. CBT is most often associated with college entrance examinations such as the Scholastic Aptitude Test (SAT), Graduate Record Examination (GRE), or licensure and certifications. They have added value in academia to assess students' learning styles, allowing educators to tailor lesson plans to meet student needs (Zwirn & Muehlenkord, 2009). CBT is the current mode of delivery for the majority of health care licensure and certification examinations, in addition to its use in other areas. Computerized psychometric tests have been used in both employment and military entrance screenings (Luecht & Sireci, 2011)

NCLEX was the first health care licensure examination to utilize computerized adaptive testing (NCSBN, 2014). CAT models generate test items in real time based on the tester's score of the previous item (Luecht & Sireci, 2011). Based on the correct (or incorrect) answer to the previous question, testing software automatically selects the next from an item bank of which the tester has a 50% chance of answering correctly. Because administered test items are adapted to the examinee's ability, this type of test is thought to provide a more reliable measure of the test taker's true competency level (NCSBN, 2014).

RECOMMENDATIONS

Continued advances in computer technology will result in continuous change and improvements in existing test-taking software and capabilities. Further research is warranted to support what types of CBT will be most beneficial to nursing students at the associate, baccalaureate, and graduate levels. Administration of CBT and utilization of progression policies should be a practice that is evidence based.

Gaps in nursing research also exist regarding implementation of CBT by nurses as a means of assessing patients' needs. For instance, physical therapists have studied the use of CBT in measuring activities of daily living (ADL) function (Hsueh, Chen, Wang, Hou, & Hsieh, 2013). This type of testing may prove valuable to nurses, not only in assessment of patients' physical needs, but as a psychometric assessment to measure efficacy of patient education interventions.

Dosch, M. P. (2012). Practice in computer-based testing improves scores on the National Certification Examination for Nurse Anesthetists. *AANA Journal, 80*(4), S60–S66.

Hsueh, I., Chen, J., Wang, C., Hou, W., & Hsieh, C. (2013). Development of a computerized adaptive test for assessing activities of daily living in outpatient with stroke. *Physical Therapy, 93*(5), 681–693.

Luecht, R. M., & Sireci, S. G. (2011). *A review of models for computer-based testing. Research Report 2011–2012.* The College Board. Retrieved from https://research.collegeboard.org/sites/default/files/publications/2012/7/researchreport-2011–12-review-models-for-computer-based-testing.pdf

NCSBN: NCLEX Examinations. (2014). *Computer Adaptive Testing (CAT).* National Council of State Boards of Nursing. Retrieved from https://www.ncsbn.org/1216.htm

Oermann, M. H., & Gaberson, K. B. (2014.) Interpreting test scores. In M. Zuccarini (Ed.), *Evaluation and testing in nursing education* (4th ed., pp. 163–164). New York, NY: Springer Publishing Company.

Zwirn, E. E., & Muehlenkord, A. (2009). Using media, multimedia, and technology-rich learning environments. In D. M. Billings & J. A. Halstead (Eds.), *Teaching in nursing: A guide for faculty* (3rd ed., pp. 339–340). St. Louis, MO: Elsevier Saunders.

Carli A. Carnish
Mary T. Quinn Griffin

CONCEPT-BASED CURRICULUM

C

DEFINITION

A concept-based curriculum is a program of study in which there is an integration of conceptual content within a situational context to promote critical thinking, improve clinical decision making, and link theory and practice (Lasater & Nielsen, 2009; Vacek, 2009). A concept-based learning curriculum meets the five components of development of critical thinking skills described by Facione (1990) that include "analysis, interpretation, inference, explanation and self-regulation."

Concept-based learning is a teaching strategy that has origins in the educational philosophy of constructivism grounded in experiential learning. Dewey (1916) first described experiential learning as learning from experience rather than from didactic methods commonly used in traditional education. *Merriam-Webster Online Dictionary* (2014) defines concept as "an idea of what something is or how it works." The exponential growth in knowledge makes it impossible to focus teaching based on content only but rather teaching learners how to think conceptually. Concepts are the building blocks of learning. These building blocks are organized and processed in a coherent structure to make the material more meaningful and support deeper understanding to the learner (Bristol, 2014; Crookes, K., Crookes, P. A., & Walsh, 2013; Nielsen, 2009; Vacek, 2009).

APPLICATION

Patients receiving care in multiple settings are older and present with higher levels of acuity. Consequently, the learning process in educating professional nurses requires a paradigm shift. Nursing education is becoming more complex as a result of a rapidly changing health care delivery system, accessibility of information through Internet technology, and exponential growth of the body of knowledge. Furthermore, due to the advances in nursing through evidence-based practice and data-driven outcomes, nursing educators are faced with challenges to deliver an active learning environment. There is a need for teaching strategies that require rethinking pedagogical techniques and adopting innovative technologies in the nursing education infrastructure. Simultaneously, there is an escalating need to address and bridge the theory-to-practice gap in nursing (Bristol, 2014; Crookes et al., 2013; Engelmann, 2010).

Case studies, simulation, and nursing grand rounds are some methods to integrate concept-based learning in a nursing education setting. For example, a case study is presented about a patient admitted to the hospital with multiple comorbid conditions. K. W. is a 46-year-old obese female who has a history of type 2 diabetes mellitus. Her condition was complicated by coronary artery disease, for which she had a coronary artery bypass graft. Postoperatively, she developed acute renal failure and Stage III pressure ulcer. Her hospital stay was complex, requiring a full integration of knowledge and skills of nursing care. After discharge at home, due to her noncompliance with medications, she also developed congestive heart failure. K. W. was readmitted within 30 days. Application of a distinct knowledge base alone would not prepare the nurse for this patient's plan of care. The interplay of multiple concepts serves as a superior teaching methodology as compared to an isolated didactic knowledge or practice of skills.

The learners will follow this patient during the course of hospitalization and discharge to home, followed by subsequent admissions and discharge to a subacute setting. Learners apply the nursing process through identifying pertinent assessment findings, making a nursing diagnosis, planning and implementing interventions, and evaluating outcomes. The integration of basic concepts, such as oxygenation, nutrition, fluid and electrolyte balance, ambulation, mobility, pain management, and risk reduction of falls and pressure ulcers, is primary. The reinforcement of the general care of a patient allows the learner to apply the concepts in a specific situational context. The learners will also be able to identify concepts that could manifest in other patient populations (Nielsen, 2009). As an example, how would the care of the aforementioned patient differ if this patient would present as an 85-year-old? The concept of geriatric care must also be integrated as an adjustment in the nursing care plan (Nielsen, 2009). Lastly, the introduction of the challenges of the health care delivery system mandates reportable events such as Stage III pressure ulcer, and readmission in 30 days can be introduced. Reflection on these entire variables of care becomes an integral component of concept-based curriculum (Engelmann, 2010; Lasater & Nielsen, 2009; Nielsen, 2009).

SYNOPSIS

The call for innovation in nursing education and the enhancement of professional nurse performance to the highest level of training have recently been addressed in the Carnegie Report and Institute of Medicine Report on the future of nursing (2010). The literature is replete with articles on concept-based learning in the academic setting. However, the application of this approach to the education of professional nurses is critical to continued professional development.

Concept-based learning outcomes identified in the literature include improved critical thinking; problem-solving skills; integration and synthesis of knowledge (Heims & Boyd, 1990; Lasater & Nielsen, 2009; Nielsen, 2009); self-direction; information retrieval; and motivation (Nielsen, 2009). Identification of learning needs (Heims & Boyd, 1990); team work; learning from peers and group process (Nielsen, 2009); creative discussion (Nielsen, 2009); connecting theory into practice (Lasater & Nielsen, 2009; Nielsen, 2009); and progression into the novice to expert continuum (Benner, 1984; Benner, Sutphen, Leonard, & Day, 2010; Nielsen, 2009) are also demonstrated with this style of teaching/learning.

RECOMMENDATIONS

Despite the limited literature available to apply concept-based learning, this has several benefits and implications for nursing education. Adjusting the way students learn translates into enhanced performance in clinical practice within the complex environment of health care in the 21st century. A balanced approach between active and passive learning to introduce new information and reinforce best practices is critical to safe, effective, and efficient health care delivery. More research is needed to evaluate concept-based curriculum using a measure of learning outcomes, such as the Lasater Clinical Judgment Rubric (Adamson, Gubrud, Sideras, & Lasater, 2012). Finally, shared outcomes, as a measure of success, will promote faculty to be creative in developing innovative teaching strategies to provide a learning environment that promotes critical thinking and clinical decision making in a nonthreatening environment (Engelmann, 2010). A concept-based learning curriculum provides a venue to build knowledge, skills, and competence through analysis and synthesis rather than recall of isolated facts. Furthermore, a concept-based curriculum builds educational experiences that strive to prepare the nursing workforce to deliver high-quality care for patients and families.

Adamson, K. A., Gubrud, P., Sideras, S., & Lasater, K. (2012). Assessing the reliability, validity, and use of the Lasater Clinical Judgment Rubric: Three approaches. *Journal of Nursing Education, 51*(2), 66–73.

Benner, P. E. (1984). *From novice to expert: Excellence and power in clinical nursing practice*. Menlo Park, CA: Addison-Wesley Pub. Co., Nursing Division.

Benner, P., Sutphen, M., Leonard, V., & Day, L. (2010). *Educating nurses: A call for radical transformation*. San Francisco, CA: Jossey-Bass.

Bristol, T. (2014). Flipping the classroom. *Teaching and Learning in Nursing, 9,* 43–46.

Crookes, K., Crookes, P. A., & Walsh, K. (2013). Meaningful and engaging teaching techniques for student nurses: A literature review. *Nurse Education in Practice, 13*(4), 239–243.

Dewey, J. (1916). *Democracy and education: An introduction to the philosophy of education.* New York: The Free Press.

Engelmann, L. (2010). Clinical learning: Do faculty teach how to learn? *Teaching and Learning in Nursing, 5,* 93–94.

Facione, P. A. (1990). Critical thinking: A statement of expert consensus for purposes of educational assessment and instruction. Retrieved from http://files.eric.ed.gov/fulltext/ED315423.pdf

Heims, M. L., & Boyd, S. T. (1990). Concept-based learning activities in clinical nursing education. *Journal of Nursing Education, 29*(6), 249–254.

Institute of Medicine. (2010). *The future of nursing: Leading change, advancing health.* Retrieved from http://www.iom.edu/~/media/Files/Report%20Files/2010/The-Future-of-Nursing/Future%20of%20Nursing%202010%20Recommendations.pdf

Lasater, K., & Nielsen, A. (2009). The influence of concept-based learning activities on students' clinical judgment development. *Journal of Nursing Education, 48*(8), 441–446.

Merriam-Webster Online Dictionary. (2014). Retrieved from http://www.merriam-webster.com/dictionary/concept

Nielsen, A. (2009). Concept-based learning activities using the clinical judgment model as a foundation for clinical learning. *Journal of Nursing Education, 48*(6), 350–354.

Vacek, J. (2009). Using a conceptual approach with concept mapping to promote critical thinking. *Educational Innovations 48*(1), 45–48.

Maria L. Vezina
Medel Salvador-Paguirigan

C

C

CONCEPT MAPS

DEFINITION

Concept maps are graphic tools in the form of drawings or diagrams that can be used to visually describe relationships between and among concepts as well as show the mental connections students make between new concepts and prior knowledge (Angelo & Cross, 1993; Oerman & Gaberson, 2014). Concept mapping requires critical thinking, knowledge, and an understanding of the interrelationships between concepts. Furthermore, concept mapping reflects the inherent cognitive hierarchical processes between new learning and prior knowledge (Hicks-Moore, 2005). Similar to a map of a city, a concept map illustrates connections between various points of interest and highlights areas of importance (Hicks-Moore, 2005).

APPLICATION

In nursing, concept mapping is used in the clinical setting, although it can be used both in the clinical and classroom settings (Billings & Halstead, 2012). In the clinical setting, concept mapping can be used as an illustration of the key concepts and relationships involved in a patient's care. In addition to drawing the concept map, students should include a written description of the depicted relationships (Oerman & Gaberson, 2014). The use of concept maps can also help students plan clinical experience by developing a map in preclinical conference and adjusting the map throughout the day based on assessment while providing patient care (Oerman & Gaberson, 2014). In fact, concept mapping can be used as an alternative to traditional nursing care plans as a way for students to demonstrate knowledge, critical thinking skills, and understanding of material (Billings & Halstead, 2012). Some students who struggle with traditional, columnar-style care plans may find it more meaningful to define relationships between data by using a concept map (Hicks-Moore, 2005).

Concept mapping may allow for a better understanding and memorization of complex phenomena, thus promoting active involvement of the student in the learning process (Billings & Halstead, 2012). It is particularly useful for courses with a high level of theoretical content because it can provide insights into the relationship between theories and concepts (Angelo & Cross, 1993). This method of learning assists faculty in clarifying students' misconceptions about relationships and concepts (Billings & Halstead, 2012). Concept mapping can be a useful teaching/learning strategy for most types of learning styles; however, it may not appeal to concrete or auditory learners. This approach is time intensive for both students and faculty (Billings & Halstead, 2012). Concept mapping may be enhanced through software available on the Internet. Although it may take time to become familiar with the software and technique, it can be a useful tool.

A concept map is best used for formative evaluation. Furthermore, it can evaluate in a written paper in which a concept is illustrated with a map (Oerman & Gaberson, 2014). A grading rubric for a concept map is helpful for students, particularly if they are new to this method of learning. The concept map can be graded based on comprehensiveness of the data, correct linkages and justifications, and a developed plan that is specific, relevant, and accurate (Oerman & Gaberson, 2014). Evaluation criteria can also include number of items included, clarity of overarching organizational structure, and categorization of concepts (Billings & Halstead, 2012).

SYNOPSIS

The utilization of concept maps in the clinical setting, in lieu of traditional care plans, is a helpful tool to facilitate data gathering, critical thinking, and carrying out a plan of care (Hicks-Moore, 2005). The concept map is also helpful for teaching new theories and concepts to students, and can be used to promote understanding by visually linking the new knowledge with what was previously known (Bastable, 2008).

RECOMMENDATIONS

Concept maps are currently being used in the clinical setting and for courses with high theoretical content. They should be considered for use in other settings where the goal is to understand the relationships between concepts. Application of concept maps can apply to all nursing courses. The map can illustrate classes of medications, adverse pharmacological effects, diagnostic categories, symptoms, and nursing implications. Concept mapping should be taught early and reinforced throughout the curriculum. Faculty need to conduct research related to the relationship between concept mapping and student learning, as well as between concept mapping and active learning.

Angelo, T. A., & Cross, K. P. (1993). *Classroom assessment techniques: A handbook for college teachers.* San Francisco, CA: Jossey-Bass.

Bastable, S. B. (2008). *Nurse as educator: Principles of teaching and learning for nursing practice* (3rd ed.). Sudbury, MA: Jones and Bartlett Publishers.

Billings, D. M., & Halstead, J. A. (2012). *Teaching in nursing: A guide for faculty.* St. Louis, MO: Saunders.

Hicks-Moore, S. L. (2005). Clinical concept maps in nursing education: An effective way to link theory and practice. *Nurse Education in Practice, 5*(6), 348–352.

Oerman, M. H., & Gaberson, K. B. (2014). *Evaluation and testing in nursing education* (4th ed.). New York, NY: Springer Publishing Company, LLC.

Sarah E. Givens
Mary T. Quinn Griffin

CONTINUING EDUCATION

DEFINITION

Continuing education is an instructional program for adults, consisting of nursing courses in a particular area of knowledge and expertise to increase the learner's knowledge and skills in order to provide competent patient care. The purpose of continuing education in nursing is to enhance knowledge, skills, and confidence of professional nurses to provide high-quality, competent, and safe patient care (Tame, 2013). The complexities of health care necessitate the professional nurse to continually obtain education.

APPLICATION

Continuing education can be provided by academic and health care institutions for the professional registered nurse (RN) to achieve the necessary education to fulfill current or prospective positions in nursing. Hospitals may require completion of a certain number of continuing education credits within a particular time frame.

Continuing education may be a requirement for state licensure and/or specialty certification. These requirements may be yearly or over the duration of the licensing and certification periods. Regional, state, and national nursing organizations may offer continuing education courses to members and nonmembers as a means to fulfill the specified requirements. The individual is given a choice of topics and scheduling options. Specialty organizations may also offer courses in specific areas to provide the individual with expertise, knowledge, and skill in the specialty domain that may not be found from other sources.

Continuing education programs and courses can be offered using various methods and media. Nurses can attend live sessions offered at conferences, workshops, and

C

short-term courses offered through colleges/ universities, professional organizations, continuing education companies, and health care organizations. Some benefits of live in-person sessions are asking real-time questions, obtaining immediate feedback, and networking. Another benefit with live in-person sessions is that a recording can be made of the session for review at another time. Some barriers to this method of instruction include lack of technology, time requirements, travel, and cost.

Some nurses may choose to utilize written methods of continuing education. This is accomplished through journal and magazine articles as well as information sent via postal mail by an organization or company. Completing the offering in a timely manner convenient to the learner is a benefit of written methods. Journal clubs have been used by health care institutions to encourage reading and synthesis of material. This form of continuing education has been reported by Nesbitt as beneficial in establishing community, incentive, confidence, and making an impact on practice. The written form of continuing education allows colleagues to network outside of the work environment and promote reflection on practice.

eLearning is one of the fastest growing methods of providing continuing nursing education. The possibilities are endless and allow for flexibility and cost-effective ways to provide the educational materials. Participants can choose from a wide variety of educational offerings including, but not limited to, live and recorded webinars, video and audio conferencing, round-table discussions, articles posted on websites, and virtual classrooms. eLearning can be combined with live in-person sessions for those who are unable to attend the live session.

Continuing education, regardless of the method of delivery, further develops the knowledge and confidence of nurses. It also facilitates collaboration with colleagues and a healthy questioning of practice by nurses, physicians, and other health care professionals (Tame, 2013). Because of the multitude of delivery methods for continuing education, nurses are able to obtain the education necessary to be current in practice.

SYNOPSIS

Technological advancements, increasing number of pharmaceuticals, and increased patient complexity have presented nursing and other healthcare professionals with professional challenges (Kowitlawakul, 2013). These challenges have led to the increased need for continuing education to increase knowledge and engage in professional development. The need for competent and safe care has also led to the requirements and mandates for continuing education for licensure, certification, and credentialing at institutions.

The state nurse practice act guides the professional nurse to provide safe, competent care by fulfilling the requirements of the state board of nursing. It also encourages familiarity with the guidelines and requirements necessary for professional practice. Such motivators are one of the impetuses to obtain continued education in nursing (Pawlyn, 2012; Russell, 2013).

Motivators to complete continuing education can be intrinsic or extrinsic. Regulatory requirements are key motivators. Schweitzer and Krassa (2010) reported extrinsic factors as weak motivators for completion of continuing education. The personal and professional benefits of continuing education were identified as key factors for success. Motivators related to success were remaining current with knowledge and skills, providing immediate practice benefits, advancing in a new position, interacting with colleagues, and applying research and evidence to practice (Nalle, Wyatt, & Myers, 2010; Schweitzer & Krassa, 2010). Nalle et al. (2010) reported personal and professional interests as being the primary reason for participation in continuing education. A combination of intrinsic and extrinsic motivators is considered to be most ideal for providing continuing education.

As there are motivators for attending courses there are also barriers. Time constraints and conflicts, family obligations, finances, fatigue, difficulty getting off work, and the intensity of the course are some of the main barriers (Baxter et al., 2013; Nalle et al., 2010; Schweitzer & Krassa, 2010). Ways to help nurses overcome barriers are imperative to successful course attendance. Flexibility through combination of offerings helps to accomplish overcoming barriers. Courses that are readily accessible, affordable, and take into consideration time constraints of individuals promote successful course completion (Baxter et al., 2013).

Continuing education leads to increased job satisfaction and decreased levels of burnout while updating professional skills (Schweitzer & Krassa, 2010). In addition, continuing education leads to increased empowerment and decreased intent to leave a current position. Higher levels of perceived empowerment among critical care and emergency nurses as well as fewer reports of intent to leave a current position among these certified nurses were reported. Continuing education is a major component of the requirements for initial and continued certification and may be a reason for these findings (Fitzpatrick, Campo, & Gacki-Smith, 2013; Fitzpatrick, Campo, Graham, & Lavendaro, 2010).

RECOMMENDATIONS

Fulfillment of mandatory requirements and patient needs, as well as meeting the personal and professional demands of practice while supporting the learner, is the goal of continuing education. Innovative methods to deliver high-quality continuing education courses need to be a priority of educators, clinicians, and professional organizations to maintain the ever-changing and expanding standards of patient care. Financial considerations can significantly impact the delivery of such programs and requires careful consideration.

Interprofessional continuing educational offerings with shared resources can help to minimize financial burdens of providing courses. Sharing of simulation labs, integration of eLearning methodologies, and multisite offerings can also help reduce the cost of educational programs.

Baxter, P., DiCenso, A., Donald, F., Martin-Misener, R., Opsteen, J., & Chambers, T. (2013). Continuing education for primary health care nurse practitioners in Ontario, Canada. *Nurse Education Today, 33*(4), 353–357. doi:10.1016/j.nedt.2012.07.018

Fitzpatrick, J. J., Campo, T. M., & Gacki-Smith, J. (2013). Emergency care nurses: Certification, empowerment, and work-related variables. Retrieved from http://www.jenonline.org/article/S0099–1767(13)00023–8/abstract.

Kowitlawakul, Y. (2013). From novice to expert: Sharing professional development experience in different practice settings. *Singapore Nursing Journal, 40*(3), 42–46.

Nalle, M. A., Wyatt, T. H., & Myers, C. R. (2010). Continuing education needs of nurses in a voluntary continuing nursing education state. *Journal of Continuing Education in Nursing, 41*(3), 107–115; quiz 116.

Pawlyn, J. (2012). The use of e-Learning in continuing professional development. *Learning Disability Practice, 15*(1), 33–37.

Russell, K. A. (2013). Nurse Practice Acts guide and govern nursing practice. *Missouri State Board of Nursing Continuing Education, 3*(3), 8–10.

Schweitzer, D. J., & Krassa, T. J. (2010). Deterrents to nurses' participation in continuing professional development: An integrative literature review. *Journal of Continuing Education in Nursing, 41*(10), 441–447; quiz 448. doi:10.3928/00220124–20100601-05

Tame, S. L. (2013). The effect of continuing professional education on perioperative nurses' relationships with medical staff: Findings from a qualitative study. *Journal of Advanced Nursing, 69*(4), 817–827. doi: 10.1111/j.1365–2648.2012.06065.x

Theresa M. Campo

C

CONVERSATION MAPPING

DEFINITION

The Conversation Map® is a tabletop display of visuals that helps participants contextualize the information they gain (Healthy Interactions, n.d.). The maps contain bright and colorful graphics and are easy to read. Conversation Maps promote learning with interaction and participation. They were developed by Merck & Company, Healthy Interactions, the American Diabetes Association, and the Canadian Diabetes Association. They are available in 35 languages and in 110 countries (Healthy Interactions, n.d.).

APPLICATION

Conversation Maps are used by trained facilitators. They were created for participants with specific diseases, most frequently diabetes mellitus. Using the maps in secondary education settings for students is novel and innovative. Several studies suggest that college-age students are team oriented, socially oriented, work well in groups, and thrive on collaborative activities (Croasdale, 2008; Matulich, Papp, & Haytko, 2008; McGlynn, 2007). Recommendations are that the learning environment should be collaborative, active, and intellectually challenging (Matulich et al., 2008). A review of the literature by Conklin (2013) recommended that faculty create learning environments by including listening, giving opportunities to talk, giving praise as feedback, being responsive to questions and comments, and acknowledging perspectives and experiences. The experiential, interactive Conversation Map teaching method emphasizes all of these recommendations. A description of using a Conversation Map with undergraduate nursing students for persons with diabetes is described by Strang, Bagnardi, and Utz (2010).

SYNOPSIS

There are three key points for the use of Conversation Maps as a teaching pedagogy. Studies have been focused on outcomes with adult patients with diabetes (Monk, 2010; Reaney, Eichorst, & Gorman, 2012; Sperl-Hillen et al., 2013). These studies have shown short-term results and participant satisfaction. Studies on the long-term effects are limited. The interactive, participative, and experiential nature of this teaching pedagogy supports the learning needs of students. Engaging students in the course material through Conversation Maps has benefits beyond the traditional classroom format.

RECOMMENDATIONS

Health care providers and health care educators are tasked with providing learning environments that meet the needs of learners. Generational factors, learning styles, and individual characteristics need to be considered. Conversation Maps are relatively new in both health care and the secondary education settings, and study results are beginning to appear in the literature. Using this tool in health-related classes serves a twofold purpose: It is well suited for active participation and exposes health care learners to a new learning tool. Conversation Maps have an exciting future; however, more use and research are needed.

Conklin, T. A. (2013). Making it personal: The importance of student experience in creating autonomy-supportive classrooms for millennial learners. *Journal of Management Education, 37*(4), 499–538.

Croasdale, M. (2008). *Med schools adjusting to millennial students.* American Medical News. Retrieved from http://www.ama-assn.org/amednews/2008/01/14/prsd0114.htm

Healthy Interactions. (n.d.). *The U.S. Diabetes Conversation Map® Program.* Retrieved from http://www.healthyinteractions.com/conversation-map-programs/

conversation-map-experience/current-programs/usdiabetes

Matulich, E., Papp R., & Haytko, D. L. (2008). Continuous improvement through teaching innovations: A requirement for today's learners. *Marketing Education Review, 18*(1), 1–7.

McGlynn, A. (2007). Millennials in college: How do we motivate them? *The Hispanic Outlook in Higher Education, 17*, 34–36.

Monk, J. (2010). It's good to talk: Using Conversation Maps in diabetes education. *Journal of Diabetes Nursing, 14*(3), 104–108.

Reaney, M., Eichorst, B., & Gorman, P. (2012). From acorns to oak trees: The development and theoretical underpinnings of diabetes Conversation Map education tools. *Diabetes Spectrum, 25*(2), 111–116.

Sperl-Hillen, J., Beaton, S., Fernandes, O., Worley, A., Vasquez-Benitez, G., Hanson, A.,...Spain, C. V. (2013). Are benefits from diabetes self-management education sustained? *American Journal of Managed Care, 19*(2), 104–112.

Strang, S., Bagnardi, M., & Utz, S. (2010). Tailoring a diabetes nursing elective course to millennial students. *Journal of Nursing Education, 49*(12), 684–686.

Sharon L. Strang

CRISIS MANAGEMENT

DEFINITION

Crisis management is a series of steps used to intervene and establish order in situations where events and stressors threaten to disrupt an equilibrium state. The threat to homeostasis could be at the individual, group, or community level, but the steps would still apply. The basic steps according to Elders (2008) are (a) assess the individual and the problem, (b) plan the intervention, (c) implement the intervention, (d) resolve the crisis, and (e) anticipatory planning (Elders, 2008).

APPLICATION

Incidents of crises can plague students as they progress in nursing school. Crisis management for students during this time is an apt approach to decrease stress and allow them to focus on discernible methods to success. To address the identified crisis, the issue or situation must be identified and defined. A team approach including faculty and students is essential; the students describe the problem and the faculty assist with a planned approach to the crisis management. Aspects of the issue need to be discovered and explored. While this may seem like a lengthy process, clues to the severity of the problem will surface, thereby defining and providing information that can guide a planned intervention. When an intervention is identified, a plan for implementation can be developed. Measures within the plan can direct any actions taken when the intervention is initiated. Having outcome objectives derived from and guided by the intervention plan will allow the student/faculty to evaluate progress. As the crisis resolves, the expected outcomes can be evaluated. If no resolution to the crisis is observed, a reassessment of the problem follows and another approach may be attempted. If the crisis is resolved, it is important to do anticipatory planning to prevent the crisis from reappearing (Reinhardt, Keller, Ochart Summers, & Schultz, 2012). There are a number of situations that can precipitate a crisis for nursing students; therefore, anticipatory planning by the faculty in schools of nursing is important.

The use of standardized high stakes testing such as standardized entrance and exit examinations in a nursing program can create crises for all students and especially students identified as at risk. The licensing examination (NCLEX-RN®) is an important consideration in educating nurses and by itself can precipitate a crisis in some. Clinical testing is another example where performance is evaluated under the observation of an instructor and can lead to a perceived crisis in a student. In essence, learning to be a nurse can be like learning a new language

C

and approach to life. The student may question all previous learning.

SYNOPSIS

The literature addresses crisis management in a number of areas. Apart from management in industry such as hotels and other business environments (Elsubbaugh, Fildes, & Rose, 2004; Hamidizadeh, Hosseini, & Anoosheh, 2011; Lalonde, 2007), theories of crisis management in health care are primarily devoted to emergency situations where lives are at risk (Kim, Neilipovitz, Cardinal, Chiu, & Clinch, 2006; Yee et al., 2005). Elder, Ayala, & Harris (1999) suggest that multiple models used in crisis management have theoretical bases in behavior modification. The Behavior Modification Model encourages remediation of coping skills and use of both positive and negative behaviors to modify behavior. The Health Belief Model addresses a reduction of environmental barriers to behavior change. Perceptions of skill use and reinforcement of behavior may direct behavior as suggested by the social learning theory. Self-changing actions emphasize the use of self-management models. Of these, social support theories stress the reinforcement found through social networks. The theory of reasoned action points out perceptions of social processes. The Transtheoretical Model requires action to match intervention in both cognitive and behavioral stages. Management in a crisis can support behavior-change efforts by ensuring that students: (a) have a positive intention; (b) face minimum barriers; (c) perceive themselves as having the requisite skills or self-efficacy; (d) believe that positive behavior will be reinforced; (e) believe that there is a positive pressure to perform and no negativity will follow the behavior change; (f) believe that the behavior is right for their self-image; (g) feel good about the behavior change; and (h) find positive encouragement in the behavior (Elder et al., 1999).

Management of a crisis is closely linked to the precipitating event causing the crisis. Crisis prevention is best approached by anticipatory planning. Forecasting related to previous events can go a long way to prevent the development of a crisis event. Disaster planning is an example of preparedness necessary in any health care setting (Lalonde, 2007; Morrison, 2007). The lessons learned when reviewing such plans can support a nursing student in developing his or her own plan of crisis prevention.

RECOMMENDATIONS

Nurses, both students and faculty, can be at risk of crises. Finding an approach to crisis management can be a shared responsibility and one from which both can gain insight and strength. Although there are a variety of approaches found in the literature, the most straightforward approach lies in first identifying the situation in the crisis, developing a plan of action, implementing that plan, then evaluating the actions taken, followed by developing any anticipated action if the crisis returns (Elders, 2008). The perceptions of crisis for students are ubiquitous to nursing education. The profession requires rigorous standards in both education and practice. Because these demands are inherent in the profession, continued perception of crisis events may surface. As a profession, nurses must be able to identify and develop interventions and coping strategies to deal with these issues as they arise. Research is needed to meet the needs of students undergoing a crisis in their education and to prevent untoward outcomes such as leaving the profession or developing barriers to learning. Programs that can improve student learning in methods that have a broad and current appeal devised to reduce stress, as well as practice questions for NCLEX-RN, have been developed and may prove useful. Research-based evaluation of these approaches will be helpful.

Elder, J. P., Ayala, G. X., & Harris, S. (1999). Theories and intervention approaches to health-behavior change in primary care. *American Journal of Preventive Medicine, 17,* 275–284.

Elders, D. (2008). Theory and intervention. In K. Fortinash & P. Holoday Worret (Ed.), *Psychiatric/mental health nursing* (4th ed.), St. Louis, MO: Mosby-Elsevier.

Elsubbaugh, S., Fildes, R., & Rose, M. B. (2004). Preparation for crisis management: A proposed model and empirical evidence. *Journal of Contingencies and Crisis Management, 12,* 112–127.

Hamidizadeh, M. R., Hosseini, S. M., & Anoosheh, A. (2011). Explanation and evaluation of a four step model for crisis management planning process. *Canadian Social Science, 7,* 103–110.

Kim, J., Neilipovitz, D., Cardinal, P., Chiu, M., & Clinch, J. (2006). A pilot study using high-fidelity simulation to formally evaluate performance in the resuscitation of critically ill patients: The University of Ottawa critical care medicine, high-fidelity simulation, and crisis resource management I study. *Critical Care Medicine, 34,* 2167–2174.

Lalonde, C. (2007). Crisis management and organizational development: Towards the conception of a learning model in crisis management. *Organization Development Journal, 25,* 17–26.

Morrison, J. Q. (2007). Social validity of the critical incident stress management model for school-based crisis intervention. *Psychology in the Schools, 44,* 765–777.

Reinhardt, A. C., Keller, T., Ochart Summers, L., & Schultz, P. (2012). Strategies for success: Crisis management model for remediation of at-risk students. *Journal of Nursing Education, 51,* 305–311.

Yee, B., Naik, V. N., Joo, H. S., Savoldelli, G. L., Chung, D. Y., Houston, P. L. , … Hamstra, S. J. (2005). Nontechnical skills in anesthesia crisis management with repeated exposure to simulation-based education. *Anesthesiology, 103,* 241–248.

Anita C. Reinhardt

CRITICAL THINKING

DEFINITION

Critical thinking is defined as having 11 affective components (such as confidence, inquisitiveness, and intellectual integrity) and 7 cognitive skills (such as analyzing, logical reasoning, and predicting and transforming knowledge). This definition was created from a study of 55 nurse experts to develop a consensus statement on critical thinking in nursing (Scheffer & Rubenfeld, 2000).

APPLICATION

Critical thinking is an important skill for competence and performance at a high level. Nurse educators must have a clear understanding of critical thinking and possess the ability to think critically themselves in order to teach it to others (Robert & Petersen, 2013). The importance of teaching critical thinking and introducing nursing students to the concept should be started early in nursing education and developed through experience and practice (Chan, 2013). Nurse educators and preceptors of students and new graduates need to make clear application of the critical reasoning process in complex patient care environments. They must also be aware that students and new graduate nurses need and desire clear guidance in application of critical thinking to clinical situations (Lasater, 2010).

One recommendation for educators and preceptors in clinical practice is to think out loud when making clinical decisions to help students gain insight into their thought process and decisions (Forneris & Peden-McAlpine, 2009; Lasater, 2010). Other strategies recommended to facilitate critical thinking include reflective writing and journaling, concept maps, and case studies (Walsh & Seldomridge, 2006). Approaches such as narrative understanding, situational learning, and interpretation

C

of clinical situations help students develop clinical imagination, which assists in understanding changes in the patient situation over time (Benner, Sutphin, Leonard, & Day, 2010).

A model to teach critical thinking is the Lasater Clinical Judgment Rubric (LCJR) (Lasater, 2010). It is a model for educators and preceptors to use in helping to develop the clinical judgment of students. The rubric has four aspects: noticing, interpreting, responding, and reflecting. For each aspect, there are multiple levels that assist the educator and preceptor in rating the student's development of critical thinking skills. In addition, the use of high-level questions promotes thinking at deeper levels. An example of a high-level question to stimulate deep thinking and learning is "What did you first notice about the patient?" (Lasater, 2010, p. 89).

Another approach to develop critical thinking is the use of case studies. Case studies can provide a low-risk opportunity for nurse educators to help students and nurses achieve skill development. Case studies help to stimulate the critical thinking process and provide challenges for students to advance in skill acquisition (Lunney, 2009).

SYNOPSIS

Nursing literature on critical thinking supports the view that educational preparation of registered nurses must include development of strong critical thinking skills to provide safe, quality care (Benner et al., 2010; Fater & Ready, 2011; Lasater, 2010; Newton & Moore, 2013). In a comprehensive literature review of critical thinking, Chan (2013) identified four categories that influenced critical thinking in nursing education: students, educator, education system, and environment. For example, students may be hindered to critically think by their cultural background or a language barrier. The educator can influence critical thinking by being supportive and approachable.

Teachers of nursing should value critical thinking and teach it as a subject with active learning opportunities. Lastly, positive learning environments, such as feeling accepted in the clinical arena, can facilitate critical thinking.

Most importantly, nurse educators may not have mastered the teaching of critical thinking; therefore, support for faculty development is a requisite. Faculty development for teaching critical thinking to students should be started early since it promotes a higher level of student performance (Chan, 2013; Fater & Ready, 2011).

RECOMMENDATIONS

The overarching goal of nursing is to provide safe, quality patient care. Critical thinking is recognized as an important nursing skill that can improve nursing practice at all levels of the professional practice environment. Nurse educators in both academia and clinical settings must be competent to teach critical thinking and measure outcomes tied directly to critical thinking. Students learn how to critically think and reason by situational experiences involving patients, such as case studies, as well as patients in clinical settings or simulation (Benner et al., 2010; Robert & Petersen, 2013).

Rather than focusing on conventional strategies of recalling content, future research in nursing education should focus on the process of thinking. This process demonstrates thinking critically about the content and asking questions related to how the content applies to the clinical situation (Forneris & Peden-McAlpine, 2009). More research is needed on how nursing students' critical thinking skills progress from an evolutionary perspective during their learning experiences (Newton & Moore, 2013). Understanding how critical thinking skills are developed and practiced at a level to produce the best patient outcomes is a fertile area for current research.

Benner, P., Sutphin, M., Leonard, V., & Day, L. (2010). *Educating nurses.* San Francisco, CA: Jossey-Bass.

Chan, Z. C. (2013). A systematic review of critical thinking in nursing education. *Nurse Education Today, 33,* 236–240.

Fater, K. H., & Ready, R. (2011). An education-service partnership to achieve safety and quality improvement competencies in nursing. *Journal of Nursing Education, 50*(12), 693–696.

Forneris, S. G., & Peden-McAlpine, C. (2009). Creating context for critical thinking in practice: The role of the preceptor. *Journal of Advanced Nursing, 65*(8), 1715–1724.

Lasater, K. (2010). Clinical judgment: The last frontier for evaluation. *Nurse Education in Practice, 11*(2), 86–92.

Lunney, M. (2009). Use of critical thinking to achieve positive health outcomes. In M. Lunney (Ed.), *Critical thinking to achieve positive health outcomes: Nursing case studies and analyses* (p. 9). Ames, IA: Wiley-Blackwell.

Newton, S. E., & Moore, G. (2013). Critical thinking skills of basic baccalaureate and accelerated second degree nursing students. *Nursing Education Perspectives, 34*(3), 154–158.

Robert, R., & Petersen, S. (2013). Critical thinking at the bedside: Providing safe passage to patients. *Medsurg Nursing: Official Journal of the Academy of Medical-Surgical Nurses, 22*(2), 85–93, 118.

Scheffer, B. K., & Rubenfeld, M. G. (2000). A consensus statement on critical thinking in nursing. *Journal of Nursing Education, 39*(8), 352–359.

Walsh, C. M., & Seldomridge, L. A. (2006). Critical thinking: Back to square two. *Journal of Nursing Education, 45*(6), 212–219.

Marie Cox

CULTURAL AWARENESS

DEFINITION

Cultural awareness is the process of examining one's feelings and thoughts in regard to the effect on interactions with others (Giger et al., 2007). Culture involves elements that are learned including lifeways, norms, symbols, and other aspects of living that are often shared from one generation to the next (Leininger & McFarland, 2002). Gender, age, religious affiliation, nationality, and other factors are described as primary characteristics of culture. Secondary characteristics of culture include education, occupation, and socioeconomic and additional factors (Giger et al., 2007). It is important to develop an awareness of one's own cultural and professional values to prevent engaging in cultural imposition and ethnocentrism. Cultural imposition is imposing on another culture one's beliefs and values (Leininger & McFarland, 2002). Ethnocentrism is the belief that one's own culture or view is superior (Douglas et al., 2011). Awareness of cultural viewpoints and the effect this has on interactions is a major step toward cultural competence.

APPLICATION

As the population of the United States becomes more diverse (United States Census Bureau, 2010), striving for cultural competence is imperative in nursing education and practice. Cultural awareness is a key construct in developing cultural competence (American Association of Colleges of Nursing [AACN], 2008). Critical reflection of one's own values, beliefs, and culture in addition to having awareness of the effect of these on culturally congruent care are part of the Standards of Practice for Culturally Competent Nursing Care (Douglas et al., 2011). The American Academy of Nursing (AAN) Expert Panel Report: Developing Cultural Competence to Eliminate Health Disparities in Ethnic Minorities and Other Vulnerable Populations indicates that eliminating health disparities must begin in educational settings, which includes curricula that integrates content to develop sensitivity and competence in health care (Giger et al., 2007).

Qualitative studies have shown that reflective journaling during international

C

cultural immersion may aid in cultural awareness (Curtain, Martins, Schwartz-Barcott, DiMaria, & Ogando, 2013; Larson, Ott, & Miles, 2010). When the resources are not available for international immersion, the teaching application of virtual communities shows promise in regard to cultural awareness (Giddens, North, Carlson-Sabelli, Rogers, & Fogg, 2012). Simulations, virtual experiences, and communities are emerging as supplements to learning in the classroom and clinical settings (Giddens et al., 2012). International video conference exchange may also aid in promoting cultural awareness (Kemppainen, Kim-Godwin, Mechling, Kanematsu, & Kikuchi, 2012). Cultural competency curricular threads should be integrated throughout the components of the program and courses (Jeffreys, 2010).

SYNOPSIS

Becoming culturally competent requires the ability to be aware of one's own values, beliefs, and perspectives in addition to understanding these aspects in others (Jeffreys, 2010). Formal education, clinical training, and ongoing continuing education are important in preparing nurses to provide and promote culturally congruent care (Douglas et al., 2011). Additional research is needed to provide more information regarding teaching, learning, and assessing cultural awareness for both the novice and experienced nurse.

RECOMMENDATIONS

Nursing faculty and students can develop cultural awareness through assessing and understanding their own cultural background. It is important to maintain a sensitive, open attitude toward others with an awareness of potential biases. Collaborating with organizations to increase the number of nurses from minority groups (Giger et al., 2007) as well as increased diversity of faculty are recommended. The quest for cultural competency begins in nursing education and needs to be modeled by nurse educators and students through living cultural awareness with those they serve as nurse. Additional research regarding cultural awareness is needed to expand evidence-based practice.

American Association of Colleges of Nursing (AACN). (2008). *Tool kit of resources for cultural competent education for baccalaureate nurses*. Retrieved from http://www.aacn.nche.edu/education-resources/toolkit.pdf

Curtain, A., Martins, D., Schwartz-Barcott, D., DiMaria, L., & Ogando, B. (2013). Development and evaluation of an international service learning program for nursing students. *Public Health Nursing, 30*(6), 548–556.

Douglas, M., Pierce, J. U., Rosenkoetter, M., Pacquial, D., Callister, L. C., Hatter-Pollara, M., . . . Purnell, L. (2011). Standards of practice for culturally competent nursing care: 2011 update. *Journal of Transcultural Nursing, 22*(4), 317–333.

Giddens, J., North, S., Carlson-Sabelli, L., Rogers, E., & Fogg, L. (2012). Using a virtual community to enhance cultural awareness. *Journal of Transcultural Nursing, 23*(2), 198–204.

Giger, J., Davidhizar, R. E., Purnell, L., Harden, J. T., Phillips, J., & Strickland, O. (2007). American Academy of Nursing expert panel report: Developing cultural competence to eliminate health disparities in ethnic minorities and other vulnerable populations. *Journal of Transcultural Nursing, 18*(2), 95–102.

Jeffreys, M. R. (2010). *Teaching cultural competence in nursing and health care* (2nd ed.). New York, NY: Springer Publishing.

Kemppainen, J., Kim-Godwin, Y., Mechling, B., Kanematsu, Y., & Kikuchi, K. (2012). Promoting cultural awareness in nursing education through international videoconferences. *International Journal of Nursing Practice, 18*, 56–61. doi:10.1111/j.1440–172X.2012.02029.x

Larson, K., Ott, M., & Miles, J. (2010). International cultural immersion: En vivo reflections in cultural competence. *Journal of Cultural Diversity, 17*(2), 44–50.

Leininger, M., & McFarland, M. (2002). *Transcultural nursing: Theories, concepts and practices* (3rd ed.). New York, NY: McGraw Hill, Inc.

United States Census Bureau. (2010). *Overview of race and Hispanic origin: 2010*. Retrieved from http://www.census.gov/prod/cen2010/briefs/c2010br-02.pdf

Susan Peck Tipperman

CULTURAL COMPETENCY

DEFINITION

Cultural competence is a set of congruent behaviors, attitudes, and policies that enable working effectively in cross-cultural situations (Cross, et al. 1989). Culturally competent care is based on cultural beliefs, heritage, behaviors, and attitudes (Giger et al., 2007). Culture is comprised of the beliefs of groups (American Nurses Association [ANA], 1991).

APPLICATION

As the population of the United States becomes more diverse (U.S. Census Bureau, 2010), striving for cultural competence is imperative in nursing education. This includes cultural assessment that takes into consideration cultural values, beliefs, and health care practices (Douglas et al., 2011). There are several models and methods that can be used in the teaching of cultural competence and for cultural assessment. The American Association of Colleges of Nursing (AACN) *Tool Kit of Resources for Cultural Competent Education for Baccalaureate Nurses* (2008) provides many resources and recommends several models that can be used. The National League of Nursing

Diversity Toolkit for Innovation in Curriculum Design (2009) provides resources for teaching strategies and curriculum. These include recommending cultural learning activities through experience, as well as providing culturally appropriate and evidence-based nursing care (National League of Nursing [NLN], 2009). Diversity is listed as one of NLN's four core values where individuals and institutions embrace the richness of individual differences. Guidelines for diversity in nursing education are provided to achieve this goal (NLN, 2009). It is important to consider that variation within cultures requires that the client be assessed as an individual. In addition, it is important for nurses to understand the need to be aware of their own culture and perspective (ANA, 1991). Transcultural, international, and service-learning experiences that involve immersion in cultures different from one's own are recommended (Douglas et al., 2011). Leininger and McFarland (2002) emphasize that the development of cultural competence requires interaction with diverse families, communities, and health care providers in addition to diverse patients. Qualitative studies have been completed and indicate that reflective journaling during international cultural immersion aids is beneficial (Curtain, Martins, Schwartz-Barcott, DiMaria, & Ogando, 2013; Larson, Ott, & Miles, 2010). When resources are not available, the teaching application of virtual communities has been shown to be effective in increasing cultural awareness (Giddens, North, Carlson-Sabelli, Rogers, & Fogg, 2012). Simulations, virtual experiences, and communities are emerging as enhancements to learning in the classroom and clinical settings (Giddens et al., 2012). International video conferences can promote cultural awareness (Kemppainen, Kim-Godwin, Mechling, Kanematsu, & Kikuchi, 2012).

SYNOPSIS

There are several key points in understanding cultural competence: (a) cultural

C

competence is a critical component in providing culturally congruent care to every patient; (b) culturally competent care requires the ability to be aware of one's own values, beliefs, and perspectives in addition to understanding these aspects in others (Jeffreys, 2010); and (c) the development of cultural competence requires interaction with diverse families, communities, and health care providers in addition to diverse patients (Leininger & McFarland, 2002).

RECOMMENDATIONS

Nursing faculty and students can develop cultural competence through assessing and becoming aware of their own cultural background. It is important to maintain a sensitive, open attitude toward others with an awareness of potential biases. The quest for cultural competency begins in nursing education and needs to be modeled by nurse educators through their own efforts to continue the process of cultural competence. Faculty continuing education programs aid in cultural competence (Douglas et al., 2011). Additional research in the teaching, learning, and assessment of cultural competence is needed to expand evidence-based practice.

American Association of Colleges of Nursing (AACN). (2008). *Tool kit of resources for cultural competent education for baccalaureate nurses.* Retrieved from http://www.aacn.nche.edu/education-resources/toolkit.pdf

American Nurses Association (ANA). (1991). *Cultural diversity in nursing practice.* Retrieved from http://www.nursing-world.org/MainMenuCategories/Policy-Advocacy/Positions-and-Resolutions/ANAPositionStatements/Position-Statements-Alphabetically/prtetcldv14444.html

Cross, T., Bazron, B., Dennis, K., & Isaacs, M., (1989). *Towards A Culturally Competent System of Care, Volume I.* Washington, DC: Georgetown University Child Development Center, CASSP Technical Assistance Center.

Curtain, A., Martins, D., Schwartz-Barcott, D., DiMaria, L., & Ogando, B. (2013). Development and evaluation of an international service learning program for nursing students. *Public Health Nursing, 30*(6), 548–556.

Douglas, M., Pierce, J. U., Rosenkoetter, M., Pacquial, D., Callister, L. C., Hatter-Pollara, M., . . . Purnell, L. (2011). Standards of practice for culturally competent nursing care: 2011 update. *Journal of Transcultural Nursing, 22*(4), 317–333.

Giddens, J., North, S., Carlson-Sabelli, L., Rogers, E., & Fogg, L. (2012). Using a virtual community to enhance cultural awareness. *Journal of Transcultural Nursing, 23*(2), 198–204.

Giger, J., Davidhizar, R. E., Purnell, L., Harden, J. T., Phillips, J., & Strickland, O. (2007). American academy of nursing expert panel report: Developing cultural competence to eliminate health disparities in ethnic minorities and other vulnerable populations. *Journal of Transcultural Nursing, 18*(2), 95–102.

Jeffreys, M. R. (2010). *Teaching cultural competence in nursing and health care* (2nd ed.). New York, NY: Springer Publishing.

Kemppainen, J., Kim-Godwin, Y., Mechling, B., Kanematsu, Y., & Kikuchi, K. (2012). Promoting cultural awareness in nursing education through international videoconferences. *International Journal of Nursing Practice, 18,* 56–61. doi:10.1111/j.1440–172X.2012.02029.x

Larson, K., Ott, M., & Miles, J. (2010). International cultural immersion: En vivo reflections in cultural competence. *Journal of Cultural Diversity, 17*(2), 44–50.

Leininger, M., & McFarland, M. (2002). *Transcultural nursing: Theories, concepts and practices* (3rd ed.). New York, NY: McGraw Hill, Inc.

National League of Nursing (NLN). (2009). *Diversity toolkit.* Retrieved from https://

C

www.nln.org/facultyprograms/
Diversity_Toolkit/diversity_toolkit.pdf
United States Census Bureau. (2010). *Overview
of race and Hispanic origin*. Retrieved from
http://www.census.gov/prod/cen2010/
briefs/c2010br-02.pdf

Susan Peck Tipperman

CULTURAL DIVERSITY

DEFINITION

Definitions of cultural diversity vary and may include differences in race, age, ethnicity, religion, and gender within a situation, group, or institution (Wood, 2003). It may also be the coexistence of different ethnic, gender, racial, and socioeconomic groups within one social unit (Wood, 2003) or the totality of socially transmitted behavioral patterns, arts, beliefs, values, customs, lifeways, and all other products of human work and thought characteristics of a population of people (Purnell & Paulanka, 2003, p. 3).

APPLICATION

Cultural diversity is a complex, multifaceted concept that is essential to the education of nurses. Its complexity is inherent in the multiple ways in which it can be viewed. For example, in the context of representation, the term is used to depict images of particular social groups, which tend to be defined by race, gender, age, or socioeconomic status. When used in the context of ideology, the term does not refer to real people, but rather to a set of beliefs for the purpose of changing people's attitudes. When an event happens and people's thoughts need to be changed, diversity training or sensitivity training can be used to affirm a different set of beliefs or justify the attempt to change a stereotype (Wood, 2003).

Students achieve understanding of cultural diversity by engaging in processes to promote their cultural awareness. The teaching strategies used most often to move students toward cultural competence include virtual patient encounters where students can apply cultural skills and knowledge to diverse patient populations in a safe manner (Rutledge et al., 2008); diversity experiences among students and faculty outside of the classroom that might involve a guest speaker (Ranzijn, McConnochie, Nolan, & Wharton, 2007); or more formal cultural diversity events aimed at examining diversity issues to increase cultural awareness (Sanner, Baldwin, Cannella, Charles, & Parker, 2010). Studying abroad and immersion experiences also promote cultural awareness and sensitivity, and decrease stereotyping (Ruddock & Turner, 2007).

SYNOPSIS

There are three key points in understanding cultural diversity. First, professional nursing organizations value cultural diversity. For example, the American Association of Colleges of Nursing (AACN, 2014) supports more faculty and student diversity in nursing programs: "racial and ethnic diversity of health professions faculty and students helps to ensure that all students will develop the cultural competencies necessary for caring for patients in an increasingly diverse nation." The National League for Nursing (NLN, 2014) supports the creation of "a culture of diversity" within nursing programs that "embraces acceptance, respect and inclusivity that is about understanding ourselves and each other and moving beyond simple tolerance to embracing and celebrating the richness of each individual. While diversity can be about individual differences, it also encompasses institutional and system-wide behavior." Finally, the National Advisory for Nursing Education and Practice stresses the need for increased numbers of minority nurses in education and leadership roles to develop models of care that meet the health care needs of minority populations. The second key point is that despite the nursing profession's valuing of diversity and putting forth strategies to increase the nursing workforce diversity, there has only been a small increase in the numbers of minority nurses while the majority of the nursing workforce remains White (The Sullivan Commission, 2007). Villarruel, Bigelow, and Alvarez (2014) purport that a disconnect exists between what the nursing profession says about the value of diversity and what it has been able to actually accomplish in increasing the nursing workforce diversity. This disconnect is of great concern because U.S. minorities will be the majority by 2042, increasing from 34% in 2008 to 54% in 2042 (U.S. Census Bureau, 2007). Furthermore, the continued increase in immigration and minority populations in the United States indicates that more nontraditional rather than traditional students are seeking nursing degrees, making the need to integrate diversity within nursing programs and the nursing profession a priority (Bednarz, Schim, & Doorenbos, 2010). A third key point is that nurse educators must shoulder the responsibility of moving students toward cultural competence and increasing cultural sensitivity so that they are qualified to provide culturally appropriate patient care.

RECOMMENDATIONS

Preparation of graduates to care for patients in culturally appropriate ways can be achieved by integrating cultural diversity into clinical and capstone experiences. Nurse educators must also be skilled at facilitating students through the steps of becoming culturally competent. There is a need for future research to focus on evaluating the effectiveness of learning activities aimed at promoting students' cultural awareness and competence and linking them to student learning outcomes.

American Association of Colleges of Nursing (AACN). (2014). *Diversity and equality of opportunity.* Retrieved from http://www.aacn.nche.edu/publications/position/diversity-equality

Bednarz, H., Schim, S., & Doorenbos, A. (2010). Cultural diversity in nursing education: Perils, pitfalls and pearls. *Journal of Nursing Education, 49*(5), 253–260.

National League for Nursing (NLN). (2014). *Global/diversity initiatives.* Retrieved from http://www.nln.org/aboutnln/globaldiversity/index.htm

Purnell, L., & Paulanka, B. (2003). *Transcultural health care: A culturally competent approach* (2nd ed.). Philadelphia, PA: F. A. Davis.

Ranzijn, R., McConnochie, K., Nolan, A., & Wharton, M. (2007). Towards cultural competence: Australian indigenous content in undergraduate psychology. *Australian Psychologist, 43*(2), 132–139.

Ruddock, H., & Turner, D. (2007). Developing cultural sensitivity: Nursing students' experience of a study abroad programme. *Journal of Advanced Nursing, 59*(4), 361–369.

Rutledge, C., Barham, P., Wiles, L., Richardean, B., Eaton, S., & Palmer, K. (2008). Integrative simulation: A novel approach to educating culturally competent nurses. *Contemporary Nurse: A Journal for the Australian Nursing Profession, 28*(1/2), 119.

Sanner, S., Baldwin, D., Cannella, K., Charles, J., & Parker, L. (2010). The impact of cultural diversity forum on students' openness to diversity. *Journal of Cultural Diversity, 17*(2), 56–61.

The Sullivan Commission. (2007). *Missing persons: Minorities in the health professions, a report of the Sullivan Commission on diversity in the health care workforce.* Retrieved from www.sullivancommission.org

U.S. Census Bureau. (2007). *Population.* Retrieved from http://www.census.gov/prod/www/abs/popula.html

Villarruel, A., Bigelow, A., & Alvarez, C. (2014). Integrating the 3Ds: A nursing perspective. *Public Health Reports, 129*(Suppl. 2), 37–44.

Wood, P. (2003). *Diversity. The invention of a concept*. San Francisco, CA: Encounter Books.

Susan Sanner

CULTURAL SAFETY

DEFINITION

Cultural safety refers to awareness and action aimed at ensuring patients from different backgrounds feel safe in their clinical encounters. It is a conscious provision of care that takes into account how power relations influence health care. This conscious provision of care aims to protect the identities of patients, particularly those from minorities and disempowered groups.

APPLICATION

Cultural safety is a key component in educating nurses to deliver humane and effective care. In order to provide culturally safe care, nurses and other caregivers need to understand the ways in which power structures influence health, and to reflect on how personal and professional power positions influence their encounters with patients (Ramsden, 2002). Cultural safety education is particularly important in diverse societies with histories or present situations of colonialism, racism, discrimination, and conflict (Arieli, Mashiach-Eizenberg, Friedman, & Hirschfeld, 2012).

Translating the concept of cultural safety into nursing education practice is complex and challenging. The major goals for educators and students include identifying conscious and subconscious perceptions of others and acknowledging how these perceptions influence the provision of care. Education focuses on transforming negative perceptions and attitudes toward others (Ramsden, 2002). Educational strategies include providing knowledge on historical and sociopolitical contexts in terms of what these contexts mean in working relationships where there is a difference (Richardson & Carryer, 2005). Other suggestions include focusing on the ways in which power is embedded in nursing practice and is inherent in the relations between nurses and patients (Jeffs, 2001).

Cultural safety education might be experienced as unsafe by both students and teachers, from both majority and minority groups, because it involves dealing with power relations and tensions, which are often threatening and raise powerful emotions of blame and guilt (Arieli, Friedman, & Hirschfeld, 2012). In order to teach cultural safety, educators have the responsibility to construct a learning environment where all students feel safe to reflect on and give expression to their cultural identities (Jeffs, 2001). Engaging in reflexivity, both as teachers and as learners, is key to cultural safety education.

SYNOPSIS

The concept of cultural safety was introduced by Ramsden, a Mauri nurse from New Zealand, in the late 1980s (Papps & Ramsden, 1996; Ramsden, 2002). In 1991, the New Zealand Nursing Council ruled that the state examination would include 20% on cultural safety. The concept of cultural safety was further developed by Ramsden and other scholars who suggested a broader meaning where culture referred not only to ethnic differences but also to differences such as gender, age group, sexual preference, religion, profession, and disability (Ramsden, 2002). Cultural safety is a key competency for professional responsibility. It includes demonstrating professional, legal, ethical, and cultural safety. These categories are examined through the application of physiological and psychosocial knowledge, as well as communication and clinical skills (Nursing Council of New Zealand, 2002/2012).

Cultural safety in nursing education is focused on educating students to be reflective of their own attitudes toward patients and their power relations with patients, rather than on their cultural customs and perspectives. While the goal of cultural competence education is to educate a professional nurse who treats patients in a culturally appropriate way (Wells & Black, 2000), the educational aim of cultural safety is a nurse who investigates the strategies, which can illuminate the factors that threaten the patients' sense of safety (Ramsden, 2002). There have been some attempts to combine the two concepts—cultural safety and cultural competence—and develop a model for an ethic of care based on both concepts (McEldowney & Connor, 2011). Cultural safety education is also an institutional responsibility, because structural conditions enable provision and/or teaching of culturally safe care (Richardson, 2010).

Cultural safety became a key concept in nursing education in the 21st century. The meanings of the concept and its application have been explored by scholars in New Zealand and Australia (Phiri, Dietsch, & Bonner 2010); Canada (Cash et al., 2013); the United States (Doutrich, Arcus, Dekker, Spuck, & Pollock-Robinson, 2012); and Israel (Arieli et al., 2012).

RECOMMENDATIONS

Integrating cultural safety in nursing education necessitates educating nursing students to perceive themselves as active social agents who endeavor to promote social justice. Nursing educators should be responsible for designing adequate cultural safety education programs that will take into consideration the specific power relation structures of each society, as well as the backgrounds of students and teachers. Because the idea of cultural safety may encounter resistance, there is a need for institutional, national, and international support for this educational perspective

Arieli, D., Friedman, V., & Hirschfeld, M. (2012). Challenges on the path to cultural safety in nursing education. *International Nursing Review, 59*(2), 187–193.

Arieli, D., Mashiach-Eizenberg, M., Friedman, V., & Hirschfeld, M. (2012). Cultural safety and nursing education in divided societies. *Nursing Education Perspectives, 33*(6), 364–368.

Cash, P. A., Moffitt, P., Fraser, J., Grewall, S., Holmes, V., Mahara, S.,…Nagel, D. (2013). Writing reflexivity to illuminate the meanings in cultural safety. *Reflective Practice, 14*(6), 825–839.

Doutrich, D., Arcus, K., Dekker, L., Spuck, J., & Pollock-Robinson, C. (2012). Cultural safety in New Zealand and the United States: Looking at a way forward together. *Journal of Transcultural Nursing, 23*(2), 143–150.

Jeffs, L. 2001. Teaching cultural safety the culturally safe way. *Nursing Praxis in New Zealand, 17*(3), 41–50.

McEldowney, R., & Connor, M. J. (2011). Cultural safety as an ethic of care: A praxiological process. *Journal of Transcultural Nursing, 22*(4), 342–349.

Nursing Council of New Zealand. (2002/2012). *Handbook for nursing departments offering programs leading to registration as an enrolled nurse or registered nurse.* Wellington: Author.

Papps, E., & Ramsden, I. (1996). Cultural safety in nursing: The New Zealand experience. *International Journal for Quality in Health Care, 8*(5), 491–497.

Phiri, J., Dietsch, E., & Bonner, A. (2010). Cultural safety and its importance for Australian midwifery practice. *Collegian, 173*, 105–111.

Ramsden, I. M. (2002). *Cultural safety and nursing education in Aotearoa and Waipounamu.* A thesis submitted to the Victoria University of Wellington for the fulfillment of the requirements for the degree of Doctor of Philosophy in Nursing.

Richardson, F. (2010). *Cultural safety in nursing education and practice in Aoterearoa New Zealand.* A thesis submitted to Massey University in partial fulfillment of the requirements for the degree of doctor of philosophy.

Richardson, F., & Carryer, J. (2005). Teaching cultural safety in a New Zealand nursing education program. *Journal of Nursing Education, 44*(5), 201–208.

Wells, S., & Black, R. (2000). *Cultural competence for health professionals.* Bethesda, MD: AOTA.

Daniella Arieli

CURRICULUM DEVELOPMENT

DEFINITION

Curriculum development is the process of designing a formal plan of study that provides the philosophical underpinnings, goals, and guidelines for the delivery of a specific educational program (Keating, 2011). Curriculum development refers to designing new programs and evaluating/revising existing programs (Kim, 2012).

APPLICATION

Nursing curriculum development, ongoing evaluation, and redesign of curriculum are the responsibility of the faculty (Ruchala, 2011). Nurse educators are responsible for formulating program outcomes and designing curricula that reflect contemporary health care trends and prepare graduates to function effectively in the health care environment (National League for Nursing [NLN], 2005). To this end, nurse educators have the multiple responsibilities of ensuring that the curriculum reflects institutional and departmental mission, vision, philosophy, and internal processes, as well as the standards of individual State Boards of Nursing and national accrediting agencies. Integration of these standards into the curriculum helps administrators and faculty to prepare for program approval or review and accreditation by ensuring that the program meets essential quality standards (Keating, 2011).

At the institutional level, curriculum development requires support of both the faculty and administration (Ruchala, 2011). Faculty engagement in the process includes utilization of knowledge, skills, and expertise; serving on curriculum committees; updating courses with current information each time the course is taught; as well as mentoring faculty who have less experience in the curriculum design process. Support from administration includes assurance of needed resources; physical, secretarial, and workload support; external consultants; and assurance that the work invested in the curriculum is valued and needed by the institution (Ruchala, 2011).

The NLN and the American Association of Colleges of Nursing (AACN) provide guidelines and competencies related to curriculum development and accreditation. NLN have been developed as suggestions for faculty as they strive to achieve a level of outstanding performance or service, relevant to all types of programs and institutions. Indicators of the curriculum as a Hallmark of Excellence in Nursing Education include an evidence-based curriculum that is flexible and reflective of current societal and health care trends. Additional indicators include research and innovation, local and global perspective, cultural learning, student values development and socialization, preparation for the roles that are essential to quality nursing practice, learning that supports evidence-based practice, and multidisciplinary approaches to care and clinical competence (NLN, 2004).

AACN curriculum standards provide a framework for positioning baccalaureate and graduate-degree nursing programs to meet the health care challenges of a new century. The AACN guidelines have been implemented in a curriculum design to produce sufficient numbers of nurses for a health system in continual change. The AACN Essentials series outlines the necessary curriculum content and expected competencies of graduates from baccalaureate, master's, and doctor of nursing practice programs, as well as the clinical support

C

needed for the full spectrum of academic nursing (AACN, 2014).

SYNOPSIS

Dynamic changes in health care, health care workforce education, and the call to better prepare students for the registered nurse and advanced practice role have generated dialogue regarding continuous curriculum review to prevent curriculum drift and ensure quality (van de Mortel & Bird, 2010) as well as curriculum development process reform and consideration of new models (Kim, 2012; Waters, Rochester, & McMillan, 2012). Significant changes occur in the discipline, context of employment, higher education, and health care sector in between accreditation cycles (Waters et al., 2012). Challenges for faculty in schools of nursing include keeping curricula relevant and current, responsive to innovations in practice and teaching and learning (Waters et al., 2012) as years pass in between accreditation and formal reaccreditation cycles (van de Mortel & Bird, 2010).

Curriculum drift, a widening gap between the accredited curriculum and the taught curriculum, occurs when changes to a course occur and the changes are not monitored. Possible reasons for this include the close protective association of the curriculum and academic freedom, faculty autonomy in development and delivery of their courses, and faculty teaching their courses in isolation (van de Mortel & Bird, 2010). Van de Mortel and Bird (2010) propose a continuous curriculum review that provides a data-informed process that addresses quality improvement of the curriculum; ensures that issues with delivery affecting the student experience are identified and addressed; contains curriculum drift while encouraging positive change; and provides opportunity for team building, development of leadership skills, holistic perspective of the curriculum, and faculty development in the form of sharing wisdom.

Outcomes-based education (also referred to in the literature as abilities-based education) has come to be associated with competency-based education. The key principle in this approach is the development of educational programs and application of learning processes, beginning with identifying outcomes expected as a result of an educational process. Competency-based education advocates for a time-independent approach. Curricular contents and learning processes are driven by outcomes/competencies specified for educational programs. In professional education, this means identification of competencies needed by graduates to meet the needs of specific professional roles determined by professions and social needs (Kim, 2012).

RECOMMENDATIONS

Integrated and comprehensive curriculum development takes into consideration appraisal of feedback from graduates and current learners, expectations of consumers of health care, recent developments in regulations and standards, and changes in higher education and health care. Nursing curriculum needs to achieve a balance between the body of nursing knowledge; skills such as communication, teamwork, and leadership: and analytical and critical thinking (Waters et al., 2012). Ensuring continuous quality in nursing education with the goal of producing graduates who show evidence of competencies in the beginning registered nurse and advanced practice roles requires ongoing dialogue on reforming the process of curriculum development and considering new models of nursing education in the context of accreditation.

American Association of Colleges of Nursing (AACN). (2014). *Education resources*. Retrieved from http://www.aacn.nche.edu/education-resources

Keating, S. (2011). Introduction to the history of curriculum development and curriculum approval process. In S. Keating (Ed.), *Curriculum development and evaluation in nursing* (2nd ed., pp. 1–4). New York, NY: Springer.

Kim, H. (2012). Outcomes-based curriculum development and student evaluation in nursing education. *Journal of Korean Academic Nursing, 42*(7), 917–927.

National League for Nursing (NLN). (2004). *Hallmarks, indicators, glossary, and references.* Retrieved from https://www.nln.org/excellence/hallmarks_indicators.htm

National League for Nursing (NLN). (2005). *Core competencies of nurse educators with task statements.* Retrieved from http://www.nln.org/profdev/corecompetencies.pdf

Ruchala, P. (2011). Curriculum development and approval process in changing educational environments. In S. Keating (Ed.), *Curriculum development and evaluation in nursing* (2nd ed., pp. 33–45). New York, NY: Springer.

van de Mortel, T., & Bird, J. (2010). Continuous curriculum review in a bachelor of nursing program: Preventing curriculum drift and improving quality. *Journal of Nursing Education, 49*(10), 592–595.

Waters, C., Rochester, S., & McMillan, M. (2012). Drivers for renewal and reform of contemporary nursing curricula: A blueprint for change. *Contemporary Nurse, 41*(2), 206–215.

Robin S. Goodrich
Kari L. Luoma

CURRICULUM EVALUATION

DEFINITION

Curriculum evaluation is an ongoing systematic process centered on continuous improvement of the nursing curriculum (Gard, Flannigan, & Clusky, 2004). Curriculum evaluation is defined as the gathering and analysis of data that match curricular objectives and using those data to make improvements in the curriculum.

APPLICATION

Continuous curriculum evaluation is essential to the maintenance of quality nursing education. Nursing programs contract with multiple stakeholders, but it is the contract with society that is most important because the public deserves the best care possible. To produce a safe, competent nurse, curricula must be assessed to determine if state-of-the-art objectives and outcomes of nursing essentials are reflected within the curricula. With the advent of technology, a new challenge to nursing curricula is the delivery of courses via web-based methods. The use of asynchronous courses and discussion boards threatens the integrity of the curriculum if its initial intent was use in the traditional classroom (Keating, 2006). The use of a theoretical framework to guide curriculum evaluation assists faculty to produce high-quality outcomes.

Multiple models for curriculum evaluation are embraced by some programs of nursing while other programs find it most beneficial to adhere to one specific model. A classic, the 1942 objectives model described by Tyler, identifies four teaching principles: defining appropriate learning objectives; establishing useful learning experiences; organizing learning experiences to have a maximum cumulative effect; and evaluating the curriculum and revising those aspects that did not prove effective (Keating, 2006). Prototype context, input, process, and product (CIPP) is a curriculum evaluation model developed by Stufflebeam and Shinkfield (2007). It consists of four evaluation types that result in four decisions: *Context* (Is there a need?); *input evaluation* (What resources are available?); *process evaluation* (Is the program implemented as planned?); and *product evaluation* (Does the data determine that the objectives were met?). This model often serves as a basis for other curriculum evaluation models in nursing education (Bradshaw & Lowenstein, 2007). It is imperative that the evaluation method matches the model on which the curriculum was built (Chavasse, 1994).

C

SYNOPSIS

Continuous curriculum assessment in nursing education is a method to inform stakeholders about the quality and standards of the program. The stakeholders include society, faculty, students, alumni, the institution, councils of higher education, and accrediting bodies (Keating, 2006). Reporting data and changes made as a result of the data increases the credibility of the school. Multiple divided opinions concerning evaluation exist (Smillie, Wong, & Arklie, 1984). However, an essential component of a quality evaluation design is a comprehensive plan for the collection of data that matches the established objectives within the curriculum. The plan determines what data will be collected, the frequency of data collection, the method of data analysis, and how to handle the findings (Giddens & Morton, 2010). One method of data collection suggested by Jacobs and Koehn (2004) is the use of questionnaires. These authors suggest that the constituents included in a survey sample are students (exit survey), alumni, and employers. This method may produce a low return rate, but the online survey technologies now available may help improve return rates.

The school, in most instances, has the power to establish the timeline of data collection. Depending on the data needed, it is suggested that data be collected every 1 to 3 years or during intervals that satisfy accreditation cycles (Keating, 2006). Data collected should be analyzed in a timely manner to facilitate improvement. It is important to then report the data and implement curriculum changes. Data and reports should be systematically stored in notebooks or electronically in secure locations.

RECOMMENDATIONS

Schools of nursing have a responsibility to create and implement a plan for curriculum evaluation. An evaluation committee consisting of faculty with experience in curricula evaluation is recommended. Appointing a curriculum coordinator with extensive knowledge to oversee the curriculum committee is imperative. It is also important that the coordinator mentors an associate coordinator to maintain continuity if the coordinator is not available. The committee should be charged with determining that the data to be collected matches the objectives, setting a timeline for data collection, collecting the data, analyzing the data, making recommendations to the faculty at large, assisting in the implementation of changes, and storing the data appropriately.

Each faculty member plays a role in the evaluation process. In addition to providing assessment data and exemplars of projects and papers from courses, faculty can assist the committee by providing information concerning rapidly changing health care policies and processes. Furthermore, faculty should provide input into new curricula design and evaluation for programs such as a new web-based curriculum. The chief nursing officer (CNO) of the school is also a significant contributor to the evaluation process. Institutional data and benchmarking data obtained from accrediting bodies may be available only to the CNO (Gard et al., 2004; Giddens & Morton, 2010). There is a need for research on curriculum evaluation as new models of education delivery continue to emerge, particularly in the area of education delivered exclusively online.

Bradshaw, M., & Lowenstein, A. (2007). *Innovative teaching strategies in nursing and related health professions* (4th ed.). Sudbury, MA: Jones and Bartlett.

Chavasse, J. (1994). Curriculum evaluation in nursing education: A review of the literature. *Journal of Advanced Nursing, 19*(5), 1024–1031.

Gard, C. L., Flannigan, P. N., & Cluskey, M. (2004). Program evaluation: An ongoing systematic process. *Nursing Education Perspectives, 25*(4), 176–179.

Giddens, J. F., & Morton, N. (2010). Report card: An evaluation of a concept-based curriculum. *Nursing Education Perspectives, 31*(6), 372–377.

Jacobs, P. M., & Koehn, M. L. (2004). Curriculum evaluation. Who, when, why, how? *Nursing Education Perspectives, 25*(1), 30–35.

Keating, S. (2006). *Curriculum development and evaluation in nursing.* Philadelphia, PA: Lippincott Williams & Wilkins.

Smillie, C., Wong, J., & Arklie, M. (1984). A proposed framework for evaluation of support courses in a nursing curriculum. *Journal of Advanced Nursing, 9*(5), 487–492.

Stufflebeam, D., & Shinkfield, A. (2007). *Evaluation theory, models, and applications.* San Francisco, CA: Jossey-Bass.

Anthony R. Ramsey

D

DECISION CASE METHOD

DEFINITION

The decision case method employs open-ended cases to stimulate and develop decision-making skills and critical thinking abilities in students. Decision cases depict actual situations taken from practice; the setting, involved practitioners, known background related to the situation, and the scenario are all described in rich detail. The facts are not altered, although the identifying information is camouflaged. Rather than depicting a situation and providing the outcome, decision cases realistically portray the often messy, ambiguous reality of practice without providing solutions.

When teaching with decision cases, providing information and lecturing on theory or content is replaced by a Socratic method, which facilitates in-depth discussion and encourages the use of analytical, critical thinking skills (Wolfer, Freeman, & Rhodes, 2001). The student is required to step figuratively into the position of the decision maker (Leenders, Mauffette-Leenders, & Erskine, 2001) and confront the challenges of practice. Students learn by actually placing themselves in real-life situations where decisions must be made.

APPLICATION

Preparing students to meet the multiple, unique challenges faced in actual practice should be a top priority for nursing education. Mastering content is not enough—graduates must be able to think like nurses

and make difficult decisions in complex, risk-laden situations.

Decision case method teaching brings clinical experience into the classroom and provides a safe venue for exploring numerous situations, solutions, and potential outcomes. This teaching/learning approach promotes evidence-based nursing through the application of research and theoretical learning to actual clinical experiences (McSherry & Proctor-Childs, 2001). Students learn not only from the professor or a single preceptor, but from each other as multiple viewpoints are explored. Potential outcomes of teaching with cases include (Delpier, 2006) development of critical thinking and judgment skills; practice making real decisions; active versus passive learning; learning integration rather than mere memorization of content; experiencing the reality of clinical topics; and creation of a stimulating interactive classroom in which students are engaged.

McSherry and Proctor-Childs (2001) note the following benefits specific to nursing education: promotion of multi-professional collaboration and teaching; involvement of patients and carers in providing real-life experiences of health care provision; development of research awareness skills in the context of practice; and acquisition of or consolidation of clinical skills in a safe environment (McSherry & Proctor-Childs, 2001). Use of decision cases can move students' thinking from a dualistic framework of right versus wrong to a generalization framework of analyzing and evaluating the complexities of a situation (Perry, 1999). Additionally, retention of concepts, details, and facts is enhanced via the use of narrative and picture memory (Moon & Fowler, 2008; Sandstrom, 2006).

D

SYNOPSIS

The Institute of Medicine report, *The Future of Nursing: Leading Change, Advancing Health*, recommended radical changes in nursing education, including the replacement of highly structured curriculums focused on content and memorization of facts with new approaches, which encourage content application in a variety of settings (Committee on the Future of Nursing, 2011). This was echoed in the report of the Carnegie Foundation for the Advancement of Teaching, *Educating Nurses: A Call for Radical Transformation* (Benner, Sulphen, Leonard, & Day, 2010). Decision case method teaching provides a mechanism for bridging the gap between knowledge and practice as recommended by these reports. It encourages evidence-based nursing practice by allowing students to apply research and theory to clinical situations (McSherry & Proctor-Childs, 2001).

Use of case studies in nursing education has a long history, but cases have most often been used as points of emphasis or examples rather than a means of instruction (Harrison, 2012). The decision case method was developed at Harvard Business School in the first decades of the 20th century as a method for providing students with education based on reality. Subsequently, problem-based learning was developed as a curriculum modality at McMaster University Medical School in the 1970s and evolved as a method for promoting critical thinking by applying content to clinical dilemmas and practice settings (Williams & Beattle, 2007).

While decision case method teaching has been touted as a means for linking content and theory to practice, there are challenges involved in using this method. Both students and teachers must make adjustments and take risks in employing a new method for teaching and learning. Students accustomed to the lecture/memorization method of learning may feel unprepared for or resistant to a new approach that encourages creative thought. The classroom environment must support open communication and intellectual curiosity, and students must feel secure in the knowledge that their ideas will be supported.

RECOMMENDATIONS

The success of the decision case method depends on both the instructor's commitment to this approach and the availability of decision cases. When using the decision case teaching method, instructors must surrender the role of the authority providing information and become a facilitator of learning who skillfully uses a combination of questioning, listening, and responding to direct the session toward defined learning objectives. Initially, the instructor may feel that he or she is on "uncharted waters," but with time this approach will become comfortable and the learning outcomes will justify the initial risks involved in trying a new approach.

Perhaps, the greatest challenge when using this method is locating or developing suitable cases. The process of recruiting cases from practitioners, interviewing and documenting details, and writing the case is labor intensive, and some persons may not be skilled in writing narrative accounts. These obstacles could be overcome by working in collaboration with a team with each member assuming certain responsibilities in the process. Students could also be involved in the process of recruiting cases from nurses in practice, assisting with interviews, and reviewing the developed case to ensure accuracy; this would not only result in decision cases for use in the curriculum but also in greater exposure of the students to actual practice scenarios (Head & Bays, 2010). Groups of faculty members might agree to work together on such efforts and share the developed cases. It is also recommended that cases be published and shared by educational institutions, thereby creating a repository of cases from which instructors can select cases appropriate for teaching specific course content.

Benner, P., Sulphen, M., Leonard, V., & Day, I. (2010). *Educating nurses: A call for radical transformation.* Stanford, CA: The Carnegie Foundation for the Advancement of Teaching.

Committee on the Future of Nursing. (2011). *The future of nursing: Leading change, advancing health.* Washington, DC: Institute of Medicine.

Delpier, T. (2006). Cases 101: Learning to teach with cases. *Nursing Education Perspectives, 27,* 204–209.

Harrison, E. (2012). How to develop well-written case studies: The essential elements. *Nurse Educator, 17*(2), 67–70.

Head, B., & Bays, C. (2010). Engaging nursing students and community partners in the development of decision cases. *Journal of Nursing Education, 49*(6), 346–350.

Leenders, M. R., Mauffette-Leenders, L. A., & Erskine, J. A. (2001). *Writing cases* (4th ed.). London, Ontario: Senton Printing.

McSherry, R., & Proctor-Childs, T. (2001). Promoting evidence-based practice through an integrated model of care: Patient case studies as a teaching method. *Nurse Education in Practice, 1,* 19–26.

Moon, J., & Fowler, J. (2008). A framework for the conception of story in higher education and professional development. *Nurse Education Today, 28,* 232–239.

Perry, W. (1999). *Forms of intellectual and ethical development in the college years: A scheme.* San Francisco, CA: Jossey-Bass.

Sandstrom, S. (2006). Use of case studies to teach diabetes and other chronic illnesses to nursing students. *Journal of Nursing Education, 45,* 229–232.

Williams, S., & Beattle, H. (2007). Problem based learning in the clinical setting—a systematic review. *Nurse Education Today, 28,* 146–154.

Wolfer, T. A., Freeman, M., & Rhodes, R. (2001). Developing and teaching an M.S.W. capstone course using case methods of instruction. *Advances in Social Work, 2*(2), 156–171.

Barbara Head

DEDICATED EDUCATION UNIT

DEFINITION

The dedicated education unit (DEU) is a collaborative clinical learning environment for nursing students that takes advantage of an existing nursing setting by a specific school of nursing. A specific school utilizes the DEU during established hours or days. It involves a commitment by all stakeholders: the academic setting, the clinical setting, and the students. The traditional roles of clinical faculty and staff nurses are revised on the DEU to allow for utilization of the unique expertise of both, specifically the clinical expertise of the staff nurse in the clinical setting and the educational expertise of the clinical faculty to promote clinical reasoning and reflection (Edgecombe, Wotton, Gonda, & Mason, 1999; Moscato, Miller, Logsdon, Weinberg, & Chorpenning, 2007). DEUs enhance student learning through the application of theory to clinical practice while under the supervision of both expert staff nurses and clinical faculty (Ranse & Grealish, 2007). DEUs are built on mutual respect, open communication, and collaborative relationships, and represent a partnered commitment to student learning (Moscato et al., 2007).

APPLICATION

The DEU was conceived and first implemented in Australia, and subsequently described in the literature (Edgecombe et al., 1999). The DEU has been the solution to a nursing shortage, a nurse faculty shortage, the dissatisfaction with clinical education on the part of students, as well as the solution to a discrepancy between employers' expectations of newly graduated nurses' skill sets and the new graduate nurses' actual readiness for practice (Edgecombe et al., 1999; Miller, 2005; Moscato et al., 2007; Pappas, 2007). The DEU has been used primarily as a clinical setting for nursing students.

D

Several settings have been utilized as DEU. An acute care setting was the location of the original Australian DEU, and acute care settings continue to be the primary locations for DEUs. DEUs also have been located in inpatient psychiatric units, skilled nursing facilities, and with school nurses in an educational service district. As DEUs are developed in new settings, the essential elements remain intact: The nurse or health care team in the setting is the expert in the type of care provided and the clinical faculty member is the expert educator.

Schools of nursing anticipated that utilizing a DEU as a clinical setting would maximize the transfer of knowledge from the classroom, to the clinical setting, and back to the classroom (Edgecombe et al., 1999). Research conducted around the implementation of the DEU model has provided qualitative and quantitative data that suggest that transfer of knowledge does occur. Additional outcomes include the following: Both students and nurse clinicians prefer the DEU placement to traditional clinical learning scenarios; nurse clinicians report being challenged in their role, which results in improved practice; there is an overall sense of improved relationships, both between the academic and health care institutions, and between students and the nurse clinicians; and students report a stronger sense of inclusion in the DEU (Gonda, Wotton, Edgecombe, & Mason, 1999).

The initial DEU settings also yielded some areas for improvement. Students found that the time commitment of the DEU along with other course work allowed little time for reflection (Gonda et al., 1999; Moscato, Kaakinen, Mitchell, Gatlin, & Miller, 2004). Nurse clinicians reported being challenged to adjust to the role of teacher and to learn the language of the evaluation tools (Moscato et al., 2004). These challenges were met eagerly by the academics and the nurse clinicians, with solutions from both parties, as the overall positive experience by all resulted in a desire to continue with the DEU model.

SYNOPSIS

The DEU is a collaborative learning model that uses existing clinical settings as an optimal learning environment for nursing students. The expertise of the academic faculty and nurse clinician is maximized in this model to allow for improved knowledge transfer for students from the classroom to the clinical setting. Nurse clinicians report a preference for the model as they have a stronger relationship with the student and the academic faculty, and they are more familiar with a specific school's goals and outcomes. Students report a stronger sense of belonging to the unit, allowing them to learn the work of the nurse and grow in their role. The DEU utilizes existing clinical settings and established relationships with service partners to enhance nurse and student satisfaction in the education of nursing students.

RECOMMENDATIONS

While the current literature indicates that the DEU is an innovative and collaborative way to address the pending nurse faculty shortage, additional research in this area is needed. Evidence in support of improved student learning remains mostly qualitative and anecdotal. Further research into the learning benefits of a DEU is recommended.

Edgecombe, K., Wotton, K., Gonda, J., & Mason, P. (1999). Dedicated education units: 1. A new concept for clinical teaching and learning. *Contemporary Nurse, 8*(4), 166–171.

Gonda, J., Wotton, K., Edgecombe, K., & Mason, P. (1999). Dedicated education units: 2. An evaluation. *Contemporary Nurse, 8*(4), 172–176.

Miller, T. W. (2005). The dedicated education unit: A practice and education partnership. *Nursing Leadership Forum, 9*(4), 169–173.

Moscato, S. R., Kaakinen, J., Mitchell, C., Gatlin, P., & Miller, J. (2004). *Dedicated education unit: Innovative strategy for optimal clinical learning.* 37th Annual

Communicating Nursing Research Conference/18th Annual WIN, Portland, OR (pp. 37–247).

Moscato, S. R., Miller, J., Logsdon, K., Weinberg, S., & Chorpenning, L. (2007). Dedicated education unit: An innovative clinical partner education model. *Nursing Outlook, 55*(1), 31–37. doi:10.1016/j.outlook.2006.11.001

Pappas, S. (2007). Improving patient safety and nurse engagement with a dedicated education unit. *Nurse Leader, 5*(3), 40–43. doi:10.1016/j.mnl.2007.03.009

Ranse, K., & Grealish, L. (2007). Nursing students' perceptions of learning in the clinical setting of the dedicated education unit. *Journal of Advanced Nursing, 58*(2), 171–179. doi:10.1111/j.1365–2648.2007.04220.x

Janet M. Banks
Mary T. Quinn Griffin

DISABILITY

DEFINITION

The World Health Organization (WHO) defines disability as an umbrella term that includes impairment (problems in body function or structure), activity limitations (difficulties encountered by an individual in executing a task or action), and participation restrictions (problems experienced by an individual in involvement in life situations; WHO, 2001). The International Council of Nurses (ICN, 2010) defines disability as a physical, mental, sensory, or social impairment that adversely affects individuals' ability to carry out normal day-to-day activities in the long term.

APPLICATION

The care of persons with disabilities, including intellectual and developmental disabilities, is an essential topic for nursing education. The biopsychosocial model of disability (U.S. Department of Health and Human Services [USDHHS], 2005) emphasizes the view that disability arises from the interaction of physical, emotional, and environmental factors. This model ensures that students learn to communicate effectively and sensitively with persons with disabilities. Students learn to consider the effect of the disability on the health condition. In addition, they also learn how treatment of the health condition affects the disability. In selecting a model of disability, a key issue is the view of the role of individuals with a disability in their health care. Other models of disability (e.g., medical and rehabilitation models) consider health care professionals as the experts on disability, without recognizing the life experiences of individuals living with the disability.

Innovative approaches are needed to ensure that nursing students have the requisite knowledge, attitudes, and skills to provide quality care for patients with disabilities across health care settings, from acute and long-term care facilities to outpatient facilities, the home, and the community (Gardner, 2012).

SYNOPSIS

The need for nursing education to address disability is based on the sizable and growing population of people with disabilities: almost 60 million people in the United States (U.S. Census Bureau, 2010) and more than a billion people worldwide (WHO and World Bank, 2011). Disability affects people across all age groups, both genders, and all socioeconomic and racial and ethnic groups, and disproportionately affects marginalized, disadvantaged, or at-risk groups, including women, older people, and people who are poor. Despite having disabilities that can be severe, most people with disabilities make significant contributions to their families, communities, and work and educational settings (National Council on Disability, 2012).

Although people with disabilities have the same health needs as those without

D

disabilities—for immunization, health promotion, preventive health screening, and high-quality health care—many encounter barriers to care. These barriers include negative attitudes and lack of knowledge of health care professionals, including nurses (Gardner, 2012; Smeltzer, Avery, & Haynor, 2012), and environmental obstacles (e.g., inaccessible buildings, rest rooms, health centers, and imaging centers; and absence of accommodations, such as height-adjustable and mammography equipment).

The Americans with Disabilities Act, enacted in 1990 and amended in 2008, prohibits discrimination because of disability U.S. Department of Labor, Office of Disability and Employment Policy (1990). However, people with disabilities report continued barriers to health care. In response, multiple national and international agencies (e.g., the U.S. Surgeon General's Office; USDHHS, 2005; ICN, 2010; WHO, 2011) have called for health care professionals to be better educated about disability. The ICN's 2000 position statement on disability, revised in 2010, explicitly states that nurses are key to the health care of people with disabilities and need to be involved in health promotion, teaching, and counseling of people with disabilities and their families (2010). Nurse educators need to ensure that students achieve competencies needed to provide care for people with disabilities.

The ICN (2010) also calls for professional nursing organizations to advocate for public policy directed toward improved health care of people with disabilities. Despite the strong and explicit position of the ICN about nurses' role and the need for nursing to address disability, the topic remains largely invisible in nursing education (Betz, 2013; Gardner, 2012; Smeltzer, Dolen, Robinson-Smith, & Zimmerman, 2005). None of the organizations that establish standards of nursing care in the United States or accredit nursing education programs identify care of people with disabilities as part of those standards or criteria on which nursing education is evaluated.

RECOMMENDATIONS

Students typically enter nursing programs with little or no experience or previous contact with people with disabilities. Their attitudes toward people with disabilities are similar to those of the general population and are often negative. Thus, strategies that expose nursing students to people with disabilities through clinical experiences, simulations of patients with disabilities, or the use of standardized patients with disabilities are recommended. Visits to persons with disabilities in their homes can open students' eyes to the ability of persons with disabilities to live and function effectively and independently in their home and community, a view that is often unexpected by students.

Use of disability days, in which students are put in situations to experience a disability for an hour or two by wearing glasses that impede vision or requiring them to move around in a wheelchair, is *not* recommended by the disability community because it can result in very negative attitudes about disability in students. Alternatively, such short-term experiences may result in an undesirable conclusion by students that having a disability is not a significant issue. Having individuals with disabilities participate in teaching of nursing students through panel discussions or simulations with carefully planned standardized patient experiences are likely to be more effective than the disability-day experiences.

Faculty members knowledgeable or at least interested in disability can serve as champions and review nursing curricula to identify where disability-related topics and experiences can be integrated. Furthermore, they can also select from the array of resources, materials that faculty can use to learn about and teach students about disability, to promote positive attitudes toward patients with disabilities in clinical practice, to provide care that is equal to that given to patients without disabilities, and to advocate for public policy to improve care for people with disabilities.

Research is needed to test different teaching approaches and their effect on care of people with disabilities.

Betz, C. L. (2013). Health care transition for adolescents with special healthcare needs: Where is nursing. *Nursing Outlook, 61*(5), 258–265. doi:10.1016/j.outlook.2012.08.009

Gardner, M. R. (2012). Preparing nurses to care for people with developmental disabilities. Perspectives on integrating developmental disabilities concepts and experiences into nursing education. *Nursing Clinics of North America, 47*(4), 517–527. doi:10.1016/j.cnur.2012.07.010

International Council of Nurses (ICN). (2010). *Prevention of disability and the care of people with disabilities.* Geneva, Switzerland: International Council of Nurses.

National Council on Disability. (2012). *Rocking the cradle: Ensuring the rights of parents with disabilities.* Washington, DC: National Council on Disability.

Smeltzer, S. C., Avery, C., & Haynor, S. (2012). Interactions of people with disabilities with nursing staff during hospitalization. *American Journal of Nursing, 112*(4), 30–37. doi:10.1097/01.NAJ.0000413454.07369.e3

Smeltzer, S. C., Dolen, M. A., Robinson-Smith, G., & Zimmerman, V. (2005). Integration of disability-related content in nursing curricula. *Nursing Education Perspectives, 26*(4), 210–216.

United States Department of Health and Human Resources (USDHHS). (2005). *Surgeon general's call to action to improve the health and wellness of persons with disabilities.* Rockville, MD: Public Health Services.

U.S. Census Bureau. (2010) *Americans with disabilities: 2010.* Retrieved from http://www.census.gov/prod/2012pubs/p70-131.pdf

U.S. Department of Labor, Office of Disability and Employment Policy (1990). American with Disabilities Act (ADA Publication L, No. 110-325; 2008). Retrieved from http://www.dol.gov/dol/topic/disability/ada.htm

World Health Organization (WHO). (2001). *International classification of functioning, disability and health.* Geneva, Switzerland: World Health Organization.

World Health Organization (WHO) and the World Bank. (2011). *World report on disability.* Geneva, Switzerland: World Health Organization.

Suzanne C. Smeltzer

DISASTER PREPARATION

DEFINITION

Disaster preparation is a process that involves developing plans to protect oneself and family before, during, and after a natural or man-made disaster. A disaster is defined as any situation that overwhelms the resources available to protect those affected. Examples of natural disasters include floods, fires, hurricanes, winter storms, tsunamis, mudslides, and volcanoes. Examples of man-made disasters include chemical spills from overturned vehicles or trains, plane crashes, or terrorist attacks.

APPLICATION

Nursing faculty prepare students to practice in a wide variety of settings, including health care facilities and in the community. Preparation includes theoretical and clinical content, designed to create competent, confident nurses prepared to function in diverse situations. It is imperative that nurse educators prepare students at all levels to prepare for and respond to disasters. Education should focus on the five phases of the disaster preparation cycle: preparedness, mitigation, response, recovery, and evaluation (Goodwin-Veenema, 2013). Disaster preparedness begins prior to a disaster. Plans should include steps to take before, during, and after a disaster, and include protecting people and property. Prior to a disaster, the

D

plan should include creating a plan specific to the individual and family circumstances, plus creating a disaster Go-bag of irreplaceable, daily-use items.

Preparation should consider two different circumstances: evacuating the location or sheltering in place. If a disaster such as an approaching hurricane makes it unsafe to stay in the current location, such as home, work, or school, plans should include identifying alternative evacuation routes in case the main route is impassable, keeping at least a half tank of fuel in the vehicle at all times, and having emergency supplies in the vehicle in case shelter is not accessible during the evacuation. Some disasters require sheltering in place, meaning that the area outside is too hazardous to allow immediate evacuation and should include water and other emergency supplies for survival until evacuation becomes safe.

Nurses may be working or called in to work as a result of the disaster, so having a plan and supplies in place will provide more peace of mind about family and pets, allowing the nurse to concentrate more on patient care. It is also important to know the disaster plans at work, including evacuation and sheltering in place. Agencies, including health care facilities, which receive federal funding for disaster preparedness, are required by the Federal Emergency Management Agency (FEMA, 2008) to be compliant with the National Incident Management System (NIMS). Any employee who plays an active role in disaster response should complete several of the NIMS courses in order to understand the role of all agencies involved in disaster response. Minimum courses include IS-100, IS-200, IS-700, and IS-800.

The next step in disaster preparedness is mitigation, defined by the FEMA as an effort to reduce the loss of life and property from natural and/or man-made disasters by avoiding or lessening the impact of a disaster and providing value to the public by creating safer communities. Examples of community mitigation include building levees in flood-prone areas, building tornado shelters, or establishing stricter codes

to reinforce buildings in earthquake- or hurricane-prone regions. Health care facilities can practice mitigation by securing shelves to prevent loss of supplies during earthquakes, identifying vendors for critical supplies from more than one area in case supply routes are disrupted, and backing up all critical files every day in an off-site location in case records are lost.

The next stage of disaster preparedness is response. This stage involves notification and communication to those actually or potentially affected by a disaster, including sirens or emergency broadcasts. Smartphone applications allow individuals to receive emergency notifications and instructions. Agencies such as the American Red Cross (ARC) or FEMA may establish shelters or service centers, or temporary health care facilities if a hospital has been destroyed in the disaster zone. If the disaster involves a chemical attack or hazardous material spill, decontamination stations may be established. Individuals with functional or access needs, including serious health conditions, will need additional response efforts targeted to their needs, such as oxygen, and replacement of medications or durable medical equipment. Individuals with developmental or mental health needs will need ongoing support, as well as additional services to help them cope with the effects of the disaster.

The recovery stage of disaster preparedness may take weeks to years, but is one of the most important stages in reestablishing communities after a disaster. It involves actions to help restore a community to a pre-disaster level. The community may never return to an identical pre-disaster state, but sufficient outreach by the government, charitable organizations, and volunteers from other communities will help the affected community to become resilient and at least meet the basic needs of its members.

The final stage is evaluation, which involves a detailed, multiagency review of all the stages of disaster preparedness to determine their effectiveness. Ideally, evaluation should be accomplished during periodic drills of disaster plans involving all community organizations described in the plan. Waiting until an actual disaster may be too late to determine major flaws in the steps of disaster preparedness.

SYNOPSIS

Nursing faculty has free, immediate access to educational materials that can be used for in-class lectures or self-study by students. FEMA and the ARC provide several resources to guide professionals in the phases of disaster education. FEMA provides free online training about the NIMS, described previously. The ARC provides printed and online materials designed for individuals, families, and organizations to assist them in preparing for disasters. For nurses who volunteer with the ARC, free educational modules (ReadyRN) were donated by Goodwin-Veenema (2013), an international nurse expert in disaster preparedness. The U.S. Government provides similar resources for individual, family, and community preparedness. The Centers for Disease Control and Prevention provide information about potential biological, chemical, and nuclear/radiological hazards.

A task force of ARC volunteer nurses created a free course for pre-licensure nursing students to prepare to serve as Red Cross volunteers under registered nurse (RN) supervision in Red Cross disaster shelters. Educators may consider adding this course to their Community Health Nursing or Leadership and Management course. Sigma Theta Tau International offers an inexpensive online continuing nursing education (CNE) course to prepare staff nurses and others for disasters.

RECOMMENDATIONS

As citizens and health care professionals, nurses should set an example for their communities by demonstrating personal, family, and professional preparedness. This includes the steps described in the preparedness stages related to the self and family. Once those resources are in place, nurses need to collaborate with their colleagues in their health care agencies to create and implement disaster preparedness plans. Nurse educators serve as a pivotal force in preparing current and future nurses to participate fully in the disaster preparedness cycle.

American Red Cross (ARC). (2014). Retrieved from www.redcross.org

Centers for Disease Control and Prevention. Retrieved from www.cdc.gov

Disaster Health and Sheltering for Nursing Students. (2014). Retrieved from www.disasterhealthandsheltering.org

Federal Emergency Management Agency (FEMA). (2008). *National response framework (2008), glossary section.* Retrieved from www.fema.gov/emergency/nrf/glossary.htm#R

Goodwin-Veenema, T. (2013). *Disaster nursing and emergency preparedness for chemical, biological, and radiological terrorism and other hazards* (3rd ed.). New York, NY: Springer Publishing.

Sigma Theta Tau International. (2014). *Disaster preparedness and response—Online course.* Retrieved from www.nursingsociety.org

Cheryl K. Schmidt

DISRUPTIVE BEHAVIOR

DEFINITION

Disruptive behavior is any inappropriate behavior, confrontation, or conflict, ranging from verbal abuse to physical or sexual harassment (Rosenstein, 2013). Disruptive behaviors include overt and covert actions that are displayed by any health care worker that threaten the performance of the health care team (Joint Commission, 2008). Disruptive behavior includes profane or discourteous language, demeaning behavior, sexual comments or overtone, racial/ethnic jokes, outbursts of anger, throwing objects,

D

criticism in front of patients or staff, comments that undermine a patient's trust, and comments that undermine a caregiver's self-confidence (Porto & Lauve, 2006).

APPLICATION

Health care workers are often exposed and desensitized to behaviors that support a non-conducive and disrespectful work environment. Nurses, as well as other health care providers, must support, establish, and maintain working environments that are safe and conducive to the provision of quality health care. Disruptive behaviors not only threaten patient safety but also the ability for health care workers to perform their job competently. Hickson (2012) identified four significant implications to decrease the incidents of disruptive behaviors: orientation/residency programs, collaborative partnerships between academia and service, zero tolerance for behaviors that undermine a culture of safety, and addressing negative behaviors.

Orientation/Residency Programs

These orientation/residency programs are intended to provide positive mentorship and preceptorship to support and promote a culture of professionalism and collegiality. According to the Quality and Safety Education for Nurses (QSEN, 2014), competency nurses, physicians, and other health care professionals are expected to function effectively within interprofessional teams, foster open communication, employ mutual respect, and share decision making to achieve quality patient care. Nurse residencies and internships further indicate a relationship between the quality and quantity of nurses' orientation and the satisfaction and retention of novice professionals (Scott, Keehner-Engelke, & Swanson, 2008). The Institute of Medicine (2010) suggested that the collaboration of state boards of nursing and accrediting bodies should support the completion of a nursing residency program upon licensure or advanced practice degree program, or the transition to new clinical practice areas.

Collaborative Partnerships Between Academia and Service

A collaborative vision and partnership between academia and the practice setting can successfully translate to increased professionalism, effective communication, optimal patient care, and substantive working relationships.

Zero Tolerance for Behaviors Undermining a Culture of Safety

Based on the Sentinel Event Alert (Joint Commission, 2008), the Joint Commission began requiring health care facilities to implement zero-tolerance policies that defined intimidating and disruptive behaviors. Zero tolerance includes, but is not limited to, intimidating and/or disruptive behaviors, especially the most egregious instances of disruptive behavior such as assault and other criminal acts (Joint Commission, 2008). It is essential to provide information and education to students, as well as to the staff of all disciplines, concerning the phenomenon of disruptive behavior: defining characteristics, understanding the effects toward individuals and an organization, identifying the system for reporting and monitoring, and the responsibility that all stakeholders hold in eliminating disruptive behavior and adhering to the organization's zero-tolerance policy. Education about zero tolerance can be offered by formal or informal means, such as coaching, mentoring, or precepting. An emphasis on individual accountability at all organizational levels, as well as organizational adoption of a culture of civility, would be required for policies to be effective (Clark, Olender, Cardoni, & Kenski, 2011).

Addressing Disruptive Behavior

Careful attention must be given to implementing effective strategies to empower newly registered nurses or experienced nurses to confront, defuse, and resist disruptive behaviors in their professional nursing practice. Griffin (2004) has delineated cognitive–behavioral techniques addressing negative behaviors, emphasizing educational awareness and cognitive rehearsal as specific interventions that new nurses can use to confront their hostile offender. Strategies identified by the Center for American Nurses (2008) include nurses adopting and modeling professional ethical behavior, recognizing and addressing bullying and disruptive behaviors in the workplace, reflecting on one's own behavior and communicating respectfully, participating in collaborative interprofessional initiative to prevent abuse, and working to ensure the mission, vision, and values of their workplaces are reflective of the Code of Ethics for Nurses and standards set by the profession in order to eliminate disruptive behavior.

The burden of responsibility for decreasing and/or eliminating disruptive behavior does not fall solely on an individual or a group, but the organization as a whole. Organizational leaders should use their constitutive capacity of persuasive influence to foster healthy and nondisruptive work environments, which ultimately create the ethical practice desired by the stakeholders of the nursing profession. It is not enough for the leaders to use their influence to reinforce a nondisruptive environment but also to commit to a role-modeling change in the preexisting culture. If organizational leaders continue to overlook the urgency of the domino effect that disruptive behavior has within health care, they steadfastly default on their vow of providing a culture of safety and promoting the standards of professionalism (Hickson, 2012).

SYNOPSIS

Eliminating disruptive behavior in the nursing profession is necessary in order to support an environment conducive to a healthy workplace. If it is to be achieved, nursing education and health care organizations must develop educational and mentorship programs that foster a healthy work environment and change the culture of nursing to one of valuing self, peers, and nursing practice (Lux, Hutcheson, & Peden, 2014). Lux et al. (2014) stressed that nurse educators must educate nursing students about

how to confront disruptive behavior before entering their profession. New graduates must leave nursing programs equipped with well-developed professional communication skills.

Dellasega (2011) identified a three-step process for decreasing the incidents of disruptive behavior in the workplace, which can be affected by nursing educators to support the transition of students to newly graduated nurses. The three steps are: educating nurses who are the victims of disruptive behavior about disruptive behavior in order to improve their understanding of the phenomenon, teaching interactive strategies to help nurses relate and reframe disruptive behaviors, and using role modeling to integrate appropriate behaviors.

RECOMMENDATIONS

Disruptive behavior can have deleterious effects on a personal or organizational level, which can no longer be ignored. Accreditation of health care facilities now depends on an organization's ability to effectively address disruptive behaviors. Organizations who operationalize and reinforce zero-tolerance policies demonstrate to their employees the promotion of a healthy work environment (Hickson, 2013). A strong commitment on the part of health care agencies to eliminate disruptive behaviors, along with cooperation from everyone in the organization, is imperative. Longo (2010) identified approaches for addressing disruptive behaviors which include the following: adopt a zero-tolerance stance, develop a code of conduct that defines acceptable and unacceptable behaviors, provide education regarding communication skills, provide coaching and mentoring, provide mediation services to resolve disputes between parties, and take disciplinary action. Rosenstein (2009) echoed similar topics as a call to action for health care environments to address disruptive behavior: strong organizational leadership, awareness and accountability, communication and team collaboration training, identifying clinical champion/

D

clinical champions, enforcing policies and procedures, and reporting an intervention process.

Center for American Nurses. (2008). *Lateral violence and bullying in the workplace.* Retrieved from http://www.mc.vanderbilt.edu/root/pdfs/nursing/center_lateral_violence_and_bullying_position_statement_from_center_for_american_nurses.pdf

Clark, C. M., Olender, L., Cardoni, C., & Kenski, D. (2011). Fostering civility in nursing education and practice: Nurse leader perspectives. *Journal of Nursing Administration, 41*(7/8), 324–330. doi:10.1097/NNA.0b013e31822509c4

Dellasega, C. (2011). *When nurses hurt nurses: Recognizing and overcoming the cycle of nurse bullying.* Indianapolis, IN: Sigma Theta Tau.

Griffin, M. (2004). Teaching cognitive rehearsal as a shield for lateral violence: An intervention for newly licensed nurses. *The Journal of Continuing Education in Nursing, 35*(6), 257–263.

Hickson, J. (2012). *Nursing hostility and job satisfaction as perceived by new graduate nurses: Magnet versus non-magnet hospitals* (Doctoral dissertation). Retrieved from ProQuest Digital Dissertations (3508503).

Hickson, J. (2013). New nurses' perceptions of hostility and job satisfaction: Magnet® versus non-Magnet. *Journal of Nursing Administration, 43*(5), 293–301. doi:10.1097/NNA.0b013e31828eebc9

Institute of Medicine. (2010). *The future of nursing focus on education.* Retrieved from http://www.iom.edu/~/media/Files/Report%20Files/2010/The-Future-of-Nursing/Nursing%20Education%202010%20Brief.pdf

Joint Commission. (2008). *Sentinel event alert: Behaviors that undermine a culture of safety.* Retrieved from http://www.jointcommission.org/assets/1/18/SEA_40.PDF

Longo, J. (2010). *Combating disruptive behaviors: Strategies to promote a healthy work environment.* Retrieved from http://www.nursingworld.org/MainMenuCategories/ANAMarketplace/ANAPeriodicals/OJIN/TableofContents/Vol152010/No1Jan2010/Combating-Disruptive-Behaviors.aspx

Lux, K. M., Hutcheson, J. B., & Peden, A. R. (2014). Ending disruptive behavior: Staff nurse recommendations to nurse educators. *Nurse Education in Practice, 14*(1), 37–42. doi:org/10.1016/j.nepr.2013.06.014

Porto, G., & Lauve, R. (2006). Disruptive clinician behaviors: A persistent threat to patient safety [Electronic version]. *Patient Safety & Quality Health Care, July/August,* 1–11. Retrieved from http://www.psqh.com/julaug06/disruptive.html

Quality and Safety Education for Nurses. (2014). *Pre-licensure KSAs: Teamwork and collaboration.* Retrieved from http://qsen.org/competencies/pre-licensure-ksas/#teamwork_collaboration

Rosenstein, A. H. (2009). Managing disruptive behaviors in the health care setting: Process, policy, prevention, and intervention. *Advances in Psychology Research, 72,* 1–14.

Rosenstein, A. H. (2013). *Bad medicine: Managing the risks of disruptive behaviors in health care settings.* Retrieved from http://www.rmmagazine.com/2013/12/01/bad-medicine-managing-the-risks-of-disruptive-behaviors-in-health-care-settings/

Scott, E. S., Keehner-Engelke, M., & Swanson, M. (2008). New graduate nurse transitioning: Necessary or nice? *Applied Nursing Research, 21*(2), 75–83. doi:10.1016/j.apnr.2006.12.002

Josiane Hickson

DISTANCE EDUCATION

DEFINITION

Distance education is defined as a formal educational process that provides instruction using technology where the students and instructor are not in the same general location. The students who are taking distance education courses are separated by geographical or physical distance from the instructor (Zerwekh, 2011). The distance education student may be in the same general location or a different country than the instructor, but there is no physical presence on campus.

APPLICATION

Distance education involves communication using some form of technology that provides learning. Beaudoin (1990) posits that distance education is learner centered where the faculty reinforces learning through explanation, references, and thoughtful questioning. The education may be in the form of online (e-learning), videoconference, audioconference, or combination of online and audioconferencing called webinar. Distance education may be offered to students in a synchronous or asynchronous format.

The distance education format that is emphasized and utilized most frequently is online (e-learning). The online format uses course management systems that are considered in the classroom. The students may be assigned several learning activities including written assignments, debates, concept maps, case studies, examinations, or journaling. Instructors may offer office hours via synchronous chat or videoconferencing. The instructor facilitates learning by using Socratic questioning in the discussion board and grading of assignments. The students must be active in the online environment, motivated, self-directed, and disciplined to complete the discussions and assignments.

Students may be assigned discussions or assignments with deadlines so that the students may complete their work on their own time within the time frame assigned. The instructor facilitates discussions using Socratic questions for deep critical thinking. Some online courses may require students to attend synchronous sessions to discuss difficult concepts. The institution where the course is being offered defines the synchronous or asynchronous learning expectations for online courses and programs.

Videoconferencing is a distance education format where the instructor is at the education site and the students are present at another location. The videoconferencing format allows for the student and instructor to be available *synchronously* but at different locations. The distance classroom has two-way monitors where students and instructors can see each other in real time. The instructor can share presentations and resources with students. The learning activities that can be used are the same that may be used in the traditional classroom. The distant site has support staff to assist with technology issues and student support.

Audioconferencing is a distant education format where the learning occurs over the telephone. The instructor is located at one place and students may be at another place or call from their home. Audioconferencing may be incorporated in a blended format with online courses or webinars. Audioconferencing is synchronous, and students and instructors are able to communicate in real time. The learning activity that may be found during audioconferencing is discussions of current topics.

Webinar is a distance education format where there is a one-way video broadcast via the Internet with the instructor at one location and students at one or more locations. The instructor presents the webinar and controls the audio and video. The students call from the computer or phone. They are able to see the video online and hear the conference, but the instructor is not able to see the students. Students are able to ask questions via the chat box and open discussion sessions. The instructors and students meet in a synchronous format. The learning activities that may be used include discussions, polling, and brainstorming.

SYNOPSIS

Distance education provides opportunities for students in rural and underserved areas who may not otherwise be able to obtain a degree due to travel, personal, or time constraints. Frith (2013) presents the advantages of distance education for students who would not have an opportunity for education, including access and flexibility for those who would not have access to education due to no local programs, work, or family schedules. The disadvantages include students who may often feel they are alone and technology issues. Distance education requires the use of technology that is ever changing.

Distance education is continually changing with the rapid technological advances. A critical component of distance education is the ability of the educational institution to adapt to the technological advances in order to facilitate student learning in the rapidly changing environment. Distance education will continue to increase due to the technology driven health care industry and evolving technologies (Jones & Wolf, 2010). With evolving technology found in the health care environment, new and emerging technologies must be incorporated in the distance education environment.

Distance education that is synchronous occurs when the student and learner are interacting at the same time but in different locations. This may occur using videoconferencing, teleconferencing, or instant messaging. The main advantage to synchronous learning is increased communication and decreased travel time. The disadvantages include technological issues and audio functionality (Zsohar & Smith, 2008). The benefits for synchronous instruction are that students and instructors are available at the same time and immediate feedback is available.

Distance education that is asynchronous allows the instructor and student the ability and flexibility to complete learning activities at different times. The students have deadlines to complete assignments. The students have the time to formulate thoughts and ideas, not interrupted by other students, and create records of discussions (Zsohar & Smith, 2008). The disadvantages are that students have no direct contact, have a loss of spontaneity, and have limitations in discussions (Zsohar & Smith,

2008). The main benefit of asynchronous learning is that students are able to complete course work at a time that is convenient to them.

RECOMMENDATIONS

Distance education provides opportunities for students who may not otherwise have an opportunity to obtain a degree. To provide the best opportunity for students, the distance education course or program must consider the learning styles of all students. Faculty must be familiar with multiple media formats that are available. There is a need for current research on emerging technologies to examine if they promote student learning.

Further research should be considered to evaluate the implementation of distant education teaching methodologies. Nursing education should examine the modalities to identify if they are meeting the needs of different learning styles (Mancuso-Murphy, 2007). If students are having difficulty with the online environment there will be high student turnover. Research should also examine student turnover in the distance education environment.

Beaudoin, M. (1990). The instructors' changing role in distance education. *The American Journal of Distance Education, 4*, 2.

Frith, K. (2013). An overview of distance education and online learning. In K. Frith & J. Clark (Eds.), *Distance education in nursing* (pp. 17–31). New York, NY: Springer Publishing.

Jones, D., & Wolf, D. (2010). Shaping the future of nursing education today using distance education and technology. *ABNF Journal, 21*(2), 44–47.

Mancuso-Murphy, J. (2007). Distance education in nursing: An integrated review of online nursing students' experience with technology-delivered instruction. *Journal of Nursing Education, 46*(6), 252–260.

Zerwekh, J. (2011). E-learning defined. In T. Bristol & J. Zerwekh (Eds.), *Essentials for e-learning for nurse educators* (pp. 1–11). Philadelphia, PA: F.A Davis.

Zsohar, H., & Smith, J. (2008). Transition from the classroom to the web: Successful strategies for teaching online. *Nursing Education Perspectives, 29,* 23–28.

Kari L. Luoma

DISTANCE EDUCATION: INTERNATIONAL

DEFINITION

Distance education is a broad term that describes teaching and learning when the student and teacher are separated by time and space. Early forms of distance education included print media (correspondence courses and independent study modules), broadcast television, videoconferencing, and audioconferencing using a dial-up telephone with multiple connecting ports. With the advent of the Internet, online teaching (full web courses or online courses blended with on-site learning experiences) and Internet videoconferencing and webinars (web seminars) have replaced these formats. Emerging technologies such as Second Life (Schmidt & Stewart, 2010) and other virtual excursions and e-simulations follow the basic concepts of distance education by promoting learning just in time regardless of the proximity of the learner and educator. Recently, massively open online courses (MOOCs) are another format for offering nursing content (Billings, 2014).

Distance education offerings can be held *synchronously*, where all members of the learning community are present at the same time by using tools such as the telephone, chat, webinar, or videoconferencing. In *asynchronous* formats, learners and faculty interact independent of time, and communicate through discussion forums, archived video "lectures," blogs, wikis, and other tool components that are provided via a learning management system (LMS). Recent developments in LMSs such as the ability to authenticate the participant and the participant's work, use of software that facilitates peer learning and peer review of participant's work, capabilities for small group work, and language translation capabilities have increased the support for global use of distance education.

APPLICATION

Distance education is used to facilitate access to education for learners who cannot easily travel to the source of instruction, to provide convenience for learners who are working during the time the instruction is offered, and to recruit new learners. Distance education is widely used in nursing education, particularly to offer graduate degrees and certificates, to provide continuing education, orient new staff, and update nurses' competencies in clinical agencies, as well as for client instruction.

Distance education is also used to internationalize learning experiences for nurses. Several examples include the increasing use of MOOCs to attract a diverse and global audience. Online courses and archived webinars can be offered globally with the course content being offered at one site and the clinical experiences and application of course concepts offered worldwide.

SYNOPSIS

One of the biggest issues is the cost involved in offering distance-delivered courses, and particularly those offered at sites that require expensive infrastructure development to participate in course offerings. The costs include purchase or lease of software and hardware, adequate bandwidth to support transmission of images, and technical support to maintain the learning system and user support for course design. Time is also required to orient users to technology and new modes of teaching and learning. The need for resources may be more acute in countries where the requisite infrastructure is not in place.

Teaching at a distance uses specific pedagogical approaches to develop courses and to facilitate them. Faculty orientation is essential as is the allocation of time for faculty to prepare for these changes and design or redesign their course (Johnson & Meehan, 2013).

Reviews of the literature confirm that distance education is effective (Mancuso-Murphy, 2007). *Learning outcomes* of distance-delivered education are the same as those when the instruction is offered on campus (Coose, 2010). Broome, Halstead, Pesut, Rawl, and Boland (2011) found that doctoral programs could be offered at a distance without compromising outcomes. Learners who participate in distance education are *satisfied* with the learning experience, particularly due to the access and convenience of remaining employed in their community while studying at a well-regarded school of nursing miles away (Leners, Wilson, & Sitzman, 2007).

Several nursing and higher education organizations have developed standards, guidelines, and peer review processes for offering quality distance-delivered courses and programs: The Alliance for Nursing's *Accreditation Statement on Distance Education Policies* (American Association of Colleges of Nursing, 2005), and the Sloan Consortium (Moore, 2011). Quality indicators include having standards comparable to those on the campus including faculty qualifications, ongoing assessment and evaluation, access to resources, student and faculty support services, and monitoring of student attainment of course and program outcomes. Schools of nursing seeking accreditation for distance education programs should meet the same standards as their on-campus programs and/or demonstrate how the distance-delivered program meets the accreditation standards. *Quality matters* (www.qmprogram.org) is a peer review service offering reviews and recommendations for improving the design of an online course.

RECOMMENDATIONS

Distance education is a proven method for providing access to academic programs and continuing education programs, and will continue to evolve as nursing education becomes more global and learning is internationalized. The following are the recommendations for future development: continue to develop hardware, software, and infrastructure that facilitates international distance education; establish consortia, partnerships, and collaborative relationships to maximize resources for offering programs; foster global awareness and respect for diversity by including a mix of students from different countries and backgrounds; develop new models of international course offerings such as cohort models with an on-site learning facilitator who participates in the course and supervises student's application of course concepts; and increase funding for developing courses with an international focus and promotion of global awareness, networking, and international collaboration.

American Association of Colleges of Nursing. (2005). *Alliance for nursing accreditation statement on distance education policies.* Retrieved from http://www.aacn.nche.edu/Education/disstate.htm

Billings, D. (2014). Understanding massively open online courses. *The Journal of Continuing Education in Nursing, 45*(2), 3–4.

Broome, M., Halstead, J., Pesut, D., Rawl, S., & Boland, D. (2011). Evaluating the outcomes of a distance accessible PhD program. *Journal of Professional Nursing, 27*(2), 69–77.

Coose, C. S. (2010). Distance nursing education in Alaska: A longitudinal study. *Nursing Education Perspectives, 31*(2), 93–96.

Johnson, A., & Meehan, N. (2013). Faculty preparation for teaching online. In K. Frith & D. Clark (Eds.), *Distance education in nursing.* New York, NY: Springer Publishing.

Leners, D. W., Wilson, V. W., & Sitzman, K. L. (2007). Twenty-first century doctoral education: Online with a focus on nursing education. *Nursing Education Perspectives, 28*(6), 332–336.

Mancuso-Murphy, J. (2007). Distance education in nursing: An integrated review of online nursing students' experiences with technology-delivered instruction. *Journal of Nursing Education, 46(6)*, 252–260.

Moore, J. C. (2011). *The Sloan Consortium quality framework and the five pillars.* Retrieved from http://sloanconsortium. org/publications/books/qualityframe-work.pdf

Schmidt, B., & Stewart, S. (2010). Implementing the virtual world of Second Life into community nursing theory and clinical courses. *Nurse Educator, 35(2)*, 74–78.

Western Interstate Commission for Higher Education (WICHE). (2011). Principles of good practice. Retrieved from http://wcet.wiche.edu/wcet/docs/tbd/TbD_PrinciplesofGoodPractice.pdf

Diane M. Billings

DOCTOR OF NURSING PRACTICE

DEFINITION

Doctor of nursing practice (DNP) is defined by the American Association of Colleges of Nursing (AACN) as the terminal academic degree for nursing practice (AACN, 2006, p. 8).

APPLICATION

Enrollment of DNP students has increased to 95% from 2006 to 2011 (Eglehart, 2013, p. 1937). Graduates of the DNP program are expert clinicians who can assess evidence and translate it into practice (Reed & Crawford, 2011, p. 37). The rapidly changing health care system requires the DNP student to be educated in leadership, client-centered care, quality improvement, multidisciplinary care provision, scientific inquiry, and evidence-based care (AACN, 2006, p. 6). The goal of DNP programs is to educate advanced practice nurses to be academic leaders and educators who also maintain a clinical practice, thereby bridging the gap between nursing education and nursing practice (DNP; Mason, Leavitt, & Chaffee, 2012). The DNP graduate is expected to function as a leader, policy maker, clinical expert, researcher, and educator (Mason et al., 2012).

AACN delineated *The Essentials for Doctoral Education for Advanced Nursing Practice* in 2006. There are 13 essentials: 8 apply to all DNPs and 5 define specialty roles of advanced practice. One thousand postbaccalaureate clinical hours also are recommended (AACN, 2006).

SYNOPSIS

In 2002, the AACN established a task force to evaluate the practice-focused doctorate degree to meet the need for curriculum changes. In 2004, the AACN voted that the educational requirement for advanced practice nurses be at the doctoral level by 2015. A task force was established for creating guidelines for curriculum, and in 2006, *The Essentials for Doctoral Education for Advanced Nursing Practice* was adopted and nursing education began its transformation.

RECOMMENDATIONS

AACN recommends that educational institutions offering DNP programs should have faculty with doctoral preparation once there is a larger population of DNP-prepared nurses. DNP-prepared faculty, through their practice experience, will exemplify rapid translation of new knowledge into practice and demonstrate to students the process of knowledge dissemination (AACN, 2006, p. 21). Nursing education will continue to evolve as the health care system changes with the continued implementation of the Affordable Health Care Act. DNP leaders need to continue to pursue policies that remove practice barriers, and allow the DNP graduates to practice to the full extent of their preparation (Glazer & Fitzpatrick, 2013)

American Association of Colleges of Nursing (AACN). (2006). *The essentials for doctoral education for advanced nursing practice.* Retrieved from http://www.aacn.nche.edu/publications/position/DNPEssentials.pdf

Eglehart, J. (2013). Expanding the role of advanced nurse practitioners' risks and rewards. *The New England Journal of Medicine, 368*(20), 195.

Glazer, G., & Fitzpatrick, J. (Eds.). (2013). Introduction. *Nursing leadership from the outside in* (pp. 1–5). New York, NY: Springer Publishing.

Mason, D. J., Leavitt, J. K., & Chaffee, M. W. (2012). *Policy & politics in nursing and healthcare* (6th ed.). St. Louis, MO: Elsevier.

Reed, P., & Crawford, N. (2011). *Nursing knowledge and theory innovation: Advancing the science of practice.* New York, NY: Springer Publishing.

Therese Hulme

E

ELECTRONIC HEALTH RECORD

DEFINITION

Traditionally, patients' health records were paper based, and nursing students learned documentation skills by entering information under the supervision of the clinical faculty (Baillie, Chadwick, Mann, & Brooke-Read, 2013). The move to electronic-based health records was legislated in the United States in the Health Information Technology for Economic and Clinical Health Act (2009). According to this legislation, a qualified electronic health record (EHR) includes patient demographic and clinical health information, such as medical history and problem lists, and has the capacity to support clinical decisions; support physician order entry; capture and query information relevant to health care quality; and exchange electronic health information with, and integrate such information from, other sources. The goal of the federal legislation was to have an EHR used for each person in the United States by 2014. Nursing students need information about different EHR systems including their strengths and limitations in accessing essential information at the point of care, communicating across disciplines and settings, coordinating care, and guiding patients through the many transitions that comprise the health care experience (Mahon, Nickitas, & Nokes, 2010). Some nursing education programs are purchasing academic EHRs that have the characteristics of a qualified EHR along with an educational component that enables assessment of the student's documentation and feedback to the student through comments and grading in the electronic format (Hanson, 2013).

APPLICATION

There are many EHRs being developed and sold in the health care marketplace. As nursing students rotate through different clinical sites during their educational program, they are exposed to different EHR systems; however, there are a number of barriers that impact on whether students are able to document using the clinical agency's EHR. Rather than being given opportunities to experience in simulated settings the mistakes and frustrations inherent in using EHRs, health professional students often embark on a haphazard and variable learning curve in patient care settings, where their EHR education is directed by faculty with differing skill levels (Milano, Hardman, Plesiu, Rdesinski, & Biagioli, 2014).

Educators have responded to the need for students to have electronic documentation skills by using academic EHR during simulation experiences that encourage critical thinking while allowing for error. Vendors supplying academic EHR include SimChart by Elsevier, Neehr Perfect®, and Cerner's Academic Education Solution (AES). Borycki, Joe, Armstrong, Bellwood, and Campbell (2011) described an open-source system, the University of Victoria Interdisciplinary Electronic Health Record Educational Portal, which allows access to a number of EHR systems for health professional students. Anest (2013) described how pre-licensure nursing students were taught medication administration using barcode technology, while interprofessional students (pharmacy, nursing, physical therapy, and physician assistant) used the MEDITECH software package (Medical Information Technology, Inc., Westwood, MA) to simulate the medication administration and documentation (Kirwin,

DiVall, Guerra, & Brown, 2013). Meyer, Sternberger, and Toscos (2011) described experiences with AES, while, to avoid the cost associated with purchasing an EHR system, Rubbelke, Keenan, and Haycraft (2014) used Google Drive, a cloud storage device that stores documents and can be synced with a free Google account. Another strategy that faculty have used is to partner with the EHR system used in the clinical setting in order to have access to the same EHR system for student practice.

SYNOPSIS

The transition from paper-based record to EHRs is a worldwide phenomenon. Use of EHR has been associated with better care coordination, continuous access to evidence, information exchange between providers, and improved client engagement in health and self-care processes (Topaz, Rao, Creber, & Bowles, 2013). The cost of using an academic EHR has been estimated to be at an expense to each student of at least US$35 to US$49 per semester (Rubbelke, Keenan, & Haycraft, 2014). Not only do faculty need to learn skills associated with using EHR, they need to communicate these skills to students who are novices in clinical practice.

RECOMMENDATIONS

Nursing faculty and students must develop competence in EHR documentation skills and establish clear systems for authorized access so that students can document during clinical placements (Baillie et al., 2013).

Health professional educational programs should collaborate as they choose academic EHR systems and develop curricula modules so that not only documentation skills are taught but also the importance of communication between members of the health care team.

Anest, R. (2013). Teaching patient safety with a functional electronic medication record. *Journal of Nursing Education, 52*(5), 303.

Baillie, L., Chadwick, S., Mann, R., & Brooke-Read, M. (2013). A survey of student nurses' and midwives' experiences of learning to use electronic health record systems in practice. *Nurse Education in Practice, 13*(5), 437–441.

Borycki, E., Joe, R., Armstrong, B., Bellwood, P., & Campbell, R. (2011). Educating health professionals about the electronic health record (EHR): Removing the barriers to adoption. *Knowledge Management & E-Learning: An International Journal, 3*(1), 51–62.

Hanson, D. (2013). *Nurse educators' consensus opinion on using an academic electronic health record: A Delphi study* (doctoral dissertation). The University of North Dakota. Retrieved from http://gateway.proquest.com/openurl%3furl_ver=Z39.88–2004%26res_dat=xri:pqdiss%26rft_val_fmt=info:ofi/fmt:kev:mtx:dissertation%26rft_dat=xri:pqdiss:3596698

Health Information Technology for Economic and Clinical Health Act. (2009). Retrieved from http://www.healthit.gov/sites/default/files/hitech_act_excerpt_from_arra_with_index.pdf, 112–164

Hoyt, R., Adler, K., Ziesemer, B., & Palombo, G. (2013). Evaluating the usability of a free electronic health record for training. *Perspectives in Health Information Management, 10*(Spring), 1b. Published online April 1, 2013.

Kirwin, J., DiVall, M., Guerra, C., & Brown, T. (2013). A simulated hospital pharmacy module using an electronic medical record in a pharmaceutical care skills laboratory course. *American Journal of Pharmaceutical Education, 77*(3). Article 62. doi:10.5688/ajpe77362

Mahon, P., Nickitas, D., & Nokes, K. (2010). Faculty perceptions of student documentation skills during the transition from paper-based to electronic health records systems. *Journal of Nursing Education, 49*(11), 615–621.

Meyer, L., Sternberger, C., & Toscos, T. (2011). How to implement the electronic health record in undergraduate nursing education. *American Nurse Today,* 6(5), 40–44.

Milano, C., Hardman, J., Plesiu, A., Rdesinski, R., & Biagioli, F. (2014). Simulated Electronic Health Record (Sim-EHR) curriculum: Teaching EHR skills and use of the EHR for disease management and prevention. *Academic Medicine, 89*(3), 399–403.

Rubbelke, C. S., Keenan, S. C., & Haycraft, L. L. (2014). An interactive simulated electronic health record using Google drive. *CIN: Computers, Informatics, Nursing, 32*(1), 1–6.

Topaz, M., Rao, A., Creber, R., & Bowles, K. (2013). Educating clinicians on new elements incorporated into the Electronic Health Record: Theories, evidence, and one educational project. *CIN: Computers, Informatics, Nursing, 31*(8), 375–379.

Kathleen M. Nokes

EMOTIONAL INTELLIGENCE

DEFINITION

Emotional intelligence (EI) is the ability to perceive and understand one's own and others' emotions and use this information to guide one's thinking and actions (Salovey & Mayer, 1990).

APPLICATION

EI is integral to every interaction nurses have with patients and families. In order to provide compassionate and quality care, nurses need to have the skills to understand, interpret, manage, and respond to not only their own emotions, but to emotions of patients and families. Research indicates that EI skills and knowledge can be increased with training (Chang, 2007). Thus, information about EI needs to be well integrated into every aspect of nursing education; it should not be an addendum, a learning module, or a didactic class.

Freshwater and Stickley (2004) described transformatory learning as an effective teaching strategy to increase EI skills in part because this approach actively involves learners in critical reflection and discussion to question assumptions. This model involves reflective learning experiences such as journal writing, which enhances self-awareness; interpersonal understanding; critical analysis; cognitive learning; and clinical reasoning skills. The process of journal writing allows students to reflect on attitudes and feelings, and expand the cognitive and affective dimension of learning. Other examples of this type of learning include using the arts like drama, art, poetry, and music to express nursing students' experiences. These expressive modalities demonstrate the notion of caring in a creative way.

The Carnegie Foundation for the Advancement of Teaching is calling for changes in how nurses are educated. One of the recommendations includes using active learning strategies such as case studies. Case studies are more effective than traditional lectures because they show nursing students the ways of using nursing science and knowledge to solve patient problems. The clinical setting provides a perfect opportunity for students to present case studies in postconference discussions following clinical experiences. This format gives faculty an opportunity to not only link theory and practice but also enhances EI skills of students.

Role modeling and mentoring by faculty are imperative to foster development and growth of nurses' EI skills. Faculty must possess these EI skills themselves in order to develop their students' EI skills. Enhancing EI skills among nurses enables them to create a caring environment and implement effective coping strategies when faced with stressful situations (Evans & Allen, 2002).

Hospitals are beginning to implement health and well-being programs for staff in an attempt to help employees improve and maintain their health and overall well-being. One New York hospital is engaging employees in their own well-being and supporting them in achieving individual health goals. This hospital is offering innovative, integrated, and easily accessible programs to

E

foster employee health and well-being such as meditation classes, relaxation techniques, cooking tips, blood pressure screening, and walking clubs. The goal is to create a culture of caring, health, and well-being in the workplace. This approach might work well in other settings as well.

SYNOPSIS

Three main theories regarding EI are addressed in the literature: the *ability model*, the *trait model*, and the *mixed model*. The *ability model* was developed by Salovey and Mayer, who introduced the term "EI" into mainstream American psychology in their landmark article "Emotional intelligence." This model identified four factors of EI: perceiving emotion, reasoning with emotion, understanding emotion, and managing emotion. In addition, Salovey and Mayer developed the Mayer–Salovey–Caruso Emotional Intelligence Test (MSCEIT) to measure EI.

The *trait model* is defined as a constellation of self-perceptions located at the lower levels of personality hierarchies (Petrides, Pita, & Kokkinaki, 2007). This model is the self-perceived ability to identify, assess, and control the emotions of oneself, of others, and of groups.

The *mixed model* was introduced by Goleman (1995) in his book, *Emotional Intelligence: Why It Can Matter More Than IQ*. Goleman argued that the current definition of human intelligence was far too narrow and showed that people with high IQs were not necessarily successful. Goleman proposed that emotional factors such as self-awareness, self-discipline, and empathy contributed to a different way of being smart. He indicated that the previous factors are not fixed at birth; they are shaped by childhood experiences and can be nurtured and shaped throughout adulthood with immediate benefits to health, relationships, and work.

According to Goleman, EI consists of five attributes: self-awareness, self-regulation, motivation, social awareness, and relationship management. The first attribute, *self-awareness*, is the ability to have insight into one's emotions, strengths, and weaknesses and to see how one's feelings affect others. *Self-regulation*, the second attribute, involves controlling one's impulses and not making judgments until enough information is gathered. People with a high degree of self-regulation are more capable of facing change. The third attribute, *motivation*, can be described as passion, a quest for challenges, a desire to learn, and pride in one's work. People who are motivated actively search for solutions to problems and pursue goals with energy and commitment. Highly motivated people consistently raise performance expectations for themselves, their team, and their organization. *Social awareness*, the fourth attribute, is the ability to understand others' feelings and emotions when making decisions. People with empathy have acute organizational awareness, possess a service orientation, and are attentive to others. The final attribute, *relationship management*, involves the ability to manage and forge relationships with others (Goleman, 1998).

There has been a vast amount of research on EI outside of nursing. Articles and books have touted the relationship between successful business leaders and high levels of EI. Akerjordet and Severinsson (2008) found that nurses who displayed high EI enhanced organizational, staff, and patient outcomes.

RECOMMENDATIONS

Nursing's newest generation learns differently. Millennials (those born after 1981) prefer interactive activities and are most comfortable with technology and multitasking. Journaling, postconference discussions, blogging, and posting questions and instructing students to respond through creating threads on an electronic platform are ways for the faculty to learn more about students and the talents the students bring to the learning environment. Discussions between faculty and students about prior life experiences in an authentic manner build a trusting relationship and enable faculty to be viewed more as coaches/mentors than teachers.

EI is important for nurses because most of what they do is interact with others (e.g., patients, families, multidisciplinary team) in environments filled with stress and change. The ability to manage one's own emotions and interpret a patient's emotions to a situation is an integral piece of true patient-centered care. Therefore, attention needs to focus on implementing strategies whereby nurses enhance their coping mechanisms so they can provide compassionate and quality care.

There is a need for current research to target studies on EI, particularly in relation to new knowledge about enhancing EI skills among nursing students. As nursing education research expands, this topic is a promising area for scholarly inquiry.

Akerjordet, K., & Severinsson, E. (2008). Emotionally intelligent nurse leadership: Literature review study. *The Journal of Nursing Management, 16*(5), 65–77.

Chang, K. B. T. (2007). Can we teach emotional intelligence? Dissertation Abstracts International Section A. *Humanities and Social Sciences, 67*(12-A), 4451.

Evans, D., & Allen, A. (2002). Emotional intelligence: Its role in training. *Nursing Times, 98*(27), 41–42.

Freshwater, D., & Stickley, T. (2004). The heart of the art: Emotional intelligence in nursing. *Nursing Inquiry, 2011*(2), 91–98.

Goleman, D. (1995). *Emotional intelligence: Why it can matter more than IQ.* New York, NY: Bantam.

Goleman, D. (1998). *Working with emotional intelligence.* New York, NY: Bantam Publishing.

Petrides, K. V., Pita, R., & Kokkinaki, F. (2007). The location of trait emotional intelligence in personality faculty space. *British Journal of Psychology, 98*, 273–289.

Salovey, P., & Mayer, J. D. (1990). Emotional intelligence. *Imagination, Cognition and Personality, 9*(3), 185–211.

Patricia Prufeta
Lauraine Spano-Szekely

EMPOWERMENT

DEFINITION

Spreitzer (1995) defines empowerment as an interpersonal factor that involves motivational and cognitive processes such as finding meaning in one's role, feeling self-efficacious to engage in the role, perceiving oneself as self-determined, and feeling as though one's contributions to the work environment have an impact. Conger and Kanungo (1988) defined empowerment as a motivational construct where individuals engage in behaviors that enable or enhance another person's belief in their abilities to achieve goals, engage in decision making, find meaning in their work, and work with a sense of autonomy within bureaucratic constraints. Bradbury-Jones, Sambrook, and Irvine (2007) define student empowerment in the practice setting as being envisioned on a continuum of more or less empowerment in terms of feeling understood, being respected and included, and being encouraged to learn. However, empowerment results from mentorship, placement continuity, and sufficient and quality time in practice. When these antecedents are available, then student outcomes can include strong self-esteem, a drive for learning, and an interest in the placement setting (Bradbury-Jones, Sambrook, & Irvine, 2007). This definition of empowerment evolved to being composed of knowledge and confidence as core structures, with influencing extrinsic spheres (such as being valued as a team member, learner, and person; having a supportive mentor; practicing in a placement that included a positive culture; and social and political factors that enabled empowerment to occur) impacting students' development of empowerment (Bradbury-Jones, Irvine, & Sambrook, 2010).

APPLICATION

Studies with nurses and nurse managers in the practice context have been linked to

E

psychological empowerment, decreased incivility and burnout (Laschinger, Grau, Finegan, & Wilk, 2010); increased organizational citizenship (Gilbert, Laschinger, & Leiter, 2010); increased recruitment and retention (Laschinger, Leiter, Day, & Gilin, 2009); and patient satisfaction (Purdy, Laschinger, Finegan, Kerr, & Olivera, 2010). Clinical instructor and student empowerment have been associated with student self-efficacy in acute care settings (Babenko-Mould, Iwasiw, Andrusyszyn, Laschinger, & Weston, 2012). Structural empowerment was associated with psychological empowerment among students in a problem-based learning program; psychological empowerment was positively associated with mentoring quality and job satisfaction and negatively related to job stress among nursing faculty (Chung & Kowalski, 2012). Empowerment was positively associated with teachers' perceptions of their own use of empowering teaching behaviors and students' perceptions of those same behaviors (Babenko-Mould et al., 2012). Student empowerment was evident when practice environments consisted of a positive culture and where mentoring relationships supported students' knowledge and confidence (Bradbury-Jones et al., 2010).

SYNOPSIS

A foundational concept analysis of the term *empowerment* has resulted in the term being conceptualized from an organizational, personal development, and emancipatory perspective (Kuokkanen & Leino-Kilpi, 2000, 2007). According to Kanter's (1977, 1993) theory of structural power in organizations, power relates to an individual's ability to achieve goals by mobilizing human and material resources. To do so, individuals need to have informal and formal power (Kanter, 1993). Informal power results from connections in the organization such as peers, employees, and mentors. Formal power is developed as a result of being engaged in a role that provides autonomy and flexibility to support feelings

of being central and relevant to the organization. When individuals have formal and informal power, they are more likely to have access to empowering structures to help them achieve organizational goals. The structures include supports, resources, information, and opportunities to develop and learn.

Research findings demonstrate that empowerment has been applied to student and faculty populations in both the classroom- and practice-based context. Empowerment has been assessed from the organizational, personal development, and emancipatory perspectives. Empowerment of self and others intersects among social, cultural, and political factors and appears to be instrumental in student professional development as well as a possible influencing factor in nurse educators' intentions to remain in the role.

RECOMMENDATIONS

Educators and students need to have a strong sense of empowerment, including how empowerment impacts practice and learning processes. When nurse educators develop and implement empowering teaching behaviors, students tend to envision that person as a role model and incorporate those behaviors in a similar way of being into their own sense of self as a soon-to-be nurse (Babenko-Mould et al., 2012). Integrating the concept of empowerment into nursing education could support the enactment of empowerment as a core element of practice in academic and in professional practice settings.

Babenko-Mould, Y., Iwasiw, C., Andrusyszyn, M. A., Laschinger, H. K. S., & Weston, W. (2012). Effects of clinical practice environments on clinical teacher and nursing student outcomes. *Journal of Nursing Education, 51*(4), 217–225. doi:10.3928/01484834–20120323-06

Bradbury-Jones, C., Irvine, F., & Sambrook, S. (2010). Empowerment of nursing students in clinical practice: Spheres of influence.

Journal of Advanced Nursing, 66(9), 2061–2070. doi:10.1111/j.1365–2648.2010.05351.x

Bradbury-Jones, C., Sambrook, S., & Irvine, F. (2007). The meaning of empowerment for nursing students: A critical incident study. *Journal of Advanced Nursing, 59*(4), 342–351. doi:10.1111/j.1365–2648.2007.04331.x

Chung, C., & Kowalski, S. (2012). Job stress, mentoring, psychological empowerment, and job satisfaction among nursing faculty. *Journal of Nursing Education, 51*(7), 381–388. doi:10.3928/01484834–20120509-03

Conger, J. A., & Kanungo, R. N. (1988). The empowerment process: Integrating theory and practice. *Academy of Management Review, 13,* 471–482.

Gilbert, S., Laschinger, H. K. S., & Leiter, M. (2010). The mediating effect of burnout on the relationship between structural empowerment and organizational citizenship behaviours. *Journal of Nursing Management, 18,* 339–348. doi:10.1111/j.1365–2834.2010.01074.x

Kanter, R. M. (1977). *Men and women of the corporation.* New York, NY: Basic Books.

Kanter, R. M. (1993). *Men and women of the corporation* (2nd ed.). New York: NY: Basic Books.

Kuokkanen, L., & Leino-Kilpi, H. (2000). Power and empowerment in nursing: Three theoretical approaches. *Journal of Advanced Nursing, 31,* 235–241.

Kuokkanen, L., & Leino-Kilpi, H. (2007). Organizational change and work related empowerment. *Journal of Nursing Management, 15,* 500–507.

Laschinger, H. K. S., Grau, A., Finegan, J., & Wilk, P. (2010). New graduate nurses' experiences of bullying and burnout in hospital settings. *Journal of Advanced Nursing, 66*(12), 2732–2742. doi:10.1111/j.1365–2648.2010.05420x

Laschinger, H. K. S., Leiter, M., Day, A., & Gilin, D. (2009). Workplace empowerment, incivility, and burnout: Impact on staff nurse recruitment and retention outcomes. *Journal of Nursing Management, 17,* 302–311. doi:10.1111/j.1365–2834.2009.00999.x

Purdy, N., Laschinger, H. K. S., Finegan, J., Kerr, M., & Olivera, F. (2010). Effects of work environments on nurse and patient outcomes. *Journal of Nursing Management, 18,* 901–913. doi:10.1111/j.1365–2834.2010.01172x

Spreitzer, G. M. (1995). An empirical test of a comprehensive model of intrapersonal empowerment in the workplace. *American Journal of Community Psychology, 23*(5), 601–629.

Yolanda Babenko-Mould

ENGAGEMENT

DEFINITION

Engagement is the way in which people feel connected in a strongly positive manner. The term can also be defined by types of people and work settings where there is an ongoing positive feeling. Faculty are expected to be committed to engagement in order to help students attain the goals of learning and be prepared as professional nurses who work directly with patients and other staff.

The Center for Advancing Health (2010, p. 2) defines engagement from the patient perspective as "actions individuals must take to obtain the greatest benefit from the health care services available to them." This definition can also be applied to engagement of professional nurses, nurse educators, and student learners. The Commission on Community-Engaged Scholarship in the Healthcare Professions (n.d.) defines community engagement as "the application of institutional resources to address and solve challenges facing communities through collaboration with these communities" (p. 12).

APPLICATION

Several studies have focused on work engagement in Magnet hospitals. Nurses who work in Magnet hospitals are more engaged than those who work in non-Magnet organizations.

E

Highly engaged nurses are described as more effective than disengaged nurses. In addition, engaged nurses have a good relationship with nursing management, a supportive work environment, a sense of empowerment, and a good work–life balance. Furthermore, they participate in decision making and professional development (Carter & Tourangeau, 2012; Fasoli, 2010) as engaged practitioners.

Factors contributing to the perception of engagement nurses have in the workplace are workload, control, reward, fairness, community, and value. Positive practice environments that influence engagement were found to have the following aspects: an empowering work environment; a shared governance structure; leadership support; adequate numbers and skill mix of staff; and value autonomy, professional development, and collegial relationships (Twigg & McCullough, 2014).

Palmer, Griffin, Reed, and Fitzpatrick (2010) studied a group of acute care nurses and found that engagement associated positively with self-transcendence. Thus, when nurses are fully engaged in their personal and professional lives, it can be concluded that their growth, development, and becoming as a person will be enhanced. In another study, a significant determinant of feeling engaged was the perception that one's work is important (Rivera, Fitzpatrick, & Boyle, 2011). Therefore, the experience of being engaged in one's work is when one finds meaning in his or her work.

SYNOPSIS

Engagement is a complex concept that has a variety of meanings from various perspectives. Reports of literature in nursing and other fields indicate a relationship between productivity and engagement, such that the more engaged—the more productive. Practices defined in a document by the American Organizations of Nurse Executives provide the underpinnings of an environment where nurses experience self as being engaged to the fullest. The practices are collaboration, accountability, shared decision making, competent leadership, qualified nurses, expert practitioners, and recognition of the value of nursing's meaningful contribution to practice.

Recommendations from the Institute of Medicine's (IOM) *The Future of Nursing* (2010) have compelled schools of nursing to redesign undergraduate nursing curricula to include judgment, inquiry, engagement, and voice (D'Antonio, Brennan, & Curley, 2013). In their work, *Educating Nurses: A Call for Radical Transformation*, Benner, Sutphen, Leonard, and Day (2010) described an urgent need to restructure nursing curricula so they actively engage learners and promote clinical reasoning. Engaging students in the classroom and clinical setting allows students to envision themselves as nurses. Activities that foster student engagement in interprofessional collaboration and communication in practice settings help students to develop confidence levels. Strategies to facilitate student and new graduate nurse engagement in interprofessional collaboration suggest better patient outcomes (Pfaff, Baxter, Jack, & Ploeg, 2013; Pollard, 2009).

RECOMMENDATIONS

Learners, faculty, direct care nurses, advanced practice nurses, and nurse leaders have the opportunity and the obligation to work to improve places where nurses work, with the goal of well-engaged nurses. Although little research has been done in nursing and health care as compared to some other fields, gaining an increased understanding of engagement can lead to professional maturity.

Benner, P., Sutphen, M., Leonard, V., & Day, L. (2010). *Educating nurses: A call for radical transformation*. San Francisco, CA: Jossey Bass.

Carter, M. R., & Tourangeau, A. E. (2012). Staying in nursing: What factors determine whether nurses intend to remain employed? *Journal of Advanced Nursing*, *68*(7), 1589–1600.

Commission on Community-Engaged Scholarship in the Healthcare Professions. (n.d.). *Linking scholarship and communities.* Retrieved from http://depts.washington .edu/ccph/pdf_files/Commission%20 Report%20FINAL.pdf

D'Antonio, P. O., Brennan, A. M., & Curley, M. (2013). Judgment, inquiry, engagement, voice: Reenvisioning an undergraduate nursing curriculum using a shared decision-making model. *Journal of Professional Nursing, 29*(6), 407–423.

Fasoli, D. R. (2010). The culture of nursing engagement: A historical perspective. *Journal of Nursing Administration Quarterly, 34*(1), 18–29.

Freeney, Y. M., & Tiernan, J. (2009). Exploration of the facilitators of and barriers to work engagement in nursing. *International Journal of Nursing Studies, 46*(12), 1557–1565.

Institute of Medicine. (2010). *The future of nursing: Leading change, advancing health.* Washington, DC: National Academies Press.

Palmer, B., Griffin, M. T. Q., Reed, P., & Fitzpatrick, J. J. (2010). Self-transcendence and work engagement in acute care staff registered nurses. *Critical Care Nursing Quarterly, 33*(2), 138–147.

Pfaff, K., Baxter, P., Jack, S., & Ploeg, J. (2013). An integrative review of the factors influencing new graduate nurse engagement in interprofessional collaboration. *Journal of Advanced Nursing, 70*(1), 4–20.

Pollard, K. (2009). Student engagement in interprofessional working in practice placement settings. *Journal of Clinical Nursing, 18,* 2846–2856. doi:10.111/j.1365–2702.2008.02608.x

Rivera, R. R., Fitzpatrick, J. J., & Boyle, S. M. (2011). Nurse outcomes in Magnet and non-Magnet hospitals. *Journal of Nursing Administration, 41*(6), 265–272. doi:10.1097NNA.0b013e31821c476c

Twigg, D., & McCullough, K. (2014). Nurse retention: A review of strategies to create and enhance positive practice environments in clinical settings. *International Journal of Nursing Studies, 51*(1), 85–92. doi:10.1016/j.ijnurstu.2013.05.015

Patricia S. Yoder-Wise
Kathryn S. Whitcomb

ENGLISH AS A SECOND LANGUAGE

DEFINITION

English as a second language (ESL) students are defined as students who attend grade school outside the United States and use language other than English on a daily basis (Scheele, Pruitt, Johnson, & Xu, 2011). ESL nursing students are a subpopulation group of minority students who are bilingual and immigrant with different cultural backgrounds.

APPLICATION

Ability to communicate effectively with classmates and faculty members is essential to achieve academic success in demanding and rigorous nursing programs. In order to enroll in nursing programs, international students are required to demonstrate sufficient English skills by tests such as the Test of English as a Foreign Language (TOEFL), or International English Language Testing System (IELTS), which are expected to be an indicator of academic success. In order to help these students, some schools recommend that international students take an extra ESL course or Basic English literature course before entering the nursing program. However, even with successful completion of these various English screening tools, researchers have found that ESL nursing students still tend to have more difficulty not only with general aspects of English but also with lack of fluency in scholastic English. This contributes to difficulty in academic performance because nursing requires a higher level of cognitive language than conversational English (Salamonson,

E

Andrew, Clauson, & Cleary, 2011). High dropout rates for ESL students have been reported. Lower passing rates on National Council Licensure Examination (NCLEX) have also been reported; the passing rate was 21% lower than that of native speakers (Choi, 2005; Olson, 2012).

It is important to address potential challenges that ESL nursing students have during academic years. ESL students encounter many problems that native English speakers do not such as reading assignment, class discussion, group projects, academic writing, and written tests.

In general, faculty members use the universal teaching methods for all students regardless of racially and ethnically diverse nursing student needs, and fail to recognize learning barriers for this unique student population. Writing notes while trying to comprehend lecture with large volumes of information is extremely challenging in a second language. ESL students tend not to ask questions or participate in discussion due to self-consciousness about their English skills or fear of failing to communicate (Olson, 2012). ESL nursing students also have challenges in completing group projects. Often ESL students are viewed as slow or submissive learners to other students and it becomes an obstacle for ESL students to find a group. ESL students tend to formulate their own small group, which may not be helpful to utilize or share resources from English-speaking students.

In the clinical setting, ESL nursing students reported facing difficulty with understanding medical terminology and abbreviations. Researchers also found that ESL nursing students experienced language difficulty with patients, family, nursing staff, and other health care providers including introducing themselves, initiating daily conversation, and interacting with other nursing staff to report clinical findings or concerns (Rogan & San Miguel, 2013). Communicating with faculty members or classmates by e-mail potentially increases misunderstanding for ESL students due to limited information, inappropriate vocabulary use, or misinterpretation of the sentences and tones.

SYNOPSIS

The ability to speak languages other than English certainly has various benefits. Several researchers have reported better compliance rates and patient outcomes when care is delivered in the patient's own language (Olson, 2012). Admitting students who are culturally and linguistically diverse in nursing programs can maximize the goal of better patient care, patient satisfaction, and outcomes with current rapid demographic change in patient population and increasing complexity of care (Choi, 2005).

Students with ESL backgrounds require a higher level of support to achieve academically during their nursing program and meet the expected level during clinical experience (Boughton, Halliday, & Brown, 2010). A number of effective teaching strategies for ESL nursing students have been proposed although current literature on the effectiveness of support or educational needs for ESL students is limited.

Early identification of students who have difficulty in class and referring them to early intervention such as a writing center, additional English courses, and language support program or peer tutoring may contribute to successful program completion. Mentorship programs driven by faculty members and international students from the same native country or in nursing programs, which included one-on-one interaction, group meetings, and student support groups, showed some promise (Choi, 2005; Condrey & Derico, 2012; Salamonson et al., 2011).

Formulating mixed study groups with ESL and native speakers showed improvement for building language skills, offering clarification, and sharing information. On the other hand, study groups among ESL nursing students showed a negative impact on their academic performance by making persistent errors in English and sharing incorrect information (Brown, 2008).

Faculty members may provide summarization of the lectures at the end of the class, facilitate cognitively demanding questions, and encourage questions from ESL students. Faculty also may implement various test methods to help ESL nursing students such as teaching test-taking strategies, reducing language complexity of multiple-choice test questions, and giving a test review.

Having students bring regional food dishes and wear their native country clothing for a "Culture Day" or "International Student Committee" meeting helps the students to reduce cultural shock, and provides an opportunity to share understandings of cultural aspects to faculty members and other students.

RECOMMENDATIONS

As the number of ESL students is growing, there is a concern regarding the lack of understanding of ESL students and their cultures. The important component of providing culturally sensitive care is effective use of language. In order to meet patients' cultural needs and diversity, it is important to prepare nursing students with ESL backgrounds to achieve their academic goals and successfully complete nursing programs.

There is limited research on education of students with an ESL background focused on challenges faced by students and faculties. There is a need for research evaluating effectiveness of various support systems for ELS students. It would be interesting to see how ESL students from different cultural backgrounds present unique educational needs and language barriers.

Boughton, M., Halliday, L., & Brown, L. (2010). A tailored program support for culturally and linguistically diverse (CALD) nursing students in a graduate entry masters of nursing course: A qualitative evaluation of outcomes. *Nurse Education in Practice, 10*(6), 355–360.

Brown, J. (2008). Developing English as a second language program for foreign born nursing students at a historically Black university in the United States. *Journal of Transcultural Nursing, 19*(2), 184–191.

Choi, L. (2005). Literature review: Issues surrounding education of English as second language (ESL) nursing students. *Journal of Transcultural Nursing, 16*(3), 263–268.

Condrey, T., & Derico, S. (2012). Strategies for success for English as second language (ESL) students in the post-secondary setting. *A Journal of the College of Education & Health Professions, 13*(1), 17–21.

Crawford, T., & Candlin, S. (2013). A literature review of the language needs of nursing students who have English as a second/other language and the effectiveness of English language support programs. *Nurse Education in Practice, 13*(3), 181–185.

Olson, M. (2012). English as a second language (ESL) nursing student success: A critical review of the literature. *Journal of Cultural Diversity, 19*(1), 26–32.

Rogan, F., & San Miguel, C. (2013). Improving clinical communication of students with English as a second language (ESL) using online technology: A small scale evaluation study. *Nurse Education in Practice, 13*(5), 400–406.

Salamonson, Y., Andrew, S., Clauson, J., & Cleary, M. (2011). Linguistic diversity as sociodemographic predictor of nursing program progression and completion. *Contemporary Nurse, 38*(1–2), 84–93.

Sanner, S., & Wilson, A. (2008). The experiences of students with English as a second language in a baccalaureate nursing program. *Nurse Education Today, 28*(7), 807–813.

Scheele, T., Pruitt, R., Johnson, A., & Xu, Y. (2011). What do we know about educating Asian ESL nursing student? A literature review. *Nursing Education Perspectives, 32*(4), 244–249.

Seatbyul Diane Lee

ePORTFOLIOS

DEFINITION

An ePortfolio is an electronic compilation of professional and career accomplishments, thus providing evidence of expertise. With the explosion of technology and focus on self-learning and development of critical-thinking skills, the ePortfolio has evolved into demonstrating clinical competence and reflective practice that can be measured over time.

APPLICATION

The ePortfolio serves many purposes. One is to supplement or complement the résumé or curriculum vitae (CV) as it details one's career over time. Professional growth is demonstrated overall or in a specific category such as leadership or education, as well as detailing clinical expertise such as critical care or advanced nursing practice competencies (Pincombe, McKellar, Weise, Grinter, & Beresford, 2010). Demonstrating skills and knowledge can support credentialing, certification, or recertification, as well as support employment issues such as securing a professional nursing position serving as an adjunct for a performance review. The ePortfolio has also been used to supplement graduate admissions criteria and can serve as a basis for promotions and awards. More recent applications of the ePortfolio have focused on the development of reflective nursing practice including the assessment of clinical competencies and professional development.

SYNOPSIS

Developing and refining one's ePortfolio is a continuous ongoing process, not a one-time endeavor. The process includes collecting the materials initially wanted in the ePortfolio, reflecting on how the materials best demonstrate the primary purpose or goal of the ePortfolio, selecting the best and most appropriate materials, and then again reflecting on the overall presentation of materials to support the intended goal. The final stage is compiling the ePortfolio and storing it in an appropriate medium or on a website best suited for its purpose. The evaluation–reflection–selection process closes the loop for quality improvement.

Oermann (2002) suggests that there are two types of portfolios, each serving a specific purpose. She identifies these as "best work" and "growth and development." Best work ePortfolios equate to those supplementing the CV or résumé, while the growth and development are more reflective in nature.

The following items should be considered for inclusion in the ePortfolio when they are used to demonstrate professional development (Jones, Sackett, Erdley, & Blyth, 2007): training or education including formal education, in-services, certificates, workshops, and seminars; licensure or certification information; specialized clinical skills; language fluency including sign language; awards and honors; references that may include letters of introduction or recommendation; and scholarly activities such as podium or poster presentations, publications, work on faculty projects, grants, and research studies.

Green, Wyllie, and Jackson (2013) assert that the ePortfolio can be used to assess cognitive, reflective, and affective skills. Garrett, MacPhee, and Jackson (2013) have used the ePortfolio to assess the clinical competence of baccalaureate nursing students. Using a self-reflection process, students were able to self-identify learning needs. Faculty were able to assess and track student progress based on the College of Registered Nurses of British Columbia (CRNBC) entry-to-practice competencies. Summative assessments of students can also be accomplished through the ePortfolio (Hill, 2012; Yanhua & Watson, 2011). These uses of the ePortfolio are predicated on constructivist learning theories (Jonassen, 1991) using experiential learning and the novice to expert model defined by Benner (1984). Reflection on personal experiences not only bridges the gap between knowledge and experience but also includes evaluating the ethics of a situation, personal beliefs and values, and self-evaluating one's personal strengths and challenges.

The ePortfolio is not without its limitations. Jones, Sackett, Erdley, and Blyth (2007) cite the amount of time spent by faculty to review ePortfolios and students' complaints of the labor intensiveness of completing the ePortfolio as barriers to its use. These sentiments were echoed by Bogossian and Kellett (2010) when implementing the ePortfolio within the framework of an actual clinical setting. Support from faculty was also cited as a limitation by Jones et al. (2007). Garrett and Jackson (2006) proposed the use of a mobile clinical ePortfolio that would be directly linked to the student's personal digital assistant (PDA). This would decrease the time for documentation of competencies.

It is important to note that the ePortfolio should be differentiated from the paper portfolio. The ePortfolio needs to be portable in order to facilitate sharing of its contents with prospective employers, graduate admissions committees, faculty, and accreditation bodies. As a most cumbersome process in paper format, the ePortfolio serves an important purpose for students as well as practicing nursing professionals.

RECOMMENDATIONS

The underpinnings of the ePortfolio, such as reflective practice, can help nurses grow both professionally and personally throughout their career. Although the ePortfolio can enhance the self-reflective and critical-thinking process, there are little empirical data to support the effectiveness of the ePortfolio for summative assessments, clinical competence, and its use in reflective practice for undergraduate students, new graduates, and advanced practice nurses. The ePortfolio may also need to be incorporated into different pedagogical approaches in nursing practice in both academic and clinical settings.

Benner, P. (1984). *From novice to expert: Excellence and power in clinical.* Menlo Park, CA: Addison-Wesley.

Bogossian, F., & Kellett, S. (2010). Barriers to electronic portfolio access in the clinical setting. *Nurse Education Today, 30*(8), 768–772.

Garrett, B. M., & Jackson, C. (2006). A mobile clinical e-Portfolio for nursing and medical students, using wireless personal digital assistants (PDAs). *Nurse Education Today, 26*(8), 647–654.

Garrett, B. M., MacPhee, M., & Jackson, C. (2013). Of an ePortfolio for the assessment of clinical competence in a baccalaureate nursing program. *Nurse Education Today, 33*(10), 1207–1213.

Green, J., Wyllie, A., & Jackson, D. (2013). Electronic portfolios in nursing education: A review of the literature. *Nurse Education in Practice, 14*(1), 4–8.

Hill, T. L. (2012). The portfolio as a summative assessment for the nursing student. *Teaching and Learning in Nursing, 7*(4), 140–145.

Jonassen, D. (1991). Evaluating constructivist learning. *Educational Technology, 36*(9), 28–33.

Jones, J. M., Sackett, K., Erdley, W. S., & Blyth, J. B. (2007). ePortfolios in nursing education: Not your mother's resume. *Annual Review of Nursing Education, 5*, 245–258.

Oermann, M. H. (2002). Developing a professional portfolio in nursing. *Orthopaedic Nursing, 21*(2), 73–78.

Pincombe, J., McKellar, l., Weise, M., Grinter, E., & Beresford, G. (2010). ePortfolio in midwifery practice: "The way of the future." *Women and Birth, 23*(3), 94–102.

Yanhua, C., & Watson, R. (2011). A review of clinical competence assessment in nursing. *Nurse Education Today, 31*(8), 832–836.

Janice M. Jones

ETHICAL DECISION MAKING

DEFINITION

Ethics is a systematic approach to understanding, analyzing, and distinguishing

E

right and wrong matters (Beauchamp & Childress, 2013). Ethical decision making is a complex dynamic process where a moral problem is revisited from evolving perspectives as one reasons through the dilemma to reach a resolution (Beauchamp & Childress, 2013; Burkhardt & Nathaniel, 2014).

APPLICATION

Moral issues are present in almost every patient interaction. Moral reasoning plays a key role in ethical decision making, as does the person's cultural background, the organizational environment, practice experience, and knowledge of ethics. Because clinical ethical issues can differ from daily life experiences, norms learned during childhood are insufficient. Through practice, nurses learn over time how to be sensitive enough to identify and address ethical dilemmas. Inability to pursue the right action due to organizational constraints, when one knows it is the morally correct action to take, leads to moral distress, a negative feeling state (Corley, 2002), which can result in burnout. To hone ethical decision-making skills, nurses are encouraged to use reflection to analyze their feelings and difficult situations they encounter. Ethical sensitivity develops as one gains the personal capacity to assess responses and feelings of others and the ability to deal with the ethical conflict (Park, Kjervik, Crandell, & Oermann, 2012).

Numerous models facilitate making ethical decisions, most of which promote a step-by-step analysis of the moral problem. Burkhardt and Nathaniel's (2014) model provides a framework similar to the nursing process that enables nurses to make decisions while requiring ongoing evaluation and assimilation of information. Steps include problem identification, information gathering to clarify issues, exploration of strategies, strategy implementation, and outcome evaluation. Use of such models promotes a systematic method to critically analyze and reflect on the ethical dilemma, but they do not take into account the ethical climate or

the nature of organizational relationships in which situations occur (Hardingham, 2004; Pavlish, Brown-Saltzman, Jakel, & Rounkle, 2012). Complementary teaching methodologies like interprofessional ethics rounds, classroom group reports, or use of case studies in problem-solving teams can foster consideration of others' values and conclusions (Garity, 2009; Robichaux, 2012).

SYNOPSIS

Ethical decision making is complex and described using multiple interchangeable terms that make understanding the process even more complicated. For nursing practice, the American Nurses Association Code of Ethics states that ethics is an integral part of the foundation of nursing and one that is not negotiable in any setting (ANA, 2001). For baccalaureate nursing, the American Association of Colleges of Nurses (AACN, 2008) *Essentials* include two objectives on ethics. These are encouraging use of an ethical framework and the ethical principles of autonomy and justice in relation to ethical conduct and prevention of unethical practices (AACN, 2008). The AACN Essentials of Masters Education for Advanced Practice Nurses, Essential III, objective 1, presses for ethical decision making and analysis of common ethical dilemmas (AACN, 1996). Therefore, nurses receive instruction on bioethical principles in curricula, but research has continuously found nurses to be ill prepared to address ethical dilemmas (Dierckx de Casterle, Izumi, Godfrey, & Denhaerynck, 2008). Laabs (2012) found that advanced practice nurses have a high level of confidence in their ability to manage clinical ethical problems, but their overall knowledge is low. Comrie (2012) found that junior and senior students did not recognize conflict as part of patient care because they believed that they did not confront individual moral issues in daily practice during clinical rotations. Concurrently, new graduates base their clinical actions on individual ethical codes, eventually changing with environmental pressure (Dierckx de Casterle et al., 2008; Ham, 2004).

Most entry-level nursing programs operate in an institutionalized environment. A lone ethics course is provided because the primary focus of baccalaureate education is to instill knowledge and technical competency for students to become generalists and pass the NCLEX. Faculty freely choose how to implement ethical principles in classes, often not having time to develop the student's moral reasoning skills. No guidelines proffer faculty qualifications to teach ethics in comparison to other program requirements.

RECOMMENDATIONS

The ability to make an ethical decision develops over time. A college course on ethics may not suffice to prepare nurses to meet the growing ethical challenges they experience at the bedside and in the workplace. Continuous education of health care personnel, to include faculty, on bioethical principles and ethical decision-making skills in relation to the nurse–patient relationship must occur throughout nursing curricula and as one's career progresses. Special attention to the transition period from graduation to clinical practice, as in a nurse residency, may address moral reasoning lapses. Faculty must also be accomplished in the study of ethics as well as experienced in ethical decision making before being selected to teach an ethics class.

The need for scholarly inquiry on moral reasoning and ethical decision making in multiple areas is vast. Interprofessional team dynamics and identification of forces influencing critical review of patient dilemmas within these teams require study. High-fidelity simulation exercises could be used to discover types of moral issues that may arise during patient care experiences and how ethical decisions are reached among health care personnel.

American Association of Colleges of Nurses (AACN). (1996). *The essentials of masters education for advanced practice nurses.* New York, NY: Author.

American Association of Colleges of Nurses (AACN). (2008). *The essentials of baccalaureate education for professional nursing practice.* New York, NY: Author.

American Nurses Association. (2001). *ANA code of ethics.* Retrieved from http://www.nursingworld.org/codeofethics

Beauchamp, T., & Childress, J. (2013). *Principles of biomedical ethics.* New York, NY: Oxford University Press.

Burkhardt, M., & Nathaniel, A. (2014). *Ethics and issues in contemporary nursing.* Stamford, CT: Cengage.

Comrie, R. (2012). An analysis of undergraduate and graduate student nurses' moral sensitivity. *Nursing Ethics, 19,* 116–127.

Corley, M. C. (2002). Nurse moral distress: A proposed theory and research agenda. *Nursing Ethics, 9,* 636–650.

Dierckx de Casterle, B., Izumi, S., Godfrey, N., & Denhaerynck, K. (2008). Nurses' responses to ethical dilemmas in nursing practice: Meta-analysis. *Journal of Advanced Nursing, 63,* 540–549.

Garity, J. (2009). Fostering nursing students' use of ethical theory and decision making models: Teaching strategies. *Learning in Health and Social Care, 8,* 114–122.

Ham, K. (2004). Principled thinking: A comparison of nursing students and experienced nurses. *Journal of Continuing Education in Nursing, 35,* 66–73.

Hardingham, L. (2004). Integrity and moral residue: Nurses as participants in a moral community. *Nursing Philosophy, 5,* 127–134.

Laabs, C. (2012). Confidence and knowledge regarding ethics among advanced practice nurses. *Nursing Education Perspectives, 33,* 10–14.

Park, M., Kjervik D., Crandell J., & Oermann, M. H. (2012). The relationship of ethics education to moral sensitivity and moral reasoning skills of nursing students. *Nursing Ethics, 19,* 568–580.

Pavlish, C., Brown-Saltzman, K., Jakel, P., & Rounkle, A. M. (2012). Nurses' responses to ethical challenges in oncology practice: An ethnographic study. *Clinical Journal of Oncology Nursing, 16(6),* 592–600.

E

Robichaux, C. (2012). Developing ethical skills: From sensitivity to action. *Critical Care Nurse, 32*, 65–72.

Gina Maiocco

ETHICS

DEFINITION

Early Greek and Roman philosophers examined the idea of a good life and what may be required to live this kind of life. Aristotle identified this good life as one of virtue (Kraut, 2014) and the basis for a form of natural law (Baltzly, 2014) that guides our thoughts and actions. These philosophical theories are the basis for the definition of ethics, the "rules of behavior based on ideas about what is morally good and bad" (Merriam-Webster, 2014), that address right and wrong behaviors. Subsequent ethical schools of thought developed by 18th- and 19th-century philosophers further define morality in reference to rules and consequences. According to Kantian ethics or deontology, the focus is on the duty to act and not on the consequences (Johnson, 2014). Conversely, through theories of utilitarianism or consequentialism, consequences must be considered and are in fact an ultimate concern when defining the ethics of a situation.

APPLICATION

The result of earlier philosophical teachings combined with the technological advances of the 20th century created the field of bioethics addressing ethics in health care. Four major ethical principles—autonomy, beneficence, nonmaleficence, and justice—provide the framework for the study of bioethics (Beauchamp & Childress, 2009). These principles are closely aligned with research codes of ethics such as the Nuremberg Code and the Declaration of Helsinki. These principles also dovetail with nursing professional codes of conduct (International Council of Nursing [ICN], 2012) established a social contract and guideline for ethical practice. Ethics is taught in a variety of formats to undergraduate and graduate nursing students. In the undergraduate study, the focus is often defining the terms, discussing values clarification as a novice nurse, and providing examples of clinical application for future reference. In graduate nursing courses, much of the work may be case based and additional topics include leadership and organizational ethics. Clinically, the issue of ethics in nursing often arises with the identification of an ethical or moral dilemma, a choice between two equally unfavorable options. For example, a hospital inpatient is found unresponsive and without a pulse. The nurses know that the patient's condition was critical, that the patient and her husband discussed her desire for no further treatment, and that do-not-resuscitate (DNR) orders were discussed and agreed on with the family and patient; however, no DNR order exists in the medical record. If the nurses initiate cardio pulmonary resuscitation (CPR), they will be going against the wishes of the patient and the family. If they do not initiate CPR, they are doing so without an order. This places the nurse in an ethical quandary as to how to proceed.

SYNOPSIS

Ethics in nursing education encompasses two broad areas: fostering a climate of professional and academic integrity and providing students with a basic understanding of ethical principles and their application in practice. The first nursing code of ethics dates back to 1950 (ANA, 2005). Throughout its nine provisions, the focus has been on service to others. In 1953, the ICN (2012) developed its code of ethics focusing on four basic responsibilities: the promotion of health, prevention of illness, restoration of health, and alleviation of suffering. These responsibilities apply to four principal elements describing the ethical conduct of care: nurses and people, practice, profession, and coworkers. Although both codes address education (ANA, 2005; ICN, 2012), an additional code of ethics was created to specifically address the issues of nurse educators with a focus on students and colleagues (Rosenkoetter, 1983; Rosenkoetter & Milstead, 2010). More recently, The National League for Nursing (NLN, 2012) developed ethical principles for nurse educators focused on caring, integrity, diversity, and excellence. Throughout these various codes and principles, the guiding themes for educators are the creation and maintenance of a climate that supports professional values and beliefs; academic integrity; a collegial creative spirit; and an autonomous, honest, open, and respectful exchange (ICN, 2012; NLN, 2012).

The second focus for ethics in nursing education is the teaching of ethical principles and their application to clinical practice. Ethics is intricately woven throughout the curricular elements *The Essentials of Baccalaureate Education for Professional Nursing Practice*, the framework for baccalaureate nursing education (American Association of Colleges of Nursing [AACN], 2008). Despite the requirement that ethics be an integral part of nursing education, little guidance is provided as to the depth, breadth, or specific content of instruction. Some state boards of nursing identify ethics content as part of the required nursing curriculum, yet only a few have been examined in the literature (Park, 2009). The manner and strategies with which ethics is taught in nursing programs are inconsistent and require further development (Numminen, Leino-Kilpi, van der Arent, & Katajisto, 2009, 2010; Numminen, van der Arent, & Leino-Kilpi, 2009; Ramos et al., 2013). Through instruction, discussion of theory, and examination of case-based ethical dilemmas, students require this necessary knowledge to provide a basis for ethical future practice.

RECOMMENDATIONS

Based on the inconsistencies in teaching methods, curriculum, and educational preparation of faculty, future research may provide further guidance in standardizing some of these key components in ethics education. The question of academic honesty and its potential impact on future ethical practice in nursing also requires additional study. Initial research in this area revealed a pattern of concern; however, more research is needed (Laduke, 2013).

American Association of Colleges of Nursing (AACN). (2008). *The essentials of baccalaureate education for professional nursing practice.* Washington, DC: Author.

American Nurses Association (ANA). (2005). *Code of ethics with interpretative statements.* Silver Springs, MD: Author.

Baltzly, D. (2014). Stoicism. In E. N. Zalta (Ed.), *The Stanford encyclopedia of philosophy.* Retrieved from http://plato.stanford.edu/archives/spr2014/entries/stoicism/

Beauchamp, T. L., & Childress, J. F. (2009). *Principles of biomedical ethics* (6th ed.). New York, NY: Oxford University Press.

International Council of Nursing (ICN). (2012). *The ICN code of ethics for nurses.* Geneva, Switzerland.

Johnson, R. (2014). Kant's moral philosophy. In E. N. Zalta (Ed.), *The Stanford encyclopedia of philosophy.* Retrieved from http://plato.stanford.edu/archives/spr2014/entries/kant-moral/

Kraut, R. (2014). Aristotle's ethics. In E. N. Zalta (Ed.), *The Stanford encyclopedia of philosophy.* Retrieved from http://plato.stanford.edu/archives/spr2014/entries/aristotle-ethics/

Laduke, R. D. (2013). Academic dishonesty today, unethical practices tomorrow? *Journal of Professional Nursing, 29*(6), 402–406.

Merriam-Webster Online Dictionary. (2014). Retrieved from http://www.merriam-webster.com/dictionary/ethic

National League for Nursing (NLN). (2012). *Ethical principles for nursing education.* Retrieved from http://www.nln.org/facultyprograms/facultyresources/ethical_principles.htm

E

Numminen, O. H., Leino-Kilpi, H., van der Arend, A., & Katajisto, J. (2009) Nursing students and teaching of codes of ethics: An empirical research study. *International Nursing Review, 56*, 483–490.

Numminen, O. H., Leino-Kilpi, H., van der Arent, A., & Katajisto, J. (2010). Nurse educators' teaching of codes of ethics. *Nursing Education Today, 30*, 124–131.

Numminen, O. H., van der Arent, A., & Leino-Kilpi, H. (2009). Nurse educators' and nursing students' perspectives on teaching codes of ethics. *Nursing Ethics, 16*, 69–82.

Park, M. (2009). The legal basis of nursing ethics education. *Journal of Nursing Law, 13*, 106–113.

Ramos, F. R. S., de Pires, D. E. P., de Farias Brehmer, L. C., Gelbcke, F. L., Schmoeller, S. D., & Ramos, J. L. (2013). The discourse of ethics in nursing education: Experience and reflections of Brazilian teachers— case study. *Nursing Education Today, 33*, 1124–1129.

Rosenkoetter, M. (1983). A code of ethics for nurse educators. *Nursing Outlook, 31*, 288.

Rosenkoetter, M., & Milstead, J. A. (2010). A code of ethics for nurse educators: Revised. *Nursing Ethics, 7*(1), 137–139.

Cheryl Ann Monturo

EVALUATION: CLINICAL

DEFINITION

Clinical evaluation is a process in which an instructor evaluates a nursing student's performance in the clinical area using specific criteria. The clinical area is where students must demonstrate acquired knowledge and apply that knowledge when caring for patients. Clinical evaluation is challenging and complex because it encompasses the three domains of learning: cognitive, affective, and psychomotor (Bradshaw & Lowenstein, 2011). The goal for each student during the clinical experience is to attain acceptable clinical performance demonstrating behavior, knowledge, and attitudes, which are fostered in a variety of clinical experiences and settings (Billings & Halstead, 2011).

APPLICATION

The purpose of clinical evaluation is to ensure that the student is performing safely and providing a high standard of care. Clinical evaluation is a subjective process influenced by the attitudes and opinions of faculty and students. The role of faculty is performing a fair and comprehensive clinical evaluation that requires constant observation and documentation of the student's cognitive thinking, feelings, and performance of psychomotor skills (Bradshaw & Lowenstein, 2011). Using criterion-referenced tools along with other sources of data to evaluate behavior and learning of a student may include observations, required written work, and evidence of participation in pre- and postconferences. Clinical educators have the responsibility to assist students in the clinical area to master and develop higher level thinking skills that will support and foster effective clinical reasoning (Kuiper & Pesut, 2004).

The fairness and accuracy of clinical evaluation are associated with important factors involving the clinical faculty. The faculty member's personal values and beliefs may influence feelings toward a student or a specific clinical situation in determining whether the clinical site is an environment supportive of learning. This evaluation process should be based on curriculum objectives and a standard of practice that includes all aspects of students' performance (Bradshaw & Lowenstein, 2011).

Evaluation of a student in the clinical area can be a very challenging process. The faculty member gathers and analyzes data from many sources and provides extensive documentation of the behavior. Formative and summative evaluations occur in the evaluation process. Each week, students should be given informal, ongoing feedback in regard to strengths and weaknesses. This can be documented weekly by the instructor on a student experience form with an additional area for students to express their perceptions of the clinical experience. As a result, students are continually learning and growing as professionals while being influenced positively by mentoring of the clinical instructor (Bonnel, Gomez, Lobodzinski, & West, 2005). Summative evaluation is the final judgment of whether the student has demonstrated the required learning objectives and determined to be a safe and competent practitioner (Gallant, MacDonald, & Smith Higuchi, 2006).

SYNOPSIS

Clinical evaluation of nursing students is a complex process. Clinical competence includes safety, application of knowledge, proper performance of nursing skills, and demonstration of a positive and professional attitude. The student nurse must be efficient in analyzing complex patient situations, solving problems, and communicating effectively with patients and other health care professionals. Furthermore, instructors provide evidence of leadership and sensitivity to the cultural and spiritual needs of patients (Mitchell, Bennett, & Manfrin-Ledet, 2006). It is important to develop a valid and reliable clinical evaluation tool to establish and convey to students what objectives must be achieved to be successful (Gallant et al., 2006).

Clinical instructors use a wide range of evaluation strategies in the clinical setting to keep decisions about clinical evaluation trustworthy and fair. Strategies may include written assignments, skill testing, reflective journals, simulations, student presentations, and peer review. Observation in various clinical situations is the most popular strategy used by faculty in nursing programs (Oermann, Saewert, Charasika, & Yarbrough, 2009). Evaluating a student can be filled with flaws relating to inconsistencies with the criteria and subjectivity by the faculty.

An effective and expert clinical teacher will guide a student's clinical performance.

The outcome of a clinical evaluation is dependent on the instructor's ability to know and respond to the students' learning needs, goals, strengths, limited knowledge, and limited clinical experiences. Knowing the student as an individual minimizes assumptions and biases by faculty, making the evaluation more reliable and valid (Gillespie, 2002).

RECOMMENDATIONS

Nursing faculty involved in the clinical education of nursing students has a responsibility to reduce inconsistencies in expected learning outcomes that are evaluated in the clinical setting. Consistent standards must be created and aligned with evidence-based teaching to assess and evaluate levels of clinical competency in the nursing program (Oermann, 2008). Research studies are needed to examine new methods of clinical evaluation that will include consistent standards while fostering professional growth and meeting the challenges of changes in the delivery of health care.

Billings, D. M., & Halstead, J. A. (2011). *Teaching in nursing: A guide for faculty* (4th ed.). St. Louis, MO: Elsevier Saunders.

Bonnel, W., Gomez, D. A., Lobodzinski, S., & West, C. D. H. (2005). Clinical performance evaluation. In D. M. Billings & J. A. Halstead (Eds.), *Teaching in nursing: A guide for faculty* (2nd ed., pp. 521–542). St. Louis, MO: Elsevier Saunders.

Bradshaw, M. J., & Lowenstein, A. J. (Eds.). (2011). *Innovative teaching strategies in nursing and related health professions* (5th ed.). Boston, MA: Jones and Bartlett.

Gallant, M., MacDonald, J. A., & Smith Higuchi, K. A. (2006). A remediation process for nursing students at risk for clinical failure. *Nurse Educator, 31,* 223–227.

Gillespie, M. (2002). Student-teacher connection in clinical nursing education. *Journal of Advanced Nursing, 37*(6), 566–576.

Kuiper, R. A., & Pesut, D. J. (2004). Promoting cognitive and metacognitive reflective

E

E

reasoning skills in nursing practice: Self-regulated learning theory. *Journal of Advanced Nursing, 45*(4), 381–391.

Mitchell, D. L., Bennett, M. J., & Manfrin-Ledet, L. (2006). Spiritual development of nursing students: Developing competencies to provide spiritual care to patients at the end of life. *Journal of Nursing Education, 45*, 365–370.

Oermann, M. H. (2008). *Annual review of nursing education: Clinical nursing education* (Vol. 6). New York, NY: Springer Publishing.

Oermann, M. H., Saewert, K. J., Charasika, M., & Yarbrough, S. S. (2009). Assessment and grading practices in schools of nursing: National survey findings Part 1. *Nursing Education Perspectives, 30*(5), 274–278.

Debra O'Shaughnessy
Mary T. Quinn Griffin

EVALUATION: CLINICAL COMPETENCIES

DEFINITION

Evaluation is an informed approach that uses a systematic, rigorous procedure to examine the worth of an entity such as a program, process, procedure, individual, or other element requiring an appraisal. Evaluation of clinical competencies in nursing is the application of a process, which may use one or multiple strategies to provide both formative and summative measures of the clinical capabilities of pre-licensure, graduate students, or a licensed nurse in clinical practice.

APPLICATION

Evaluation methods for the appraisal of clinical competencies are used throughout the pre-licensure educational process. Judgments are made regarding a student's performance in the clinical setting during and at the conclusion of each clinical course. Determination of the student's ability to provide professional competent client-centered care is the central objective of the appraisal. Clinical evaluation is a decisive element in the educational process and has significant implications for students and public safety. Evaluation of clinical competency is equally important for graduate students preparing for advanced practice. Competent advanced practice requires that the graduate student has succeeded in acquiring new skills, possesses the procedural knowledge and psychomotor ability to execute them, and possesses the schematic knowledge that directs when and why to implement specific patient care measures. Determination of clinical competency provides assurance that the graduate-advanced practice nurse is prepared for entry into practice (Cook, Marienau, Wildgust, Gerbasi, & Watkins 2013; Phelen, O Connell, Murphy, McLoughlin, & Long, 2014).

SYNOPSIS

Competency in nursing is the ability to perform a skill or carry out an activity to a prescribed standard that has been instituted to ensure safety and prevent harm. Evaluation of clinical competencies is concerned with what individuals can do in addition to what they know (Garrett, MacPhee, & Jackson, 2013). The translation of knowledge into the practice of nursing by the student-engaged indirect patient care is the target of the evaluation. The process of clinical evaluation is a two-tier sequence conducted on multiple occasions during the course of the educational process in nursing. Formative evaluation of clinical competency involves observation of the student's performance, identification of strengths and/or weaknesses, and the provision of feedback regarding the student's progress on achieving the objectives. Time is allotted to learn a skill, practice a skill, and incorporate constructive feedback into the successful execution of the skill. The observations for formative evaluations are documented by the faculty as narrative notes or on a rating scale and may include assignments submitted by students regarding their clinical experience. Formative evaluation is generally not graded, but rather is used to evaluate patterns of clinical performance and continuous learning efforts as well as interval accomplishments.

The summative evaluation of clinical competency is directed at validating the acquisition of a skill or set of skills at the end of an instructional unit or level in the program. A grade is issued that indicates if the clinical competency has been achieved. Summative evaluations are often documented on a clinical evaluation tool, a numerically ranked score that denotes a successful or a failed attempt to acquire the designated competencies. The dominant strategy for evaluating clinical performance in all nursing programs is faculty observation of the student's interactions. A clinical evaluation tool was identified by 98% of nursing faculty as the instrument used to record the summative observations and rank the performance of students (Oermann, Yarbrough, Ard, Saewert, & Charasika, 2009). Faculty in undergraduate nursing programs have developed instruments for clinical evaluation using elements from the *Essentials of Baccalaureate Education for Professional Nursing Practice* (American Association of Colleges of Nursing [AACN], 2008), which identifies the expected student outcome for baccalaureate-level education. Other indicators reported by faculty that are employed to complement their direct observations of a student's clinical performance are activities demonstrated during clinical postconference such as case study analysis, values clarification exercises, and presentations on relevant clinical topics (Oermann et al., 2009).

Individuals who are in an advanced practice graduate program are prepared for a role in direct patient care. Core competencies for advanced practice specialties are determined by each specialty's professional organizations. Clinical evaluation instruments used for the systematic appraisal of graduate student's clinical competencies in the advanced practice programs have been developed using the *Essentials of Master's Education for Advanced Practice Nursing Education* (AACN, 1996), the *Essentials of Doctoral Education for Advanced Practice Nursing Education* (AACN, 2006), and the respective specialties' accreditation council standards.

The use of a clinical evaluation instrument for the determination of an individual's ability to competently practice is contingent on the properties of the instrument. The items in the instrument must be consistent with the desired outcome competency. Students at each level must be clear regarding what the successful demonstration of a particular skill includes. Trustworthiness of the tool to contain the necessary items for evaluation is indispensable if the instrument is to be a valid indicator of clinical competencies. The score on the instrument used for evaluation should be a true representation of the observed behavior. The instrument must also perform in a reliable manner; thus, the same results can be obtained when the tool is used by different faculty and with different students (Collins & Callahan, 2014; Courtney-Pratt, Fitzgerald, Ford, Johnson, & Wills, 2013).

Other measures identified in the literature to evaluate clinical competency include the Objective Structure Clinical Examination (OSCE). The instrument affords the opportunity to generate an unbiased objective review of performance in a controlled setting, not in an actual patient care setting. A key value of OSCE is that it can be used for review and practice of skills that are of a highly critical nature, yet are used infrequently; for example, disaster readiness (Rushforth, 2007).

RECOMMENDATIONS

There is a lack of information on the properties of the instruments used for the evaluation of clinical competency. Validity and reliability assessment of existing instruments are needed to guarantee confidence that the scores calculated using the clinical evaluation tool are a true representation of the observed behavior. Faculty observations are a cornerstone for the evaluation of clinical competency. The criteria to demonstrate skills at all levels must be clearly communicated, and efforts to minimize bias must be incorporated into the evaluation process.

American Association of Colleges of Nursing. (1996). *Essentials of master's education for professional nursing practice.* Washington, DC: Author.

American Association of Colleges of Nursing. (2006). *Essentials of doctoral education for professional nursing practice.* Washington, DC: Author.

American Association of Colleges of Nursing. (2008). *Essentials of baccalaureate education for professional nursing practice.* Washington, DC: Author.

Collins, S., & Callahan, M. F. (2014). Call for change: Clinical evaluation of student registered nurse anesthetists. *American Association of Nurse Anesthetists, 82*(1), 65–72.

Cook, K. A., Marienau, M. S., Wildgust, B., Gerbasi, F., & Watkins, J. (2013). Assessment of recent graduate preparedness for entry into practice. *American Association of Nurse Anesthetists, 81*(5), 341–345.

Courtney-Pratt, H., Fitzgerald, M., Ford, K., John, C., & Wills, K. (2013). Development and reliability testing of the quality clinical placement evaluation tool. *Journal of Clinical Nursing, 23*, 504–514.

Garrett, B. M., MacPhee, M., & Jackson, C. (2013). Evaluation of ePortfolio for the assessment of clinical competence in a baccalaureate nursing program. *Nurse Education Today, 33*, 1207–1213.

Oermann, M. H., Yarbrough, S. S., Ard, N., Saewert, K. J., & Charasika, M. (2009). Clinical evaluation and grading practices in schools of nursing. National survey findings Part II. *Nursing Education Perspectives, 30*, 352–357.

Phelen, A., O Connell, R., Murphy, M., McLoughlin, G., & Long, O. (2014). A contextual clinical assessment for student nurse midwives in Ireland. *Nurse Education Today, 34*, 292–294.

Rushforth, H. E. (2007). Objective structured clinical examination (OSCE): Review of literature and implications for nursing education. *Nurse Education Today, 27*(5), 481–490.

Anne Marie Mitchell

EVALUATION: OBJECTIVES VERSUS OUTCOMES

DEFINITION

Evaluation means to draw a conclusion about the value or worth of something (Oxford Dictionaries, 2014a). Objectives refer to a goal or purpose, something to attain (Oxford Dictionaries, 2014b). Outcomes refer to an end result or a consequence (Oxford Dictionaries, 2014c). Both objectives and outcomes provide a measure for evaluation.

APPLICATION

Evaluation is essential in nursing education and involves a variety of aspects of the education experience. When conducting an evaluation, it is very important to determine between objectives and outcomes. Courses have objectives and a variety of teaching and learning strategies that are used to help students to meet the course objectives. Additionally, the students have a goal of attaining a high grade in the course. The grade is an evaluation measure of how well the student achieved the course objectives. Students are evaluated based on their performance in the clinical setting that provides a measure of how well the student has achieved the objectives for the clinical course. Moreover, courses and clinical experiences are evaluated by students according to how well the course or clinical experience met their learning needs and helped them to achieve the objectives. Outcomes refer to an end result, which in nursing education is graduating from the program and passing the NCLEX-RN® licensure examination. Therefore, nursing programs are primarily evaluated by the outcome measures of graduation rates and first-time NCLEX-RN pass rates. Both course objectives and program outcomes are developed based on accreditation standards and school goals. Both course objectives and program outcomes are critical to the overall evaluation plan for the school. Course objectives provide a formative evaluation of each course and give the faculty member important feedback about the course, which can be used to improve the course to enhance the student's learning experience. In addition, program outcomes provide a summative evaluation of the program. This information allows faculty to use data about the program overall to make important decisions about the curriculum. Both formative and summative evaluations are necessary for schools of nursing to ensure that their curriculum is meeting accreditation standards and students' needs.

SYNOPSIS

Current trends in the literature related to evaluation are measuring first-time NCLEX-RN pass rates, attrition and graduation rates, and the impact of simulation on student success in achieving course objectives and program outcomes. Many schools of nursing use first-time NCLEX-RN pass rates as an outcome indicator to measure how well their program is preparing students for practice (Pennington & Spurlock, 2010; Penprase & Harris, 2013; Simon, McGinniss, & Krauss, 2013). Furthermore, schools of nursing often examine graduation/attrition rates as an important measure of how well their program is preparing students to meet both course objectives and program outcomes (Abele, Penprase, & Ternes, 2013; Dante, Valoppi, Saiani, & Palese, 2011; Fowler & Norrie, 2009; Harris, Rosenberg, & O'Rourke, 2014; O'Donnell, 2009, Penprase & Harris, 2013). Additionally, simulation is an important topic in the nursing literature in relation to evaluation. Simulation has been shown to improve students' success in assimilating into a registered nurse (RN) position (Liaw et al., 2014) and improve students' test scores on knowledge and skill examinations, but mixed results exist in how well simulation improves clinical performance (Shinnick, Woo, & Evangelista, 2012; Yuan, Williams, Fang, & Ye, 2012).

RECOMMENDATIONS

It is critical that faculty members in schools of nursing participate in ongoing evaluation of their courses (formative) and the program (summative). Moreover, it is essential that faculty use this information from the evaluation to improve their program and increase students' success in their goal of becoming licensed RNs. Furthermore, it is important that faculty members evaluate course objectives and program outcomes on a regular basis and revise them as necessary to be consistent with current standards and guidelines. This process will help ensure that each school of nursing is preparing the strongest nurses who are up-to-date with current trends in health care and are prepared to be successful nurses in today's ever-changing health care environment. Finally, an important area of continued nursing research is studying the effects of simulation on improving student's clinical skills and abilities.

Abele, C., Penprase, B., & Ternes, R. (2013). A closer look at academic probation and attrition: What courses are predictive of nursing student success? *Nurse Education Today, 33*(3), 258–261.

Dante, A., Valoppi, G., Saiani, L., & Palese, A. (2011). Factors associated with nursing students' academic success or failure: A retrospective Italian multicenter study. *Nurse Education Today, 31*(1), 59–64.

Fowler, J., & Norrie, P. (2009). Development of an attrition risk prediction tool. *British Journal of Nursing, 18*(19), 1194–1200.

Harris, R. C., Rosenberg, L., & O'Rourke, M. E. (2014). Addressing the challenges of nursing student attrition. *Journal of Nursing Education, 53*(1), 31–37.

Liaw, S. Y., Koh, Y., Dawood, R., Kowitlawakul, Y., Zhou, W., & Lau, S. T. (2014). Easing student transition to graduate nurse: A SIMulated Professional Learning Environment (SIMPLE) for final year student nurses. *Nurse Education Today, 34*(3), 349–355.

O'Donnell, H. (2009). The emotional impact of nursing student attrition rates. *British Journal of Nursing, 18*(12), 745–747, 750, 752.

E

Oxford Dictionaries. (2014a). *Evaluation*. Retrieved from http://www.oxford-dictionaries.com/definition/english/evaluation?q=evaluation

Oxford Dictionaries. (2014b). *Objectives*. Retrieved from http://www.oxforddic-tionaries.com/definition/english/objective?q=Objectives#objective__8

Oxford Dictionaries. (2014c). *Outcomes*. Retrieved from http://www.oxford-dictionaries.com/definition/english/outcome?q=Outcomes

Pennington, T. D., & Spurlock, D. (2010). A systematic review of the effectiveness of remediation interventions to improve NCLEX-RN pass rates. *Journal of Nursing Education, 49*(9), 485–492.

Penprase, B. B., & Harris, M. A. (2013). Accelerated second-degree nursing students: Predictors of graduation and NCLEX-RN first-time pass rates. *Nurse Educator, 38*(1), 26–29.

Shinnick, M. A., Woo, M., & Evangelista, L. S. (2012). Predictors of knowledge gains using simulation in the education of prelicensure nursing students. *Journal of Professional Nursing, 28*(1), 41–47.

Simon, E. B., McGinniss, S. P., & Krauss, B. J. (2013). Predictor variables for NCLEX-RN readiness exam performance. *Nursing Education Perspectives, 34*(1), 18–24.

Yuan, H. B., Williams, B. A., Fang, J. B., & Ye, Q. H. (2012). A systematic review of selected evidence on improving knowledge and skills through high-fidelity simulation. *Nurse Education Today, 32*(3), 294–298.

Carrie Buch

EVALUATION: STUDENT

DEFINITION

Evaluation is a multidimensional process of gathering data to inform judgment as to the value of something or someone. Specific to students, the evaluation process is most often related to either an assignment of grades based on a student's performance or the identification of gaps in student understanding, allowing for improvement. The teacher assesses the student's knowledge or achievement of specified objectives, determines the proportional value, and provides essential feedback for development.

APPLICATION

In nursing education, evaluation of students is complex. Students must be evaluated in the classroom and the clinical setting. Evaluation of theory is typically composed of the accumulation of points for assignments and tests, allowing a more objective determination of grade (Oermann & Gaberson, 2014). Clinical performance has historically been evaluated solely by the observation of the student in the clinical setting. The instructor must then use these observations to make judgments on the abilities of the student. Based on the subjectivity of this type of clinical evaluation, there are concerns related to reliability of the assessment.

Evaluation in nursing education is most often categorized as formative or summative evaluation (Vonderwell & Boboc, 2013). Summative evaluation is the process where value judgments are made based on the student's performance or achievement of objectives. It is often more of a static depiction of student performance. Formative evaluation is the dynamic view of a student's progress during the educational process. Based on the formative evaluation, the instructor can identify areas of needed improvement in the student's performance. This allows the instructor to provide feedback with the goal of student improvement. It typically does not result in a grade, or points being given. Instead, it allows students to be informed of the gaps in their understanding or performance of clinical skills (Vonderwell & Boboc, 2013).

Evaluation must be well planned. It should be included in the design of nursing curricula. There needs to be a clear identification of what the evaluation is for, who should be involved in conducting the evaluation, and how it is to be performed. If the students are identified as the primary stakeholders, it must be determined how they will use the evaluation information (Murdoch University, 1999). There should also be clearly defined learning outcomes in place so that the evaluator can determine if there has been a change in behavior or knowledge.

SYNOPSIS

A review of the recent literature shows a lack of research over the last 5 to 7 years devoted to evaluation of students in nursing education. Hunt and Hutchings (2014) identified the need for development of improved methods of evaluation in nursing education. Corrigan and Hardham (2011) recommended use of more innovative methods for evaluation of students and, based on their study, advocated use of student self-evaluation in the learning process. It is expected that by development of self-evaluation, we are not only enhancing students' ability to critically analyze their performance, but we are assisting the students in developing habits that will improve practice. In their study of online learning, Vonderwell and Boboc (2013) identified a number of strategies related to enhancing conventional evaluation methods to support teaching and learning. They identified a need for a partnership between the student and instructor in the online learning environment to ensure that students are meeting the educational goals.

Clinical evaluation also presents challenges in nursing education. Across multiple disciplines in a variety of health care settings, the reliability of assessment has been questioned (Hawker & Walker, 2010). Hawker and Walker (2010) indicated that there needs to be a more objective system in place to ensure that evaluation in the clinical setting is reliable. They discussed the use of Objective Structured Clinical Examination (OSCE) as a method of clinical evaluation. Han, James, and McClain (2013) recommended use of student peer evaluation in the clinical setting to enhance both formative and summative

evaluation. All of these researchers concur that little research is available regarding clinical evaluation (Hall, 2013; Han, James, & McClain, 2013; Hawker & Walker, 2010). Hall (2013) asserted that even though the majority of student time in undergraduate nursing education is spent in the clinical setting, little is really known in regard to how this evaluation occurs. Students in the United States do not perform any clinical examination for entry into practice, so the progression of students through a program and into the workforce relies heavily on the clinical instructors' skills in evaluation.

RECOMMENDATIONS

There is a lack of research on evaluation of students in nursing education. Evaluation is a critical element in the educational process as it provides the information necessary for improving instructional design, narrowing the gap in student understanding, and facilitating the development of a competent nursing workforce in our health care system.

Corrigan, R., & Hardham, G. (2011). Use of technology to enhance student self-evaluation and the value of feedback on teaching. *International Journal of Therapy and Rehabilitation, 18*(10), 579–590.

Hall, M. A. (2013). An expanded look at evaluating clinical performance: Faculty use of anecdotal notes in the U.S. and Canada. *Nurse Education in Practice, 13*(4), 271–276.

Han, Y., James, D. H., & McClain, R. M. (2013). Relationship between student peer and faculty evaluations of clinical performance: A pilot study. *Journal of Nursing Education & Practice, 3*(8), 170–178.

Hawker, J., & Walker, K. (2010). An objective structured clinical examination to assess preclinical skills. *Nutrition & Dietetics, 67*, 102–105.

Hunt, J. A., & Hutchings, M. (2014). Innovative group-facilitated peer and educator assessment of nursing students' group presentations. *Health Science Journal, 8*(1), 22–31.

E

Murdoch University. (1999). *Handbook section 1b: What is evaluation?* Retrieved from http://www.tlc.murdoch.edu.au/archive/cutsd99/handbook/section 1b.html

Oermann, M. H., & Gaberson, K. (2014). *Evaluating and testing in nursing education* (4th ed.). New York, NY: Springer Publishing.

Vonderwell, S. K., & Boboc, M. (2013). Promoting formative assessment in online teaching & learning. *TechTrends: Linking Research and Practice to Improve Learning, 57*(4), 22–27.

Amy Jones
Mary T. Quinn Griffin

EVIDENCE-BASED PRACTICE

DEFINITION

Evidence-based practice (EBP), sometimes referred to as evidence-based nursing, is a problem-solving approach to clinical care that utilizes current best evidence from well-designated studies, a clinician's expertise, and patient values and preferences.

APPLICATION

When EBP is applied in the context of caring—that is, considering patient preferences and values—the results are high-quality clinical decisions for the outcomes of patients (Melnyk & Fineout-Overholt, 2011). The process of EBP consists of six consecutive steps. The first step is asking the clinical question in the PICO format, where P is patient population, I is intervention or area of interest, C is comparison intervention or comparison group, and O is outcome. A searchable clinical question is the driver for the second step, the search process, and provides a basis for searching the electronic databases to retrieve relevant articles. Key words and phrases are used to narrow the search for relevant evidence in databases. There are six hierarchy levels of evidence for answering clinical questions, ranging from the highest level of systematic reviews of studies, such as the Cochran Reviews, to level 7, which is evidence obtained from the opinion of authorities and/or reports of expert committees. The third step is critically appraising the evidence uncovered in the literature. One needs to query: Are the results valid, reliable, and pertinent to my patient? Step 4 is a utilization of clinical judgment, patient preferences, and values to decide on final management strategies (Brenner & Leonard, 2005). These are important components of EBP, which can be highly influenced by institutional and clinical variables. A resource shortfall like budget restraints may hinder the realization of EBP. The fifth step is to carefully evaluate the outcome of the implementation of evidence in the clinician's institution. What worked, and what did not? Monitoring of data on the change in patient care and quality measures can pinpoint flaws unique to the environment and identify which patient population can benefit most. The final step is to effectively distribute the information locally through grand rounds and in-services, and nationally through publications and conference presentations. It is important to share EBP initiatives with colleagues to avoid duplication of efforts and promote integration of EBP as the standard for the clinical decision-making process.

SYNOPSIS

There has been a major emphasis on utilizing EBP. The reason for this change is multifold. First, there has been an explosion of information with over 25,000 randomized controlled studies published last year (trust-theevidence.net). It takes an average of 17 years to translate research findings into clinical practice. Methods to hasten its use have been supported by major professional and health care organizations. The 2001 Institute of Medicine's (IOM) report: *Crossing the Quality Chasm: A New Health System for the 21st Century*, stressed evidence-based decision making for health care management.

The IOM has set a 2020 goal that 90% of clinical decisions be evidence based (IOM, 2003). The National Organization of Nurse Practitioner Faculty (2012) recommends that EBP is a core competency for the nurse practitioner's approach to client management. To obtain Magnet designation, a hospital must demonstrate quality nursing care through EBP (American Nurses Credentialing Center [ANCC], 2013). In order to accelerate the EBP movement, federal agencies in the United States such as the Agency for Healthcare Research and Quality have funded EBP centers to answer important clinical questions for the ultimate purpose of improving health care delivery and patient outcomes. When used, EBP leads to improved patient outcomes by reducing mortality, morbidities, medical errors, and geographic variations (Pravikoff, Pierce, & Tanner, 2005).

Nursing has not fully adopted EBP because of professional/personal, organizational, and educational barriers. A 2005 study indicated that some nurses are not familiar with or see the value of EBP. Nurses reported that their colleagues did not use research in their practice or were not taught how to use electronic databases to find answers to clinical questions (Pravikoff et al., 2005). Most nurses ask their nursing or medical colleagues or use a drug reference book or manuals when they have a query. The concept of "tradition" or "We have always done it this way" also plays a part in decision making. Some practices have remained unit specific even though there is no evidence to support these practices. Nurses have cited lack of time and inability to understand statistical terms as other barriers for not considering research studies.

More recently, Melnyk and Fineout-Overholt (2012) found that nurses were aware and interested in EBP, but identified nurse leaders as barriers. An organizational culture that does not value EBP will hinder the use. Administration support is necessary to provide staff with the computer access, mentors, and dedicated time for EBP activities. If there are excessive demands in the clinical day, such as managing increasing numbers of patients, EBP activities cannot be pursued. The institution must be committed to fostering research efforts and then practice change activities. Nurse leaders must engage in EBP as role models, which will facilitate evidence-based care and encourage the use of EBP among staff members.

A barrier in nursing education has been that it has traditionally focused on basic research and the rigorous methods of how to conduct it. This can result in minimal interest in conducting research once nurses graduate. Education programs have started to implement EBP in their teaching methods with curriculums in undergraduate and graduate programs to provide a strong foundation in EBP. Students in these programs have to be taught a rapid approach to effectively and critically appraise research and then put it to use in their clinical practice. This will require knowledgeable and skilled instructors who can teach EBP, along with preceptors as role models/mentors in the clinical setting that can reinforce this practice (Ciliska, 2005).

According to the 2013 survey conducted by the National Council of State Boards of Nursing and The Forum of State Nursing Workforce Centers, 55% of the registered nurse (RN) workforce is aged 50 years or older (Budden, Zhong, Moulton, & Cimiotti, 2013). Seventy percent of nurses graduated from nursing programs before 1990. This presents a challenge in practice where nurses have never had the opportunity to develop the skills of EBP. Nurse educators within hospital settings need to develop workshops that would introduce these nurses to EBP and mentor nurses who have never been exposed to EBP.

RECOMMENDATIONS

For the nursing profession to embrace EBP, four populations must be targeted: nursing faculty, nursing students, nurse educators (hospital based), and existing nursing staff. Bachelors and master curriculum should be evaluated to shift from teaching basic research to incorporating EBP in all aspects of the programs. Nurse faculty has to be skilled

E

and knowledgeable in the EBP process so they can act as role models. The framework of EBP then must be intertwined throughout both didactic and clinical courses. Nursing students must be given the opportunity to use EBP as a foundation for discussion and during clinical experiences. Hospital-based nurse educators need to establish programs such as journal clubs that include review of current research, clinical guidelines, and EBP skill development workshops for less-experienced nurses. And all nurses must accept the professional responsibility of life-long learning.

American Nurses Credentialing Center. (2013). *Magnet recognition program overview.* Retrieved from http://www.nursecredentialing.org/magnet/programoverview

Brenner, P., & Leonard, V. (2005). Patient concerns, choices, and clinical judgement in evidence-based practice. In B. M. Melnyk & E. Fineout-Overholt (Eds.), *Evidence-based practice in nursing and healthcare: A guide to best practice* (pp. 39–70). Philadelphia, PA: Lippincott Williams & Wilkins.

Budden, J. S., Zhong, E. H., Moulton, P., & Cimiotti, J. P. (2013). Supplement: The National Council of State Boards of Nursing and the Forum of State Nursing Workforce Centers 2013 National Workforce of Survey of Registered Nurses. *Journal of Nursing Regulation, 4*(2), 5–14.

Ciliska, D. (2005). Educating for evidence-based practice. *Journal of Professional Nursing, 21*(6), 345–350.

Heneghan, C. (2010). *How many randomized trials are published each year.* Retrieved from http://blogs.trusttheevidence.net

Institute of Medicine (IOM). (2001). *Crossing the quality chasm: A new health system for the 21st century.* Retrieved from http://www.iom.edu/-/media/Files/Reoprt%20Files/2001?Crossing-the-Quality-Chasm%20Chasm&202001%20%20report%20brief.pdf

Institute of Medicine (IOM). (2003). *Health professions education: A bridge to quality.* Washington, DC: The National Academy of Press.

Melnyk, B. M., & Fineout-Overholt, E. (2011). *Evidence-based practice in nursing & healthcare. A guide to best practice* (2nd ed.). Philadelphia, PA: Wolters Kluwer/ Lippincott Williams & Wilkins.

Melnyk, B. M., & Fineout-Overholt, E. (2012). The state of evidence-based practice in US nurses. *Journal of Nursing Administration, 42*(9), 410–417.

National Organization of Nurse Practitioner Faculty. (2012). *Nurse practitioner competencies.* Retrieved from http://c.ymcdn.com/ sites/www.nonpf.org/resource/resmgr/ competencies

Pravikoff, D. S., Pierce, S. T., & Tanner, A. (2005). Evidence-based practice readiness study supported by academy nursing informatics expert panel. *Nursing Outlook, 53*(1), 49–50.

Janet H. Johnson

EVIDENCE-BASED PRACTICE: EDUCATION ISSUES

DEFINITION

Evidence-based practice (EBP) in nursing education is a vigilant, exhaustive process of selecting the best practice to achieve the highest standards of education to meet the planned objectives in a cost-effective manner, which prepare nursing students with what they need to practice safely.

APPLICATION

Nursing education is still in its early steps in formulating a specific EBP framework. Similar to nursing practice, the adoption of EBP in nursing education is essential to promote better quality education that reflects best practice, and creates positive attitudes among students toward the use of EBP at work. Decisions in EBP nursing education imply the adoption of best evidence in educational dialect elements, including content, strategies of teaching, and student evaluation.

It is the responsibility of nurse educators, researchers, and experts to present evidence to guide student learning and practice. Students need to spend more time on understanding the role of evidence in promoting better quality care, enhancing patient safety, and minimizing unnecessary resource waste. Students (and nurses) adhere better to EBP when they acknowledge that EBP improves time utilization, decreases job-related stress and burnout, and enhances work outcome (Scott & McSherry, 2009).

EBP is inherently present within the process of formulating nursing care plans. Students perform a comprehensive patient assessment, and, based on the data from this assessment, they set nursing diagnoses that best reflect patients' needs. Hence, students use the best available evidence from patient data to structure their nursing care. Nursing students need to be oriented to the principles of EBP so that they become part of the development, a more integrative EBP in nursing, which could occur by adopting strategies in education that allow for this engagement to occur. For instance, the use of technologies (e.g., patient simulation and computer-based modules) to improve students' knowledge, attitudes toward EBP, decision making, and clinical reasoning demonstrated positive outcomes (Hart et al., 2008).

Additionally, setting examples of what EBP can bring to students' daily activities and how this practice would save their efforts might be one way of encouraging students to engage in EBP. These examples could be presented in classrooms, laboratories, and clinical settings.

SYNOPSIS

The attention in EBP nursing education should be directed to the major components of the learning situation. These components are nurse educator, content, teaching–learning strategy, and students. The decision to adopt EBP rests on nursing educators. There are, however, factors that influence this adoption,

including knowledge in educational principles, finding and reviewing evidence, faculty practices, change in education strategies/practices, and finding and judging evidence (Al Hadid & Al Barmawi, 2012). Addressing these issues would improve nurse educators' adherence to principles of EBP.

Theory as well as practice gaps are inherently present in nursing education. Theory content provided in classrooms often reflects knowledge within textbooks; by the time this content is used, it may contain outdated information. Clinical courses usually have similar issues, and are often even more outdated. Although checklists and procedure guidelines are in the core of EBP in nursing, their review does not usually take place on a regular basis. It is, therefore, crucial that revisions for theoretical and practical content be made on a regular basis to avoid outdated information. They should also reflect community and client needs.

The process of devising, implementing, and evaluating teaching plans is essential for EBP models to be successful. This area concerns mainly the educators, who assume the role of defining the objectives, material (content), methods of delivering this material, minimal level of standards to pass, and evaluation methods. It is important for educators to be aware of all required steps to move through this process according to EBP principles.

In order to improve EBP implementation, teaching strategies need to adopt more collaborative models in theory and clinical courses (Salminen, Minna, Sanna, Jouko, & Helena, 2013). These models include computer-based and interactive teaching strategies (Hart et al., 2008) and developing collaborative partnerships between academics and clinicians (Spiel & Strohmeier, 2012).

Modifying students' attitudes toward EBP is a priority in nursing. Researchers have reported negative students' attitudes resulting from lack of knowledge and mythical assumptions about EBP (Kim, Brown, Fields, & Stichler, 2009). Frequent exposure to concepts of EBP produces a sense of familiarity, thus minimizing the negative attitudes.

Engaging students in the process of generating evidence and formulating best educational practices during their study fosters learning, solving problems, and clinical decision making (Bender, 2007).

RECOMMENDATIONS

Nurse educators are responsible for providing students with the best learning experiences. The adoption of EBP in nursing education promotes the realization of this responsibility. Elements composing the learning–teaching process should be addressed to build a successful model of EBP in nursing education.

Al Hadid, L., & Al Barmawi, M. (2012). Factors influencing the adoption of evidence-based principles in nursing education: A Jordanian perspective. *Journal of Nursing Education and Practice, 2*(2), 71–79.

Bender, D. G. (2007). Experiencing the effect of teaching and learning styles on skill mastery. *Journal of Nursing Education, 46*(3), 147–148.

Hart, P., Eaton, L., Buckner, M., Morrow, B. N., Barrett, D. T., Fraser, D. D.,…Sharrer, R. L. (2008). Effectiveness of a computer-based educational program on nurses' knowledge, attitude, and skill level related to evidence-based practice. *Worldviews on Evidence-Based Nursing/Sigma Theta Tau International, Honor Society of Nursing, 5*(2), 75–84.

Kim, S. C., Brown, C. E., Fields, W., & Stichler, J. F. (2009). Evidence-based practice-focused interactive teaching strategy: A controlled study. *Journal of Advanced Nursing, 65*(6), 1218–1227.

Salminen, L., Minna, S., Sanna, K., Jouko, K., & Helena, L. K. (2013). The competence and the cooperation of nurse educators. *Nurse Education Today, 33*(11), 1376–1381.

Scott, K., & McSherry, R. (2009). Evidence-based nursing: Clarifying the concepts for nurses in practice. *Journal of Clinical Nursing, 18*(8), 1085–1095.

Spiel, C., & Strohmeier, D. (2012). Evidence-based practice and policy: When researchers, policy makers, and practitioners learn how to work together. *European Journal of Developmental Psychology, 9*(1), 150–162.

Lourance Abdul Razzaq Enad Alzyarah Al Hadid

F

Faculty Development

DEFINITION

Faculty development is the planned course of action for the professional training of faculty (Finke, 2009). Faculty development is defined as the process by which novice, mid-career, and experienced faculty focus on career planning in the faculty roles and responsibilities including educational approaches, educational environments, nursing education leaders, and scholarship.

APPLICATION

Faculty development is essential for professional growth as an educator. Felver et al. (2010) posit that faculty development should be a lifelong learning process that is developed to be intentional, planned, and proactive. Faculty development is a planned process that is used for faculty career planning. Faculty are encouraged to examine the National League for Nursing (NLN) Core Competencies for Nurse Educators to analyze competencies required for nurse faculty development.

The NLN Core Competencies for Nurse Educators were developed by the Task Group on Nurse Educator Competencies (NLN, 2005). These competencies can provide the framework for faculty development. The eight core competencies are facilitating student learning; facilitating learner development and socialization; using assessment and evaluation strategies; participating in curriculum design and evaluation of program outcomes; functioning as a change agent and

leader; pursuing continuous quality improvement in the nurse educator role; engaging in scholarship; and functioning within the educational environment (NLN, 2005). The eight core competencies include 66 task statements that have been identified to be important in the nurse educator role. They may be used to create a faculty development program that is tailored to the needs of the nursing faculty. The NLN Core Competencies for Nurse Educators offers a comprehensive view of the faculty role to guide faculty development over time.

Faculty development requires a process that consists of learning activities that add to the nurse educator's knowledge base, with increasing skills and competencies that expand the effectiveness in the faculty role. Faculty development may be delivered by educational conferences, webinars, courses, workshops, online modules, mentoring programs, peer support systems, or centers for teaching excellence. Faculty development begins on hire with an orientation to the educational institution and opportunities for facilitation of student learning.

Once faculty have a solid foundation in student learning, including assessment and evaluation, focus should be on learning about the curriculum development and evaluation, developing as a leader, and developing as scholars in the faculty role. Faculty should have a faculty development plan that is reflective, examines what they currently know, and identifies development opportunities. Brookfield (1995) and Tanner (2006) describe the reflective practice as an essential element for faculty development. Reflective practice allows faculty to identify further faculty development opportunities.

F

SYNOPSIS

The responsibility for faculty development is shared with the faculty member, department chair, academic administrators, and college or university (Finke, 2009). According to Barksdale et al. (2011), it is essential to have a faculty development program to prepare novice educators and for faculty to remain current and relevant with new teaching strategies. Felver et al. (2010) suggest that faculty development is a lifelong process to assist faculty with transforming their teaching in the hope of retaining faculty, supporting professional growth, and assisting with faculty promotion. Faculty development is essential for professional growth and retention as a nurse educator.

Faculty development activities should be designed to motivate faculty and decrease the stress of learning the roles and responsibilities. Brazeau and Woodward (2012) discussed that instructors have high expectations of themselves, and unclear roles and expectations place stress on them. A formalized faculty development program developed by Foley et al. (2003) provided opportunities for professional development to increase skills in the faculty role with the hopes of recruiting and retaining nursing faculty. Faculty development takes into consideration individual goals and development needs of an individual faculty.

It is essential for novice, mid-career, and expert nurse educators to design a formalized faculty development plan. Once faculty have experience in facilitating teaching and learning, focus should include other areas based on the individual faculty goals related to the roles and responsibilities. Barksdale et al. (2011) designed a faculty development program that was offered to novice faculty and focused on instructional development; it also included mentoring in the academic and educator role and career development. It is essential to work closely with faculty to design an individual professional development plan that is based on each faculty member's needs that can assist him or her to be successful in the nurse faculty role.

Nursing faculty are responsible for beginning and continuing competency in the nurse educator role, including facilitating student learning; teaching strategies, assessment, and evaluation; curriculum development; faculty scholarship; continuing professional development; educational institution roles and responsibilities; and leadership development. Faculty development involves the planned activities that facilitate the professional growth of faculty as they progress in their role.

RECOMMENDATIONS

Further faculty development should be considered in the area of nursing leadership within the educational environment. Nurses must be proactive to keep current and relevant with the changes that occur in the academic institution. It is recommended that academic institutions consider faculty development as a priority to realize the ultimate goal of retaining students and fostering institutional and individual excellence. Further research should focus on faculty development activities that have been utilized and examine if the activities are working or should be revised. There is a need for further research related to new and emerging technologies that would support faculty development activities.

Furthermore, considerations include personalized faculty development programs; these may include a specific focus on assisting with the promotion in academic rank, including individualized faculty development opportunities for promotion. Consideration for faculty development includes individualized faculty goals and career plans. Personalized faculty development programs should be unique to each institution and engage faculty in developing a personalized faculty development plan related to the mission, vision, and goals of the organization. A faculty development needs assessment should be completed at each organization to design a planned process for faculty development.

Barksdale, D., Woodley, L., Page, J., Bernhardt, J., Kowlowitz, V., & Oermann, M. (2011). Faculty development: Doing more with less. *The Journal of Continuing Education in Nursing, 42*(12), 537–544.

Brazeau, G., & Woodward, J. (2012). Rethinking faculty career development strategies. *American Journal of Pharmaceutical Education, 76*(6), 1–2. doi: 10.5688/ajpe766101.

Brookfield, S. (1995). *Becoming a critically reflective teacher.* San Francisco, CA: Jossey-Bass.

Felver, L., Gaines, B., Heims, M., Lasater, K., Laustsen, G., Lynch, M., . . . Tanner, C. (2010). *Best practices in teaching and learning in nursing education.* New York, NY: National League for Nursing.

Finke, L. (2009). Teaching in nursing. In D. Billings & J. Halstead (Eds.), *Teaching in nursing: A guide for faculty.* St. Louis, MO: Saunders.

Foley, B. J., Redman, R., Horn, E., Davis, G., Neal, E., & Van Riper, M. (2003). Determining nursing faculty development needs. *Nursing Outlook, 51,* 227–232.

National League for Nursing (NLN). (2005). *The scope of practice for academic nurse educators.* New York, NY: National League for Nursing.

Tanner, C. (2006). Thinking like a nurse: A research-based model of clinical judgment in nursing. *Journal of Nursing Education, 45*(6), 204–211.

Kari L. Luoma
Robin S. Goodrich

FACULTY REFLECTION

DEFINITION

Faculty reflection is the thoughtful consideration and critical analysis of an educator's actions, thoughts, and feelings. Faculty reflection involves time spent analyzing an educational situation before, during, or after the encounter. This thoughtful examination of teaching may lead to the exploration of methods to resolve issues and development of new perspectives or ideas, which may bring about change in teaching or improved performance (Freshwater, Horton-Deutsch, Sherwood, & Taylor, 2005; Schön, 1983; Shellenbarger, Palmer, Labant, & Kuzneski, 2005).

APPLICATION

Faculty reflection is an important part of practice for nurse educators as it enhances personal and professional development in the role of educator. This self-improvement process requires faculty to examine a situation and recognize and record salient events, actions, and activities. Faculty reflection can be enhanced through a number of self-monitoring activities, many of which involve the creative expressions of ideas. Activities that can be used for reflection include writing/journaling; creating audio, video, or digital recordings; drawing; poetry; or other personal expressions that allow for the review of teaching. Faculty reflection can be an individual activity done in isolation, but it can also be enhanced through dialogue with others. The use of discussion and questioning by others can help faculty explore their thoughts and feelings. Colleagues can pose questions for faculty to examine their educational behavior and practice. Educators can consider questions as follows: What did you do or say? Why did you do it? What does it mean? What were you feeling? or What will you change? The use of these questioning approaches and further dialogue about the teaching allows for the exploration of what happened, who was involved, what role the faculty played, and the feeling related to the experience. Regardless of reflection being done in isolation or with peers, it must involve a critical analysis of the activities so that faculty can examine knowledge, challenge assumptions, explore alternatives, and create new ideas (Bridgen & Purcell, 2013).

Faculty may face a number of barriers when engaging in faculty reflection. Those barriers include the unfamiliar aspect of

F

reflection, lack of time, lack of structure, lack of support, or conflict with cultural norms and expectations. Faculty can implement a number of approaches that will promote reflection. These include being mindful of teaching, remaining open to ideas, expressing ideas freely and without restraint, allowing spontaneity, and engaging with colleagues to promote and support a culture of reflection (Taylor, 2006). Additionally, setting structured time aside to reflect is important so that reflection occurs. It is also important to complete faculty reflection activities soon after a teaching session so that ideas are clear and other distractions do not interfere with the reflection (Reflection, 2010). After critical examination and thoughtful consideration of the actions, thoughts, and feelings involved in teaching, faculty may choose to make changes to their practice or may continue with effective current approaches.

SYNOPSIS

Dewey (1933) described reflection as the active, persistent, and careful consideration of any belief or knowledge (p. 9). He also suggested that faculty may not be motivated to reflect unless there is an issue or dilemma that needs to be addressed. Additional scholars have expanded upon Dewey's work, suggesting that faculty reflection is a process of looking at a situation with careful thought, inquiry, and attention (Mezirow, 1998; Schön, 1987). Others suggest that faculty reflection involves critique of assumptions and analysis of the experience from different viewpoints (Brookfield, 1995; Mezirow, 1998). There are three phases of faculty reflection: awareness of feelings and thoughts, critical analysis of the situation, and development of new perspectives (Freshwater et al., 2005; Freshwater, Taylor, & Sherwood, 2008). The literature discusses the timing of the reflection activities and refers to reflection-before-action, or thinking in advance; reflection-in-action, used in the moment; or reflecting-on-action, reflection that occurs after an event (Sherwood & Horton-Deutsch,

2012). Successful faculty reflection should be structured, guided, purposeful, regularly occurring, intentional, focused, and involve active inquiry and critical thought. Faculty reflection may lead to professional growth and awareness of educator actions and interactions. Through reflection, faculty may gain a sense of meaning and purpose while also helping to create personal solutions to teaching problems.

RECOMMENDATIONS

Much of the literature related to faculty reflection is based on personal experience and individual activities. Educators do not have a strong evidence base to direct and support the use of faculty reflection activities. Research related to faculty reflection is essential to guide professional educator practice. Studies can be aimed at understanding the usefulness of faculty reflection strategies and best practices for faculty reflection. Additional research could also evaluate faculty reflection and its relationship with educator practice improvements, thus answering the question: Does faculty reflection lead to effective practice changes? Further work is also needed to understand the optimal timing and approaches of reflective activities. The literature suggests that faculty reflection influences teaching and professional development but further research is needed to evaluate this concept.

Bridgen, D., & Purcell, N. (2013). Focus: Becoming a reflective practitioner. *The Higher Education Academy*. Retrieved from www.heacademcy.ac.uk/resources

Brookfield, S. D. (1995). *Becoming a critically reflective teacher*. San Francisco, CA: Jossey-Bass.

Dewey, J. (1933). How we think. *A restatement of the relation of reflective thinking to the educative process*. Boston, MA: D. C. Health.

Freshwater, D., Horton-Deutsch, S., Sherwood, G., & Taylor, B. (2005). *The scholarship of reflective practice*. Indianapolis, IN: Sigma Theta Tau International. Retrieved from http://nursingsociety.org/ABOUTUS/

POSITIONPAPERS/Pages/poisition_resource-papers.aspx

Freshwater, D., Taylor, B. J., & Sherwood, G. (2008). *International textbook of reflective practice in nursing.* West Sussex, UK: Blackwell Publishing.

Mezirow, J. (1998). On critical reflection. *Adult Education Quarterly, 48*, 185–199.

Reflection. (2010). *Learning development with Plymouth University.* Retrieved from http://www.learningdevelopment.plymouth.ac.uk/LDstudyguides/pdf/11Reflection.pdf

Schön, D. A. (1983). *The reflective practitioner: How practitioners think in action.* New York NY: Basic Books.

Schön, D. A. (1987). *Educating the reflective practitioner.* San Francisco, CA: Jossey-Bass.

Shellenbarger, T., Palmer, E., Labant, A. L., & Kuzneski, J. L. (2005). Use of faculty reflection to improve teaching. In M. Oermann & K. Heinrich (Eds.), *Annual review of nursing education* (Vol. 3, pp. 343–357). New York, NY: Springer Publishing.

Sherwood, G. D., & Horton-Deutsch, S. (2012). *Reflective practice: Transforming education and improving outcomes.* Indianapolis, IN: Sigma Theta Tau International.

Taylor, B. J. (2006). *Reflective practice for healthcare professionals.* Berkshire, England: Open University Press.

Teresa Shellenbarger

FACULTY WORKLOAD

DEFINITION

Faculty workload refers to all professional duties and responsibilities of faculty related to teaching, research, scholarship, service to the institution and the community, and professional development (Allen, 1998; Townsend & Rosser, 2007; Yuker, 1984). Faculty workload refers to all the duties and responsibilities of faculty to meet the needs of their students, of the educational institution where they work, and of their self-development. These include but are not limited to teaching, research, service, professional development, and administrative duties.

APPLICATION

The Committee on Colleges and University Teaching, Research, and Publications of the American Association of University Professors (AAUP, 2000) published the *Statement on Faculty Workload* that provides guidelines for institutions. Because there is no single formula to ensure equitable and fair faculty workload, AAUP proposed three guiding principles for institutions to consider in developing policies and procedures: define maximum teaching loads at the undergraduate and graduate levels that ensure teaching effectiveness; describe the procedure to be followed in establishing, administering, and revising policies related to faculty workload; and identify actual and potential sources of inequity in workload distribution. AAUP proposed a preferred teaching load of 9 hours per week for undergraduate teaching, 6 hours per week for graduate teaching, and a maximum workload of 12 hours for undergraduate teaching and 9 hours for graduate teaching. AAUP recommended flexibility in assigning workload and consideration of factors such as difficulty of course; content of course; class size; requirements for research and publication; and other noninstructional responsibilities such as student counseling, committee work, participation in professional societies, and administrative duties. A key to allocate faculty responsibility is to sustain and ensure consistent quality in teaching and scholarship.

Faculty workload is linked to job satisfaction and attrition. In addition, workload is viewed as a contributing factor in nurse faculty shortage (Kaufman, 2007). In 2006, the National League for Nursing and the Carnegie Foundation partnered to study key factors that contribute to the faculty shortage. This partnership resulted in a survey of 8,498 nurse faculty members nationwide.

F

Nurse educators reported working about 56 hours per week while school was in session and more than 24 hours per week during breaks. In addition, those with administrative responsibilities work an extra 2 hours per week. In this study, one in four nurse educators expressed the likelihood of leaving his or her job unless workload was reduced.

Online teaching involves more faculty time compared to face-to-face teaching (Mupinga & Maughan, 2008). A study of faculty workload in distance learning by Anderson and Avery (2008) showed that online teaching requires up to 46 hours of instruction per credit compared to about 39 hours for face-to-face instruction. AAUP (2000) recommends consideration of online faculty involvement in designing the course, class preparation, increased student contacts, synchronous or asynchronous teaching formats, and other administrative duties in calculating faculty workload in distance education.

SYNOPSIS

Faculty workload is an important issue in academia that has been under scrutiny in the climate of economic duress (Dennison, 2012). In 1919, the classic landmark study on faculty workload by Koos (American Association for Higher Education-Education Resources Information Center [AAHE-ERIC]/Higher Education Research Report, 1974) led to publication of a monograph by the Bureau of Education of the United States Department of Interior. Later studies (AAHE-ERIC/Higher Education Research Report, 1974; AAUP, 2000; Cohen, Hickey, & Upchurch, 2009; Durham, Merritt, & Sorrell, 2007) proposed numerous methods to measure faculty workload. The variety of ideas on acceptable faculty activities to include in calculating workloads has resulted in lack of a standard method. Therefore, faculty workload policies vary from institution to institution.

RECOMMENDATIONS

The issue of faculty workload may be a source of conflict and dissatisfaction among faculty members that can affect teaching effectiveness and performance. Increasing collaboration between university leadership and faculty governance can ensure that a clear, equitable, and fair policy is formulated and implemented. It is essential that the faculty have a mechanism to discuss or grieve workload issues. More research is needed to address the workload allocation for nursing faculty to increase teaching effectiveness and promote job satisfaction.

Allen, H. L. (1998). *Faculty workload and productivity: Gender comparisons.* NEA 1998 Almanac of Higher Education (pp. 25–42). Washington, DC: National Education Association.

American Association for Higher Education-Education Resources Information Center [AAHE-ERIC]/Higher Education Research Report. (1974). The measurement of faculty workload. *ASHE-ERIC Higher Education Report, 3*(6), 8–14. doi: 10.1002/12h2.3640030606.

American Association of University Professors (AAUP). (2000). Interpretive comments on statement on faculty workload (Committee on Colleges and University Teaching, Research, and Publications). *Academe, 8*(5), 69–72.

Anderson, K. M., & Avery, M. D. (2008). Faculty teaching time: A comparison of web-based and face-to-face graduate nursing courses. *International Journal of Nursing Scholarship, 5*(1), 1–12.

Cohen, M. Z., Hickey, J. V., & Upchurch, S. L. (2009). Faculty workload calculation. *Nursing Outlook, 57*(1), 50–59.

Dennison, G. M. (2012). Faculty workload: An analytical approach. *Innovations in Higher Education, 37,* 297–305. doi:10.1007/s10755–011-9211-y

Durham, S., Merritt, J., & Sorrell, J. (2007). Implementing a new faculty workload formula. *Nursing Education Perspectives, 28*(4), 184–190.

Kaufman, K. (2007). Introducing the NLN/Carnegie national survey of nurse educators: Compensation, workload, and teaching practice. *Nursing Education Perspectives, 28*(3), 164–167.

Mupinga, D. M., & Maughan, G. R. (2008). Web-based instruction and community college faculty workload. *College Teaching, 56*(1), 17–21.

Townsend, B. K., & Rosser, V. J. (2007). Workload issues and measures of faculty productivity. *The NEA Higher Education Journal, Fall 2007,* 7–20.

Yuker, H. E. (1984). *Faculty workload: Research, theory and interpretation. ASHE-ERIC Higher Education Research Report No. 10, 1984.* Washington DC: Association for the Study of Higher Education.

Maria A. Mendoza

Focus Groups

DEFINITION

The focus group is a form of qualitative research used to organize group discussions around a specific topic or set of issues that will yield focused experiences, opinions, or points of view that are deliberated on during group interactions. Topics such as the causes of societal stigma about mental illness or examination of a public health announcement for cultural and developmental sensitivity are examples of its utility (Kitzinger, 1994). Focus groups are widely used in marketing, social research, and, in recent years, health care, including nursing. The key elements that differentiate focus groups from other types of inquiry are the insights and data that are produced during interactions among participants (Kitzinger, 1994).

APPLICATION

Focus groups provide an excellent approach for determining why and how people think the way they do about specific phenomena. Focus groups can be used to explore how individuals understand health and disease, treatment, and alternative approaches to care. Data that are generated by focus groups may not be easily obtainable through other methods, such as surveys, face-to-face interviews, or questionnaires. Beliefs and practices about health and disease can be deliberated on within the context of a group of individuals who share knowledge and experiences about various phenomena, and a large cluster of data can be generated in a short period of time (Fern, 2001; James, McGlone West, & Madrid, 2013).

There are some methodological requirements that should be considered when using focus groups; typically, they are 90 to 120 minutes in duration and consist of 7 to 12 individuals (Fern, 2001). The inherent nature of focus groups suggests that they should be well-planned and tightly organized events with a stated purpose and a specific outcome use for the data. A set of soundly written research questions that are based on the current state of knowledge that is being explored should serve as the basis for the questions, which guide a discussion (Gibbs, 1997; Merton & Kendall, 1946).

Recent research studies suggest that focus groups are widely used to explore approaches to improving health outcomes. Focus groups can be advantageous when there are divergent opinions and differences among people who must make important decisions regarding a variety of issues, such as those that confront nursing and health care (Higgins, Porter, & O'Halloran, 2014; Then, Rankin, & Ali, 2014). Matters that could be explored with this methodology might include identifying health disparities in rural and underserved populations, or exploring the needs of patients with severe mental illness and their caregivers (Then et al., 2014). Even though educators and researchers might be aware that these disparities or needs exist, the opulent and/or candid information that focus group data provide can allow for more accurate identification of specific areas for intervention, or barriers to care that might not otherwise be revealed (Angelo, Egan, & Reid, 2013; James et al., 2013; Kreuger & Casey, 2009; Then et al., 2014).

F

Importantly, the challenge to accurately identify and respond to the health needs of America's dramatic demographic population shifts could be enhanced through the use of focus groups (Angelo et al., 2013; McDonald, Kidney, & Patka, 2013). When working with people from varied racial/ethnic backgrounds and perspectives, focus groups can provide powerful methods for exploring cultural influence on morbidity, mortality, and well-being. Focus groups can help to galvanize trust among health care workers and individuals with chronic or terminal illnesses and their families. This method can help patients and families unravel personal experiences with specific disease conditions in the service of improving health care, or structuring salient research questions for future exploration, or addressing changes in nursing curricula.

SYNOPSIS

Whether addressing health disparities or overall improvements in care, the rich details afforded by this data collection approach has led to an increase in the use of focus groups in health care research over the last several decades (Then et al., 2014). Focus groups provide a forum through which the needs and perspectives of all involved parties are identified and on which future inquiry and evidence-based practice can be generated (Ryan, Lillie, Thwaites, & Adams, 2013). Another distinct advantage of focus groups is that they give people with limited literacy a chance to express concerns within the group milieu, where a comfortable and welcoming environment can be established and maintained by the leader. However, the researcher must be aware of some of the disadvantages of focus groups: guidelines about how confidentiality will be handled should be addressed, and some group members might decide to remain quiet because of disagreement with the decisions that the group could make or because they feel their thoughts are not within the mainstream of the themes that

are being generated by the group (Higgins et al., 2014; Kitzinger, 1994).

RECOMMENDATIONS

Focus groups can be powerful tools in nursing when data are needed about attitudes, perceptions, behaviors, and motivations about a particular phenomenon such as health and disease. They are also useful when working with groups that have limited literacy and might otherwise be excluded from other types of research protocols. Technological advances make the method more accessible to nurse educators and researchers through the use of audio- and video-recording devices that capture the essence of discussions, and computer software that can aid in data analyses. However, the essence of the value of the focus group is embedded in the interpretation and application of the information that can be gleaned from group interactions. The application of the findings from a focus group should be carefully employed. Within the context of focus group methods and data generation, the 15 National Standards for Culturally and Linguistically Appropriate Services (CLAS) in research and clinical practice might provide guidance for the advancement of health equity and the improvement of health outcomes for all people (U.S. Department of Health and Human Services, 2012).

ACKNOWLEDGMENT

Ms. Lindsey Irwin has assisted with the development of this chapter. She has added an additional dimension to this chapter. Her knowledge and expertise are deeply appreciated.

Angelo, J., Egan, R., & Reid, K. (2013). Essential knowledge for family caregivers: A qualitative study. *International Journal of Palliative Nursing, 19*(8), 383–388.

Fern, E. E. (2001). *Advanced focus group research.* Thousand Oaks, CA: Sage.

Gibbs, A. (1997). Focus groups. *Social research update* (University of Surrey, UK). Retrieved from http://sru.soc.surrey.ac.uk/SRU19.html

Higgins, A., Porter, S., & O'Halloran, P. (2014). General practitioners' management of the long-term sick role. *Social Science and Medicine, 107*, 52–60. doi:10.1016/j.socscimed.2014.01.044

James, R. D., McGlone West, K., & Madrid, T. M. (2013). Launching native health leaders: Reducing mistrust of research through student peer mentorship. *American Journal of Public Health, 103*(12), 2215–2219. doi:10.2105/AJPH.2013.301314

Kitzinger, J. (1994). The methodology of focus groups: The importance of interaction between research participants. *Sociology of Health, 16*(1), 103–121. doi:10.1111/1467-9566.ep11347023

Kreuger, R. A., & Casey, M. A. (2009). *Focus groups: A practical guide for applied research.* Thousand Oaks, CA: Sage.

McDonald, K. E., Kidney, C. A., & Patka, M. (2013). "You need to let your voice be heard": Research participants' views on research. *Journal of Intellectual Disability Research, 57*(3), 216–225. doi:10.1111/j.1365-2788.2011.01527.x

Merton, R. K., & Kendall, P. L. (1946). The focused interview. *American Journal of Sociology, 51*(6), 541–557. doi:10.1086/219886

Ryan, S., Lillie, K., Thwaites, C. M., & Adams, J. (2013). "What I want clinicians to know"—experiences of people with arthritis. *British Journal of Nursing, 22*(14), 808–812.

Then, K. L., Rankin, J. A., & Ali, E. (2014). Focus group research: What is it and how can it be used? *Canadian Journal of Cardiovascular Nursing, 24*(1), 16–22.

U.S. Department of Health and Human Services Office of Minority Health. (2012). *National CLAS standards.* Retrieved from https://www.thinkculturalhealth.hhs.gov/Content/clas.asp

Faye Gary

F

G

GLOBAL LEARNING

DEFINITION

Global learning in nursing education is an integrated comprehensive framework that provides students with multiple ways of learning, including theoretical, experiential, and reflexive learning. Global learning is "a critical analysis of and an engagement with complex, interdependent global systems and legacies (such as natural, physical, social, cultural, economic, and political) and their implications for people's lives and the earth's sustainability" (Rhodes, 2010). Through reflective and critical thinking, global learning provides students with a deeper understanding of themselves and members of the global community, both "around the corner and across the globe."

APPLICATION

Nurses need to be educated as global citizens who have a moral responsibility and professional competency to care and promote health beyond their local communities and national institutions (Chavez, Peter, & Gastaldo, 2008). The new global interdependence calls for all persons across the globe to extend their thinking about moral responsibility and health beyond their local communities and national citizenship and to become citizens of the world (Crigger, Brannigan, & Baird, 2006). Nussbaum (1997) describes three capacities necessary for the cultivation of global citizenship. The first is reflexivity, the capacity to examine our

beliefs, traditions, habits, and ourselves critically. Nussbaum's second capacity for global citizenship entails the notion of "moral cosmopolitanism," meaning adopting the fundamental view of all persons as fellow citizens who have equal moral worth and deserve equal moral consideration. Narrative imagination is the third capacity. This requires the ability to imagine what it might be like to be a person different from oneself, and to allow such imagination to inform understanding of the other person's experiences, emotions, and desires (Nussbaum, 1997). Being exposed to other cultures and people is one aspect of developing this kind of narrative imagination (Chavez, Bender, & Gastaldo, 2011).

A theoretical framework in global learning, specifically postcolonial framework, provides an analytic lens to look at the impact of health with the intersecting factors of power, race, gender, and social class. Postcolonial feminism represents an opportunity for nurses to acknowledge their multiple locations as individuals and health care professionals. It challenges deeply held certainties about the "right way" to provide care and values all knowledge as being situated within a given place and within the power relations therein. Using this perspective enables us to consider multiple perspectives on meanings of health and illness (Anderson & McCann, 2002), as well as the complex issues associated with the global locations of nursing practice.

Through global learning, nursing students become sensitized to their own culturally established perspectives on health care and become capable of identifying and challenging underlying values and assumptions

G

of their nursing education and practice. They are able to examine how social inequalities are located and constructed within a political, historical, cultural, and economic context.

SYNOPSIS

Over a decade ago, Thorne (1997) argued that nursing education has traditionally fostered social awareness within a limited local sphere of influence. At that time, the literature reflected an ongoing interest in international nursing and an inherent goodness of educational exchange programs. However, there was little analysis of what motivates students or, beyond simply providing "practical" experience, how leaders/teachers promote an attitudinal shift in students involved in such programs (Thorne, 1997). Studying the experiences of globally aware nurses, Thorne specifically explored the origins of their global awareness and their analysis of nursing as a whole in relation to the larger global perspective, in order to shed light on these more critical questions. Findings raised two key points regarding nursing education specifically. First, most of these nurses reported little or no formal learning in their nursing programs on topics they considered relevant to a global perspective. Second, some noted that their desire to incorporate preexisting interest in global health into their clinical learning was generally not supported, either by faculty or peers. Nursing education that recognizes the importance of cultural sensitivity in cultivating global consciousness ought to encourage "critical analysis of the status quo in health care and the larger society" (Thorne, 1997, p. 440). In this vein, international exchange programs offer particularly rich learning with regard to alternative (i.e., non-Western) health and social structures. She concluded by calling for a reexamination of uncritical approaches to international nursing work with their roots in colonial paternalism, those framed simplistically as charitable efforts to assist needy nations.

Some of the recurring benefits that appear in international nursing studies can inform the impact of global learning. Benefits of international experiences include changed values, increased consciousness of social justice and global health issues, significantly improved communication skills, learning to think unconventionally about other cultures, development of confidence, growth in competency, and the therapeutic use of self (Evanson & Zust, 2006; Lee, 2004; Mill, Yonge, & Cameron, 2005; Sloand, Bower, & Groves, 2008).

RECOMMENDATIONS

While there is increasing emergence and investment in many forms of global learning interchangeably used for global service learning, global health practica, international placements/exchange, and so on, systematic evaluation receives comparatively less attention. While nursing researchers have begun to evaluate the effectiveness of student learning within local contexts, a challenge exists in applying their findings to international settings, settings that represent a complexity of factors that influence learning in particular ways (Stufflebeam, 2001). There is a need for more tested strategies to evaluate learning and practice related to international experiences and global learning. Evaluation results will contribute to a growing body of evidence supporting the integration of global learning in nursing education. Evaluation of Critical Perspectives in Global Health (CPGH) reinforces many of the common themes reflective of transformative learning. CPGH, like many global learning initiatives, can only accommodate limited numbers of students and continue to be an elective course instead of a credit course. This begs the question as to why many nursing curricula do not integrate global learning as a required or foundational course.

Anderson, J. M., & McCann, E. K. (2002). Toward a post-colonial feminist methodology in nursing research: Exploring the convergence of post-colonial and black feminist scholarship. *Nurse Researcher, 9*(3), 7–27.

Chavez, F., Bender, A., & Gastaldo, D. (2011). Global health. In V. Tschudin & A. Davis (Eds.), *Community health nursing: A Canadian perspective* (pp. 480–491). Toronto, Ontario: Pearson Education Canada.

Chavez, F., Peter, E., & Gastaldo, D. (2008). Nurses as global citizens. In V. Tschudin (Ed.), *The globalisation of nursing: Ethical, legal and political issues* (pp. 175–186). Oxon, England: Radcliffe Publishing Ltd.

Crigger, N. J., Brannigan, M., & Baird, M. (2006). Compassionate nursing professionals as good citizens of the world. *Advances in Nursing Science, 29*(1), 15–26.

Evanson, T. A., & Zust, B. L. (2006). "Bittersweet knowledge": The long-term effects of an international experience. *Journal of Nursing Education, 45*(10), 412–419.

Lee, N. J. (2004). The impact of international experience on student nurses' personal and professional development. *International Nursing Review, 51*(2), 113–122.

Mill, J. E., Yonge, O. J., & Cameron, B. L. (2005). Challenges and opportunities of international clinical practica. *International Journal of Nursing Education Scholarship, 2*, Article 18, 1–13.

Nussbaum, M. (1997). *Cultivating humanity: A classical defense of reform in liberal education.* Cambridge, MA: Harvard University Press.

Rhodes, T. L. (Ed.). (2010). *Assessing outcomes and improving achievement: Tips and tools for using rubrics.* Washington, DC: Association of American Colleges and Universities.

Sloand, E., Bower, K., & Groves, S. (2008). Challenges and benefits of international clinical placements in public health nursing. *Nurse Educator, 33*(1), 35–38.

Stufflebeam, D. (2001). Evaluation models. *New Directions for Evaluation, 89*, 7–97.

Thorne, S. (1997). Global consciousness in nursing: An ethnographic study of nurses with an international perspective. *Journal of Nursing Education, 36*(9), 437–442.

Freida Chavez
Tamara Hertenstein McKinnon

GLOBAL SERVICE LEARNING

DEFINITION

Global service learning (GSL) refers to experiential educational programs in which students are immersed in another community and culture, providing meaningful service in collaboration with a partner community. GSL can take place "around the corner and across the globe." Emphasis is placed on both the learning (student-focused) and service (community partner–focused) aspects of programs.

APPLICATION

GSL programs are high-impact educational programs (Kuh, 2008) that involve collaboration among schools of nursing (SON), partner communities, and participants/students. Driving forces for GSL participation include benefits to participants, service to the partner community, and alignment with university/institutional mission and vision. Although nurses have a long history of providing service at both the local and international levels, the term GSL is new to nursing education. Defining GSL and its application in nursing education are critical as nursing establishes its role in service to the global community.

There has been an increase in interest and participation in global programs in SON over the past decade (McKinnon & McNelis, 2013). GSL educators work with administrators, colleagues, students, and partner communities, demonstrating competency in the areas of program development, relationship building, and coursework adaptation. Coursework may be an extension of an existing class or may be specially designed for a non-SON credit course. Educators are challenged to find a balance between the educational needs of students and service needs of the partner community.

Global experiences are not defined by geographic boundaries but are inclusive of experiences in which participants are

G

immersed completely in another community and culture. Global partners include culturally, and often linguistically, distinct communities within one's home country, as well as internationally. Most often, GSL programs focus on low-resource/marginalized communities. In order to ensure relevance and sustainability of programs, community members must drive the focus of service activities and are involved in each step of program planning and implementation. Smith, Fitzpatrick, and Hoyt-Hudson (2011) emphasize the importance of stakeholder involvement in global program development, stating, "local knowledge is a crucial input to the design and implementation of interventions" (p. 258).

Learners in GSL programs may include students in nursing programs and/or practicing nurses participating in continuing education programs. GSL provides a means of enhancing students' ability to become productive and engaged members of the global community (Tremethick & Smit, 2009). The ever-increasing multicultural population in the United States poses a significant challenge to nurses providing individualized and holistic care to their patients. This requires nurses to recognize and appreciate cultural differences in health care values, beliefs, and customs (Maier-Lorentz, 2008). GSL participation leads to beneficial outcomes such as increased cultural awareness, enhanced civic engagement (Edmonds, 2012), self-efficacy, and a global nursing perspective.

An example of a local GSL experience is as follows: Nursing students in a community health practicum are assigned to work in an inner-city program for recent immigrants. Collaborating with community leaders and local resource agencies, students address childhood nutrition issues by providing the following services: implementing a "train-the-trainer" program for indigenous healers; enlisting the efforts of local stores to provide options for culturally relevant, low-cost nutritional foods; engaging representatives from the local food bank and farmer's market; and coordinating a health fair with representation from agencies such as after-school activity programs.

An example of an international GSL experience is as follows: Senior-level students are assigned to work alongside students in the partner community's SON research and identify appropriate long-term interventions for addressing the emerging issue of caregiver role strain. Students from both institutions collaborate to design a plan for support groups in the community. Technology is used to support the sustainability of the program.

SYNOPSIS

Global programs in SON range from study-abroad to service programs. The distinction between GSL and study-abroad programs is the provision of service. Service is the act of providing something valuable to the partner community. The partner community identifies specific issues to be addressed by students in the GSL program and the participant's function within their scope of practice, working collaboratively with community members to provide meaningful service with a focus on sustainability and capacity development.

Experience alone does not lead to learning. Kolb (1984), integrating the writings of Dewey, Lewin, and Piaget, defined experiential learning as "the process whereby knowledge is created through the transformation of experience" (p. 38). GSL faculty create an environment that allows the transformation of a GSL experience into valuable learning. A comprehensive approach to learning must be in place in order for the global experience to lead to increased knowledge about course content, the partner community and culture, and oneself. This includes teaching theoretical content and role development prior to the global experience, ensuring opportunities for integration (e.g., journaling, case conference) during the experience, and a comprehensive overview and debriefing once the program is complete.

RECOMMENDATIONS

Measurement of outcomes on partner community is both a research and ethical imperative for nursing. Although research is available on the impact of GSL participation on students, little is known about the effects on partner communities. Measuring the outcomes of GSL programs on partner communities is the only way to ensure ethical, evidence-based programs.

McKinnon and Fealy (2011) propose core principles for GSL programs. Core principles, referred to as the "Seven Cs," include compassion, curiosity, courage, collaboration, creativity, capacity building, and competence. According to McKinnon and Fealy, "the articulation of core principles provides for consistency across programs while allowing individual programs to maintain their uniqueness at the level of program content and focus. Incorporating these principles provides for enhanced communication among programs, increased opportunity for collaborative research, and consistency of evaluation criteria" (p. 99).

Credit toward major (CTM) refers to the provision of school-of-nursing credit for coursework. A study by McKinnon and McNelis (2013) identified a lack of clarity among schools regarding regulations pertaining to provision of CTM for international practicum experiences. This uncertainty has been identified as a significant barrier to adoption of GSL programs by SON. As a result, many schools have resorted to creating high unit courses and applying extra units for the international experience. The extra units in these "work-around" offerings present a barrier to students who cannot afford to pay the additional fees, thus creating exclusionary programs. Providing CTM for global clinical courses creates opportunities for increased student participation (cost and time) and sustainability of programs (cost and faculty time), which ultimately lead to higher-quality programs.

Enhanced use of technology presents unique opportunities for GSL partners. The use of simulation to train students prior to the immersion experience, using modalities such as Skype to communicate with global partners during the planning phase, and connecting students on-site during the immersion with students in the classroom at the home institution are all examples of ways in which technology can enhance the GSL experience for all partners.

Edmonds, M. L. (2012). An integrative literature review of study abroad programs for nursing students. *Nursing Education Perspectives, 33*(1), 30–34. doi:10.5480/1536–5026-33.1.30

Kolb, D. A. (1984). *Experiential learning: Experience as the source of learning and development.* Englewood Cliffs, NJ: Prentice Hall.

Kuh, G. D. (2008). *High-impact educational practices: What they are, who has access to them, and why they matter.* Washington, DC: Association of American Colleges and Universities.

Maier-Lorentz, M. (2008). Transcultural nursing: Its importance in nursing practice. *Journal of Cultural Diversity, 15*(1), 37–43.

McKinnon, T. H., & Fealy, G. (2011). Core principles for developing global service-learning programs in nursing. *Nursing Education Perspectives, 32*(2), 95–100. doi:10.5480/1536–5026-32.2.95

McKinnon, T. H., & McNelis, A. M. (2013). International programs in United States schools of nursing: Driving forces, obstacles, and opportunities. *Nursing Education Perspectives, 34*(5), 323–328.

Smith, B., Fitzpatrick, J., & Hoyt-Hudson, P. (2011). *Problem solving for better health: A global perspective.* New York, NY: Springer Publishing.

Tremethick, M. J., & Smit, E. M. (2009). Preparing culturally competent health educators: The development and evaluation of a cultural immersion service-learning program. *International Electronic Journal of Health Education, 12,* 185–193.

Tamara Hertenstein McKinnon

GRADE INFLATION

DEFINITION

Scholars define grade inflation as an increase in student grades without a concomitant increase in ability (Cacamese, Elnicki, & Speer, 2007; Donaldson & Gray, 2012; Fazio,

G

Papp, Torre, & DeFer, 2013; Scanlan & Care, 2004, 2008). Although the issue of grade inflation has been a concern in academia for more than four decades, grade inflation is still rampant across disciplines and universities (O'Flynn-McGee & Clauson, 2013; Scanlan & Care, 2004, 2008; Weaver, Humbert, Besinger, Graber, & Brizendine, 2007).

APPLICATION

The issue of grade inflation is important to nurse educators as gatekeepers to a practice profession (Fazio et al., 2013; O'Flynn-McGee & Clauson, 2013; Roman & Trevino, 2006; Scanlan & Care, 2008; Sowbel, 2011). According to these authors, the purpose of grades is to provide the student with information regarding the ability to master knowledge of nursing, as well as the application of knowledge to practice. If students have over-inflated perceptions of their knowledge and competence as a nurse, the concern for safe practice is real. Furthermore, in a consumer-driven era, students may focus on attaining high grades, rather than learning (Duane & Satre, 2014; O'Flynn-McGee & Clauson, 2013; Scanlan & Care, 2004). Nurse educators experience uneasy feelings when a marginal student graduates. The question faced is "What will be the long-term impact on patient care for a student whose practice was, at best, marginal?"

In universities, student evaluations of teaching performance and course delivery are integral factors considered in promotion and tenure decisions; there is widespread belief that higher grades lead to better teaching evaluations (Fazio et al., 2013; Germain & Scandura, 2005; O'Flynn-McGee & Clauson, 2013; Scanlan & Care, 2004, 2008). Faculty question the validity and reliability of standardized evaluation tools (Donaldson & Gray, 2012; Germain & Scandura, 2005), an issue that is particularly critical when clinical practice is graded. For example, if tools designed to evaluate classroom teaching are mandated for use by students in clinical practice courses, student feedback may not be useful. Nonetheless, fear of poor student evaluations may underlie faculty practices to assign higher clinical grades in the belief that these higher grades will lead to better student evaluations of teaching effectiveness.

Another factor related to grade inflation is the use of part-time faculty as preceptors for students in clinical practice (Bickes & Schim, 2010; Roman & Trevino, 2006; Scanlan & Care, 2008). These nurses, while skillful practitioners, are not familiar with the nursing curriculum, intended clinical outcomes, nor the theoretical underpinnings of evaluation. In addition, the relationship with the student can interfere with the preceptor's ability to make a reasoned judgment (Bickes & Schim, 2010; Donaldson & Gray, 2012; O'Flynn-McGee & Clauson, 2013; Scanlan & Care, 2008; Sowbel, 2011). More importantly, these part-time faculty lack experience and the confidence to make a determination that the student does not have the requisite knowledge and understanding to pass the course (Heaslip & Scammell, 2012).

SYNOPSIS

In reviewing the literature, there are consistent themes regarding the reasons for grade inflation that include rising consumerism among students, institutional policies such as mandatory teaching evaluations and threat of appeal, use of part-time faculty, lack of faculty understanding regarding evaluation practices, and completion of assigning a grade-to-clinical practice (Bickes & Schim, 2010; Germain & Scandura, 2005; O'Flynn-McGee & Clauson, 2013; Scanlan & Care, 2004, 2008; Schneider, 2013; Weaver et al., 2007). Although there are some empirical studies (Bickes & Schim, 2010; Donaldson & Gray, 2012; O'Flynn-McGee & Clauson, 2013; Scanlan & Care, 2004, 2008), there is no sustained body of empirical evidence that addresses grade inflation in nursing, particularly in clinical practice.

Grade inflation in clinical practice is particularly important to nurse educators as gatekeepers of the profession. The underlying factors of use of part-time clinical teachers, lack of understanding of evaluation practices, and university policies contribute to grade inflation and allow marginal students to graduate.

There is a reluctance to fail students clinically, especially in the first year of clinical practice because faculty may believe it is important to give students a second chance (Heaslip & Scammell, 2012; Scanlan & Care, 2004, 2008). Clinical evaluations are further compromised when one considers the complexity of professional values and the impact of regulatory requirements inherent in nursing practice (O'Flynn-McGee & Clauson, 2013). Without genuine feedback, students may proceed with the program without addressing underperforming issues.

University policies contribute to the potential for grade inflation (Donaldson & Gray, 2012; Fazio et al., 2013; Scanlan & Care, 2004, 2008). Students who perform poorly in a course may voluntarily withdraw late in the term. More troubling is the threat that a student may appeal to a low grade. Students view themselves as consumers and believe that hard work equals a high grade (Germain & Scandura, 2005; Scanlan & Care, 2004). When the grade desired is not forthcoming, students can appeal the grade. Rather than face the prospects of an appeal, faculty find it easier to assign a higher grade in keeping with the grade the student expects (Bickes & Schim, 2010; Fazio et al., 2013; Scanlan & Care, 2004, 2008). An unintended consequence of assigning higher grades when not warranted is that the grade scale becomes compressed and truly good work and effort are not rewarded (O'Flynn-McGee & Clauson, 2013; Scanlan & Care, 2004, 2008). Students quickly learn that minimal effort is all that is required for a "good" grade.

RECOMMENDATIONS

There are few solutions to grade inflation that have not been discussed in the discourse concerning grade inflation, including faculty development regarding evaluation practices, use of valid and reliable evaluation tools, and review of university policies (Cacamese et al., 2007; Heaslip & Scammell, 2012; O'Flynn-McGee & Clauson, 2013; Scanlan & Care, 2004, 2008). Clear criteria that address clinical practice outcomes could ameliorate grade inflation in clinical practice courses. In an effort to address grade inflation in clinical grades, nurse educators have moved to a pass/fail in clinical courses. However, as Heaslip and Scammell (2012) contend, even pass/fail clinical evaluations are subjective and not value free. The evaluations depend on an assessment by the evaluator.

Conceptually, the definition of grade inflation as described is the accepted definition in the literature across a wide range of university disciplines. However, is there conceptual clarity regarding grade inflation? Are the studies in the current literature studying the same phenomenon? A rigorous concept analysis of grade inflation would add clarity to the literature.

Nurse educators teach the nurses of tomorrow. As the entry point to the profession, it is incumbent upon nurse educators to ensure that feedback to students is genuine and reflects nursing practice abilities. Ongoing research addresses the issues necessary to ensure that graduates of nursing programs are clearly able to provide safe and competent nursing care.

Bickes, J. T., & Schim, S. M. (2010). Righting writing: Strategies for improving nursing student papers. *International Journal of Nursing Education Scholarship, 7*(1), Article 8.

Cacamese, S. M., Elnicki, M., & Speer, A. J. (2007). Grade inflation and the internal medicine subinternship: A national survey of clerkship directors. *Teaching and Learning in Medicine: An International Journal, 19*(4), 343–346.

Donaldson, J. H., & Gray, M. (2012). Systematic review of grading practice: Is there evidence of grade inflation? *Nurse Education in Practice, 12,* 101–114.

Duane, B. T., & Satre, M. E. (2014). Utilizing constructivism learning theory in collaborative testing as a creative strategy to promote essential nursing skills. *Nurse Education Today, 34,* 31–34.

Fazio, S. B., Papp, K. K., Torre, D. M., & DeFer, T. M. (2013). Grade inflation in the internal medicine clerkship: A national survey. *Teaching and Learning in Medicine, 25*(1), 71–76.

Germain, M. L., & Scandura, T. A. (2005). Grade inflation and student individual differences as systematic bias in faculty evaluations. *Journal of Instructional Management, 32*(1), 58–66.

Heaslip, V., & Scammell, J. M. E. (2012). Failing underperforming students: The role of grading in clinical practice assessment. *Nurse Education in Practice, 12,* 95–100.

O'Flynn-Magee, K., & Clauson, M. (2013). Uncovering nurse educators' beliefs and values about grading academic papers: Guidelines for best practices. *Journal of Nursing Education, 52*(9), 492–499.

Roman, B. J. B., & Trevino, J. (2006). An approach to address grade inflation in a psychiatry clerkship. *Academic Psychiatry, 30*(2), 110–115.

Scanlan, J. M., & Care, W. D. (2004). Grade inflation: Should we be concerned? *Journal of Nursing Education, 43,* 475–478.

Scanlan, J. M., & Care, W. D. (2008). Issues with grading and grade inflation in nursing education. In M. H. Oermann (Ed.), *Annual review of nursing education* (Vol. 6, pp. 173–188). New York, NY: Springer Publishing.

Schneider, G. (2013). Student evaluations, grade inflation and pluralistic teaching: Moving from customer satisfaction to student learning and critical thinking. *Forum for Social Economics,* 122–134.

Sowbel, L. R. (2011). Gate keeping in field performance: Is grade inflation a given? *Journal of Social Work Education, 47*(2), 367–377.

Weaver, C. S., Humbert, A. J., Besinger, B. R., Graber, J. S., & Brizendine, E. J. (2007). A more explicit grading scale decreases grade inflation in a clinical clerkship. *Academic Emergency Medicine, 14*(3), 283–286.

Judith M. Scanlan

GRADING

DEFINITION

Grading involves assigning a level of merit to a student's work. A grade can be a letter, a number, or pass/fail, and represents the student's effort and abilities on an assignment or in a course. Letter and number grades are on a ratio scale, which allows comparison between students.

APPLICATION

In nursing, grades are assigned in both theory and clinical courses. It is generally thought that theory course grades are more objective than clinical course grades. In a recent national survey of nursing faculty, the grade for a theory course was primarily comprised of test grades, and then papers and projects (Oermann, Saewert, & Charasika, 2009). The survey also assessed how nursing faculty assign grades in clinical courses, which are primarily pass/fail as opposed to letter or number grades, and found that most faculty use a rubric that is often the same across courses, but altered slightly to address the specific learning goals of each course (Oermann, Yarbrough, Saewert, Ard, & Charasika, 2009).

Three key themes are present in the nursing literature around grading: grade inflation, disparity between clinical and theory course grades, and challenges in assigning failing clinical grades.

Grade inflation refers to giving higher grades for lower levels of effort and ability over time. Some reasons for grade inflation are due to faculty concerns around receiving good student evaluations that determine their rank and tenure and ensuring high enrollment in their courses (Shoemaker & DeVos, 1999). Another reason cited is that when a C grade is considered the lowest acceptable grade rather than D, there is upward pressure on grades (Walsh & Seldomridge, 2005). One of the biggest concerns with grade inflation is ensuring nurses who graduate are able to provide safe and skilled care to patients, and elevated grades may make it difficult to determine who will pass the National Council Licensure Examination (NCLEX) as well as who is adequately prepared for graduate studies (Shoemaker & DeVos, 1999). One solution to address grade inflation involves training faculty to improve grading practices (Shoemaker & DeVos, 1999).

Grade inflation may be related to the increasing disparity between theory and clinical grades, whereby clinical grades are helping to inflate course grades. It is assumed that theory underlies excellent nursing practice; therefore, a correlation is expected between grades in theory and corresponding clinical courses (Walsh & Seldomridge, 2005). In a study comparing clinical and theory grades, the authors found that clinical grades were higher than theory grades (Walsh & Seldomridge, 2005). The reasons cited for the disparity primarily involve the challenging nature of clinical grading.

Clinical grades are seen as more subjective than theory grades, and are therefore more challenging to determine. In a qualitative study of clinical faculty, faculty admitted overseeing students who did not meet safe patient-handling standards in clinical settings, but were reluctant to fail them (Luhanga, Yonge, & Myrick, 2008). Some reasons for not failing unsafe students included concern for how the failing grade might affect the student right before he or she was to graduate, feeling they did not have enough time to observe the student in clinical, and empathy for the amount of money spent on the course (Luhanga et al., 2008).

One way to objectify clinical grades is to create clear evaluation standards and share these with students ahead of time. As Isaacson and Stacy (2009) suggest, creating a rubric that clearly explains what clinical skills students are to demonstrate to meet the course objectives is one way to assist clinical faculty in ranking student performance. However, clinical evaluation tools have been criticized for their lack of differentiation among students, allowing marginal students to pass. For instance, some areas of the evaluation may be seen as more important to clinical performance; however, all areas are weighed the same, so if a student does well in the less important areas, he or she may still be able to satisfactorily complete clinical courses (Walsh & Seldomridge, 2005). Another issue with rubrics is that clinical experiences are varied; instructors cannot ensure that each student will have the opportunity to exhibit all of the skills listed on the rubric (Walsh & Seldomridge, 2005).

One option explored by a university in the United Kingdom was allowing clinical faculty to use an evaluation tool with a grade scale for clinical practice rather than using a pass/fail system (Heaslip & Scammell, 2012). Although most faculty (64.2%) reported they liked the tool and grading on a scale allowed for greater differentiation of students' performance, 67.9% wanted more training on how to grade and 59.8% reported wanting more training on how to work with failing students (Heaslip & Scammell, 2012).

Because failing students for poor clinical performance is such a difficult endeavor for preceptors, it is important to consider what can be done to support them in the grading process. The consensus from preceptors is that patient safety is the key criterion in assessing student clinical performance (Amicucci, 2012). One possibility would be to make patient safety carry more weight on clinical rubrics. Some suggestions that came out in a qualitative study of preceptors were to have clinical liaisons who are supportive and listen to a preceptor's concerns regarding student safety, speak to the student with the preceptor, and follow up with the preceptor after failing a student (Hrobsky & Kersbergen, 2002).

SYNOPSIS

Grading in nursing education is a complex matter that has differing challenges in theory and clinical courses. Some key themes in the literature involve grade inflation, lack of failing grades for poor clinical performance,

G

and the disparity between theory and clinical grades.

RECOMMENDATIONS

The practice of grading in nursing would be aided by research on alternative methods of clinical grading, including finding ways to assess varied clinical experiences while ensuring that students provide safe patient care. Due to the complexity involved in clinical grading, it would be helpful for nurse researchers to examine innovative clinical grading scenarios to evaluate their effectiveness in capturing student learning and patient safety. Studies of faculty development around grading practices are also needed.

Amicucci, B. (2012). What nurse faculty have to say about clinical grading. *Teaching and Learning in Nursing, 7,* 51–55. doi:10.1016/j.teln.2011.09.002

Heaslip, V., & Scammell, J. M. E. (2012). Failing underperforming students: The role of grading in practice assessment. *Nurse Education in Practice, 12,* 95–100. doi:10.1016/j.nepr.2011.08.003

Hrobsky, P. E., & Kersbergen, A. L. (2002). Preceptors' perceptions of clinical performance failure. *Journal of Nursing Education, 41*(12), 550–553.

Isaacson, J. J., & Stacy, A. S. (2009). Rubrics for clinical evaluation: Objectifying the subjective experience. *Nurse Education in Practice, 9,* 134–140. doi:10.1016/j.nepr.2008.10.015

Luhanga, F., Yonge, O. J., & Myrick, F. (2008). "Failure to assign failing grades": Issues with grading the unsafe student. *International Journal of Nursing Education Scholarship, 5*(1), 1–14.

Oermann, M. H., Saewert, K. J., & Charasika, M. (2009). Assessment and grading in schools of nursing: National survey findings part I. *Nursing Education Perspectives, 30*(5), 274–278.

Oermann, M. H., Yarbrough, S. S., Saewert, K. J., Ard, N., & Charasika, M. (2009). Clinical evaluation and grading practices in schools of nursing: National survey findings part II. *Nursing Education Perspectives,* 352–357.

Shoemaker, J. K., & DeVos, M. (1999). Are we a gift shop? A perspective on grade inflation. *Journal of Nursing Education, 38*(9), 394–398.

Walsh, C. M., & Seldomridge, L. A. (2005). Clinical grades: Upward bound. *Journal of Nursing Education, 44*(4), 162–168.

Kathryn E. Phillips

GRADING CLINICAL PRACTICE

DEFINITION

Grading clinical practice is a process in which a clinical nurse faculty assesses the nursing student in a clinical setting and then assigns a grade that deems whether or not that student has met clinical course objectives and is safe to practice (Amicucci, 2012).

APPLICATION

Evaluating a student's level of performance involves monitoring the student's progression toward learning goals and then making a decision on that student's performance, which is reflected in the student's final grade (Oermann, Yarbrough, Saewert, Ard, & Charasika, 2009). The current standard of grading clinical practice is based on the evaluation of clinical competency. Safe practice is one aspect of competency along with analyzing complex patient situations, problem solving, and effective communication with other health care providers, as well as the patient (Oermann et al., 2009). Nurse educators have failed to clearly define competency (Oermann et al., 2009; Watson, Stimpson, Topping, & Porock, 2002). According to Watson, Stimpson, Topping, and Porock (2002, p. 423), "competence may be achieved by a general level of performance being assessed or it may be achieved by having a number of component parts of competence, so called competencies, being performed." Competencies are determined by and distributed through national organizations of nursing, accrediting bodies in nursing, schools of nursing, and clinical nurse faculties.

SYNOPSIS

Clear guidelines for grading clinical practice in nursing education have not been established. When grading clinical practice, multiple strategies should be incorporated in making a decision on a student's clinical performance (Oermann et al., 2009). Strategies and tools reported in the literature include clinical evaluation forms/checklists, student contribution to clinical conferences, case presentations, skills laboratory, simulation, and rubrics (Ashcraft et al., 2013; Coralli, 2006; Himes & Ravert, 2012; Houghton, Casey, Shaw, & Murphy, 2012; Oermann et al., 2009).

Due to the lack of a clear definition, it is not surprising that there also is a lack of valid and reliable instruments to assess clinical competency. The tools and strategies mentioned above may be used but "the likelihood that vital concepts are excluded and irrelevant concepts are included in existing clinical competence assessment instruments is very high…when developed, there remains the issue of what level of performance indicates competence and…at what level a student can be deemed incompetent" (Watson et al., 2002, p. 423).

Graded versus pass/fail assessment is another topic of debate when assessing clinical practice. Use of pass/fail when grading clinical practice represents either "acceptable" or "nonacceptable" standards of nursing practice (Andre, 2000). Thus, application of a pass/fail grading system does not represent the efforts of the high-achieving student and "pass/fail" does not accurately describe these efforts to future employers, scholarship, and postgraduate committees (Andre, 2000). The grading process provides insight to both the teacher and student on the student's standing as well as what the

student needs to do to improve that standing (Biggs, 1992).

In contrast, proponents for pass/fail propose that pass/fail encourages self-reflection and self-regulated learning. According to the proponents, overall performance and motivation among students is no less when using pass/fail as opposed to grading; pass/fail fosters a less competitive learning environment; pass/fail results in better group cohesion as well as increased collaboration among students; and use of pass/fail can lead to improved well-being, better mood, and lower stress in students (Robins et al., 1995; Rohe et al., 2006; Spring, Robillard, Gehlbach, & Simas, 2011; White & Fantone, 2010).

Irrespective of the grading system chosen, grades in clinical practice are affected by leniency and subsequent grade inflation (Donaldson & Gray, 2012; Seldomridge & Walsh, 2006). Grade inflation occurs when clinical scores exceed actual student performance and is made obvious by class evaluations demonstrating many high grades and a few average grades in the clinical setting (Seldomridge & Walsh, 2006). Reasons for grade inflation include student–instructor relationships, inexperience of faculty, pressure from students for good grades, avoiding conflict associated with failing a student, and tool design (Donaldson & Gray, 2012).

RECOMMENDATIONS

The literature is rife with discussion on the problems of clinical evaluation, but sparse in terms of solutions. Clinical nurse faculty has a professional responsibility to fairly and accurately determine if a student is competent and safe to practice. There is a need for research in grading clinical practice, specifically in the following areas: (a) defining clinical competency; (b) developing valid and reliable instruments to determine competence; (c) choosing between graded versus pass/fail assessment; and (d) reducing grade inflation. As the role and opportunities for nursing practice continue to expand, optimizing accuracy in grading clinical practice

G

will help to ensure that nursing students are prepared for the challenges of clinical practice.

Amicucci, B. (2012). What nurse faculty have to say about clinical grading. *Teaching and Learning in Nursing, 7,* 51–55.

Andre, K. (2000). Grading student clinical practice performance: The Australian perspective. *Nurse Education Today, 20,* 672–679.

Ashcraft, A. S., Opton, L., Bridges, R. A., Caballero, S., Veesart, A., & Weaver, C. (2013). Simulation evaluation using a modified Lasater Clinical Judgment Rubric. *Nursing Education Perspective, 34,* 122–126.

Biggs, J. (1992). A qualitative approach to grading students. *HERDSA News, 14,* 3–6.

Coralli, C. H. (2006). Effective case presentations—an important clinical skill for nurse practitioners. *Journal American Academy Nurse Practitioners, 18,* 216–220.

Donaldson, J. H., & Gray, M. (2012). Systematic review of grading practice: Is there evidence of grade inflation? *Nurse Education Practise, 12,* 101–114.

Himes, D. O., & Ravert, P. K. (2012). Situated peer coaching and unfolding cases in the fundamentals skills laboratory. *International Journal of Nursing Education Scholarship, 9,* 1–19.

Houghton, C. E., Casey, D., Shaw, D., & Murphy, K. (2012). Staff and students' perceptions and experiences of teaching and assessment in Clinical Skills Laboratories: Interview findings from a multiple case study. *Nurse Education Today, 32,* e29–e34.

Oermann, M. H., Yarbrough, S. S., Saewert, K. J., Ard, N., & Charasika, M. E. (2009). Clinical evaluation and grading practices in schools of nursing: National survey findings part II. *Nursing Education Perspective, 30,* 352–357.

Robins, L. S., Fantone, J. C., Oh, M. S., Alexander, G. L., Shlafer, M., & Davis, W. K. (1995). The effect of pass/fail grading and weekly quizzes on first-year students' performances and satisfaction. *Academic Medicine, 70,* 327–329.

Rohe, D. E., Barrier, P. A., Clark, M. M., Cook, D. A., Vickers, K. S., & Decker, P. A. (2006). The benefits of pass-fail grading on stress, mood, and group cohesion in medical students. *Mayo Clinical Proceedings, 81,* 1443–1448.

Seldomridge, L. A., & Walsh, C. M. (2006). Evaluating student performance in undergraduate preceptorships. *Journal of Nursing Education, 45,* 169–176.

Spring, L., Robillard, D., Gehlbach, L., & Simas, T. A. (2011). Impact of pass/fail grading on medical students' well-being and academic outcomes. *Medical Education, 45,* 867–877.

Watson, R., Stimpson, A., Topping, A., & Porock, D. (2002). Clinical competence assessment in nursing: A systematic review of the literature. *Journal of Advanced Nursing, 39,* 421–431.

White, C. B., & Fantone, J. C. (2010). Pass-fail grading: Laying the foundation for self-regulated learning. *Advances in Health Sciences Education: Theory and Practice, 15,* 469–477.

Suzy Mascaro Walter

H

HANDHELD TECHNOLOGY

DEFINITION

Handheld technology refers to a device that is highly portable and small enough to be held and operated in one's hand or hands. Most commonly, this term is used interchangeably with the terms *mobile device* or *handheld computer* and is generally pocket sized with a display screen and an input–output interface. Usually, these are multifunctional, integrated devices that have operating systems that run programs; can browse the Internet; capture, manipulate, and display data; and so on. Frequently, these functionalities are integrated with mobile phones and are referred to as *smartphones*.

APPLICATION

In 1994, the Psion I was introduced as the world's first handheld computer. It was about the size of a pack of cigarettes and had limited functionality. While it was a very simple personal organizer, it became a catalyst for rapid innovation leading to the landmark launching of the Palm Pilot™ in 1996. The Palm Pilot was a totally new handheld device that used a data entry system by means of a stylus and specialized handwriting software. This device transformed handheld technology. Palm's open source platform encouraged independent development of third-party add-ons and software. The underlying premise was that the more accessories and applications, the greater the versatility and hence greater demand for the devices. Since those early days, the field has become highly competitive with more and more powerful devices with greater functionalities becoming widely available.

Consequently, handheld technology has established a strong foothold in contemporary society. The use of these devices transcends age, class, gender, nationality, race, and ethnicity barriers. Handheld technology is replacing bulky desktop computers, landline telephones, and other "hard wired" and "fixed" technologies, and has stimulated an astounding shift from the wired to the wireless world that would not have been possible without the introduction of handheld devices. The benefits of handheld technology include: (a) "Complete office functionalities" in a mobile environment so that individuals are not bound to their desks in order to be productive and connected; (b) convenience; (c) greater connection and access to information; (d) enhanced and immediate communication capabilities via phone, instant messaging, e-mail, and so on; (e) global positioning; and (f) remote sensing and data collection, and much more.

For health care providers, handheld technology offers the ability to store, organize, process, and permit instant retrieval of information swiftly and easily at the *point of care/point of need*. It is because of this capability that handhelds have emerged as useful and often indispensable tools to support professional practice—as essential as the stethoscope. These small computers can store clinical reference books and tools, permit input and management of clinical databases, and access web-based clinical resources, thus making information more easily accessible while delivering care in any setting, including the bedside (Doran et al., 2007; Mickan, Tilson, Atherton, Roberts, & Heneghan, 2013;

Ruland, 2002). In addition, these devices offer the health care provider a means to access "just enough information, just in time," a clear benefit at the point of care (Cornelius, Haslam, & Dreher, 2009). Contemporary health professionals are using handheld technology to improve accuracy, save time, streamline workflow, improve patient safety, and improve patient outcomes as well as "facilitate the transformation of documentation of assessments, interventions, and outcomes into evidence-based decision making resources" (Hardwick, Pulido, & Adelson, 2007, p. 251).

SYNOPSIS

Handheld technology has made notable contributions to nursing education by providing opportunities to expand the scope and functionality of inquiry activities, as well as by creating unique educational opportunities (Slotta & Aleahmad, 2002). Evolving handheld technology allows for a more integrative approach to teaching nursing, spanning beyond the classroom and providing opportunities to support learning outside of the classroom (Suplee, Cornelius, & Gallagher Gordon, 2009). The use of handheld technology fits well with the use of constructivist and situated learning approaches. The constructivist approach uses previously acquired knowledge as the foundation on which to scaffold new learning. This approach is strengthened by the integration of handheld technology as it permits learning to take place "on the go." The situated learning approach would utilize handheld technology to support social interaction and collaborative learning, and would permit incorporation of authentic tasks and activities for students in the process of knowledge creation. The role of the nurse educator is to help students construct knowledge via "real-life problem solving including ill-structured goals and opportunity for the detection of relevant versus irrelevant information" (Young, 2002, p. 2). Handheld technology supports that endeavor. As a student learning tool, handheld technology can enrich nursing education, provide the foundation

for lifelong practice, and have far reaching impact on patient care (Cornelius et al., 2009; Koeniger-Donohue, 2008; Krauskopf & Farrell, 2011).

Accrediting agencies and organizations endorse nursing students' acquiring skills in technology, information management, and information literacy. The National League of Nursing (NLN), American Association of Colleges of Nursing (AACN), and the National Organization for Nurse Practitioner Faculties (NONPF) have identified these skills as essential competencies at the baccalaureate, masters, and doctoral level. Nursing curricula should be designed to integrate technology in order to promote lifelong learning and prepare students for their future roles in the profession. It is imperative that nurse educators strive to improve the preparation of nurses—at all levels—with the goal of developing proficiencies so they will flourish in a technology-driven health care industry (Suplee et al., 2009).

RECOMMENDATIONS

Strategies to incorporate handheld technology into authentic learning activities include:

1. Identifying desired resources and tools that can support achievement of established learning objectives.

2. Constructing structured learning activities that are relevant and meaningfully linked with the specialty content being taught.

3. Designing activities to model realistic point-of-care/point-of-need information access one might experience in an actual clinical setting.

    a. Basic information seeking, such as pharmacology challenges, are utilized.

    b. Case studies can be more complex, requiring triangulation of information resources.

    c. Simulations provide a more realistic experience by creating a "live" experience using simulation manikins.

Given the dynamic nature of the classroom and clinical learning environments, faculty can rely on handheld technology as a tool that supports development of student competencies by making the most of "teachable moments." Leveraging handheld technology in nursing education will enhance and promote lifelong learning. It is essential that nursing programs provide students with the essential skills and competencies that will prepare them to function effectively in a "high-tech" health care environment. "The pace of innovation in healthcare will only accelerate; therefore, it is imperative that both faculty and students develop a level of comfort and openness to future technological advances. Doing so will not only help us improve our practice, but will ultimately improve patient outcomes" (Suplee et al., 2009, p. 4).

Cornelius, F. H., Haslam, E., & Dreher, H. D. (2009). *Handheld technology and nursing education: Utilization of handheld technology in development of clinical decision-making in undergraduate nursing students.* EDULEARN09 Proceedings: Barcelona, Spain.

Doran, D. M., Mylopoulos, J., Kushniruk, A., Nagle, L., Laurie-Shaw, B., Sidani, S.,…McArthur, G. (2007). Evidence in the palm of your hand: Development of an outcomes-focused knowledge translation intervention. *Worldviews on Evidence-Based Nursing/Sigma Theta Tau International, Honor Society of Nursing, 4*(2), 69–77.

Hardwick, M. E., Pulido, P. A., & Adelson, W. S. (July/August, 2007). The use of handheld technology in nursing research and practice. *Orthopaedic Nursing, 26*(4), 251–255.

Koeniger-Donohue, R. (2008). Handheld computers in nursing education: PDA pilot project. *Journal of Nursing Education, 47*(2), 74–77.

Krauskopf, P. B., & Farrell, S. (2011). Accuracy and efficiency of novice nurse practitioners using personal digital assistants. *Journal of Nursing Scholarship, 43*(2), 117–124.

Mickan, S., Tilson, J. K., Atherton, H., Roberts, N. W., & Heneghan, C. (2013). Evidence of effectiveness of health care professionals using handheld computers: A scoping review of systematic reviews. *Journal of Medical Internet Research, 15*(10), e212.

Ruland, C. M. (2002). Handheld technology to improve patient care: Evaluating a support system for preference-based care planning at the bedside. *Journal of the American Medical Informatics Association: JAMIA, 9*(2), 192–201.

Slotta, J., & Aleahmad, T. (2002). Integrating handheld technology and web-based science activities. In P. Barker & S. Rebelsky (Eds.), *Proceedings of world conference on educational multimedia, hypermedia and telecommunications* (pp. 25–30). Retrieved from http://www.editlib.org/p/9282

Suplee, P. D., Cornelius, F. H., & Gallagher Gordon, M. (2009). *Developing lifelong learning skills through integration of mobile devices in women's health education.* EDULEARN09 Proceedings: Barcelona, Spain. ISBN: 978–84-612–9802-0.

Young, D. (2002). *Second year medical resident amazed with potential of PDAs, pdaMD.com.* Retrieved from http://www.pdamd.com/vertical/features/MedResAmz.xml

Frances H. Cornelius

HEALTH LITERACY

DEFINITION

In *Healthy People 2010*, health literacy is defined as, "the degree to which individuals have the capacity to obtain, process, and understand basic health information and services needed to make appropriate health decisions" (U.S. Department of Health and Human Services, 2000, Section 11, p. 20).

H

APPLICATION

People with poor literacy skills have much higher medical costs and more hospitalization than literate people. Poor health literacy results in increased morbidity and mortality, more emergency department visits, less likelihood of the use of preventive services, and less likelihood that a person will take medications as instructed (Bastable, Meyers, & Poitevent, 2014).

Nurses are in a unique position as patient advocates and educators to help their clients obtain, process, and understand health information to make appropriate health decisions (Bastable et al., 2014). Whether in hospitals, long-term facilities, clinics, or public health settings, nurses provide care to more than 90 million Americans who struggle to locate, understand, and appropriately use health information (Zarcadoolas, Pleasant, & Greer, 2006).

The American Association of Colleges of Nursing (2008) in its *Essentials of Baccalaureate Education for Professional Nursing Practice* identifies health literacy as an important content area for all baccalaureate programs. "Nurse educators recognize the need for curriculum standards in the area of health literacy" (Smith & Zsohar, 2011, p. 48). Nursing education programs best prepare students by focusing on current health literacy topics including the definitions of literacy and health literacy, the scope of the problem, at-risk populations, the relationship between health literacy and poor health outcomes, how to identify people with low literacy skills, e-health literacy (appraising information from electronic sources), and ways to optimize the readability of patient education materials. Plain language communication, interpersonal skills, cultural sensitivity, at-risk populations, and observed client behavior related to low literacy are often included in health literacy education programs (Smith & Zsohar, 2011).

Nurse educators can use active teaching strategies to help students integrate health literacy skills into practice (Smith & Zsohar, 2011). Nursing students can view video vignettes and then demonstrate skills. Patient education materials can be tested for readability and then rewritten at more appropriate reading levels.

SYNOPSIS

Research in health literacy has focused on the development of standardized tests nurses can use to measure reading and health literacy skills of patients. These tests include the Wide Range Achievement Test (WRAT), the Rapid Estimate of Adult Literacy in Medicine (REALM), the Test of Functional Health Literacy in Adults (TOFHLA), the Newest Vital Sign (NVS), the eHealth Learning Scale (eHEALS), and the Literacy Assessment of Diabetes (LAD; Bastable et al., 2014). The dental/medical health literacy screen (REALMD-20) is now available for adult dental and medical patients (Gironda, Der-Martirosian, Messadi, Holtzman, & Atchison, 2013).

Administration of health literacy screening tests can be awkward for nurses to use in practice and the results can be hard to use. According to Chew, Bradley, and Boyko (2004), an easier way to identify inadequate health literacy skills is to ask three questions: (a) "How often do you have someone help you read hospital materials?" (b) "How confident are you filling out medical forms by yourself?" and (c) "How often do you have problems learning about your medical condition because of difficulty understanding written information?"

Bastable et al. (2014) summarize the literature and present practical strategies for nurses to use when in the role of an educator. These strategies include establishing a trusting relationship before starting the learning process, using the smallest amount of information to accomplish behavioral objectives, teaching one step at a time, using multiple methods and tools requiring fewer literacy skills, allowing patients the opportunity to restate information in their own words and demonstrating procedures, recognizing patient progress to keep motivation high, tailoring new regimens into daily schedules of clients, and utilizing repetition by saying the same thing in different ways.

Nurses often rely on the classic work of Doak, Doak, and Root (1996) for ideas on preparing written materials. Bastable et al. (2014) consolidate the literature and provide a comprehensive list of 27 strategies to use in writing easy-to-read patient education materials. Suggestions include ideas on text and sentence construction, format, layout, and the use of graphics. Specific writing ideas include the following: use conversational style, use short words, use headers, have sufficient white space, use short sentences, define technical words, use simple and realistic drawings, use simple type style at 14 to 16 font size, and aim at or less than the 6th-grade reading level. In addition, all written materials should be readability tested using a formula such as SMOG (estimate of the years of education a person needs to understand written material) or FRY (evaluates readability) and be pretested.

RECOMMENDATIONS

The role of an educator has always been an important part of nursing practice. Nurses are communicators and interpreters of health information. As stated by Bastable et al. (2014), "Nurse educators need to know how to identify clients with literacy problems, assess their needs, and choose appropriate interventions that create a supportive environment directed toward helping those with poor reading and comprehension skills to better and more safely care for themselves" (p. 303).

Nurses are in the ideal position to improve the quality of care delivered to clients. As the health care system becomes increasingly diverse and populations more heterogeneous, it becomes critical for nurses to learn and implement health literacy concepts and skills to help clients with the many problems associated with poor health literacy.

American Association of Colleges of Nursing. (2008). *The essentials of baccalaureate education for professional nursing practice.* Retrieved from www.aacn.nche.edu/Education/pdf/BaccEssentials08.pdf

Bastable, S. B., Meyers, G. M., & Poitevent, L. B. (2014). Literacy in the adult client population. In S. B. Bastable (Ed.), *Nurse as educator: Principles of teaching and learning for nursing practice* (4th ed., pp. 255–311). Burlington, MA: Jones & Bartlett Learning.

Chew, L. D., Bradley, K. A., & Boyko, E. J. (2004). Brief questions to identify patients with inadequate health literacy. *Family Medicine, 36*(8), 588–594.

Doak, C. C., Doak, L. G., & Root, J. H. (1996). *Teaching patients with low literacy skills* (2nd ed.). Philadelphia, PA: J. B. Lippincott.

Gironda, M., Der-Martirosian, C., Messadi, D., Holtzman, J., & Atchison, K. (2013). A brief 20 item dental/medical health literacy screen (REALM-20). *Journal of Public Dentistry, 75,* 50–55.

Smith, J. A., & Zsohar, H. (2011). Teaching health literacy in the undergraduate curriculum: Beyond traditional methods. *Nursing Education Perspectives, 32*(1), 48–50.

U.S. Department of Health and Human Services. (2000). *Healthy People 2010: Understanding and improving health* (2nd ed.). Washington, DC: U.S. Government Printing Office.

Zarcadoolas, C., Pleasant, A. F., & Greer, D. S. (2006). *Advancing health literacy: A framework for understanding and action.* San Francisco, CA: Jossey-Bass.

Jackie A. Smith

HEALTH POLICY

DEFINITION

Policy is the deliberate course of action chosen by an individual or group to deal with a problem (Anderson, 2008). "Health policy refers to decisions, plans, and actions that are undertaken to achieve specific health

H

care goals within a society. An explicit health policy can achieve several things: it defines a vision for the future, which in turn helps to establish targets and points of reference for the short and medium term. It outlines priorities and the expected roles of different groups; and it builds consensus and informs people" (World Health Organization, 2014).

APPLICATION

Health policy crosses all aspects of nursing. It guides and directs patient care at the individual, community, national, and global levels. Nurses need to understand the role of health policy in relation to delivery systems, quality standards, reimbursement, and finance. Core concepts need to be included in all levels of nursing education. Educating nurses in health policy is a mandate found in the American Association of Colleges of Nursing (AACN, 2014).

Students need to understand the current health policy. Health policy is integrated at all levels of the curriculum, including reimbursement guidelines, insurance, and laws guiding professional practice. Guidelines, standards, and laws direct nursing practice. Health policy decisions are guided by the principle of quality and safe patient care. Nurses need to be knowledgeable about health policy, and willing to sit at the table with other decision makers to discuss health policy. Nurses are in the best position to be engaged in policy making and decisions at the local, state, national, and international level.

Coursework should include core concepts such as health policy process and analysis; community, state, and national health care trends; disparities and quality outcomes; health care financing and delivery systems; leadership principles; and practice management.

SYNOPSIS

Nursing has been engaged in promoting health policy since the time of Florence Nightingale. Nurses have long held patient advocacy as a central tenet of nursing practice. While nurses view their role as a patient advocate, advocacy is a poorly understood concept in nursing (McSteen & Peden-McAlpin, 2006). Nurses are the largest segment of the health care workforce, and are at the closest contact to patients. Research demonstrates that the quality of nursing care is directly related to patient outcomes (Needleman, 2008).

The literature explores various roles and viewpoints of nurses engaging in health policy. One view is that the sphere of influence includes the community, workforce and workplace, government, professional organizations, and special interest groups (Chaffee, Mason, & Leavitt, 2012). Research studies show that nurses can develop their own political conscience by learning about and engaging in the policy and political process. Several strategies for nurses to become stronger advocates and develop a political conscience include the direct experiences of volunteering, campaigning, joining professional organizations, and seeking internships and fellowships in areas related to health policy. Other activities for developing health policy expertise include political sophistication, moving to the public arena, and leading the way to health policy change (Yoder-Wise, 2011). Health care is changing with the implementation of the Patient Protection and Affordable Care Act (2010). Therefore, it is imperative that nurses become more politically savvy.

RECOMMENDATIONS

Nurses focus on delivering quality care and using evidence to continually improve care. Understanding the relationship between health care financing and quality outcomes that direct treatment protocols and length of stay is essential in providing care. There needs to be a strong emphasis in nursing education linking the relationship between health policy and safe patient care.

In the informatics age, there are resources available for easy access to health care and policy information. Internet sites such as the Centers for Medicare and Medicaid (CMS) have online information regarding quality, safety, and standard compliance along with financial tracking data. The Agency for Healthcare Research and Quality offers comprehensive information regarding standards, health care statistics, and research funding. Lastly, nurse educators can partner with legislators and other decision makers in education, research, practice, and policy improvements. Nurses need to use their strong voice and be involved in areas where health policy decisions are made in shaping health policy.

American Association of Colleges of Nursing (AACN). (2014). Retrieved from http://www.aacn.nche.edu

Anderson, J. (2008). *Public policy making: An introduction* (6th ed.). Boston, MA: Houghton Mifflin.

Chaffee, M. W., Mason, D. J., & Leavitt, J. K. (2012). A framework for action in health policy and politics. In D. J. Mason, J. K. Leavitt, & M. W. Chaffee (Eds.), *Policy & politics in nursing and healthcare* (5th ed., pp. 1–12). St Louis. MO: Elsevier Saunders.

McSteen, K., & Peden-McAlpin, C. (2006). The role of nurse as advocate in ethically difficult care situations with dying patients. *Journal of Hospice and Palliative Nursing*, 8(5), 259–269.

Needleman, J. (2008). Is what is good for the patient what is good for the hospital? Aligning incentives and the business case for nursing. *Policy, Politics & Nursing Practice, 9*(2), 80–87.

Patient Protection and Affordable Care Act. (2010). *Act of 2010, HR 3590, 110th Congress*. Retrieved from https://www.govtrack.us/congress/bills/111/hr3590/text

World Health Organization. (2014). *Health policy*. Retrieved from http://www.who.int/topics/health_policy/en/

Yoder-Wise, P. (2011). *Leading and managing in nursing*. St. Louis, MO: Elsevier Mosby.

Claudia Grobbel

HEALTH PROFESSIONS EDUCATION

DEFINITION

Health professions education is a team approach to preparing health professions from a range of health care disciplines, including nursing. In health professions education there is an emphasis on providing care through a team approach. The team consists of varied health care professionals with the patient at the center. Care is provided in an interprofessional environment, with an emphasis on evidence-based practice, quality improvement, and informatics.

APPLICATION

Within the care delivery environment there has been an emphasis on family- and patient-centered care, evidence-based practice, and interprofessional collaboration. This emphasis has evolved from the work done by the Institute of Medicine (IOM) and various commissions developed to evaluate all aspects of the American and global health care systems (Frenk, 2011; Greiner & Knebel, 2003). Within this framework of care delivery, there is also an emphasis on interdependence among the health professions in education and on transformative learning (Frenk, 2011). Transformative learning is the process of effecting change in a frame of reference (Cranton, 1994; Mezirow, 1991).

The IOM committee on health professions education delineated five core competencies that all clinicians should possess, regardless of their discipline (Hundert, Hafferty, & Christakis, 1996). These five core competencies are: (a) provide patient-centered care; (b) work in interprofessional teams; (c) employ evidence-based practice; (d) apply quality improvement; and (e) utilize informatics.

SYNOPSIS

There is an emphasis on three key points when considering the education of the health professions: (a) the five core competencies defined by the IOM education summit committee (b) a global outlook as it pertains to health care and education (Frenk, 2011); and (c) transformative learning (Frenk, 2011). Providing patient-centered care incorporates respect, cultural differences, and relief of pain and suffering. Listening, informing, communicating, educating, shared decision making, and wellness and disease prevention are the guideposts. Working in interprofessional teams fosters cooperation, collaboration, and communication, and integration of care ensures continuity and reliability. Employing evidence-based practice integrates research, clinical expertise, and patient values to provide the best care. Applying quality improvement helps health care professionals to identify errors, implement safety design principles, and measure quality of care and outcomes that are patient and community centered. Utilizing informatics helps to improve communication, increase knowledge, prevent errors, and support decision making. Each discipline of the health professions has unique contributions to make. Those contributions will be best delivered when the professionals are in clinical settings that value interprofessional care.

RECOMMENDATIONS

Nurses are uniquely prepared to take care of patients, paying particular attention to the patient and family as an entity. The education of nurses is centered on knowing the cultural background, treating the patient as a whole being, and navigating between nursing and medical diagnoses as well as promoting an environment of health promotion and wellness. Nursing education now needs to focus on collaboration and team building. Thus, nurses can assume a unique and important role in the interprofessional management and care of patients and families.

Cranton, P. (1994). *Understanding and promoting transformative learning: A guide for educators of adults.* San Francisco, CA: Jossey-Bass.

Frenk, J. (2011). *Health professionals for a new century: Strengthening 21st century global health systems: Investing strategically in the health care workforce. Education of health professionals for the 21st century: A global independent commission.* New York City: Global Health Workforce Alliance.

Hundert, E. M., & Wakefield, M. (2003). *Health professions education: A bridge to quality.* Washington, DC: The National Academies Press.

Hundert, E. M., Hafferty, F., & Christakis, D. (1996). Characteristics of the informal curriculum and trainees ethical choices. *Academic Medicine, 71*(6), 624–642.

Mezirow, J. (1991). *Transformative dimensions of adult learning.* San Francisco, CA: Jossey-Bass.

Mary C. Lemp

HIGH-RISK STUDENTS

DEFINITION

High-risk students are individuals who have limited social supports, resources, or cognitive abilities that add to their proclivity for poor academic performance or failure. High-risk students are academically disadvantaged and commonly characterized by their ethnic minority status, gender, socioeconomic status, levels of self-esteem, disability status, behavioral dysfunction, or prior academic performance (Egerton, 1968; Jones & Watson, 1990).

APPLICATION

The identification and allocation of resources to high-risk nursing students is central to retention, diversity, and development of future nurses. In the United States, there is a projected shortage of registered nurses that will be compounded by a growing cohort of older Americans who will require nursing care (Janiszewski Goodin, 2003). As a consequence of a shortage in registered nurses, the proportion of high-risk students admitted to schools of nursing is proportionately on the rise. For nurse educators, the early identification of high-risk students is critical and necessary to optimize the congruence between the instructional methods and these students' learning needs to enhance their likelihood of academic success. As the numbers of high-risk nursing students increase, it is important for nurse educators to identify and support these students to ensure academic success, diversify the nursing workforce, and address the public health concerns regarding the shortage of registered nurses.

There are a variety of methods that facilitate the early identification of high-risk students. The evaluation of a student's risk for academic success usually entails the analysis of academic and nonacademic variables (Hopkins, 2008). Academic variables, such as standardized test scores and cumulative high-school grade point average (GPA), are used as indicators of a student's likelihood of academic success (Abrams & Jernigan, 1984; Hopkins, 2008). Nonacademic variables, such as quality of the individual's high-school education, self-efficacy, and levels of anxiety or stress, have also been examined as indicators of academic success. There are a variety of academic and nonacademic variables that are associated with the risk of poor academic performance and failure. Yet, research in this area continues to be focused on academic success (e.g., passing the National Council Licensure Examination for Registered Nurses [NCLEX-RN®], course grades, cumulative GPA), which limits the translation of this evidence to nursing practice outcomes.

SYNOPSIS

There are three key points in understanding how to identify and support high-risk nursing students: (a) Early identification of high-risk students requires a comprehensive evaluation of preadmission characteristics, and the assessment of academic and nonacademic variables associated with academic success (Grossbach & Kuncel, 2011; Hopkins, 2008); (b) high-risk students may come from communities that are economically depressed, and may feel disenfranchised or stigmatized by others, which result in a lack of confidence, lower academic motivation, and a heightened propensity for academic failure (Schunk & Mullen, 2012; Syed, Azmitia, & Cooper, 2011). Often high-risk students will not seek out the support from faculty but can significantly benefit from additional educational, social, financial, emotional, and culturally sensitive support to promote academic success; and (c) effective strategies for high-risk students have focused on self-directed activities, congruence between instructional methods and learning styles, as well as formative feedback in a supportive climate (Lockie, Van Lanen, & Mc Gannon, 2013; Pizzolato, 2004; Reyes, Brackett, Rivers, White, & Salovey, 2012). To date, there are no prevailing theoretical frameworks or strategies for early identification of high-risk students in nursing.

RECOMMENDATIONS

High-risk students represent a significant challenge to nurse educators. With a projected estimate of a shortage of registered nurses, nurse educators must recognize high-risk students early in their nursing education and provide evidence-based strategies to enhance their academic success. Nurse educators who wish to conduct evaluations to identify high-risk students must have a sound understanding of their student population, as well as the academic and nonacademic variables that may have influence on their likelihood of academic success. Attention to the definition of academic success varies significantly in nursing education. As highlighted by several studies, academic success and performance can be measured by an individual's performance in a fundamental nursing

H

course, cumulative college GPA, or passing the NCLEX-RN examination. Strategies that enhance academic success among high-risk students should be initiated early, personalized, and provide holistic support.

There is a significant need for longitudinal and interventional research to develop and test strategies for early identification and practices that fortify academic success among high-risk students. As nursing education research advances, examination of social determinants, cognitive processing, learning styles, experiential learning, coaching, and the use of interactive educational technologies hold significant promise to improve the learning outcomes of nursing students who are academically disadvantaged (Ashley & O'Neil, 1991; Lockie & Burke, 1999).

Abrams, H. G., & Jernigan, L. P. (1984). Academic support services and the success of high-risk college students. *American Educational Research Journal, 21*(2), 261–274.

Ashley, J., & O'Neil, J. (1991). The effectiveness of an intervention to promote successful performance on NCLEX-RN for baccalaureate students at risk for failure. *Journal of Nursing Education, 30*(8), 360–366.

Egerton, J. (1968). *Higher education for "high risk" students*. Atlanta, GA: Southern Education Foundation.

Grossbach, A., & Kuncel, N. R. (2011). The predictive validity of nursing admission measures for performance on the National Council Licensure Examination: A meta-analysis. *Journal of Professional Nursing, 27*(2), 124–128.

Hopkins, T. H. (2008). Early identification of at-risk nursing students: A student support model. *Journal of Nursing Education, 47*(6), 254–259.

Janiszewski Goodin, H. (2003). The nursing shortage in the United States of America: An integrative review of the literature. *Journal of Advanced Nursing, 43*(4), 335–343.

Jones, D. J., & Watson, B. C. (1990). *High-risk students and higher education: Future trends*.

ASHE-ERIC Higher Education Report No. 3: ERIC.

Lockie, N. M., & Burke, L. J. (1999). Partnership in Learning for Utmost Success (PLUS): Evaluation of a retention program for at-risk nursing students. *Journal of Nursing Education, 38*(4), 188–192.

Lockie, N. M., Van Lanen, R. J., & Mc Gannon, T. (2013). Educational implications of nursing students' learning styles, success in chemistry, and supplemental instruction participation on National Council Licensure Examination-Registered Nurses Performance. *Journal of Professional Nursing, 29*(1), 49–58.

Pizzolato, J. E. (2004). Coping with conflict: Self-authorship, coping, and adaptation to college in first-year, high-risk students. *Journal of College Student Development, 45*(4), 425–442.

Reyes, M. R., Brackett, M. A., Rivers, S. E., White, M., & Salovey, P. (2012). Classroom emotional climate, student engagement, and academic achievement. *Journal of Educational Psychology, 104*(3), 700.

Schunk, D. H., & Mullen, C. A. (2012). Self-efficacy as an engaged learner. In S. L. Christenson, A. L. Reschly, & C. Wylie (Eds.), *Handbook of research on student engagement* (pp. 219–235). New York, NY: Springer.

Syed, M., Azmitia, M., & Cooper, C. R. (2011). Identity and academic success among underrepresented ethnic minorities: An interdisciplinary review and integration. *Journal of Social Issues, 67*(3), 442–468.

Ronald L. Hickman

HOLISTIC NURSING CARE

DEFINITION

Holistic nursing care is defined as "all nursing practice that has healing the whole person as its goal" (Thornton, n.d., p. 1). The process of holistic nursing care takes into account complementary and alternative approaches within the provision of health care to address the totality of the individual. Brady (2013) characterized the definition of holistic care as "the inter-relationship of body, mind, and spirit, and the promotion of psychological, physiological, and socio-logical well being" (p. 31). Each of these definitions integrates the ideas of managing the care of the individual from all vantage points—mind, body, and soul. In provid-ing holistic nursing care, the nurse seeks to identify and incorporate the individual's unique understanding of health, health beliefs, and values. Thornton (n.d.) acknowl-edges that holistic nursing is a mind-set, a way of life, and a method of conducting care. Every individual is valued as a unique person who is seen as having multiple com-ponents to embrace in the management of the health care plan.

APPLICATION

A concept basis to holistic nursing is salu-togenesis. This concept is defined as "culti-vating wellness through a healthy work-life balance and advocates for good health at three levels of existence: physical, soulful, and spiritual" (Hudson, 2013, p. 12). Applying this concept in nursing education requires self-determination and commitment to part-nerships in the learning process. Students along with faculty advocate for indepen-dence and autonomy for the patient. Key to this process is multidimensional approaches that influence and promote health and well-ness. Understanding that health and wellness take on unique meanings for each individual is crucial. Students can be encouraged to guide patients to identify self-care measures for enjoying life.

Another component required in the pro-vision of holistic nursing care is the idea of effective communication. According to Buck (2013), straight talk with patients necessitates making peace with the patients' involvement in the plan of care; planning ahead for chal-lenges; communicating with all members of the team; prioritizing the aspects that are of paramount importance to the patient; and getting help when the need arises. Each of these ideas is an important part in the pro-cess of engaging in holistic nursing care. Furthermore, discussing verbal and non-verbal communication strategies should include these elements to help the student be successful.

A final area of application is compas-sionate care. According to Price (2013), "com-passionate care attends to the perceived needs and situations of patients; it draws on their existing knowledge and experi-ence, and includes nurse expertise" (p. 53). Many aspects discussed in compassion-ate care and relationship-based care mirror the ideas included within holistic nursing care.

The art of listening is vital to the pro-vision of holistic nursing care. By actively listening to what the patient is saying and not saying, nurses can ascertain a better picture of the patient's needs and oppor-tunities to provide holistic nursing care. Time is vital to providing holistic care, and is a finite commodity. Nurses are pulled in many different ways while providing care. Learning how to listen is critical to under-standing the primary aspects important to the patient, which results in holistic nursing interventions.

SYNOPSIS

Wright and Neuberger (2012) address the topic of engaged spirituality. This is connect-ing with the spiritual side of a patient. The physical and social sides of a person tend to be linked. The spiritual and/or mind/soul part of the patient may be harder to incorpo-rate in the plan of care. According to Wright and Neuberger (2012), "spirituality culti-vates a deepening of our understanding of what it is to be human, of resources we can draw on to connect with and serve others" (p. 20). Understanding how to connect the mind, body, soul, and social realms into one plan of care requires careful, thoughtful engagement with multiple individuals on the team.

H

Byrne (2013) suggests that "quality holistic care requires that we understand the person we are caring for, but all too often these days, with shorter hospital stays and less nurse-patient contact, we do not get to know those we care for as well as we used to" (p. 28). Batcheller, Davis, and Yoder-Wise (2013) investigated the spiritual aspect of patients in the workplace. Several strategies were given to support the management of spirituality at work. The strategies included huddles, rituals, partnerships, self-care, reflection, and tranquility rooms. Each of these strategies provides a foundation for addressing the total patient, thereby providing holistic care.

RECOMMENDATIONS

The American Holistic Nurses Association (Jackson, 2012) has identified core values for holistic nursing care. Along with the core values, the association publishes Standards of Holistic Nursing Practice while providing a certification in the discipline. Jackson (2012) discusses several core values. These are personal awareness, maturity, research, resource utilization, cost-effectiveness, caring, evidence-based practice, collegiality, collaboration, communication, therapeutic environment, cultural diversity, humor, leadership, and quality. Each of these core values is integrated into the practice of holistic nursing care to ensure that the total individual is cared for as they desire.

Nurses have a mandate to keep an open mind and seek to address the total needs of the individual. Through the commitment to strive to understand the different facets of an individual—mind, body, soul, and social—the uniqueness of the person can be understood. At times, care of the physical side may be more needed, while at other times the social or mind/soul side needs more attention. By striving to help the individual gain balance, the nurse helps the patient gain control of his or her situation.

Research into these different aspects of holistic nursing care must be considered, identified, and carried out. Much of the differences within these areas are not known. The relationships among the body, mind, soul, and spirit must be investigated.

Batcheller, J., Davis, J., & Yoder-Wise, P. S. (2013). Hope for the future: Intensifying spirituality in the workplace. *Nursing Administration Quarterly, 37*(4), 309–316.

Brady, M. (2013). The nature of health and social care partnerships. *Nursing Management, 19*(9), 30–35.

Buck, H. G. (2013). Help family caregivers in the "sandwich generation." *Nursing, 43*(11), 19–20.

Byrne, G. (2013). Listening is a vital part of care, but how many of us have the time? *Nursing Standard, 27*(51), 28.

Hudson, K. (2013, November). Salutogenesis: The origin of health. *Nursing Management, 44*(11), 12–13.

Jackson, C. (2012). Doing more with less: Using core values and standards of holistic nursing to expand practice in an era of shrinking resources. *Holistic Nursing Practice, 26*(5), 238–242.

Price, B. (2013). Promoting compassionate care through learning journeys. *Nursing Standard, 27*(48), 51–57.

Thornton, L. (n.d.). *What is holistic nursing?* Retrieved from http://ahna.org/About-Us/What-is-Holistic-Nursing

Wright, S., & Neuberger, J. (2012). Why spirituality is essential for nurses. *Nursing Standard, 26*(40), 19–21.

Carol Boswell

HONORS PROGRAM

DEFINITION

An honors program is an academic program or curriculum designed to provide a qualitatively different educational experience and learning environment for exceptional students (National Collegiate Honors Council [NCHC], 2014). The first honors program in higher education began in 1922, based on the principles of student freedom and choice, more focused topics, and the use of discussion-based courses as opposed to traditional lectures (Oleson, 1988). The first mention of a nursing honors program in the literature was in 1964 (Stanley, 1964). Early reports included nursing honors programs based on an undergraduate research model.

APPLICATION

The primary aim of an honors program is to recruit and retain students of high scholastic intellectual aptitude, to nurture their specific needs, and to raise the academic profile of the institution. Some enduring themes in promoting a nursing honors program are to attract high-achieving, gifted students who may not have considered nursing as a profession of study (Hartshorn, Berbiglia, & Heye, 1997); to provide a fertile ground to cultivate future nursing leaders in research and clinical practice (Buckner, 2008; Reutter et al., 2010; Schumann & McNeill, 2008; Stanford & Shattell, 2010); and to usher exceptional students toward pursuing advanced degrees in nursing practice, research, and education (Gillis, 2003; Williams & Snider, 1992).

SYNOPSIS

Nursing honors is an example of departmental honors, or honors in the major, culminating in recognition at graduation *with honors in nursing*. Departmental honors complements a university honors program, providing opportunities for honors thesis development (Buckner, 2004).

The targeted student population for a nursing honors program is defined by a clear set of admission criteria, which typically includes grade point averages (GPAs), scholastic achievement test scores, written essays, and/or satisfactory completion or progress in other coursework (NCHC, 2014). On entry, whether as a pre-nursing student or student entering the nursing program, honors students should receive specific honors-related academic advising from qualified faculty throughout the duration of the program (NCHC, 2014).

In addition to seminars and/or other experiential learning courses, honors programs in nursing have traditionally emphasized research projects as a major learning outcome. Several research models have been used to guide honors projects, including undergraduate research (Buckner, 2004); fellowship programs (Vessey & DeMarco, 2008); independent study (Stanford & Shattell, 2010); and research assistantships/apprenticeships (Reutter et al., 2010). Despite the prior focus on research-intensive experiences, learning outcomes may be achieved through other student-led projects and activities, such as service-learning projects, study-abroad experiences, new course development, and quality improvement projects (Buckner & Holcomb, 2013; Ross & Buckner, 2009). Student projects and research have been presented at the National Conference on Undergraduate Research (NCUR); The Honor Society of Nursing, Sigma Theta Tau International; the annual conference of the NCHC; and others. Buckner (2004) related student development during the dissemination process to the highest levels in the affective domain, organization, and characterization of the values of the profession (Buckner, 2004).

Challenges and opportunities in nursing honors programs can be categorized into system, faculty, and student factors. When developing and implementing an honors program, it is imperative to have committed administrators who understand the resources and faculty commitment that are needed for the sustainability and longevity of the program (Oleson, 1988). Faculty overseeing and teaching in honors programs must not only be qualified, but should also have their participation in program activities counted in their workload. In addition, students may have concerns regarding the workload and its impact on their GPA (Hartshorn et al., 1997).

RECOMMENDATIONS

To be able to attract exceptional students into an honors program in nursing, the school or college must have a clear mission and vision regarding what the program wishes to achieve. Curriculum elements integrate the *Essentials of Baccalaureate Education* from the American Association of Colleges of Nursing (AACN) with active and experiential learning comprising the core of the honors program. The faculty will assume various roles as facilitators, coaches, preceptors, mentors, supporters, and role models. However, it is the student's unique talents and interest that should drive the process.

Despite honors programs being considered an excellent testing ground for piloting educational innovations (Duckett, Brand, & Fairbanks, 1990), there is scant research on the systematic evaluation of honors programs. Williams and Snider (1992) conducted a comparative analysis of the long-term impact among graduates in honors programs compared to non-honors program counterparts with 4 to 6 years postgraduation. Enrollment in advanced nursing programs was the strongest outcome indicator of being an honors program participant. Similar educational research and outcomes studies are needed to gain greater insight into the merits of honors programs in pre-licensure nursing education.

Buckner, E. B. (2004). Honors research in nursing: Integration of theory and evidence-based practice using multiple modalities of thinking. *Journal of the National Collegiate Honors Council, 5*(1), 53–60.

Buckner, E. B. (2008). Nursing theory in inquiry-based education: Formative experiences for novice nursing students. *Self-Care, Dependent-Care & Nursing, 16*(1), 5–6.

Buckner, E. B., & Holcomb, L. (2013). Chapter 14: Nursing honors and study abroad: Building a partnership for collaboration in nursing research in Honduras. In M. K. Mulvaney & K. Klein (Eds.), *Preparing tomorrow's global leaders: Honors international education* (pp. 275–287). Lincoln, NE: National Collegiate Honors Council.

Duckett, L. J., Brand, K. P., & Fairbanks, D. (1990). Recruiting the brightest and best for nursing—an honors program can help. *Nurse Educator, 15*(1), 12–16.

Gillis, A. J. (2003). Honours education: Releasing leadership potential. *Nursing Leadership, 16*(3), 69–78.

Hartshorn, J. C., Berbiglia, V. A., & Heye, M. (1997). An honors program: Directing our future leaders. *Journal of Nursing Education, 36*(4), 187–189.

National Collegiate Honors Council (NCHC). (2014, June 19). *Basic characteristics of a fully developed honors program.* Retrieved from http://nchchonors.org/faculty-directors/basic-characteristics-of-a-fully-developed-honors-program/

Oleson, M. (1988). To be or not to be: Honors programs in baccalaureate nursing education. *Nurse Educator, 13*(4), 26–29.

Reutter, L., Paul, P., Sales, A., Jerke, H., Lee, A., McColl, M.,…Visram, A. (2010). Incorporating a research apprenticeship model in a Canadian nursing Honors Program. *Nurse Education Today, 30*(6), 562–567.

Ross, J. A., & Buckner, E. B. (2009, November). *Service learning as a model for nursing honors experiences.* Paper presented at the biennial convention of Sigma Theta Tau International, The Honor Society of Nursing, Indianapolis, IN.

Schumann, R., & McNeill, J. (2008). Honors programs as a way to grow the discipline. *International Journal for Human Caring, 12*(2), 54–56.

Stanford, D., & Shattell, M. (2010). Using an honors program to engage undergraduate students in research. *Nursing Education Perspectives, 31*(5), 325–326.

Stanley, M. K. (1964). Honors programs in nursing education. *Nursing Outlook, 12,* 28–32.

Vessey, J. A., & DeMarco, R. F. (2008). The undergraduate research fellows program: A unique model to promote engagement in research. *Journal of Professional Nursing,* 24(6), 358–363.

Williams, P. D., & Snider, M. J. (1992). Honors program participation and performance postgraduation. *Journal of Nursing Education,* 31(2), 65–69.

Fidelindo A. Lim
Larry Z. Slater
Ellen B. Buckner

HUMOR

DEFINITION

Humor is an interpersonal, culturally determined communication intended to elicit a response of amusement (Robinson, 1991). This communication is context dependent, can be planned or spontaneous in creation, and can be positive or negative in purpose (Chapman & Foot, 2004; McCreaddie & Wiggins, 2008).

APPLICATION

In nursing education, humor has four facets: humor as an overall teaching style, humor as a pedagogical technique, humor as a nursing socialization technique, and humor as a therapeutic nurse–patient communication technique. Much interest in humor in nursing education was motivated by the hypothesis that humor improves health, but such links have been tenuous (Martin, 2004; McCreaddie & Wiggins, 2008).

Humor as a teaching style is a part of the teacher's personality and demeanor presented to students. It is related to the teacher's sense of humor, the willingness to engage in humor, and the ability to formally or spontaneously create humorous stories or responses. Positive humor that is uplifting, self-deprecating, or insightful is preferred. Avoid a derogatory or tendentious style (Chabeli, 2008). Shared cultural experiences, knowledge of the language, ability to engage in word play, and awareness of what is contextually acceptable are also part of a humorous teaching style. A humorous style can relieve stress, create a positive student–teacher relationship, and improve student engagement in learning (Lukehart, 2009).

Humor as a pedagogical technique is the deliberate use of humor to enhance learning. This can be planned or spontaneous. It is distinct from teaching style in its purpose to teach students a topic, concept, or skill in an engaging manner. Humor can make learning fun, be a learning device or mnemonic, and stimulate creativity (Berk, 2002). Additionally, humor can stimulate critical thinking through a relaxed classroom atmosphere, illustration of affective and cognitive conflicts, and stimulation of creative approaches to a problem (Johnson, 1990).

Humor as a socialization technique helps establish group cohesion, delineates roles, and enforces group norms (Robinson, 1991). Nursing students enter a world that can be scary for the uninitiated. Students may have no experience with issues of life, death, and ethical decision making. Finding humor in tragedy, or "gallows humor," can provide an outlet for fear, relieve tension, and act as a coping mechanism (McCreaddie & Wiggins, 2008; Robinson, 1991). Self-deprecating humor or funny clinical stories by the teacher can also humanize the experience for students who may worry about their ability to handle the stresses of practice (Johnson, 1990; Lukehart, 2009). Teachers must be especially careful in this facet of humor to not dehumanize students or patients with negative humor.

Humor in nursing can also be a learned communication technique with patients. Just as humor can relieve students' stress, it can, when used appropriately, aid in patients' well-being. Patient teaching can be enhanced with humor for the same reasons it helps nursing students in the classroom. It can keep the patient engaged in learning, help remember new concepts, and enhance the nurse–patient relationship (Robinson, 1991). Nurse educators must teach students the boundaries of appropriate and inappropriate

H

patient interactions. Students must also be aware of how cultural differences can influence perception of humor (Chiang-Hanisko, Adamle, & Chiang, 2009).

SYNOPSIS

Humor is a mysterious and complex human quality that has been debated and studied for thousands of years (Perks, 2012). The ancient Greeks and Romans saw the balance of "humors" as indicative of one's mood or temperament. Even the Bible makes references to the benefits of humor. The development of humor as an innate trait is evident in that infants are quick to smile and laugh (Chapman & Foot, 2004). Prevailing theories have been categorized as cognitive perceptual, social behavioral, and psychoanalytical (Apte, 1985; Johnson, 1990). These categories reflect the theories of humor as arising from the unexpected and incongruous, its liberating effects of being playful, or relief from anxious or tense situations (Robinson, 1991). The traditional theory of superiority proposes that humor is found in situations or stories that make us feel superior to others, but this theory is considered an inappropriate basis for educational humor (Chapman & Foot, 2004).

Much interest in humor in health care is derived from popular literature and film in the 1970s and 1980s promoting the hypothesis that health was connected to humor (Robinson, 1991). Numerous subsequent studies failed to show a connection (Martin, 2004; McCreaddie & Wiggins, 2008).

Humor has been identified as an important characteristic of good teaching (Chabeli, 2008; Eason & Corbett, 1991). Teachers identified as having a good sense of humor are rated more highly by students (Bryant, Comisky, Crane, & Zillman, 1980; Ulloth, 2002). Humor can create a classroom conducive to learning, as well as promote spontaneity and individuality (Lukehart, 2009). Humor can also be seen as a therapeutic intervention between teacher and student (Chiarello, 2010).

Humor can help socialize students on ways to cope with situations that are outside the norm of usual experience (Robinson, 1991). McCreaddie and Wiggins (2008) cite examples of how humor is seen as a coping method among nurses to prevent burnout and act as a stress moderator. They also note that much humor research in nursing is done without a foundation in theory. Humor can be brought to class to not just aid learning but to also model therapeutic communication (Chiarello, 2010; Johnson, 1990).

RECOMMENDATIONS

Much of the literature on humor in nursing reports findings or theories from other disciplines such as psychology, sociology, and anthropology. Nurse educators need to explore the concept of the sense of humor in students and faculty, and particularly investigate gender and cultural differences.

The link between humor and learning has been studied but in nursing there is a need to investigate possible links among humor, critical thinking, cognitive learning, retention, and affective learning. An anthropological approach to the socialization of nursing is needed in relation to gender and cultural influences on students as they progress through their education. While the humor–health relationship has been elusive there should be further study of what types of humor are conducive to improving the nurse–patient relationship (Johnson, 1990). Gender and cultural influences on the use of humor in patient care is another area in need of study.

Apte, M. L. (1985). *Humor and laughter: An anthropological approach.* Ithica, NY: Cornell University Press.

Berk, R. A. (2002). *Humor as an instructional defibrillator: Evidence-based techniques in teaching and assessment.* Sterling, VA: Ithica, NY.

Bryant, J., Comisky, P. W., Crane, J. S., & Zillman, D. (1980). Relationship between college teachers' use of humor in the classroom and students' evaluations of their teachers. *Journal of Educational Psychology,* 72(4), 511–519.

H

Chabeli, M. (2008). Humor: A pedagogical tool to promote learning. *Curationis, 31*(3), 51–59.

Chapman, A. J., & Foot, H. C. (2004). *Humor and laughter: Theory, research, and applications.* New Brunswick, NJ: Transaction Publishers.

Chiang-Hanisko, L., Adamle, K., & Chiang, L. C. (2009). Cultural differences in therapeutic humor in nursing education. *The Journal of Nursing Research, 17*(1), 52–61.

Chiarello, M. A. (2010). Humor as a teaching tool. Use in psychiatric undergraduate nursing. *Journal of Psychosocial Nursing and Mental Health Services, 48*(8), 34–41.

Eason, F. R., & Corbett, R. W. (1991). Effective teacher characteristics identified by adult learners in nursing. *Journal of Continuing Education in Nursing, 22*(1), 21–23.

Johnson, H. A. (1990). Humor as an innovative method for teaching sensitive topics. *Educational Gerontology, 16*, 547–555.

Lukehart, D. E. (2009). *The use of humor as a teaching strategy in nursing education.* Capella University, PhD UMI Dissertations Publishing 3366285.

Martin, R. A. (2004). Sense of humor and physical health: Theoretical issues, recent findings, and future directions. *Humor, 17*(1/2), 1–19.

McCreaddie, M., & Wiggins, S. (2008). The purpose and function of humour in health, health care and nursing: A narrative review. *Journal of Advanced Nursing, 61*(6), 584–595.

Perks, L. G. (2012). The ancient roots of humor theory. *Humor, 25*(2), 119–132.

Robinson, V. M. (1991). *Humor and the health professions: The therapeutic use of humor in health care* (2nd ed.). Thorofare, NJ: Slack.

Ulloth, J. K. (2002). The benefits of humor in nursing education. *Journal of Nursing Education, 41*(11), 476–481.

Brent W. Thompson

I

INFORMATICS

DEFINITION

Informatics is the scholarly study of computer science and includes "the collection, classification, storage, retrieval, and dissemination of recorded knowledge" (Campbell, 2013, p. 29). Nursing informatics (NI) encompasses the study of nursing, information, and computer science (McGonigle & Mastrain, 2012). As technology has evolved, so has the definition of NI, first expressed as the application of computer technology to all fields of nursing (Scholes & Barber, 1980). Then, it was expanded to include the management and processing of data, information, and knowledge in nursing to support patient care (Graves & Corcoran, 1989). Internet applications, communication, personal data assistants (PDAs), and laptop computers, commonplace in the 1990s, led to recognition of NI as a nursing specialty and not just a term (Zytkowski, 2003).

To emphasize NI's supportive role for patients, nurses, and other providers, the American Nurses Association (ANA) expanded its definition of NI in 2008 to include the word *wisdom* and defined NI as a specialty that combines nursing science, computer science, and information science to manage and communicate data, information, knowledge, and wisdom into nursing practice (Hart, 2008). In 2009, the International Medical Informatics Association (IMIA) fine-tuned the definition to, "... (the) science and practice integrates nursing, its information and knowledge and their management, with information and communication technologies to promote the health of people, families and communities worldwide" (Murphy, 2010, p. 204).

APPLICATION

Preparing student nurses for practice requires awareness of the NI role. There are two distinct but separate roles for NI in nursing: nurses who utilize informatics in patient care and NI specialists who help to develop, guide, and implement use in practice. Clinical nurses routinely use NI in practice through charting, communication, and the execution of patient care. NI specialists are highly skilled nurses who have extensive knowledge and training in NI, hold a graduate or postgraduate degree in informatics, and often seek official certification (American Nurses Credentialing Center [ANCC], 2014). NI specialists work in positions beyond the electronic health record (EHR) including administration, information technology, analysis, quality management, consulting, development, education, and in ever-emerging and yet-unthought-of areas where technology, data, and patient care do and will fuse.

The ANCC has developed an NI certification examination. Applicants must hold an active registered nurse (RN) license, a minimum education of a bachelor's degree, 2 years of practice experience as a nurse, 30 hours of continuing education in informatics, and one more of a list of specific requirements, which can be found through the ANCC website (ANCC, 2014).

The Technology Informatics Guiding Education Reform (TIGER) initiative was formed in 2004 in collaboration among key stakeholders. TIGER includes a set of basic technological components that all nurses should master in three areas: competencies, information literacy, and information management. Phase III of the TIGER initiative is underway to make tools to learn Health Information Technology (HIT), such as EHRs, computerized physician order entry (CPOE) systems, and virtual learning environments, more readily available for nurses, faculty, and nursing students (TIGER Initiative, 2014).

NI entails knowledge, evidence, and trends in bedside technologies. The practice of NI includes the use of handheld and medical devices, EHRs, computers, and any aspect of information science within the health care setting. Bedside technologies include everything from computerized intravenous pumps and point-of-care laboratory testing, to smartphone apps to improve and individualize patient care, all of which hold promise and are points of ethical and legal discussion (Schmitt, 2013). For example, mobile handheld devices have the potential to eliminate computer shortages and nurses' station congestion, to connect provider and patient, and to personalize health care. Yet cost, Food and Drug Administration (FDA) approval, and knowledge of use remain barriers (Schmitt, 2013).

The Internet and information access continues to usher rapid changes requiring examination of old and previously unconceived legal, ethical, and moral applications of technology. The following are key areas all educators and nurses should be aware of in regard to NI.

Health Insurance Portability and Accountability Act (HIPAA)

Title II of the 1996 HIPAA legislation, also called the Administrative Simplification provisions, first protected patient health information (PHI) by directing the Department of Health and Human Services to set guidelines for the electronic transmission of PHI. HIPAA requires covered entities, such as hospitals and health systems, to put safeguards into place for protecting the confidentiality, integrity, and availability of PHI (U.S. Department of Health and Human Services, 2013).

The Health Information Technology for Economic and Clinical Health Act and Meaningful Use

The Health Information Technology for Economic and Clinical Health (HITECH) Act, part of the American Recovery and Reinvestment Act of 2009, mandates universal implementation of EHRs through financial incentives and new standards for electronic privacy, updating HIPAA. HITECH directs the goals, stages, and core requirements of meaningful use in EHR capabilities and the exchange of health information. Data input by nurses will comprise the data set from which evidence-based care is analyzed. Consistency, access, accuracy, and interfaces must be accurate. In addition to improving the quality of care, the goal of meaningful use is to promote EHRs for improvements in health care outcomes.

NI is used at the bedside, in new learning platforms, nursing education, and in the exploration of new learning technologies. Learning management systems (LMS) offer new ways to educate, engage, and track student learning. Likewise, the explosion of communication technology offers new ways to connect, learn, and educate students (Schmitt, Sims-Giddens, & Booth, 2012). Nurse educators need to implement teaching strategies to accommodate the 21st-century tech-savvy learners. One creative teaching strategy encompasses the use of Go Animate, an innovative Web 2.0 tool that allows faculty and students to simulate and animate nursing scenes through creatively staged information (Lilly & Hunt, 2013).

SYNOPSIS

The nursing profession needs to adopt and universally utilize NI competencies and a universal definition for NI (Flood, Gasiewicz, & Delpier, 2010). The growth of NI and technology requires high-level understanding and application of technology through changes in how nurses are educated.

RECOMMENDATIONS

With the evolution of technology, so the demand for high-quality evidence in both application and how nurses are educated in regard to technology grows. More evidence is needed in the following areas of NI and nursing education:

- Universal integration of NI competencies into nursing curriculum and its effect on professional practice and patient outcomes.

- Measurement of specific competencies used to evaluate NI skills among nurses and nursing students.

- Understanding and application of legislation guiding technology use in practice.

- The use and application of various forms of computer and communication technology in nursing education and impact on learning outcomes.

- Best practices for more effectively teaching NI at all levels of nursing education.

Technology will continue to be one of the largest driving forces in health care and education. EHRs will be the core hub of information for reporting on quality patient care. Competencies must be developed in NI. Nurses in every profession must be fully equipped to use these technologies and to prepare nurses to be equipped to embrace these technologies with NI now and in the future.

American Nurses Credentialing Center (ANCC). (2014). *Informatics nursing certification eligibility criteria*. Retrieved from http://www.nursecredentialing.org/Informatics-Eligibility.aspx

Campbell, R. J. (2013). Defining health informatics. *Journal of AHIMA, 84*(2), 28–30, 32.

Flood, L. S., Gasiewicz, N., & Delpier, T. (2010). Integrating information literacy across a BSN curriculum. *Journal of Nursing Education, 49*(2), 101–104.

Graves, J. R., & Corcoran, S. (1989). The study of nursing informatics. *Image–The Journal of Nursing Scholarship, 21*(4), 227–231.

Hart, M. (2008). Informatics competency and development within the US nursing population workforce. *CIN: Computers, Informatics, Nursing, 29*(4), 256–262.

Lilly, K., & Hunt, D. (2013). Innovative web 2.0 teaching tool: Go animate. *Nursing Education Perspectives*, in press.

McGonigle, D., & Mastrain, K. (2012). *Nursing informatics and the foundation of knowledge*. Burlington, MA: Jones and Bartlett.

Murphy, J. (2010). Nursing informatics: The intersection of nursing, computer, and information sciences. *Nursing Economics, 28*(3), 204–207.

Schmitt, T. (2013). Smartphone healthcare apps: Tricorder quality yet? *Online Journal of Nursing Informatics, 17*(3). Retrieved from http://ojni.org/issues/?p=2854

Schmitt, T., Sims-Giddens, S., & Booth, R. (2012). Social media use among nurse educators. *Online Journal of Issues in Nursing, 17*(3). Retrieved from http://www.nursingworld.org/MainMenuCategories/ANAMarketplace/ANAPeriodicals/OJIN/TableofContents/Vol-17–2012/No3-Sept-2012/Social-Media-in-Nursing-Education.html

Scholes, M., & Barber, B. (1980). Towards nursing informatics. *Medinfo*. Amsterdam, The Netherlands: North-Holland, The Netherlands (pp. 70–73).

TIGER Initiative. (2014). *Informatics competencies collaborative team*. Retrieved from http://www.tigersummit.com/Competencies_New_B949.html

U.S. Department of Health and Human Services. (2013). *HIPAA administrative simplication*. Retrieved from http://www.hhs.gov/ocr/privacy/hipaa/administrative/combined/hipaa-simplification-201303.pdf

Zytkowski, M. E. (2003). Nursing informatics: The key to unlocking contemporary nursing practice. *AACN Clinical Issues, 14*(3), 271–281.

Kezia Lilly
Terri L. Schmitt

INTERNATIONAL PROGRAM

DEFINITION

An international program is a structured component of a U.S. school of nursing curriculum that provides a focus on global health, including an awareness and appreciation of the importance of culture, issues of globalization, and the diversity of the human condition (Hinrichs, 2003). These programs vary by duration, purpose, and complexity. The duration of an international program may include short-term, 1- to 3-week faculty-led programs or longer-term immersion experiences and include both single episode experience and long-term program development. The purpose of international programs may be focused on education, or on travel/study. Travel/study programs are designed to help students learn about international sites, culture, health system and health challenges, and service-oriented programs that are providing direct service or capacity building in an underserved area. International programs may involve a one-way outreach of students and/or faculty or two-way exchanges that involve students and faculty in multilevel complex interactions.

APPLICATION

Impetus for the development of international programs in nursing education has been grounded in an awareness of the rapidly changing landscape in which the next generation of nurses will practice. The changing landscape includes transformations in population mobility, communication, information technology, social media, and increasing diversity. A nursing workforce with the cultural awareness, sensitivity, and appreciation necessary to provide competent care is the goal.

Civic engagement through international programs provides a mechanism for teaching the social responsibility of nursing including the role of advocacy for the health of populations, development of health policy, social justice, and fulfilling nursing's social contract with society (Nicholas, Corless, Fulmer, & Meedzan, 2012). The addition of academic service learning (ASL) to international programs provides experiential learning opportunities to develop the assessment and caregiving skills needed to provide culturally competent care to diverse populations. ASL programs contribute to teaching international leadership, clinical reasoning, professional role development, and interprofessional teamwork (Kaddoura, Puri, & Dominick, 2014).

SYNOPSIS

Issues identified in the literature are focused in three main categories: the value of developing international programs and obstacles to doing so; impact of the programs on students; and impact on the international sites.

In an early survey of study-abroad baccalaureate programs in the United States, Linquist (1986) reported that 14% of the 319 schools responding currently had a study-abroad program as part of the curriculum. Despite growing support for international programs in nursing education, in a recent survey, still less than half of the schools of nursing in the United States were identified as having international programs (McKinnon & Fitzpatrick, 2012). In addition, there are significant obstacles to developing international programs (McKinnon & McNelis, 2013). Major obstacles include a limited number of faculty prepared to develop and lead international programs, as well as constraints on including the program as part of the required curriculum. When the program is not part of the regular curricula, there is a reduction in resources available to support the program. In addition, adding an elective course may not be considered a significant part of faculty work so that time spent in developing or leading the program may increase demands on faculty. Memmott et al. (2010) highlight the importance of developing an international program in congruence with the overall mission of the school by articulating the contribution of the international program to learning outcomes in order for it to be an integral part of the curriculum.

Although participation in an international program is viewed as a valuable student experience, a review of the literature reveals relatively little evaluation beyond personal and anecdotal reports of the value of international programs (McAuliffe & Cohen, 2005). Studies are primarily descriptive and focus primarily on the students' increased understanding and appreciation of other cultures, as well as a deeper appreciation of their own culture. Experiences were described as transformational and life changing (Levine, 2009). In a qualitative study, Evanson and Zust (2006) studied former baccalaureate students 2 years after an international experience. The overarching theme of Bittersweet Knowledge was identified. Three subthemes were: coming to understand, representing positive feelings of increased cultural awareness, and long-term connections; unsettled feelings, representing questions about the value of the experience to the site and guilt over the economic disparities that existed; and advocating for change, reflecting the subject's sense of a long-term changed life view and a sense of responsibility to advocate for changes at personal, local, and global levels.

A significant issue in sustaining an international program is balancing the benefit of the host site with sporadic, short-term service.

RECOMMENDATIONS

International programs can be a valuable part of a school of nursing program and, as the process of globalization of society continues, an increasingly essential one. The following recommendations contribute to the sustainability of an international program. The program should be congruent with the overall mission of the school of nursing and/or the college or university and contribute to the learning objectives of the school of nursing curriculum; theoretical and evidence based as part of the required curriculum rather than an elective in order

to have sufficient resources and be a regular part of a faculty workload; developed in collaboration with the host site personnel, identifying specific outcomes to be achieved for the host site as well as learning outcomes for the students, along with an evaluation plan; and evaluated with short- and long-term goals that are planned prior to initiating the program.

American Association of Colleges of Nursing (AACN). (2008). *The essentials of baccalaureate education for professional nursing practice*. Retrieved from www .aacn.nche.edu/education-resources/ BaccEssentials08.pdf

Evanson, T. A., & Zust, B. L. (2006). "Bittersweet knowledge": The long-term effects of an international experience. *Journal of Nursing Education, 45*(10), 412–419.

Hinrichs, J. (2003). A comparison of levels of international understanding among students of the international baccalaureate diploma and advanced placement. *Journal of Research in International Education, 2,* 331–348.

Kaddoura, M., Puri, A., & Dominick, C. A. (2014). International academic service learning: Lessons learned from students' travel experiences of diverse cultural and health care practices in Morocco. *Journal of Nursing Education, 53*(1), 45–47.

Levine, M. (2009). Transforming experiences: Nursing education and international immersion programs. *Journal of Professional Nursing, 25*(3), 156–169.

Linquist, G. J. (1986). Programs that internationalize nursing curricula in baccalaureate schools of nursing in the U.S. *Journal of Professional Nursing, 2,* 143–150.

McAuliffe, M. S., & Cohen, M. Z. (2005). International nursing research and educational exchanges: A review of the literature. *Nursing Outlook, 53*(1), 21–25.

McKinnon, T., & Fitzpatrick, J. (2012). *Global service learning in nursing*. New York, NY: National League for Nursing.

McKinnon, T. H., & McNelis, A. M. (2013). International programs in United States schools of nursing: Driving forces, obstacles, and opportunities. *Nursing Education Perspectives, 34*(5), 323–328.

Memmott, R. J., Coverston, C. R., Heise, B. A., Williams, M., Maughan, E. D., Kohl, J., & Palmer, S. (2010). Practical considerations in establishing sustainable international nursing experiences. *Nursing Education Perspectives, 31*(5), 298–302.

Nicholas, P. K., Corless, I. B., Fulmer, H., & Meedzan, N. (2012). Preparing nursing students for education in the global village. *MCN. The American Journal of Maternal Child Nursing, 37*(6), 367–372.

Marilyn J. Lotas

INTERPROFESSIONAL COMMUNICATION

DEFINITION

Interprofessional communication is the use of verbal and nonverbal methods to engage in collaborative practice with multiple health care professionals for the benefit of patients, families, and communities. Interprofessional communication is defined by the use of effective methods for communicating in teams, with the goals of safe and effective patient-centered practice (Canadian Interprofessional Health Collaborative [CIHC], 2010).

APPLICATION

Interprofessional communication is foundational to establishing collaborative practice. The seminal Institute of Medicine (IOM) report, *To Err Is Human*, highlighted the scope and severity of patient safety errors, and identified ineffective communication among health care providers as a leading contributor to those errors (IOM, 2000). As a result, health care facilities began work on safe patient handoff procedures such as Situation-Background-Assessment-Recommendations (SBAR), which is a best practice in today's

health care facilities (Institute for Healthcare Improvement [IHI], 2014). Furthermore, communication standards were added to National Patient Safety Goals (NPSG), which are updated yearly by The Joint Commission (TJC, 2014).

A subsequent 2003 IOM report challenged health profession educators to avoid educating health professionals in silos in an effort to reduce patient safety errors in practice (IOM, 2003). Educating health profession students together while they are in their curricula supports the culture of safety cultivated by many health care institutions (Agency for Healthcare Research and Quality [AHRQ], 2012).

To advance interprofessional communication development in health professions students, educators have devised several strategies. One rapidly growing strategy is the use of low- or high-fidelity simulation to create an experience for teams of students. The range of opportunities using simulation is seemingly unlimited. Educators may construct simulations to develop patient handoff skill sets in a nonthreatening environment, or challenge students with a patient stressor where the team must communicate immediately to provide safe patient care (Reising, Carr, Shea, & King, 2011). Along similar lines, standardized patients may be used as a method to promote interprofessional communication for student teams.

Whether using simulation or standardized patients, student teams are placed in an environment where they must simultaneously interact with the patient and family, while also collaborating with one another on the best plan of action. Joint or coeducation is also being used to foster interprofessional communication. In the case of coeducation, students from more than one health professions discipline enroll in a course together, and study subjects that are relevant to both (or several) disciplines.

Many different topics may serve as the "theme" to educate and help students develop interprofessional communication skills. These themes may be specialty oriented, such as labor and delivery or behavioral health, or process oriented such as managing and delegating patient care. One growing area of education involves error disclosure by health care professionals. Given that patient errors continue to occur, error disclosure best practices are critical to effective communication. Scenarios that include all relevant health care professions allow student teams to practice error disclosure prior to a real situation and provide a valuable learning experience (University of Washington, 2011).

Regardless of the strategy or topics being addressed, proper training in interprofessional communication is essential. An evidence-based strategy developed by AHRQ and the United States Department of Defense (USDOD) is the TeamSTEPPS® program. TeamSTEPPS provides a structure and process for education regarding safe team communication. One of the most meaningful parts of the program is that students learn specific words they may use when encountering a difficult situation such as an errant order or an incorrect procedure. Providing training such as TeamSTEPPS to health professional students as a group is an ideal method for creating more comfort in an area of great discomfort. Program materials are fully available online (AHRQ, 2013).

Educators have resources in the construction of interprofessional communication competencies. Two main resources are *Core Competencies for Interprofessional Collaborative Practice* (Interprofessional Education Collaborative Expert Panel, 2011) and a *National Interprofessional Competency Framework* (CIHC, 2010). Additionally, competencies in informatics that also relate to interprofessional education are accessible: *TIGER Informatics Competencies Collaborative (TICC) Final Report* (Technology Information Guiding Education Reform [TIGER], 2009).

SYNOPSIS

Educational innovations incorporating tools for interprofessional communication have been reported. For example, as a version of SBAR patient handoffs, a standardized interprofessional tool was integrated throughout an undergraduate curriculum. The new tool was used as a consistent method for students to report on patients to both faculty and other care providers (Enlow, Shanks, Guhde, & Perkins, 2010). In a study of medical, nursing, pharmacy, and physician assistant students, a 4-hour joint training that included a component of TeamSTEPPS was evaluated for its impact on interprofessional communication. The results indicate that the joint training session significantly, and positively, influenced ratings with regard to communication in general and interprofessional communication (Brock et al., 2013).

Faculty have used roundtables, simulation, and standardized patients to develop interprofessional communication skills. In one study, researchers found that simulation experiences in medical and nursing student teams were superior to roundtables for the advancement of interprofessional communication skills (Reising et al., 2011). In another study, using standardized patients for health professions students improved confidence in communication skills (Solomon & Salfi, 2011). Health professions faculty have also integrated interprofessional communication competencies into stand-alone communication courses, as well as courses that focus on interprofessional communication (Doucet, Buchanan, Cole, & McCoy, 2013).

RECOMMENDATIONS

Nurse educators must emphasize the importance of the entire health care team in the protection of patients. Developing evidence-based interpersonal and interprofessional communication skills is foundational to ensuring sound practice that will promote patient quality and safety. Coeducation or training is strongly recommended in health professions' curricula. The literature on the many different and innovative methods to develop interprofessional communication skills is rapidly expanding. Nurse educators should seek opportunities with other health professions faculty to further advance teamwork skills, and are encouraged to

I

publish and present their innovations and experiences.

Agency for Healthcare Research and Quality (AHRQ). (2012). *Safety culture.* Retrieved from http://psnet.ahrq.gov/primer .aspx?primerID=5

Agency for Healthcare Research and Quality (AHRQ). (2013). *TeamSTEPPS®: National implementation: About the national implementation plan.* Agency for Healthcare Research and Quality. Retrieved from http://teamstepps.ahrq.gov/aboutnationalIP.htm

Brock, D., Abu-Rish, E., Chiu, C. R., Hammer, D., Wilson, S., Vorvick, L.,…Zierler, B. (2013). Interprofessional education in team communication: Working together to improve patient safety. *BMJ Quality & Safety, 22*(5), 414–423.

Canadian Interprofessional Health Collaborative (CIHC). (2010). *A national interprofessional competency framework.* Vancouver, BC: Her Majesty the Queen in Right of Canada.

Doucet, S., Buchanan, J., Cole, T., & McCoy, C. (2013). A team approach to an undergraduate interprofessional communication course. *Journal of Interprofessional Care, 27*(3), 272–273.

Enlow, M., Shanks, L., Guhde, J., & Perkins, M. (2010). Incorporating interprofessional communication skills (ISBARR) into an undergraduate nursing curriculum. *Nurse Educator, 35*(4), 176–180.

Institute for Healthcare Improvement (IHI). (2014). *SBAR technique for communication: A situational briefing model.* Retrieved from http://www.ihi.org/ knowledge/Pages/Tools/SBARTechnique forCommunicationASituationalBriefing Model.aspx

Institute of Medicine (IOM). (2000). *To err is human: Building a safer health care system.* Washington, DC: The National Academies Press.

Institute of Medicine (IOM). (2003). *Health professions education: A bridge to quality.* Washington, DC: The National Academies Press.

Interprofessional Education Collaborative Expert Panel. (2011). *Core competencies for interprofessional collaborative practice: Report of an expert panel.* Washington, DC: Interprofessional Education Collaborative.

The Joint Commission (TJC). (2014). *National patient safety goals.* The Joint Commission. Retrieved from http://www.jointcommission.org/standards_information/npsgs .aspx

Reising, D. L., Carr, D. E., Shea, R. A., & King, J. M. (2011). Comparison of communication outcomes in traditional versus simulation strategies in nursing and medical students. *Nursing Education Perspectives, 32*(5), 323–327.

Solomon, P., & Salfi, J. (2011). Evaluation of an interprofessional education communication skills initiative. *Education for Health, 24*(2), 616.

Technology Information Guiding Education Reform (TIGER). (2009). *TIGER informatics competencies collaborative (TICC) final report.* Retrieved from http://tigercompetencies.pbworks.com/f/TICC_Final.pdf

University of Washington. (2011). *Video example of error disclosure* (video). Retrieved from http://collaborate.uw.edu/educators-toolkit/error-disclosure-toolkit/ video-example-of-error-disclosure.html

Deanna L. Reising

INTERPROFESSIONAL EDUCATION

DEFINITION

As students and faculty from multiple health professions begin to work together in teams, there is a need to have a common language and understanding of interprofessional education (IPE) and collaborative practice. In 2002, the United Kingdom's Centre for the Advancement of Interprofessional Education (CAIPE) defined IPE as more than students studying together (CAIPE, 2002). The CAIPE definition of IPE is the most accepted one used in health professions education and interprofessional practice. IPE includes purposeful activities designed so that students can learn from, with, and about each other and work toward the ultimate goal of providing collaborative, team-based care focused on quality of care (CAIPE, 2002). It is not just about students from different disciplines taking the same courses together.

APPLICATION

Two national initiatives affecting how nurses are educated to address the need for IPE and collaborative practice are the Institute of Medicine's (IOM, 2011) report *The Future of Nursing: Leading Change, Advancing Health* and the 2010 Lancet Commission Report *Health Professionals for a New Century: Transforming Education to Strengthen Health Systems in an Interdependent World* (Frenk et al., 2010). These two reports include recommendations that have implications for nursing education. One of the recommendations from the Future of Nursing report (2011) was that nurses should be full partners with physicians in redesigning health care. This recommendation was not specifically about IPE but was about empowering nurses to be leaders to participate with physicians and other health professionals in the design, implementation, and evaluation of reforms in health care. The implication for nursing education was to train nurses to be leaders and collaborative partners in addressing health care system reform. In order for nurses to be full partners, they need to gain knowledge in process improvement, health care systems, health care financing, patient safety initiatives, and health care policies. Leadership training that promoted collaboration and mutual respect was also recommended, so that nurses could work effectively with other members of the health care team to make decisions and act independently. The recommendations for nurse leaders were very much aligned with the subsequent "Team and Teamwork" subcompetencies recommended for health

profession students (Interprofessional Education Collaborative [IPEC] Expert Panel Report, 2011):

> Specific Team and Teamwork Competency #5—Apply leadership practices that support collaborative practice and team effectiveness; and Specific Team and Teamwork Competency #7—Share accountability with other professions, patients, and communities for outcomes relevant to prevention and health care. (p. 25)

SYNOPSIS

In the last 10 years, there have been numerous external forces influencing changes in health professions education that have resulted in a renewed focus on IPE. These forces include: (a) the establishment of national and international organizations and institutes supporting IPE; (b) changes in accreditation standards requiring IPE (Zorek & Raehl, 2013); (c) health care reform that aligns financial incentives for team-based care with a focus on quality and not volume of care (Patient Protection and Affordable Healthcare Act, 2010); (d) discipline-specific and international reports and forums dedicated to improving health and the delivery of health care in a more efficient and equitable manner; and (e) funding of a national center through private and public partnerships to coordinate IPE and collaborative practice (University of Minnesota's National Center for Interprofessional Practice and Education; http://nexusipe.org/).

The relationship between IPE and collaborative practice was described in a 2010 World Health Organization (WHO) report: *Framework for Action on Interprofessional Education and Collaborative Practice,* which stated:

> After almost 50 years of enquiry, the World Health Organization and its partners acknowledge that there is sufficient evidence to indicate that effective interprofessional education enables effective collaborative practice. Collaborative practice strengthens health systems and improves health outcomes. (p. 7)

In 2010, six national health profession associations formally joined together to

I

create the IPEC. The IPEC's founding organizations include the American Association of Colleges of Nursing, the Association of American Medical Colleges, the American Association of Colleges of Osteopathic Medicine, the American Dental Education Association, the American Association of Colleges of Pharmacy, and the Association of Schools of Public Health. In 2011, the IPEC published a report describing four competency domains and 38 subcompetency statements for interprofessional collaborative practice (IPEC, 2011). Increasingly, professional organizations and accrediting bodies have recognized the importance of IPE, which has led to accreditation standards for including IPE. The four, broad-based IPE domains for which most health professional students are held accountable are values/ethics for interprofessional practice, roles/responsibilities, interprofessional communication, and teams and teamwork.

The Lancet Commission Report (Frenk et al., 2010) was a seminal article in health professions education and of great importance for nurse educators. One outcome of this article was the creation of an international global forum (IOM Global Forum on Innovations in Health Professions Education) involving educational leaders from academia and practice, as well as professional organizations and governments, to share perspectives and discuss needed institutional and instructional reforms that were addressed in the report. Summaries of each forum can be found at www.iom.edu/Activities/Global/InnovationHealthProfEducation.aspx

Two of ten instructional and institutional reforms proposed by the Lancet Commission for the purpose of advancing the transformations needed in health professions education to enhance patient and population-centered care (2010) had direct implications for nursing education:

> "Promotion of interprofessional and transprofessional education that breaks down professional silos while enhancing collaborative and non-hierarchical relationships in effective teams" (reform #2) and promote a new professionalism that uses competencies as the objective criterion for the classification of health professionals, transforming present conventional silos. (reform #6; p. 1951)

RECOMMENDATIONS

The recommendations from the two reports (*Future of Nursing* [2011] and the Lancet Commission Report [2010]) address the changes needed in nursing education and nursing organizations (purposeful leadership training and IPE) that will lead to competent nursing leaders who can engage in decision making with other professionals in health care reform and competent nursing students who are "collaborative-practice-ready" to provide high-quality and safe, patient- or population-centered care as a member of a team on graduation.

To realize these recommendations in day-to-day practice, nurses at all levels, from deans to pre-licensure students, need to demonstrate leadership. Nursing deans need to collaborate with other health science deans to provide infrastructure support for IPE and resources to develop IPE-competent faculty. Nurse educators need to create opportunities for students to be educated with other health professional students as part of their core curriculum. Nursing students need to be engaged and lead IPE student activities to break down the professional silos. Through leadership and participation at all levels, nurses will be able to demonstrate competency in IPE and collaborative practice.

Centre for the Advancement of Interprofessional Education (CAIPE). *Defining IPE*. Retrieved from http://caipe.org.uk/resources/defining-ipe

Frenk, J., Chen, L., Bhutta, Z. A., Cohen, J., Crisp, N., Evans, T.,…Zurayk, H. (2010). Health professionals for a new century: Transforming education to strengthen health systems in an interdependent world. *Lancet, 376*(9756), 1923–1958.

Institute of Medicine (IOM). (2010). *The future of nursing: Leading change, advancing health.* Washington, DC: National Academies Press.

Interprofessional Education Collaborative (IPEC) Expert Panel. (2011). *Core competencies for interprofessional collaborative practice: Report of an expert panel.* Washington, DC: Interprofessional Education Collaborative.

Patient Protection and Affordable Care Act, 42 U.S.C. § 18001 et seq. (2010).

World Health Organization (WHO). (2010). *Framework for action on interprofessional education & collaborative practice.* Retrieved from http://www.who.int/hrh/resources/ framework_action/en/index.html

Zorek, J., & Raehl, C. (2013). Interprofessional education accreditation standards in the USA: A comparative analysis. *Journal of Interprofessional Care, 27*(2), 123–130.

Brenda K. Zierler
George E. Thibault

I

J

JOURNALING

DEFINITION

Journaling is the act of writing or recording one's thoughts, feelings, and experiences in a journal, a process that can be achieved by hand or electronically. It may be marked or graded, and may contain scholarly references and structured questions designed to guide the writer.

APPLICATION

In education in general and nursing education in particular, journaling is used primarily as a tool for research to enhance the learning experience of students. As a research tool, the journal contributes to data collection and is analyzed against the research question. For learning purposes, the journal is assigned as part of the expected course work. Students, however, may choose to continue to journal on completion of the course, particularly if they found it useful and helpful in their learning.

The process of journaling implies multiple entries. The actual number and length of the entries, however, is contingent on the expectations of the instructor and/or the purpose of the journal. The journal might only be read by the instructor; by the instructor and other students; or not at all by anyone but the writer. For example, the student might be required to generate a number of journal entries, as well as write a subsequent reflection about the journaling experience that is then marked.

SYNOPSIS

As a teaching and learning strategy, journaling has been supported by numerous renowned theorists including Dewey (1916), Kolb (1984), and Schon (1987). Dewey characterized experience as either active (undertaking an activity) or passive (undergoing the consequences). He believed reflective patterns of thought must be taught and learning and growth take place only through the cycle of reflecting and drawing on past experiences. Kolb (1984) developed a cycle of learning whereby a student learns by doing, reflects on these actions, and then assesses performance with the guidance of his or her preceptor. Schon's (1987) seminal book on reflective journaling spurred nurse educators to use more journaling assignments as a way to promote reflection.

There are several studies on the quality of the content in student journals, their level of reflection, their ability to think critically, and the process in which they engage to link theory and practice experiences (Epp, 2008; Harrison & Fopma-Loy, 2010). Benefits of journaling identified include decreasing stress, increasing satisfaction with learning, enhancing emotional competence, and learning about ethics (McMillian-Coddington, 2013). Overall, it has been found that the use of journaling is more beneficial than detrimental to student learning.

RECOMMENDATIONS

Journaling is an excellent tool to enhance student learning. Educators, however, need to be aware that there are a variety of issues that must be considered. First, there are differences of opinion as to whether journals should be marked or graded. Given that the journal is designed to be a safe learning tool with which the student can reflect on his or her own development as a nurse, it can be premature or even inappropriate to assign a mark/grade. Moreover, students may not feel safe in their reflections and instead write what they think the instructor would like to read. Furthermore, when students are expected to answer specific questions and to provide references, the journal becomes a formal assignment that resembles an essay. Second, the formal assignment of journaling increases the marking time for the educator; thus, some educators may ask students to share their journal with each other for the purpose of providing peer feedback. This act, although well meaning, can have ethical consequences if the journal contains self-disclosures. Third, educators are expected to write and reflect on their own experiences as part of scholarly teaching. Educators should develop and integrate journaling activities into their own teaching practice. If the educator decides to use journaling as an assignment, it is important to consider *all* the factors that must be considered for student-centered learning.

Dewey, J. (1916). *Democracy and education.* New York, NY: The Macmillan Company.

Epp, S. (2008). The value of reflective journaling in undergraduate nursing education: A literature review. *International Journal of Nursing Studies, 45*(9), 1379–1388.

Harrison, P., & Fopma-Loy, J. (2010). The value of reflective journaling in undergraduate nursing education: A literature review. *International Journal of Nursing Studies, 45*(9), 1379–1388.

Kolb, D. (1984). *Experiential learning: Experiences as the source of learning and development.* Englewood Cliffs, NJ: Prentice-Hall.

McMillian-Coddington, D. (2013). Reflection through journal writing to educate registered nursing students on patient care. *Teaching & Learning in Nursing, 8*(2), 63–67.

Schon, D. (1987). *Educating the reflective practitioner: Toward a new design for teaching and learning in the professions.* San Francisco, CA: Jossey-Bass.

Olive Yonge
Florence Myrick
Sandra Davidson

L

LEADERSHIP

DEFINITION

Leadership is a social process in which one individual influences the behaviors of others without the use of threats or violence (Huczynski & Buchanan, 1991). It is the ability to describe a vision and focus both individuals and groups toward this vision while engaging them, encouraging teamwork and commitment, and being effective.

APPLICATION

Effective leadership is essential to nursing, as the Institute of Medicine (IOM) 2010 report, *The Future of Nursing: Leading Change, Advancing Health*, states, "The nursing profession must produce leaders throughout the health care system, from the bedside to the boardroom, who can serve as full partners with other health professionals and be accountable for their own contributions to delivering high-quality care while working collaboratively with leaders from other health professions" (IOM, 2010, p. 221). The teaching of leadership skills both in and out of the classroom is essential for advancing nursing. Nursing requires teamwork; to have an effective team, a leader needs to possess the essential leadership skills.

Students need to be engaged in the theoretical foundations and the conceptual principles of nursing leadership, gain the essential skills to practice leadership competently in the rapidly changing health care environment, and begin to define their own leadership style. The student needs to develop awareness of his or her leadership style and can utilize the Leadership Practice Inventory (LPI) or the Multifactor Leadership Questionnaire (MLQ) for assessment. The LPI assesses individuals' leadership behaviors and provides feedback for developing and enhancing leadership skills (Kouzes & Posner, 1990). The MLQ is designed to measure transactional, transformational, and laissez-faire leadership performance (Bass & Avolio, 2005).

The Magnet® model has transformational leadership as one of its four model components (American Nurses Credentialing Center, 2014). This model is an essential part of any nursing education curriculum in leadership.

SYNOPSIS

There are many identified styles of leadership in the literature. *Democratic leadership* encourages open communication and staff participation in decision making. Staff is given accountability and responsibility as well as feedback on their performance. The focus is on relationship building between the leader and the individual in order to improve upon the quality of the system and process rather than to place blame on the individual. *Servant leadership* motivates and influences others by developing the skills of each individual and motivating him or her. The entire team has influence on organizational decision making based on the values and ideals of the institution. The servant leader possesses the following qualities: listening, persuasion, access to intuition and foresight, use of language, and pragmatic measurements of outcomes (Greenleaf, 1977). *Laissez-faire leadership* is one in which the leader provides little to no supervision or direction and takes a hands-off approach. Consequently, few decisions

L

are made and minor changes occur. This is often referred to as passive leadership. This type of leadership usually occurs at the beginning of one's career, when there is inexperience, or at the very end of a career, when one is aware that his or her replacement will make any necessary changes. *Authoritarian or autocratic leadership* occurs when the leader makes all decisions without any input from his or her employees. There is a system of punishment that is used to enforce the rules of the organization. In this type of leadership, knowledge is power; therefore, information that the individual and team may need is withheld. Errors and mistakes are not tolerated and there is a culture of blame placed on the individual rather than considering the process at fault. This type of leadership is useful to enforce policy and procedures, but does not build a culture of trust or teamwork. *Transactional leadership* occurs when the followers are in a relationship of mutual dependence in which the contributions of both sides are acknowledged and rewarded (Kellerman, 1984). Additionally, Burns (1978) believed that transactional leaders tend to focus on task completion and employee compliance and rely heavily on organizational rewards and punishment to influence employee performance. Transactional leadership occurs when the leader rewards or disciplines the follower, depending on the adequacy of the follower's performance (Bass & Riggio, 2006). In contrast, *transformational leadership* occurs when leaders create and sustain significant change in performance, morale, motivation, and dedication of their followers, supporters, organizations, and within themselves. There is a shared vision and mission. The major characteristics of transformational leadership include engendering trust, admiration, loyalty, and respect among followers through application of charismatic vision and behavior (Nayab, 2010). These leaders encourage their followers to pursue goals that go beyond their immediate self-interests. Transformational leaders motivate followers and other constituencies to do more than they originally expected to do as they strive for higher order outcomes

(Burns, 1978). Burns published his seminal works in 1978, which introduced the concepts of transformational and transactional leadership and defined transformational leadership as a "process whereby leaders and followers raise one another to higher levels of morality and motivation" (Burns, 1978, p. 19). Transformational leadership was further developed by Bass and Avolio (1994) and is considered one of the most effective models of leadership. Transformational leadership consists of four constructs known as the "4 I's": idealized influence, inspirational motivation, intellectual stimulation, and individual consideration. Idealized influence involves building trust and confidence by becoming admired and respected. Inspirational motivation creates enthusiasm toward a convincing vision of the future. Leaders also challenge followers toward high goals, expectations, and standards in an effort for the individual to reach his or her full potential. Through intellectual stimulation, the leader promotes change by challenging and reassessing the status quo. Leaders encourage excitement and implement innovative and creative ways to resolve routine functions or recurrent issues. Individual consideration acknowledges that each person has unique needs, abilities, and goals. It is imperative for leaders to listen attentively, support, provide opportunities for growth, educate, and mentor their followers.

Kouzes and Posner (2012) identified *five* core practices that are necessary for leaders: (a) model the way, (b) inspire a shared vision, (c) challenge the process, (d) enable others to act, and (e) encourage the heart. A leader models the way he or she is behaving in a way that is consistent with the shared values of the group. When challenging the process, leaders do not settle for the status quo; they always are striving for excellence. When they inspire a vision, they communicate a unique view of the future. When leaders enable others to act, they promote mutual goals, seek fresh solutions, and build trust in the relationship. Encouraging the heart builds self-confidence through high expectations and rewarding performance by recognizing the individual and rewarding performance.

RECOMMENDATIONS

There is a need for nurse researchers to examine leadership styles and describe the leadership characteristics that improve outcome. These leadership characteristics can then be emphasized to nurses at all levels of education and practice. The linkages between leadership styles and nurse satisfaction, retention, and engagement are important areas for future research. Future research also can be developed to address the nurse, system, and patient outcomes in relation to leadership styles practiced within organizations.

American Nurses Credentialing Center. (Ed.). (2014). *Application manual: Magnet recognition program*. Silver Spring, MD: Author.

Bass, B., & Avolio, B. (1994). *Improving organizational effectiveness through transformational leadership*. Thousand Oaks, CA: Sage Publications.

Bass, B. M., & Riggio, R. E. (2006). *Transformational leadership*. Mahwah, NJ: Lawrence Erlbaum Publisher.

Burns, J. M. (1978). *Leadership*. New York, NY: Harper & Row.

Greenleaf, R. (1977). *Servant leadership: A journey into the nature of legitimate power and greatness*. New York, NY: Paulist Press.

Huczynski, A., & Buchanan, D. (1991). *Organizational behaviour: An introductory text* (2nd ed.). London, England: Prentice Hall.

Institute of Medicine (IOM). (2010). *The future of nursing: Leading change, advancing health*. Retrieved from http://www .thefutureofnursing.org/sites/default/ files/Future%20of%20Nursing%20 Report_0.pdf2010

Kellerman, B. (1984). *Leadership: Multidisciplinary perspectives*. Englewood Cliffs, NJ: Prentice Hall.

Kouzes, J., & Posner, B. (1990). *Leadership practices inventory (LPI): A self-assessment and analysis*. San Diego: Pfeiffer.

Kouzes, J., & Posner, B. (2012). *The leadership challenge: How to make extraordinary things happen in organizations* (5th ed.). San Francisco, CA: Jossey-Bass.

Nayab, N. (2010). *Characteristics of transformational leadership*. Retrieved from http:// www.brighthub.com/office/home/articles/71743.aspx

Robin S. Krinsky

LEADERSHIP DEVELOPMENT

DEFINITION

Leadership development is the multifaceted process of identifying a goal, motivating other people to act, and providing support and motivation to achieve mutually negotiated goals (Porter-O'Grady, 2003). A leader's role is to encourage effective performance from others through the development of shared values, vision, and expectations to enhance the organization's planned goals and pathway to success (Feather, 2009).

APPLICATION

Leadership development is paramount to the future of nursing education. An increasing need for new and innovative nursing leaders is emerging as massive retirement of nursing leaders is predicted to occur throughout the globe within the next decade. Just as nursing education is now based on evidence, leadership development must be grounded in leadership theories and frameworks (Doody & Doody, 2011, 2012). It is vital that nursing education prepares strong nursing leaders for the future of health care delivery. The clinical environment of today is characterized by cultural diversity and increasing patient acuity, thus calling for knowledgeable nurse leaders (Perry Schoenfelder & Gaffney Valde, 2009). Traditionally, nurses have been managed by leaders who have had minimal formal leadership development. However, the workforce of today is faced with unprecedented clinical care challenges that require educated nurse leaders to move and progress into the leadership roles of the future.

Nursing educators must incorporate leadership development into undergraduate and graduate programs. It is essential that the foundational knowledge of leadership theories conceptualized in terms of transactional, transformational, authentic, quantum, and servant leadership be included in all levels of nursing programs (Duygulu & Kublay, 2011). Health care organizations are complex with constant daily change requiring flexible leadership to meet the many challenges. Nursing educators can facilitate the development of future nurse leaders by appealing to higher ideals and moral values when facing the challenges of complex organizations (Barbuto, 2005; Bass, 1998).

SYNOPSIS

Leadership development is minimally introduced during basic nursing education and varies according to nursing program, educational setting, and country of origin. Duygulu and Kublay (2011) concluded that a focus on leadership development for unit charge nurses should be mandatory to develop strong leaders in clinical settings. In addition, transformational leadership programs had a positive impact on both the charge nurses and the unit staff nurses. Effective clinical leadership has been found to be the key to healthy, functional, and supportive work environments (Mannix, Wilkes, & Daly, 2013).

Leadership development educational programs have focused on the concept of emotional intelligence, which prepares leaders to become aware of not only their own emotions in managing staff, but in understanding the emotional level of the staff in their workday environment (Walton, 2012). Giltinane (2013) found that supportive emotional behaviors by the nurse leader were achieved by maintaining effective communication and emotional support

with followers. Leaders with emotional intelligence help staff to be successful with patient care.

Ethical nursing leadership development is another realm of leadership education that is important for educators to impart on future nursing leaders for managing the complexities of today's health care issues and challenges. Expectations for ethical leadership are that individuals take responsibility to engage in ethical behavior and provide leadership in building a moral community in the clinical setting (Storch, Makaroff, Pauly, & Newton, 2013). Ethical values should be clear and direct ethical action within the clinical environment.

RECOMMENDATIONS

Mentoring leadership development programs are extremely successful in preparing nursing leaders. Kelly and Hagerman (2013) developed a 6-week mentoring program with novice and experienced nurse leaders that was successful in the preparation of new nurse leaders. Nursing educational leadership development for future nurse leaders is needed to prepare nurses for the dynamics of the evolving health care world of today and the future. Leadership development courses and modules may be offered at colleges, universities, hospitals, and through leadership continuing education offerings. Research demonstrates that where leadership development has been taught and integrated into nursing, it has a positive impact on leadership, skills, and practice (Curtis, Sheerin, & de Vries, 2011). Nursing leadership development is the key to creating empowered nursing leaders to meet the daily struggles of the future.

Barbuto, J. E. (2005). Motivation and transactional, charismatic and transformational leadership: A test of antecedents. *Journal of Leadership Organizational Studies, 11*(4), 26–40.

Bass, B. M. (1998). *Transformational leadership: Industry, military and educational impact.* Newark, NJ: Lawrence Erlbaum.

Curtis, E. A., Sheerin, F. K., & de Vries. (2011). Developing leadership in nursing: The impact of education and training. *British Journal of Nursing, 20*(6), 344–352.

Doody, C. M., & Doody, O. (2011). Introducing evidence into nursing practice: Using the IOWA model. *British Journal of Nursing, 20*(11), 661–664.

Doody, O., & Doody, C. M. (2012). Transformational leadership in nursing practice. *British Journal of Nursing, 21*(20), 1212–1218.

Duygulu, S., & Kublay, G. (2011). Transformational leadership training programme for charge nurses. *Journal of Advanced Nursing, 67*(3), 633–642. doi:10.1111/j.1365–2648.2010.05507.x

Feather, R. (2009). Emotional intelligence in relation to nursing leadership: Does it matter? *Journal of Nursing Management, 17*(3), 376–382.

Giltinane, C. (2013). Leadership styles and theories. *Nursing Standard, 27*(41), 35–39.

Kelly, M., & Hagerman, L. (2013). Growing tomorrow's leaders. *Canadian Nurse, 109*(5), 26–29.

Mannix, J., Wilkes, L., & Daly, J. (2013). Attributes of clinical leadership in contemporary nursing: An integrative review. *Contemporary Nurse: A Journal for the Australian Nursing Profession, 45*(1), 10–21. doi:10.5172/conu.2013.45.1.10

Perry Schoenfelder, D., & Gaffney Valde, J. (2009). Creative practicum leadership experiences in rural settings. *Nurse Educator, 34*(1), 38–42.

Porter-O'Grady, T. (2003). A different age for leadership, part I: New context, new content. *Journal of Nursing Administration, 33*(2), 105–110.

Storch, J., Makaroff, K., Pauly, B., & Newton, L. (2013). Take me to my leader: The importance of ethical leadership among formal nurse leaders. *Nursing Ethics, 20*(2), 150–157. doi:10.1177/0969733012474291

Walton, D. (2012). *Introducing emotional intelligence: A practical guide*. London, England: Icon Books.

Sharon Elizabeth Metcalfe

LEADERSHIP: TRANSFORMATION

DEFINITION

The concept of transformational leadership was originally developed by Burns in 1978 (Marshall, 2011). Transformational leaders inspire and motivate people to follow them in ways that far surpass other types of leaders.

Transformational leaders are generally described as having four characteristics (referred to as the four I's): inspirational motivation, idealized influence, intellectual stimulation, and individualized consideration (Marshall, 2011). Inspiring others through motivation involves visioning. Transformational leaders create compelling vision for the future. The vision is so clear and convincing that people want to follow the leader to achieve the vision. Transformational leaders influence others by articulating a clear sense of purpose and talking about ideals and values so that people can see how the vision can be realized. Followers can see how they fit into the new vision. This level of change requires people to challenge the assumptions they hold. Transformational leaders must be able to intellectually show followers the path to the new vision and compel them to follow that path. In addition, transformational leaders provide focus to individuals by coaching and mentoring them to achieve the new vision (Grant, 2012).

Transformational leaders are admired, trusted, and respected by others. They are considered to be principled leaders and others want to follow them. Transformational leaders inspire others to greatness. Schools and colleges of nursing are facing turbulent times with massive changes in health care delivery that will push changes in academia. Deans and directors of nursing colleges, schools, and departments need to become transformational leaders during these turbulent times. Academic leaders must create the new vision and make it compelling enough so that faculty want to take this journey we are facing.

APPLICATION

Nursing education is at a pivotal point not seen in the past. Health care reform is advancing. Education leaders are expected to prepare nursing graduates for roles that do not currently exist; these roles can only be envisioned. Nursing leaders in academia are challenged to form partnerships with service leaders to test new care delivery models focused on wellness instead of illness, change the traditional focus on acute care at the baccalaureate level and find new primary care models that include nurses as care managers and coordinators, and ensure nurse practitioners are steeped in nursing theory and nursing frameworks as they fill the ever-expanding void in primary care.

Deans and directors in academia must create vision with faculty that can be carried on to students. Academic leaders must help faculty become transformational leaders with their students. Nursing leaders and faculty in higher education have a unique opportunity to influence the future. Students are at a stage in their lives when they are ready to make transitions (Ingleton, 2013). Students look at faculty as experts and role models. As such, faculty need to help students see the need to be prepared for roles not currently used in practice (Boglar, Caspi, & Roccas, 2013). Leaders in nursing education have a responsibility to create future leaders who will continue the journey of transforming health care (Mathis, 2013).

Yet, faculty are not prepared for the role of being transformational leaders. Faculty arrive in their roles as expert practitioners or expert researchers. Deans, directors, and chairs have this dual role in higher education leadership of transforming the environment and convincing faculty of the need to prepare students differently. Therefore, faculty need to be mentored and coached to become transformational leaders.

Being a transformational leader in the higher education environment has challenges. Nursing academic leaders face faculty who are tenured in a system of higher education that has traditionally valued stability and tradition. Thus, structures in higher education may be detrimental to change. Rewards and incentives may be more focused on obtaining grant monies than on recreating education and practice structures. Institutions of higher education have been faced with reductions in budgets and nursing faculty shortages that may hamper the creativity needed for transformational leaders (Basham, 2012).

Nursing deans, directors, and chairs rise to the challenge by creating a vision for the future that is compelling so that faculty realize it is essential to change. This vision can guide faculty to see how they can be successful in the new landscapes in higher education and in health care. Leaders must be fearless and principled as they develop new paths and lead others to follow.

SYNOPSIS

Transformational leaders create vision and convince others to follow. Transformational leaders are principled and fearless as they help others to realize the new vision. Academic leaders face changes in health care with rapid transformations in higher education. Higher education is steeped in tradition and nursing leaders face unique challenges such as faculty shortages and the need for graduates to function in roles that do not yet exist.

RECOMMENDATIONS

Nursing leaders in higher education can take the opportunity to learn as much as they can about transformational leadership, strategic planning, and change management. Think tanks can be formed to create new practice models following changes in higher education to ensure a prepared workforce for tomorrow. Deans, directors, and chairs can hone their mentoring and coaching skills to be expert role models for the faculty. Research on transformational leadership needs to continue a focus on academic leadership in preparing the next generation.

Basham, L. (2012). Transformational and transactional leaders in higher education. *SAM Advanced Management Journal, 77*(2), 15–37.

Boglar, R., Caspi, A., & Roccas, S. (2013). Transformational and passive leadership: An initial investigation of university instructors as leaders in a virtual learning environment. *Educational Management Administration and Leadership, 41*(3), 372–392.

Burns, J. (1978). *Leadership.* New York, NY: Harper & Row.

Grant, A. M. (2012). Leading with meaning: Beneficiary contact, prosocial impact, and the performance effects of transformational leadership. *Academy of Management Journal, 55*(2), 458–476.

Ingleton, T. (2013). College student leadership development: Transformational leadership as a theoretical foundation. *International Journal of Academic Research in Business and Social Sciences, 3*(7), 219–229.

Marshall, E. (2011). *Transformational leadership in nursing: From expert clinician to influential leader.* New York, NY: Springer.

Mathis, S. (2013). Nursing leadership from the outside in. In G. Glazer & J. Fitzpatrick (Eds.), *Nursing leadership: As it should be* (pp. 151–158) New York, NY: Springer.

Pam Springer

LEARNER CENTERED

DEFINITION

"Learner-centered" teaching and learning combine a focus on: (a) individual learners, taking into account their experiences, perspectives, backgrounds, talents, interests, capacities, needs; and (b) the best available knowledge about learning and how it occurs. The incorporation of these teaching and learning practices is most effective in promoting the highest levels of motivation, learning, and achievement for all learners.

This dual focus then informs and drives educational decision making. Learner-centered activities involve active cognitive processes, such as creating, problem solving, reasoning, decision making, and evaluation. In addition, students are fundamentally motivated to learn due to the meaningful nature of the learning environment and activities (Billings & Halstead, 2012; Oermann, 2015).

APPLICATION

Traditionally, approaches that are labeled as teacher centered define teachers as the disseminators of knowledge and students as passive recipients. By contrast, the learner-centered approach seeks to engage students in an active manner in their learning in appropriate ways that are relevant to them in their lives outside the classroom (Peyton, Moore, & Young, 2010).

In an effort to clarify, the definition of learner-centered teaching (Weimer, 2013) identified five characteristics:

1. **Learner-centered teaching engages students in the hard, messy work of learning.** Students engage in dialogue with each other and with the teacher. Teachers talk and listen more to their students.

2. **Learner-centered teaching includes explicit skill instruction.** Critical thinking and problem-solving skills are enhanced, and learning skills develop faster if they are taught with the content.

3. **Learner-centered teaching encourages students to reflect on what they are learning and how they are learning it.** Assignments actively engage students in reflection to analyze what they are learning and how they are learning it.

4. **Learner-centered teaching motivates students by giving them some control over learning processes.** Teachers find responsible ways to share power with students. For example, they might give students choices about assignments and deadlines.

5. **Learner-centered teaching encourages collaboration; classrooms are considered**

communities of learners. Learner-centered teachers believe that students learn from and with each other. This gives encouragement to students who do not find it easy to participate (phrases in boldface are from Weimer, 2013).

New technological advances introduced into the classroom continue to expand and offer diverse and creative ways to further nursing education. Technological advances have led to rapid changes in the nature of classroom instruction as well. Mixed media forms of instruction (PowerPoint, jpeg images, mpg, mp3 files, and the World Wide Web) have spread widely, as has the utilization of distance learning formats. Learner-centered education requires a focus on student learning, but not all learners are equally invested. Regardless of how we teach and what technology we bring into the classroom or outside the classroom, we need to assess, through various forms of feedback, the extent to which learner-centered education is working and meeting our goals.

Web-based instruction can be a powerful means of enhancing the learning experience, including the posting of online quizzes and links to other websites for further enrichment. It also provides a means for video streaming of lectures, podcasting, and interactive (live) linking between classes at different and/or distant institutions. Some learner-centered courses have experienced student-led creation of class blogs, wikis, and other websites, allowing independent student interaction regarding varied aspects of class-related studies, including exam review.

SYNOPSIS

The learner-centered approach means creating a learning environment that is authentic, where students are directed toward how to set realistic goals and take responsibility for their learning as they build new knowledge connected to old (Billings & Halstead, 2012).

The learner-centered approach requires faculty to set clear course objectives and provide students with feedback on their own learning strategies to meet those course objectives. Learner-centered nursing education needs a supportive, considerate, positive environment if learners are to thrive.

In a learner-centered classroom, teachers and students reflect on the learning process. Teachers learn to shift the focus to the learners and encourage them to share responsibility for their learning.

The following are characteristics of a teacher conducting a learner-centered classroom:

- Seeks background information about students to guide in planning instructional lessons
- Sets instructional goals with learners' needs, backgrounds, and interests in mind
- Differentiates instructions based on learners' needs
- Uses a variety of student groupings to encourage target language communication among students
- Sets goals that are purposeful and meaningful from the students' point of view
- Makes lesson plans flexible to accommodate students' needs
- Assures classroom environment is warm, open, and encourages students to participate
- Arranges the classroom in a manner that is easy for students to work together in pairs or groups and also easy for the teacher to move around to facilitate conversations among student groups
- Uses authentic, practical, and realistic activities for language performance
- Adjusts teaching based on formative assessment results
- Provides maximum opportunities for students to use authentic materials

- Uses a variety of resources beyond the textbook
- Establishes short-term benchmarks to monitor students' progress

These characteristics enhance learner-centered learning for the students by ensuring:

- Students feel comfortable asking questions and
- Students have maximum opportunity to interact and communicate

RECOMMENDATIONS

To effectively engage students in the learning process, nurse educators need to understand multiple factors in the teaching–learning process. Nursing faculty members must also be able to teach students how to learn and how to be successful in their coursework. Having a classroom that is engaged with students actively participating is the challenge. Nurse educators can accept this challenge by finding innovative ways to teach and reach all students and, in this way, create motivated nurses for the future.

Billings, D. M., & Halstead, J. A. (2012). *Teaching in nursing: A guide for faculty, fourth edition* (pp. 160–169). St. Louis, MO: Elsevier Saunders.

Oermann, M. H. (Ed.). (2015). *Teaching in nursing and role of the educator. The complete guide to best practice in teaching, evaluation, and curriculum development* (pp. 35–57). New York, NY: Springer Publishing.

Peyton, J. K., Moore, S. C., & Young, S. (2010). *Evidence-based, student-centered instructional practices, CAELA network brief.* Washington, DC: Centre for Applied Linguistics. Retrieved from http://www.cal.org/adultesl/pdfs/student-centered-instructional-practices.pdf

Weimer, M. (2013). *Learner-centered teaching: Five key changes to practice* (2nd ed., pp. 59–168). San Francisco, CA: John Wiley.

Irena L. Kenneley

LIBRARY PARTNERSHIPS

L

DEFINITION

Library partnerships in nursing education are defined by close working relationships, collaborative teaching and research, and consultation between nursing students, their educators, and library professionals. Partnerships between library professionals and nurses of all levels (practitioners, educators, and students) enable nurses to improve patient care through finding and incorporating evidence-based practice information into the care they deliver (Arndt, 2009). Librarians and nurse educators together can help students with information navigation and evaluation expertise and combine this with pedagogical knowledge and subject area skill (Dewey, 2001).

APPLICATION

Nursing education–library partnerships bring those involved in, or benefiting from, nursing education together with the various resources a library offers. "Library" describes both a collection of materials (electronic, print, photographs, other media, etc.) and the facility that houses these materials. Libraries may serve municipalities, educational institutions, hospitals, corporations, or private citizens. Depending on the type, libraries may receive funding from public or private entities, or a combination thereof. There are multiple types of library employees with differing specializations. Professionals, or librarians, usually hold master's degrees in library or information sciences. Paraprofessionals often have special training to assist professionals in their work or in other library-related services. Library professionals and paraprofessionals may work in different capacities in research, reference, and information services; material preparation and circulation; building function and safety; material categorization or cataloging; technology; and a host of other areas. Librarians employed by health care-focused libraries and as subject specialists within other types of libraries often have professional and/or educational backgrounds in health care.

Educators of pre- and post-licensure practicing nurses partner with libraries by first accepting overtures from library employees who offer to provide them service or by seeking out assistance and partnership from the library that serves them. Nurse educators who work with post-licensure colleagues at hospitals and other health care centers may be served by and partner with:

- An individual library or information management resource serving a particular hospital or health care system;
- State-specific Area Health Education Center (AHEC) library focused on meeting information needs of practicing health care professionals. Contact information for AHECs can be found by consulting the AHEC Directory through the National AHEC Organization (www.nationalahec .org/). Although not all state AHECs offer library support, many do provide electronic resources and/or physical collections and support;
- Public library reference services. Larger public libraries may have employees specializing in health information. Most general reference librarians can also provide assistance with training opportunities, finding health care resources, and conducting searches;
- Academic library serving a community college or 4-plus-year institution. Depending upon contractual agreements with publishers and resource providers, the library may restrict resource usage or services to institution affiliates.

Nurse educators and librarians may partner to:

- Increase or improve educational opportunities for pre- and post-licensure nurses. Nursing educators can incorporate librarians' information finding and evaluation expertise into research methods and evidence-based practice classes and any coursework requiring students to find and use information. Incorporation methods include instructional visits to the class by the librarian, task and assignment-specific searching guides, and co-teaching.
- Conduct research. Librarians, particularly those specializing in research and reference or with expertise in relevant subjects, can assist nursing educators and students in conducting advanced searches of the literature, identifying survey tools and analysis procedures, and performing various other research-related capacities.
- Pool human, monetary, space, and other resources. Nursing educators and librarians can draw from each other's skill sets to improve libraries' nursing resource collections and services to nursing students and other library users. Nursing educators may host professional gatherings, in-person continuing education sessions, and displays in library physical spaces, while nursing educators may facilitate librarians' presentation of information finding and evaluation sessions for health care consumers in a care setting.

SYNOPSIS

Primary benefits of collaboration between nursing education and libraries are strengthening of the information literacy skills in current and future nurses (Miller, Jones, Graves, & Sievert, 2010) and improving patient care through fostering effective evidence-based nursing practice (Winsett & Moutseous, 2012). Librarians' skill set makes them uniquely able to sift through large amounts of primary and secondary research across formats and disciplines to help identify evidence most cogent to practice. Nurse educators should connect with librarians to gather authoritative and current literature on evidence-based teaching (Cannon & Boswell, 2012, p. 20) to increase effectiveness and efficiency of teaching methods, just as those educators who encourage students to draw from timely and accurate evidence-based practice literature to improve patient care (Winters & Echeverri, 2012). Modeling such partnerships at the educator level sets a valuable precedent for student nurses when they begin work and can draw from the knowledge management expertise of librarians serving care settings (Marshall et al., 2013) and maintain lifelong professional learning (Dee & Reynolds, 2013).

RECOMMENDATIONS

Despite the availability of resources online, librarians make available other materials that are not freely accessible and information that they are uniquely able to navigate and evaluate. By partnering with libraries and their employees, nurse educators can improve their teaching practice, research, and the care they provide to patients.

Arndt, R. M. (2009). Library and information literacy. *Journal of Emergency Nursing, 35*(4), 360–362.

Cannon, S., & Boswell, C. (2012). *Evidence-based teaching in nursing: A foundation for educators.* Sudbury, MA: Jones & Bartlett Learning.

Dee, C. R., & Reynolds, P. (2013). Lifelong learning for nurses building a strong future. *Medical Reference Services Quarterly, 32*(4), 451–458.

Dewey, B. I. (Ed.). (2001). *Library user education: Powerful learning, powerful partnerships.* Lanham, MD: Scarecrow Press.

Marshall, J. G., Sollenberger, J., Easterby-Gannett, S., Morgan, L. K., Klem, M. L., Cavanaugh, S. K.,…Hunter, S. (2013). The value of library and information services in patient care: Results of a multisite study. *Journal of the Medical Library Association, 101*(1), 38–46.

Miller, L., Jones, B., Graves, R., & Sievert, M. (2010). Merging silos: Collaborating for information literacy. *Journal of Continuing Education in Nursing, 41*(6), 267–272. doi: 10.3928/00220124-20100401-03

Winsett, R. P., & Moutseous, M. (2012). Collaborating with hospital librarians to engage nurses in evidence-based practice education. *Journal of Hospital Librarianship, 12*(4), 309–316. doi:10.1080/15323269.2012.719188

Winters, C. A., & Echeverri, R. (2012). Teaching strategies to support evidence-based practice. *Critical Care Nurse, 32*(3), 49–54.

Ann Hallyburton

LIFELONG LEARNING

DEFINITION

Lifelong learning is: "A cradle to the grave involvement of the individual with his or her learning and working environment. It implies a growth of all skills and a cumulative interweaving of knowledge and experience" (Benedict, Collier, Masar, & Wilkinson, 1984, p. 25). In nursing, a current definition of lifelong learning is a dynamic formal and informal learning process involving the continued evaluation of ideas to gain new perspectives concerning one's environment and interaction (Davis, Taylor, & Reyes, 2014). "The most essential characteristics of a lifelong learner are reflection, questioning, enjoying learning, understanding the dynamic nature of knowledge, and engaging in learning by actively seeking learning opportunities" (Davis et al., 2014, p. 444).

APPLICATION

Lifelong learning in nursing can be implemented through mandatory educational requirements including continuing education units and certifications (postgraduate). Mandatory requirements would be applicable in all states with the support of the state boards of nursing and credentialing agencies. In addition, mandatory educational requirements would embrace the importance of a nursing culture that encompasses "the relationship between professionalism, knowledge expansion, and enhancement of educational curiosity" (Eason, 2010, p. 157). Certifications would be twofold: One is a formal celebration for the nurse passing a competency examination and the second is where a nurse is involved in seeking higher standards to provide quality care (Eason, 2010).

Within the professional nursing bodies, there is a need to "develop programs and initiatives that support the ongoing academic progression of staff, enabling them to expand their competencies and implement new roles" (National League for Nursing [NLN] Board of Governors, 2011, p. 3). A new curriculum toward self-directed learning to be taught by nursing faculty in nursing programs is essential to ensure that the student nurses develop habits of study that are self-directed and lifelong in practice.

SYNOPSIS

A review of the literature shows an unclear view of the concept of lifelong learning in nursing. In the nursing literature, it shows that both the definition and implementation are not well articulated. The literature also points out that lifelong learners need to develop critical thinking skills. Self-directed learning is also a necessary attribute for lifelong learners (Winch, 2008). In addition, the literature shows a lack of measurement of outcomes after educational experiences. According to Maslin-Prothero (1997), "If courses provided by nurse education are examined, the emphasis continues to be on 'input'…rather than on 'output.' There is a need to follow up learners to evaluate the outcome of any education. There is little research examining individuals in their practice to establish any changes in practice following education" (p. 434).

RECOMMENDATIONS

There is a need for development of a systemic program for continuing education to encourage nurses to pursue lifelong learning. This program should be developed and executed by highly skilled professional nurses who are both educators and practitioners. Continuing education units should be mandatory throughout the United States. Benchmark studies should be executed to measure both learning and application (input and output).

A second recommendation is to develop partnerships with educators to construct nursing programs (college and graduate) to include self-directed learning skills in nursing practice. These new programs should be designed to assure practice in current and future nursing environments. In conjunction with these new programs, faculty should be trained to teach in the mode of self-directed education.

Benedict, D., Collier, F., Masar, B., & Wilkinson, L. (1984). *Learning a living in Canada* (Vol. 1). Quebec, Canada: Report to the Minister of Employment and Immigration.

Davis, L., Taylor, H., & Reyes, H. (2014). Lifelong learning in nursing: A Delphi study. *Nursing Education Today, 34*(3), 441–445.

Eason, T. (2010). Lifelong learning: Fostering a culture of curiosity. *Creative Nursing, 16*(4), 155–159.

Maslin-Prothero, S. E. (1997). A perspective on lifelong learning and its implications for nurses. *Nurse Education Today, 17*(6), 431–436.

National League for Nursing (NLN) Board of Governors. (2011). *Academic progression in nursing education*. NLN Vision Series.

Winch, C. (2008). Learning how to learn: A critique. *Journal of Philosophy of Education, 42*(3–4), 649–665.

Sheryl Kirk

M

MENTORING

DEFINITION

Mentoring is a process by which guidance is provided by a more-experienced person to a less-experienced person with the goal of having the less-experienced person develop competencies. Vance and Olson (1998) defined mentoring as a "developmental, empowering, and nurturing relationship extending over time in which mutual sharing, learning, and growth occur in an atmosphere of respect, collegiality and affirmation" (p. 5). Mentoring can be formal or informal. Mentoring can be with an individual or groups of individuals.

APPLICATION

Mentoring in nursing education takes place between many different types and levels of individuals or groups. It can help to facilitate relationships and interactions among faculty, and assist faculty members on the path to tenure. Mentoring is an influential factor in retaining new faculty members as it provides them with support and guidance. It may help to increase job satisfaction and reduce the stress associated with teaching and an academic career. Mentoring may help the mentee to develop new skills related to teaching, research, leadership, and scholarship. Mentoring may be formal or informal, but must be performed with the intention to ensure success. New faculty members in education can benefit from the experience of other educators in nursing through formal programs established by their schools of nursing. In two studies, researchers described results of focus groups with novice and expert nurse educators in a formal mentoring program developed for novice faculty (White, Brannan, & Wilson, 2010; Wilson, Brannan, & White, 2010). The program included two off-campus retreats and four all-day workshops, a significant investment of dedicated time. Each mentee was assigned a formal mentor, and biweekly contact between the mentor and mentee was encouraged. Mentees had positive feedback and included guidance and support, journaling, and openness in communication among their perceived benefits (White et al., 2010). The mentors were positive about the significance of the relationship and the communication with the mentees (Wilson et al., 2010). However, they felt they lacked the time to engage in meaningful activities with the mentees, and felt there was potential for a power imbalance (Wilson et al., 2010).

Mentoring has been identified as a critical attribute for faculty success and leadership development. Many professional organizations had developed resources to support mentorship initiatives. The National League for Nursing (NLN, 2008), which is dedicated to excellence in nursing education, has created the Mentoring of Nursing Faculty Tool Kit to promote mentoring among nurse faculty. The American Association of Colleges of Nursing (AACN) recognizes the importance of mentoring as evidenced by their creation of the New Dean Mentoring Program that links an experienced AACN-member dean to a member who is new to the role (AACN, n.d.). Sigma Theta Tau International (STTI), the honor society of nursing, is dedicated to mentoring and has developed a Center of Excellence in Nursing Education with

M

dedicated programs for nurse faculty leadership and mentoring (STTI, n.d.).

SYNOPSIS

The concept of mentoring became more visible in nursing education literature in the 1980s when mentoring was focused on clinical education. For the past few decades, an increased focus on mentoring worldwide has occurred, spurred on by the shortage of skilled health care professionals and nursing educators (Seekoe, 2013). Eller, Lev, and Feurer (2014) in a qualitative study identified key components of an effective mentoring relationship at 12 U.S. universities with 117 mentor–mentee dyads attending 12 workshops. The key components included open communication, goals, passion and inspiration, role modeling, and mutual respect and trust (Eller et al., 2014). The components of the mentoring process and the relationship between the mentor and mentee as listed by Zachary (2009) include reciprocity, collaboration, partnership, mutually defined goals, learning, and development for both mentor and mentee.

New mentoring models are emerging that include multiple mentors, junior partner reciprocally mentoring the senior individual, and peer-mentoring networks. These new models are all products of the classic mentor–mentee relationship. The thought is that those who have benefited from a good mentoring relationship are those who are "well balanced with personal and work issues as well as successful in their professional careers" (Grossman, 2013, p. 23).

RECOMMENDATIONS

As academia experiences shortages of nurse faculty, the importance of mentoring programs becomes vital. The development of best practice programs can help new faculty to be successful in their role (Nick et al., 2012). For student mentoring, adequate resources, education, and preparation of mentors are needed if transition from student to professional nurse is to occur.

Interdisciplinary/interprofessional teams, as reported in *Teaching IOM* (Finkelman & Kenner, 2012), are required as patient-centered care needs to continue to be collaborative and collegial. The mentoring of students and nurses is essential so that gaining the knowledge and experience with working on teams is clear and realistic.

Research recommendations include further investigation of peer mentoring, as well as identification of different forms of mentoring to meet specific learning needs as well as needs of diverse faculty and students. A culture of mentoring needs to be developed in nursing, a collaborative network that nurtures partnering with others (Grossman, 2013). Nurses have a professional responsibility to provide mentoring to their students and colleagues. Inexperienced nurses need to be mentored by those nursing leaders who are interested in the development of future leaders in nursing.

American Association of Colleges of Nursing (AACN). (n.d.). *New dean mentoring program.* Retrieved from https://www.aacn.nche.edu/membership/new-dean-mentoring-program

Eller, L. S., Lev, E. L., & Feurer, A. (2014). Key components of an effective mentoring relationship: A qualitative study. *Nurse Education Today, 34*(5), 815–820. doi:http://dx.doi.org/10.1016/j.nedt.2013.07.020

Finkelman, A., & Kenner, C. (2012). Incorporating the core competencies into nursing education. *Teaching IOM: Implications of the Institute of Medicine reports for nursing education* (3rd ed., pp. 119–130). Silver Springs, MD: Nursebooks.org.

Grossman, S. (2013). *Mentoring in nursing: A dynamic and collaborative process* (2nd ed.). New York, NY: Springer.

National League for Nursing (NLN). (2008). *The mentoring of nursing faculty tool kit.* Retrieved from http://www.nln.org/facultyprograms/MentoringToolkit/

Nick, J. M., Delahoyde, T. M., Del Prato, D., Mitchell, C., Ortiz, J., Ottley, C.,...Siktberg, L. (2012). Best practices in academic mentoring: A model for excellence. *Nursing Research and Practice, 2012,* 937906. Retrieved from http://dx.doi.org/10.1155/2012/937906

Seekoe, E. (2013). A conceptual framework for a mentoring model for nurse educators. *African Journal for Physical, Health Education, Recreation and Dance, 13,* 142–151.

Sigma Theta Tau International (STTI). (n.d.). *Center of excellence in nursing education.* Retrieved from http://www.nursingsociety.org/Education/Pages/CENE.aspx

Vance, C., & Olson, R. (1998). *The mentor connection in nursing.* New York, NY: Springer.

White, A., Brannan, J., & Wilson, C. B. (2010). A mentor–protégé program for new faculty, part I: Stories of protégés. *Journal of Nursing Education, 49*(11), 601–607.

Wilson, C. B., Brannan, J., & White, A. (2010). A mentor–protégé program for new faculty, part II: Stories of mentors. *Journal of Nursing Education, 49*(12), 665–671.

Zachary, L. (2009). *The mentee's guide: Making mentoring work for you.* San Francisco, CA: Jossey-Bass.

Patricia L. Schrull
Mary T. Quinn Griffin

MENTORING: MENTOR AND PROTÉGÉ RELATIONSHIP

DEFINITION

The traditional concept of mentoring is described as an interpersonal process between a seasoned expert and a novice protégé. The relationship is multidimensional, accounts for cultural differences, and can be either formal or informal. It evolves over time according to the needs and desires of the mentor and protégé. The mentor provides emotional support, shares knowledge and experience, acts as a role model, and gives professional and personal guidance for the protégé (Mijares, Baxley, & Bond, 2013; Stokes, 2010).

Contemporary perspectives have expanded the concept of mentoring into a more collaborative model that uses peer mentoring. Peer mentoring has been described as a more-experienced peer showing the ropes to a less-experienced colleague. Peer mentoring gives recognition to the fact that even novices have valuable knowledge and experiences to share. It encourages them to participate in peer-mentoring relationships where information and expertise can be pooled and mutual support is received. These reciprocal relationships allow for input from a number of sources rather than the traditional interaction between mentor and protégé.

Successful mentoring requires institutional support through administrative, collegial, and financial investments (National League for Nursing [NLN], 2006; Nick et al., 2012). Jakubik (2008) went so far as to include the organization in the definition of mentoring, making it a triad. The triad consists of a mentor who acclimates a protégé within an organization to attain specific outcomes.

APPLICATION

The literature clearly documents that there are not enough qualified nurse educators to provide education to the next generation of nurses (American Association of Colleges of Nursing [AACN], 2014). Mentorship has been identified as an influential factor to recruit and retain new nursing faculty. The NLN (2006) advocated mentoring as a primary strategy to facilitate the ongoing career development of nurse educators across the career continuum. Mentoring relationships have the potential to offer guidance, socialization, and role development of new faculty (Diekelmann, 2004). The literature suggests that mentoring is mutually beneficial to both mentor and protégé. Therefore, mentoring is a topic that is relevant to all members of the academic nursing community.

M

SYNOPSIS

Four functional outcomes of mentoring in nursing education have been identified as: (a) orientation to faculty role; (b) socialization to the academic community; (c) development of teaching, research, and service skills; and (d) facilitation of the growth of future leaders in nursing and nursing education (NLN, 2006). Using these four outcomes as the foundation, Nick et al. (2012) identified six major themes of best practices from the literature to develop a model for excellence in establishing mentoring programs for academic nurse educators. The major themes are: (a) achieve appropriately matched dyads; (b) establish clear mentorship purpose and goals; (c) solidify the dyad relationship; (d) advocate for and guide the protégé; (e) integrate the protégé into the academic culture; and (f) mobilize institutional resources. The model is designed to assist faculty in a variety of settings to create and evaluate the effectiveness of mentoring programs.

The literature indicates that mentoring has many benefits and positive outcomes such as easing the transition of novice nurse faculty from clinical into the academic environment (Turnbull, 2010). Mentored faculty experience a decrease in the degree of role ambiguity and role conflict (Specht, 2013). Increased professional identity and a more committed professoriate are added benefits (Gwyn, 2011). Not surprisingly, institutions have benefited from sponsoring faculty mentoring programs by experiencing improved retention rates and increased productivity in the workplace (Hart, 2009).

RECOMMENDATIONS

Nursing education in the 21st century has been challenged to embrace mentoring as a strategy to facilitate the ongoing career development of nurse faculty. The literature provides discussion of various mentoring models to prepare neophyte educators to understand the multifaceted roles of an academician. However, little is known about what approach works best and what are the experiences of clinical nurses transitioning to academia. To recruit and retain clinical nurses for the education arena, further research is necessary to explore their experience. Future research should focus on the most effective mentoring methods to optimize outcomes. Because mentoring is an abstract concept of the subjective experience of both mentor and protégé, more qualitative research is needed.

American Association of Colleges of Nursing (AACN). (2014). *Nursing faculty shortage fact sheet*. Retrieved from http://www.aacn.nche.edu/Media/FactSheets/FacultyShortage.htm

Diekelmann, N. (2004). Experienced practitioners as new faculty: New pedagogies and new possibilities. *Journal of Nursing Education, 43*(3), 101–103.

Gwyn, P. G. (2011). The quality of mentoring relationships' impact on the occupational commitment of nursing faculty. *Journal of Professional Nursing, 27*(5), 292–298.

Hart, W. (2009). Nurturing relationships have many benefits. *Leadership in Action, 29*(9), 17–19.

Jakubik, L. D. (2008). Mentoring beyond the first year: Predictors of mentoring benefits for pediatric staff nurse protégés. *Journal of Pediatric Nursing, 23*(4), 269–281.

Mijares, L., Baxley, S., & Bond, M. L. (2013). Mentoring: A concept analysis. *The Journal of Theory Construction and Testing, 17*(1), 23–28.

National League for Nursing (NLN). (2006). Position statement: Mentoring of nurse faculty. *Nursing Education Perspectives, 27,* 110–113.

Nick, J. M., Delahoyde, T. M., Del Prato, D., Mitchell, C., Ortiz, J., Ottley, C.,…Siktberg, L. (2012). Best practices in academic mentoring: A model for excellence. *Nursing Research and Practice, 2012,* 937906.

Specht, J. A. (2013). Mentoring relationships and the levels of role conflict and role ambiguity experienced by novice nursing faculty. *Journal of Professional Nursing, 29*(5), e25–e31.

Stokes, E. (2010). Faculty to faculty mentoring. In L. Caputi (Ed.), *Teaching nursing: The art and science* (pp. 514–525). Glen Ellyn, IL: College of Du Page Press.

Turnbull, B. (2010). Scholarship and mentoring: An essential partnership? *International Journal of Nursing Practice, 16*(6), 573–578.

Mary A. White

MENTORING: TRANSITION TO ADVANCED PRACTICE ROLE

DEFINITION

Mentoring in nursing has been defined as a non-evaluated experience that empowers the mentor and mentee to develop personally and professionally within the auspices of a caring, collaborative, and respectful environment (Rosser, Rice, Campbell, & Jack, 2004). Mentoring can be a source of support in the transition of practice from a registered nurse (RN) role to an advanced practice nurse (APN) role (Poronsky, 2013; Rauckhorst, 2005).

APPLICATION

Transition to the APN role evolves over time, beginning with rigorous graduate-level academic preparation that includes acquisition of new knowledge and skills, and leading to major changes in function and scope of practice. For experienced RNs, this transition includes a change in role from that of a competent and expert RN to a novice APN. The changes and upheavals inherent with transition can bring about a wide array of feelings, including disorientation, distress, and anxiety, as well as elation and happiness.

Mentoring can be a source of support for guiding, nurturing, and facilitating novice APNs with balancing their transition into advanced practice. Mentoring has been identified as a way to assist newcomers into and advancing in the profession of nursing (American Academy of Nurse Practitioners,

2006). However, there is no one universal model of mentoring. The mentoring relationship may be a one-to-one dyad with an individual mentor, or a group-mentoring relationship. The setting can be in person, face-to-face, or virtual in cyberspace. The mentoring relationship can be informally established and initiated voluntarily between the mentor and mentee; it can also be formally established, initiated within an institution or academic setting by an administrator or senior manager (Harrington, 2011; Vance, 2002). In an informal mentoring model, a voluntary one-to-one relationship is created between two people based on a spoken or unspoken commitment to the relationship and to each other. Formal mentoring takes place in a structured program in which the mentor and protégé are assigned to one another, typically for a specified amount of time.

The mentoring relationship, whether it is informal or formal in structure, unfolds as an apprenticeship, competency, or reflective prototype (Oliver & Aggleton, 2002). In the apprenticeship model, the mentor offers guided supervision to the mentee. In the competency model, the mentor acts as a coach who monitors and evaluates practice of a defined set of behaviors or competencies. In the reflective model, the mentor guides the mentee to develop professional identity.

SYNOPSIS

APN students and novice APNs may experience anxiety, conflict, loss of confidence in clinical skills, and feelings of incompetence when making their transition into practice (Brykczynski, 2009). Although transition is part of life, the capacity to balance transition is dependent on multiple factors including the nature of the transition itself and the surrounding environment, an individual's personality, and available resources and supports (Goodman, Schlossberg, & Anderson, 2006). One resource for balancing the stress of transition can be mentoring. Harrington (2011) found that a mentoring relationship could positively affect new nurse practitioners in four areas of practice: quality of care,

M

productivity, job satisfaction, and longevity in practice.

Successful mentoring relationships require advance preparation for both the mentor and the mentee. Mentoring programs that prepare the mentor and mentee to understand the nature of the relationship, set realistic expectations and goals, and monitor the progress of the relationship between compatible mentors and mentees can improve professional growth, productivity, and competence (Barker, 2006).

RECOMMENDATIONS

Recommendations for academic and health care institutions include creating a mentoring culture and establishing formal mentoring programs that include training for mentors. There is a need for new APNs to smoothly transition into practice. Nurse practitioners play a key role in providing care and have demonstrated their ability to increase access to cost-effective, comprehensive, and high-quality care (American College of Nurse Practitioners, 2009).

Formal mentoring programs for student and novice APNs may foster their transition to APN practice. Adequate preparation of both the mentor and protégé is essential for success (Barker, 2006). Mentoring of novice APNs and APN students may enhance their transition from RN to APN.

American Academy of Nurse Practitioners. (2006). *Mentoring assessment.* Presented May 2, 2006, at the American Academy of Nurse Practitioners Invitational Think Tank. Retrieved from http://www .aanp.org/NR/rdonlyres/0A3FD4FD-9EF4–4AF1-B7C3-D9E1B65D4E62/0/MentoringAssessment.pdf

American College of Nurse Practitioners. (2009). *What is a nurse practitioner?* Retrieved from http://www.acnpweb .org/files/public/What_is_a_Nurse_Practitioner.pdf

Barker, E. R. (2006). Mentoring—A complex relationship. *Journal of the American Academy of Nurse Practitioners, 18*(2), 56–61.

Brykczynski, K. A. (2009). Role development of the advanced practice nurse. In A. B. Hamric, J. A. Spross, & C. M. Hanson (Eds.), *Advance practice nursing: An integrative approach* (4th ed., pp. 95–120). St. Louis, MO: Saunders/Elsevier.

Goodman, J., Schlossberg, N. K., & Anderson, M. L. (2006). *Counseling adults in transition: Linking practice with theory* (3rd ed.). New York, NY: Springer Publishing.

Harrington, S. (2011). Mentoring new nurse practitioners to accelerate their development as primary care providers: A literature review. *Journal of the American Academy of Nurse Practitioners, 23*(4), 168–174.

Oliver, C., & Aggleton, P. (2002). Mentoring for professional development in health promotion: A review of issues raised by recent research. *Health Education, 102*(1), 30–38.

Poronsky, C. B. (2013). Exploring the transition from registered nurse to family nurse practitioner. *Journal of Professional Nursing, 6*(6), 350–358. Retrieved from http://dx.doi.org/10.1016/j.profnurs.2012.10.011

Rauckhorst, L. (Ed.). (2005). *Mentoring: Ensuring the future of NP practice and education.* Washington, DC: National Organization of Nurse Practitioner Faculties.

Rosser, M., Rice, A. M., Campbell, H., & Jack, C. (2004). Evaluation of a mentorship programme for specialist practitioners. *Nurse Education Today, 24*(8), 596–604.

Vance, C. (2002). Mentoring: A professional obligation. Interview by Mae McWeeny. *Creative Nursing, 8*(3), 4–6, 8.

Cathlin Buckingham Poronsky

MINORITY STUDENT RETENTION

DEFINITION

Retention is defined as students remaining enrolled in an institution of higher education until they graduate with a degree (Hagedorn, 2005). As an institutional measure, retention is an indicator of quality, fiscal responsibility, and accountability by boards of higher education, state and federal governments, and accreditation agencies. Minority students are typically one of the following groups, as defined by the U.S. Census guidelines: American Indian or Alaska Native, Asian, Black, Hispanic, and Native Hawaiian or Other Pacific Islander (U.S. Census Bureau, 2012). Minority student retention is the center of the threefold process of recruitment, retention, and graduation needed to achieve diversity in the nursing profession. To address minority student retention, a variety of strategies have been developed by colleges and universities in general and nursing programs in particular.

APPLICATION

Retention of minority students in nursing education programs has consequences for health care as greater numbers of nurses from racial and ethnic minorities are needed to care for an increasingly diverse population (American Association of Colleges of Nursing [AACN], 2014). More workforce diversity is likely to lead to improved public health, primarily through greater access to care for underserved populations and better interactions between patients and health care providers (Institute of Medicine [IOM], 2011).

The issues of increased demand for nurses, lack of diversity in the nursing workforce, and high costs of academic preparation make minority student retention a crucial matter for nursing programs. The first step to ensure representation in the profession is recruitment of minority groups into nursing education programs. Gaining admittance may be more difficult for minority students, in light of screening criteria imposed by many programs. Yet, current evidence indicates that growing enrollments of minority students are making the composition of the student body more racially and ethnically diverse than

that of the nursing workforce (National League for Nursing [NLN], 2013).

Effective retention depends on the commitment the institution has to quality education and maintenance of an environment conducive to learning (Tinto, 1993). The commitment to minority student retention includes valuing cultural competence, reducing barriers to education, and making it the responsibility of the program to embrace diversity in all areas, including the website, the catalog, the curriculum, and the classroom. Other inclusive policies for nursing education programs are supportive student organizations and recognition of the assets of a diverse student body (Read, Vessey, Amar, & Cullinan, 2013).

SYNOPSIS

Many student variables have been linked to student retention and degree attainment, such as skills and abilities, grade point average (GPA), standardized test results, previous learning, and financial resources (Baker, 2010; Tinto, 1993). Certain variables have more influence than others on minority students. These are financial resources, family support, social integration, and the academic environment (Evans, 2013; Syed, Azmitia, & Cooper, 2011). From the evidence, several studies addressing students' perspectives and positive interactions with nursing faculty were among the most important determinants of student success in nursing programs (Baker, 2010).

Successful completion of nursing programs may be impeded by insufficient academic preparation, financial constraints, ineffective study skills, and poor English-language skills (Igbo et al., 2011). Retention strategies have been developed to address these variables and improve student retention. Examples include mentoring, tutoring, special advising, financial assistance, study groups, faculty advising and counseling, peer mentoring, program orientation, and student nurse clubs (Baker, 2010; Dapremont, 2013). The literature consistently showed these multifaceted interventions were used in retaining minority students in nursing programs.

RECOMMENDATIONS

While retention strategies are implemented for the purpose of maintaining student enrollment through degree attainment, the key outcome measure for minority nursing student retention is the number of racial/ethnic nurses entering the health care workforce. The challenge remains to identify and measure retention strategies that help students progress to graduation (Gilliss, Powell, & Carter, 2010).

Many retention strategies are combined into comprehensive retention programs that address multiple student needs, making it difficult to know which particular components may be valuable and which are not effective. Well-designed research that evaluates the effectiveness of individual retention strategies are missing in the literature. Retention research is needed in nursing education in the areas of online classes, test preparation, and value of pre-entrance programs. Additional research could investigate the efficacy of social media networks, student peer groups, and academic role models.

The goal of retention should be second only to education (Tinto, 1993). As diversity continues to be pursued within the nursing profession, retention strategies must be powerful enough to engender change in the nursing workforce. It is in the public interest to ensure that the health care workforce is diverse and that all population groups are well served.

American Association of Colleges of Nursing (AACN). (2014). *Fact sheet: Enhancing diversity in the workforce.* Retrieved from http://www.aacn.nche.edu/media-relations/fact-sheets/enhancing-diversity

Baker, B. H. (2010). Faculty ratings of retention strategies for minority nursing students. *Nursing education perspectives, 31*(4), 216–220.

Dapremont, J. (2013). A review of minority recruitment and retention models implemented in undergraduate nursing programs. *Journal of Nursing Education and Practice, 3*(2), 112–119.

Evans, D. B. (2013). Examining the influence of noncognitive variables on the intention of minority baccalaureate nursing students to complete their program of study. *Journal of Professional Nursing: Official Journal of the American Association of Colleges of Nursing, 29*(3), 148–154.

Gilliss, C. L., Powell, D. L., & Carter, B. (2010). Recruiting and retaining a diverse workforce in nursing: From evidence to best practices to policy. *Policy, Politics & Nursing Practice, 11*(4), 294–301.

Hagedorn, L. (2005). How to define retention: A new look at an old problem. In A. Seidman (Ed.), *College student retention: Formula for student success* (pp. 1–30). Westport, CT: Praeger.

Igbo, I. N., Straker, K. C., Landson, M. J., Symes, L., Bernard, L. F., Hughes, L. A., & Carroll, T. L. (2011). An innovative, multidisciplinary strategy to improve retention of nursing students from disadvantaged backgrounds. *Nursing Education Perspectives, 32*(6), 375–379.

Institute of Medicine (IOM). (2011). *The future of nursing: Leading change, advancing health.* Washington, DC: The National Academies Press.

National League for Nursing (NLN). (2013). *Annual survey of schools of nursing, Fall, 2012.* Retrieved from www.nln.org/research/slides/index.htm

Read, C. Y., Vessey, J. A., Amar, A. F., & Cullinan, D. M. (2013). The challenges of inclusivity in baccalaureate nursing programs. *Journal of Nursing Education, 52*(4), 185–190.

Syed, M., Azmitia, M., & Cooper, C. R. (2011). Identity and academic success among underrepresented ethnic minorities: An interdisciplinary review and integration. *Journal of Social Issues, 67*(3), 442–468.

Tinto, V. (1993). *Leaving college: Rethinking the causes and cures of student attrition* (2nd ed.). Chicago, IL: University of Chicago Press.

U.S. Census Bureau. (2012). *2012 National population projections.* Retrieved from http://www.census.gov/population/projections/data/national/2012.html

Barbara H. Baker

MOBILE TECHNOLOGY

DEFINITION

Mobile technology refers to any computing device that is portable and can access wireless local area networks (WIFI). The most common forms of mobile technologies are tablets, smartphones, and reading devices. Mobile technologies are continuously evolving and some are now small enough to wear in a watchband. The rapid proliferation of mobile technology and their capacity coupled with high-speed WIFI creates opportunities in health care.

APPLICATION

Mobile technology devices used in health are often referred to as mobile health or mHealth. Mobile health is used to advance life sciences research, health professions education, public health, and patient care (American Medical Informatics Association [AMIA], 2011). The first generations of mobile technology, such as personal digital assistants, were used by health care providers to access health information. As mobile technologies penetrated the general public with easy-to-use functions and interface, mobile health became a central mechanism for consumers to access information and health care teams to communicate and collaborate. In the most technology-rich environments, mHealth is used to connect patients and providers in a variety of ways: social media, patient monitoring, disease management, and wellness (American Nursing Informatics Association [ANIA], 2014).

Today, mHealth applications for tablets and smartphones are exploding in number. There are more than 5,000 mobile health applications (Atienza & Patrick, 2011), and 6 billion users of mobile technology worldwide. This accounts for nearly 87% of the global population (Labrique, Vasudevan, Chang, & Mehl, 2013). This is astounding when one considers the infrastructure required to support wireless networks. Mobile health technologies use conventional methods to access and retrieve (push and pull) data through secure networks, but mHealth applications are also using more novel approaches to "push and pull" data by incorporating biosensors that collect and gather information about a consumer's health practices. For example, pedometers are now available that measure distances walked, the number of calories burned, and even sleep habits. These data can be synchronized to a repository monitored by health care providers.

A growing number of studies are examining the impact of mobile health on patient outcomes such as patient adherence to treatments, attrition to follow-up visits, patient interaction with health care providers, and access to information on demand. Many of these studies report promising results (Ben-Zeev, Drake, Corrigan, Rotondi, & Nilsen, 2012; Burke et al., 2012; Petrie, Perry, Broadbent, & Weinman, 2012).

SYNOPSIS

Mobile technology is advancing very rapidly; thus, the limitations of mobile technology and associated functions are not yet realized. To date, the most common ways mobile technology supports health care are through: (a) access to health data within and across institutions, (b) patient monitoring, (c) health and wellness support, (d) treatment adherence, and (e) communication between providers and with patients. The ease of use, convenience, portability, and advanced functions of mHealth contribute to their growing popularity. In fact, consumer-based mHealth is growing more rapidly than our ability to evaluate the tools. Standards and evaluation criteria for mobile health applications are priorities among federal agencies, mobile health leaders, and health information technology professional organizations (Barton, 2012; U.S. Food and Drug Administration [USFDA], 2013).

Attempts at creating standards, however, have fallen short. One of the first known standards for Internet-based health content is the Health on the Net Foundation or HONCode. The foundation offers certification, a HONCode Seal, to those health-related sites that follow the recommended guidelines and criteria developed by the foundation. The standards still exist, but many sites that are reputable and offer scientific evidence on health topics are not HONCode certified (Health on the Net Foundation [HONCode], 2014). Happtique, a for-profit organization designed to oversee health applications, developed standards for mobile health applications that were released in spring 2013. The purpose of these standards is to help regulate products, establish criteria for the booming mobile health application industry, and offer certification to mHealth devices and applications. The standards and certification have failed performance and security requirements, forcing Happtique to suspend their certification program (Misra, 2014). The lessons for health care providers, including nurses, are the responsibility of establishing standards and ensuring the quality and accuracy of information in applications falls on all health care workers. No one organization, industry, foundation, or regulatory body can or will guarantee the quality of health-related content and applications. To further advance the quality and validity of mHealth, nurses must engage in meaningful discussions with key organizations and regulatory bodies, direct or participate in research that measures patient outcomes, and partner with mobile health developers as content experts. All mobile technology and applications for health must be validated for quality and accuracy of content and based on evidence that provides services to patients and those in the health care industry. Ensuring quality

is our collective responsibility as health care providers and consumers.

RECOMMENDATIONS

Nurse educators have the unique opportunity to influence the mobile health industry through today's nursing students who are tomorrow's nurse leaders. Nursing students without knowledge about mHealth and associated tools cannot be informants to patients. This is a paramount role of the nurse since the general public consumes more mHealth and associated applications than health care providers. It is neither feasible nor possible for any one nurse or nurse educator to know the gamut of mHealth, but it is plausible to have a basic understanding of technologies that support health (smartphones, tablets, biosensors, cloud-based content sharing), industry standards and guidelines, and how to determine the credibility and quality of content. Further, practicing nurses, nursing students, and nurse educators must be aware of the limitations of mHealth tools, the proliferation of these tools without evidence and current standards, and the easy access to these tools by health care providers and health consumers. While one cannot be an expert on all topics and their associated mHealth applications, one must know how to determine the credibility of mHealth tools and applications and how to advise consumers.

American Medical Informatics Association (AMIA). (2011). *What is biomedical and health informatics?* AMIA Position Statement. Retrieved from http://www.amia.org/sites/amia.org/files/What-is-Informatics-Fact-Sheet-04–08-11.pdf

American Nursing Informatics Association (ANIA).* (2014). *Mobile Health 2. Oh! The mouse has left the house. ANIA Webinar Series.* Retrieved from http://www.pro-libraries.com/ania/?select=webinar_register

Atienza, A. A., & Patrick, K. (2011). Mobile health: The killer app for cyberinfrastructure and consumer health. *American Journal of Preventive Medicine, 40*(5 Suppl. 2), S151–S153.

Barton, A. J. (2012). *The regulation of mobile health applications: A commentary. Biomedical Central Medicine.* Retrieved from http://www.biomedcentral.com/content/pdf/1741–7015-10–46.pdf

Ben-Zeev, D., Drake, R. E., Corrigan, P. W., Rotondi, A. J., & Nilsen, W. (2012). Using contemporary technologies in the assessment and treatment of serious mental illness. *American Journal of Psychiatric Rehabilitation, 15,* 357–376.

Burke, L. E., Styn, M. A., Sereika, S. M., Conroy, M. B., Ye, L., Glanz, K.,...Ewing, L. J. (2012). Using mHealth technology to enhance self-monitoring for weight loss: A randomized trial. *American Journal of Preventive Medicine, 43*(1), 20–26.

Health on the Net Foundation (HONCode). (2014). Medical information you can trust. *Health on the Net.* Retrieved from http://www.hon.ch/home1.html

Labrique, A., Vasudevan, L., Chang, L. W., & Mehl, G. (2013). H_pe for mHealth: More "y" or "o" on the horizon? *International Journal of Medical Informatics, 82*(5), 467–469.

Misra, S. (2014). *Happtique's recent setback shows that health app certification is a flawed proposition.* iMedical Apps. Retrieved from http://www.imedicalapps.com/2014/01/happtiques-setback-future-app-certification/

Petrie, K. J., Perry, K., Broadbent, E., & Weinman, J. (2012). A text message programme designed to modify patients' illness and treatment beliefs improves self-reported adherence to asthma preventer medication. *British Journal of Health Psychology, 17*(1), 74–84.

U.S. Food and Drug Administration (USFDA). (2013). *Mobile medical applications.* USFDA Medical Devices. Retrieved from http://www.fda.gov/medicaldevices/products andmedicalprocedures/connectedhealth/mobilemedicalapplications/default.htm

Tami H. Wyatt

MORAL INTEGRITY

M

DEFINITION

Moral integrity is knowing what is right and what is wrong, acting on that knowledge even at personal cost, verbalizing that one is acting on what is known to be the right thing to do, and doing it with a high degree of consistency (Laabs, 2007). Moral integrity is a concern of each individual nurse and is necessary to maintain a wholeness of character and an unassailability that is free from corrupting influences or motives.

APPLICATION

There is a high expectation of moral integrity in the profession of nursing, which is built on a firm foundation of values and codes reflecting high moral integrity and an obligation to society. Accountability for personal nursing practice including professional, social, and personal responsibility have been emphasized from Florence Nightingale to the current day *Code of Ethics for Nurses With Interpretive Statements* from the American Nurses Association (ANA, 2010). Integrity is so important that according to the ANA (2010) it is "essential to professional practice" (p. 7).

Although nursing consistently receives top scores in the Gallup poll, *Honesty/Ethics in Professions* (Gallup, 2013), nurses bring an array of value systems into the profession. The actions of many nurses do not consistently reflect the foundation of high moral integrity upon which the profession was built. For example, in the last quarter of 2013 alone, there were in excess of 250 disciplinary actions taken by the Ohio Board of Nursing (2013).

Moral integrity is the expectation of all nurses even when facing pressure to act otherwise (ANA, 2010). When under compulsion to compromise, nurses have a responsibility to "express their conscientious objection to participation" (ANA, 2010, p. 20). In light of this and the knowledge of the moral slide in society, it is incumbent upon nurse educators to promote a standard of high moral integrity. As the Greek philosopher Plato, who believed the purpose of education was to "form moral character" (Le Vasseur, as cited in Lachman, 2009, p. 7), so too, nurse educators today must recognize the importance of instilling the ethical component of moral integrity into nursing curriculum. Nightingale advocated for moral courage in her nurses (Lachman, 2009); this advocacy must continue within the profession both to maintain the standards of previous generations of nurses and to meet the expectation from society in general.

In addition, nurses have a responsibility to themselves to maintain moral integrity. Nurses who are unable to act in ways they think are morally right due to constraints of external forces report moral distress (Laabs, 2007). This may manifest as feelings of "anger, guilt, powerlessness, and frustration" (Laabs, 2007, p. 795) and can result in burnout. When faced with threats to integrity, nurses have the duty to preserve both personal and professional values and only accept integrity-preserving compromise, which safeguards the dignity of the nurse and others (ANA, 2010).

SYNOPSIS

Moral integrity is knowing what is right and what is wrong and doing right at all times, even at personal cost. According to Eby et al. (2013), "nursing has been spared the ethical scandal of many other professions, but issues of compromised moral integrity are growing in practice and education" (p. 1). The need for consistent application of integrity among the profession of nursing is imperative for the profession to fulfill its duty to the public and to maintain the trust of populations. Without moral integrity, nursing will cease to be the ethical profession it is perceived to be.

RECOMMENDATIONS

Literature reports a normalizing of dishonest behavior among students (Arhin, 2009). Both the character of the student and that of the teaching institution influence the decision to deviate from acceptable practice (Balik, Sharon, Kelishek, & Tabak, 2010). In contrast to this, faculty stated they felt a sense of ownership for the education of integrity (Rosenkoetter & Milstead, 2010). If this is true, there is a need for creation of an institutional context that promotes positive change in belief of the need for moral integrity (Balik et al., 2010). Faculty must modify both classroom characteristics and content delivered (Balik et al., 2010) to instill a sense of value and high moral standards in the students they teach.

Demonstrating a similar pattern of decline in nursing academic arenas, McCabe (2009) reported a higher rate of cheating and dishonesty among nursing students than among other disciplines studied. The concern raised by faculty in the McCabe (2009) study suggested a correlation between those students who are dishonest (e.g., plagiarism, misrepresentation, and falsification, McNabb and Olmstead as cited in McCabe) in academics and those who go on to be dishonest in practice as nursing professionals. To combat this, nurse educators need to develop expertise in the concepts of moral literacy, in best practices for teaching moral integrity, and in designing classroom experiences that bring students to a deeper level of understanding of moral integrity in nursing practice (Gray, 2008).

Nursing educators "model and develop professional ethics in students" (Gray, 2008, p. 333). In support of this role, there is a need for research on the concept of moral integrity and of best practice for teaching moral integrity in nursing education. The health of the profession of nursing may depend on educators, who are the standard-bearers of professional and ethical behavior for future members of the nursing profession (McCabe, 2009).

American Nurses Association (ANA). (2010). *Code of ethics for nurses with interpretive statements*. Silver Spring, MD: Author.

Retrieved from http://www.nursing-world.org/codeofethics

Arhin, A. Q. (2009). A pilot study of nursing student's perceptions of academic dishonesty: A generation Y perspective. *The ABNF Journal, 20,* 17–21.

Balik, C., Sharon, D., Kelishek, S., & Tabak, N. (2010). Attitudes towards academic cheating during nursing studies. *Medicine and Law, 29*(4), 547–563.

Eby, R. A., Hartley, P. L., Hodges, P. J., Hoffpauir, R., Newbanks, S., & Kelley, J. H. (2013). Moral integrity and moral courage: Can you teach it? *Journal of Nursing Education, 52*(4), 229–233.

Gallup. (2013). *Honesty/ethics in professions.* Retrieved from http://www.gallup.com/poll/1654/honesty-ethics-professions.aspx

Gray, M. T. (2008). Nursing leaders' experiences with the ethical dimensions of nursing education. *Nursing Ethics, 15*(3), 332–345.

Laabs, C. A. (2007). Primary care nurse practitioners' integrity when faced with moral conflict. *Nursing Ethics, 14*(6), 795–809.

Lachman, V. (2009). *Ethical challenges in health care: Developing your moral compass.* New York, NY: Springer Publishing.

McCabe, D. L. (2009). Academic dishonesty in nursing schools: An empirical investigation. *Journal of Nursing Education, 48*(11), 614–623.

Ohio Board of Nursing. (2013). Board disciplinary actions. *Momentum, 11*(4), 23–30. Retrieved from http://www.nursing.ohio.gov/PDFS/Mom/2013FallMom.pdf

Rosenkoetter, M. M., & Milstead, J. A. (2010). A code of ethics for nurse educators: Revised. *Nursing Ethics, 17*(1), 137–139.

Ruth A. Eby
Patricia Hartley
Patricia Hodges

N

NARRATIVE PEDAGOGY

DEFINITION

Narrative pedagogy is a method of teaching where there is a focus on reflection and learning through reflective writing about one's experience (Diekelmann, 2001). It involves creating and receiving stories; narrative in nursing has roots in Nightingale, where the power of her reflective writing continues to inspire our discussions and nursing directions today. Narrative offers a humanistic approach to health care, as participants derive shared meaning from the interpretation of stories (Walsh, 2011) through writing, art, and other creative practices. The narrative process often occurs in a planned, structured situation with defined goals and guidelines including a safe, confidential space for sharing. Health care team members are provided with a prompt/creative practice (e.g., literature, poetry, film, and art), which stimulates them to reflect on information about self, patients, and/or colleagues. The participants then write for a prescribed amount of time, and finally share, if desired, while others listen respectfully. The trained leader is a facilitator, creating a safe space for participants to share and their voices to be heard. Goals of a program using a narrative pedagogy have been described as facilitating reflection, enhancing the quality of relationships, and promoting professionalism (Hofstra-North Shore LIJ School of Medicine, 2011). New knowledge and perspectives are often attained as a result of the sharing and reflection, along with a decrease in isolation, individualism, competition, and faculty centeredness (Andrews et al., 2001).

Reflection is the act of considering something, giving it serious thought, or the process of looking back. Critical reflection is the "analysis of personal experience to enhance learning and improve future professional behavior and outcomes" (Aronson, Niehaus, Hill-Sakurai, Lai, & O'Sullivan, 2012). The use of critical reflection supports one as a reflective practitioner (Schon, 1983) and may involve two processes: reflection in action and reflection on action. Reflection in action is described as a practitioner reshaping what he or she is doing, while doing it, using past experience as a guide; this is a mindful practitioner, totally in the moment. Reflection on action refers to reflecting on a past event, often used in clinical situations, in journaling, or when one is seeking personal growth or problem solving. Reflection on action may help practitioners assess current practice or identify areas of strength, feelings, and opportunities for growth.

APPLICATION

Narrative pedagogy, rooted in the tradition of learning from stories through the use of reflection, is now being combined with competency and content-focused curriculum in both medicine and nursing education. As students, teachers, and clinicians interpret and share their experiences, as well as express and analyze feelings and reactions, communication skills are enhanced and connections are increased. As narrative gains popularity in academia, selective institutions are incorporating this pedagogy into their curriculum, forming narrative interprofessional committees, programs, electives, and workshops to foster reflection,

N

interpersonal skills, job satisfaction, retention, and empathy.

The goals of the narrative in various programs are similar. One nursing education institute described goals as enhancing self-awareness, facilitating critical reflection and problem solving, promoting patient-centered care and safety, and identifying learning needs (Lumley, 2012). Reflection in education has been reported to improve learning and competency performance, including professionalism and clinical reasoning (Aronson, 2011). Narrative pedagogy helped nursing students and their teachers to pool wisdom, challenge preconceptions, and develop new ideas surrounding patient-centered care (Ironside, 2006). In medicine, one trait of professionalism enhanced by narrative is empathy, a skill that previously took years of experience to attain (Charon, 2001). Through reflective writing, participants are provided with a mechanism to voice emotions, concerns, and feelings that we previously did not recognize.

While practitioners reflect on patient encounters, educators must critically reflect on teaching behaviors to potentially improve the teaching practice. Visual arts, media, and creative arts may be used in conjunction with written narrative and to enhance the reflective process. In one study, faculty participants felt viewing abstract paintings changed their mood and emotionally prepared them for reflective writing. The art and narrative increased participant's ability to access feelings, promoted examination of educational challenges, and led to compassion for self and others. Finally, sharing of narrative was helpful for fostering active listening and appreciating multiple perspectives (Karkabi, Wald, & Cohen, 2013).

Key points in the narrative pedagogy process include teaching the learners about reflection prior to the activity, goals for the exercise, guidelines for the reflection and sharing, appropriate method for the reflection, prompt a plan for dealing with concerns raised (Peterkin, 2010), and a mechanism for follow-up or assessment. The writing may or may not be subjected to a rubric for formative evaluation. Thus, narrative pedagogy can foster the development of students, practitioners, and faculty in an ongoing manner, as self-development requires ongoing attention.

SYNOPSIS

With the increased focus on practitioner and educator self-development, patient-centered care, health promotion, and wellness, various strategies are being sought to enhance both education and practice. The application of narrative in both life and learning is limited only by the creativity of the individual, institution, or university.

The literature supports the many varied endeavors at narrative in both education and practice, including incorporation of this pedagogy into curriculum, electives, programs, and workshops. Narrative pedagogy aligns with many of the National League for Nursing Core Competencies for Nurse Educators including facilitating learning, development and socialization, assessment and evaluation strategies, curriculum development, and change agent (Halstead, Green, Speziale, & Tomasic, 2005). Narrative pedagogy is one method of teaching where the learner is an active participant in a reflective process, and the goals of enhancing critical reflection, respect, empathy, collegiality, cultural diversity, communication, and evidence-based practice are enhanced. The development of these skills fosters self-development, lifelong learning, and patient-centered care.

The many forms and possibilities of narrative partner with the complicated scenarios of the health care provider's practice. The focus of the narrative may be an actual experience, or involve prompts and the use of modalities such as poems, close readings of short stories, art, film, and music. As the use of narrative increases, rubrics have been developed (Reis et al., 2010), and attempts to measure outcomes are being highlighted in both quantitative and qualitative research studies.

RECOMMENDATIONS

As patient populations and health care teams increase in cultural diversity, and we face ongoing challenges with ethical dilemmas, educational leaders are seeking learning opportunities for students and faculty development that provide knowledge, skills, and attitudes to meet these challenges. Narrative pedagogy is one way in which health care professionals can learn techniques to enhance their personal development, improve patient care, and collaborate with the health care team or faculty. Incorporating narrative pedagogy in educational programs as part of the honored curriculum, in structured settings, with knowledgeable faculty who provide essential feedback is critical to its success (Aronson, 2011).

Further research is warranted to support current practices and identify new best practice models. Areas such as interprofessional collaboration, development of empathy skills, and the use of technology for narrative warrant attention. Future directions may also include research on teaching methods and evaluation tools for the various forms of narrative. Finally, the link between self-development of the educator and practitioner and health-promoting outcomes, job satisfaction, and retention need further investigation. As practitioners and educators increase the use of narrative, the opportunity for increased use in patient care, for both individual and groups, may be realized and utilized.

Andrews, C. A., Ironside, P. M., Nosek, C., Sims, S. L., Swenson, M. M., Yeomans, C.,...Diekelmann, N. (2001). Enacting narrative pedagogy. The lived experiences of students and teachers. *Nursing and Health Care Perspectives, 22*(5), 252–259.

Aronson, L. (2011). Twelve tips for teaching reflection at all levels of medical education. *Medical Teacher, 33*(3), 200–205.

Aronson, L., Niehaus, B., Hill-Sakurai, L., Lai, C., & O'Sullivan, P. S. (2012). A comparison of two methods of teaching reflective ability in Year 3 medical students. *Medical Education, 46*(8), 807–814.

Brown, S. T., Kirkpatrick, M. K., Mangum, D., & Avery, J. (2008). A review of narrative pedagogy strategies to transform traditional nursing education. *Journal of Nursing Education, 47*(6), 283–286.

Charon, R. (2001). Narrative medicine a model for empathy, reflection, profession, and trust. *Journal of American Medical Association, 286*(15), 1897–1901.

Diekelmann, N. (2001). Narrative pedagogy: Heideggerian hermeneutical analyses of lived experiences of students, teachers and clinicians. *Advances in Nursing Science, 23*(3), 53e71.

Halstead, J., Green, P., Speziale, H., & Tomasic, D. (2005). Core competencies of nurse educators with task statements. *National League for Nursing.*

Hofstra-North Shore LIJ School of Medicine. (2011). *Narrative reflection for medical students toolkit.* Hempstead, NY: author.

Ironside, P. M. (2006). Using narrative pedagogy: Learning and practising interpretive thinking. *Journal of Advanced Nursing, 55*(4), 478–486.

Karkabi, K., Wald, H. S., & Cohen, C. (2013). The use of abstract paintings and narrative to foster reflective capacity in medical educators; a multinational faculty development workshop. *Medical Humanities, 40*(1), 44–48. November 22. doi:10.1136/m3dhum-2013–010378

Lumley, L. (2012). *Narrative pedagogy toolkit.* North Shore Long Island Jewish Health System, Institute for Nursing.

Peterkin, A. (2010). Using reflective writing with students: Ten tips. *Canadian Association for Medical Education (CAME) Newsletter.* Special Edition May 2010.

Reis, S. P., Wald, H. S., Monroe, A. D., & Borkan, J. M. (2010). Begin the BEGAN (The Brown Educational Guide to the Analysis of Narrative)—A framework for enhancing educational impact of faculty feedback to students' reflective writing. *Patient Education and Counseling.*

Schon, D. A. (1983). *The reflective practitioner. How professionals think in action.* New York, NY: Basic Books.

Walsh, M. (2011). Narrative pedagogy and simulation: Future directions for nursing education. *Nurse Education in Practice, 11*(3), 216–219.

Deborah McElligott

NCLEX SUCCESS

DEFINITION

NCLEX success is passing the National Council Licensure Examination. There are two National Council Licensure Examinations, the NCLEX-RN® and the NCLEX-PN®. The NCLEX-RN is for graduates of entry-level registered nurse (RN) programs and the NCLEX-PN is for graduates of practical nurse programs. Each test is designed to protect the public by assessing the competencies of new nurse graduates and whether they can perform safely and effectively in their respective roles. The National Council of State Boards of Nursing (NCSBN) publicly reports data on first-time, repeat, U.S., and internationally educated test takers (NCSBN, 2013). Data on NCLEX success are also reported to its member boards and nursing programs.

APPLICATION

NCLEX success has a number of important applications, including determining eligibility for licensure. NCLEX is considered a high-stakes examination because (a) failure has serious consequences for test takers, (b) low pass rates have serious consequences for nursing programs, (c) clear distinctions exist between passing and failing, and (d) test takers invest considerable personal and financial resources (Sullivan, 2014). NCLEX success provides information for (a) hiring decisions, (b) internal program evaluation, (c) evaluation of external program effectiveness, (d) school comparisons made by potential applicants, and (e) new graduates preparing to enter the workforce.

SYNOPSIS

The NCLEX pass rates for U.S.-educated first-time test takers for the RN examination averaged 87.89%, 90.34%, and 80.50% for 2011, 2012, and 2013, respectively (NCSBN, 2013). For the PN examination, pass rates for U.S.-educated first-time test takers were 84.83%, 84.23%, and 84.63% for 2011, 2012, and 2013, respectively (NCSBN, 2013). Some nursing board jurisdictions have provisions for allowing new graduates to practice with a temporary permit; no jurisdiction allows practice after notification of a candidate's failure on the NCLEX. In the few jurisdictions that have temporary permits, their use has been limited as employers of new graduates are increasingly reluctant to invest time and resources in orienting new graduates until they have successfully passed the NCLEX-RN or NCLEX-PN.

Nurse educators have made numerous efforts to improve and maintain NCLEX success rates. These include efforts focused on identifying factors predictive of NCLEX success in order to make programmatic improvements and identify strategies to assist students at risk. Studies examining predictors of NCLEX success have most commonly been conducted within a single school or school system; most have been focused on baccalaureate programs. A meta-analysis of nursing school admission and program measures of 31 samples ($N = 7,159$) indicates that admission tests (SAT and ACT), and preadmission grade-point average (GPA) are predictors; GPA and grades earned during the second year were the strongest predictors (Grossbach & Kuncel, 2011). These findings are similar to that of an earlier meta-analysis indicating that grades in nursing and science courses were the strongest predictors of NCLEX success; parental education and age were the strongest demographic predictors (Campbell & Dickson, 1996). For associate degree programs, preadmission GPA, as well as grades in the sciences and psychology, are strong predictors (Yin & Burger, 2003). For practical nursing students, positive predictors are nursing GPA and science test scores (Ostrye, 2001).

Nursing programs expend considerable resources to improve the NCLEX success of their graduates. However, comprehensive reviews of intervention studies designed to improve NCLEX success rates indicate that identifying specific causes of improvements has been difficult, with most studies being descriptive in nature (DiBartolo & Seldomridge, 2005; Pennington & Spurlock, 2011). Reports of efforts to improve the NCLEX success of minority graduates have been limited (Sutherland, Hamilton, & Goodman, 2007).

Common strategies to improve NCLEX success have been the use of review courses, study materials, and standardized examinations designed to assist students and recent graduates in success on the NCLEX. The standardized test industry for NCLEX preparation has experienced considerable growth in the last 15 years. These tests are used at the completion of major content areas of a program as well as a predictor of NCLEX success at or near the conclusion of a program. The Health Education Systems, Inc. (HESI), Kaplan Nursing, and ATI™ Nursing Education are major providers of standardized tests predicting the likelihood of NCLEX success. HESI has published the results of its validation studies in the literature (Zweighaft, 2013), whereas data about other standardized tests are generally made available to schools purchasing various test preparation products.

The use of standardized tests as predictors of NCLEX success has led to a proliferation of curricular policies designed to improve the NCLEX success of first-time test takers. A number of RN programs, and to a lesser extent PN programs, have instituted policies that require students to pass a standardized exit examination as a prerequisite to graduation from a program, or as a prerequisite for the program's approval of a graduate's candidacy for the licensure examination, or for progression within a program (National League for Nursing [NLN], 2012). This practice has come under criticism because standardized tests may be able to predict which students will pass

the NCLEX, but they are not as reliable in predicting who will fail the NCLEX (Yeom, 2013). In response to this issue, the NLN has developed *Fair Testing Guidelines* to provide faculty in nursing programs with guidance in the use of tests and evaluative procedures for high-stakes testing with regard to the selection of appropriate tests, informing test takers, test administration and scoring, and reporting/interpretation of results, as well as recommendations for achieving a fair-testing environment (NLN, n.d.).

Program NCLEX success is closely monitored externally by boards of nursing as well as accreditation agencies. For example, schools with NCLEX success rates of less than 80% for three consecutive years may be placed upon provisional approval, requiring a detailed plan for improvement. This potentially jeopardizes the ability of the school to continue to operate, as well as receive initial or continuing accreditation. These, in turn, may jeopardize the ability of the school to recruit qualified candidates, which then may further impact the NCLEX success rate. Potential applicants may be aware of the need to request information about a school's NCLEX success rate, but may be less familiar with the need to learn about attrition rates, progression policies, and high-stakes exit examination requirements.

NCLEX success rates provide information about the number of new nurses educated in the United States and internationally who are eligible to enter the workforce as well as valuable trend data. However, it does not provide specifics of employment (type of setting or role, full or part time, etc.), since hiring typically occurs after the achievement of NCLEX success.

RECOMMENDATIONS

Predictors of NCLEX success for the RN examination have been well established for baccalaureate programs and are somewhat similar for associate degree and practical nurse programs. With one in five or six NCLEX U.S.-educated candidates unable to pass the NCLEX on the first attempt,

N

and with only about half the repeat U.S.-educated NCLEX-RN and a little more than a third of NCLEX-PN test takers passing on subsequent attempts (NCSBN, 2013), additional efforts should be made to address the needs of students who have invested considerable resources of time and money without success. While NCLEX success is important as a program outcome, NCLEX success rates need to be placed in the context of a program's attrition rate, progression policies, and use of high-stakes exit examinations. Increased emphasis needs should be placed on examination of factors related to NCLEX success for minority students. High-quality, large-scale multisite studies are needed on interventions designed to increase NCLEX success to identify interventions that have the most value.

Campbell, A. R., & Dickson, C. J. (1996). Predicting student success: A 10-year review using integrative review and meta-analysis. *Journal of Professional Nursing, 12*(1), 47–59.

DiBartolo, M. C., & Seldomridge, L. A. (2005). A review of intervention studies to promote NCLEX-RN success of baccalaureate students. *Nurse Educator, 30*(4), 166–171.

Grossbach, A., & Kuncel, N. R. (2011). The predictive validity of nursing admission measures for performance on the National Council Licensure Examination: A meta-analysis. *Journal of Professional Nursing, 27*(2), 124–128.

National Council of State Boards of Nursing, Inc. (NCSBN). (2013). *NCLEX pass rates*. Retrieved from https://www.ncsbn.org/1237.htm

National League for Nursing (NLN). (n.d.). *NLN fair testing guidelines*. New York, NY: Author.

National League for Nursing (NLN). (2012). *NLN vision: Fair testing imperative in nursing education*. New York, NY: Author.

Ostrye, M. E. (2001). Predicting NCLEX-PN performance for practical nursing students. *Nurse Educator, 26*(4), 170–174.

Pennington, T. C., & Spurlock, D. Jr. (2011). A systematic review of the effectiveness of remediation interventions to improve NCLEX-RN pass rates. *Journal of Nursing Education, 49*(9), 485–492.

Sullivan, D. (2014). A concept analysis of "high stakes testing." *Nurse Educator, 39*(2), 72–76.

Sutherland, J. A., Hamilton, M. J., & Goodman, N. (2007). Affirming at-risk minorities for success (ARMS): Retention, graduation, and success on the NCLEX-RN. *Journal of Nursing Education, 46*(8), 347–353.

Yeom, Y. J. (2013). An investigation of predictors of NCLEX-RN outcomes among nursing content standardized tests. *Nurse Education Today, 33*(12), 1523–1528.

Yin, T., & Burger, C. (2003). Predictors of NCLEX-RN success of associate degree nursing graduates. *Nurse Educator, 28*(5), 232–236.

Zweighaft, E. L. (2013). Impact of HESI specialty exams: The ninth HESI exit exam validity study. *Journal of Professional Nursing, 29*(2 Suppl. 1), S10–S16.

Margarete L. Zalon

NURSE EDUCATOR CERTIFICATION

DEFINITION

Nurse educator certification is defined as voluntary, periodic certification for academic nurse educators (National League for Nursing [NLN], 2012, p. 1). Academic nursing education is a specialty area and an advanced practice role within professional nursing (NLN Certification Commission, 2012, p. 4). This practice discipline has a defined practice setting and demonstrable standards of excellence (NLN, 2008), and projects a level of expertise that demonstrates the holder is highly qualified for the practice of teaching.

APPLICATION

Nurse educator certification advances the science of nursing by creating a means for faculty to demonstrate their expertise in this advanced practice role. The research conducted during the development of the certification delineated the full scope and practice of academic nurse educators. Likewise, it is the only professional credential that recognizes excellence in the advanced specialty role of the academic nurse educator (Ortelli, 2008).

In the initial publication on research related to the core competencies (Halstead, 2007, p. 13), a task group used the competencies and related task statements to organize the existing body of research on nursing education and discovered gaps in the research literature. Using the core competencies as a framework for relating new nursing education knowledge is an essential step in the advancement of the science of nursing education.

The certification core competencies are being used by faculty to organize promotion and tenure documents; additionally, graduate programs have used the competencies as the framework for curricula specializing in nursing education (Kalb, 2008). Subsequently, the identification of the core competencies has given the science of nursing education a model and has made excellence in the practice of nursing education quantifiable.

SYNOPSIS

The NLN developed the certification program in 2005, which was patterned after certification programs in advanced clinical practice. The NLN Certification Commission administered the first examination in 2005 at the annual Summit. In 2013, the historical events surrounding the development of the Academic Nurse Educator Certification Program were documented (Nick, Sharts-Hopko, & Leners, 2013).

During this process of developing evidence, the NLN identified eight core competencies in the practice analysis: (a) facilitate learning; (b) facilitate learner development and socialization; (c) use assessment and evaluation strategies; (d) participate in curriculum design and evaluation of program outcomes; (e) pursue continuous quality improvement in the nurse educator role; (f) function as a change agent and leader; (g) engage in scholarship; and (h) function within the institutional environment and the academic community (Ortelli, 2006). A more recent practice analysis, in 2010, revealed very minor changes to the task statements and core competencies (NLN Certification Commission, 2012, p. 4), thus providing validity and reliability to this evidence-based list. These competencies, infused with education and pedagogy, are characteristics Hagler, Poindexter, and Lindell (2014) acknowledged as necessary for successful nursing faculty members.

To become certified, candidates take a computerized examination that is offered throughout the United States through a third-party computer testing service. Eligibility requirements include holding a master's or doctoral degree in nursing with (a) a major emphasis on nursing education or (b) 2 years of experience as a full-time educator (NLN, 2012, p. 3). The pass rate for the certification examination has consistently been around 84% (Ortelli, 2008), slightly higher than exemplar clinical certification pass rates (American Association of Critical-Care Nurses, 2012) and similar to nurse practitioner pass rates (American Academy of Nurse Practitioners, n.d.). Candidates who pass the rigorous standardized examination use the certification mark Certified Nurse Educator (CNE) after their name. Certification is valid for 5 years; similarly, recertification is granted for 5 years by demonstrating currency in academic teaching practice in addition to meeting requirements for continuous professional development.

Interest in the CNE credential has been demonstrated by nurse educators in all career stages, as well as by those who teach in all program types (Ortelli, 2008). As the number of CNEs continues to increase, myriad research opportunities exist that will assist maturation in the practice of nursing education.

RECOMMENDATIONS

Nurse educators have a professional responsibility to demonstrate excellence in practice by creating a learning environment where students thrive while impacting the science of nursing. Leaders focusing on identifying the impact of certification on student success indicators will contribute to nursing science and the validation of this certification program. Determining differences in teaching environments between certified and non-CNEs will provide continuing evidence for best practice. And, as the demographic characteristics of nursing students change, tracking modifications in tasks embedded within each core competency is necessary for the certification to remain relevant.

There is a need to document the effect of certification on success indicators of departments, such as changes in cohesion, scholarship, philosophies of teaching, and socialization efforts. Determining the impact of certification on individual faculty maturation, such as role fulfilment, promotion and tenure, salary differential, and role expansion, continues to be important. Research documents professional benefits experienced by certified clinical nurses (Fitzpatrick, Campo, Graham, & Lavandero, 2010). It is important to investigate the benefits realized from becoming a CNE.

The NLN understands that not all nurse educators implement all eight competencies in the course of their duties—factors such as the mission of the institution, academic preparation, and type of program all affect how broadly these competencies are practiced (Halstead, 2007, p. 13; NLN Certification Commission, 2012, p. 13). Ascertaining which tasks and related competencies are the most and least practiced would help nursing departments or professional nurse educator organizations tailor faculty development programs. With certification standards now set, there is an evidence-based, detailed, systematic role identified for U.S. nurse educators.

American Academy of Nurse Practitioners. (n.d.). *American Academy of Nurse Practitioners certification program.* Retrieved from http://www.aanpcert.org/ptistore/control/certs/pass

American Association of Critical-Care Nurses. (2012). *Exam statistics.* Retrieved from http://www.aacn.org/wd/certifications/content/statistical.pcms?menu=certification

Fitzpatrick, J. J., Campo, T. M., Graham, G., & Lavandero, R. (2010). Certification, empowerment, and intent to leave current position and the profession among critical care nurses. *American Journal of Critical Care, 19*(3), 218–226.

Hagler, D., Poindexter, K., & Lindell, D. (2014). Integrating your experience and opportunities to prepare for nurse educator certification. *Nurse Educator, 39*(1), 45–48.

Halstead, J. A. (2007). *Nurse educator competencies: Creating an evidence-based practice for nurse educators.* New York, NY: National League for Nursing.

Kalb, K. A. (2008). Core competencies of nurse educators: Inspiring excellence in nurse educator practice. *Nursing Education Perspectives, 29*(4), 217–219.

National League for Nursing (NLN). (2008, March 25). *NLN news releases: Certified nurse educator credential deemed valuable in professional advancement by nurse educators along entire faculty spectrum.* Retrieved from http://www.nln.org/newsreleases/CNEonNEP_release_032508.htm

National League for Nursing (NLN). (2012). *Certified academic nurse educator (CNE) 2012–2013 candidate handbook.* Carbondale, IL: National League for Nursing Customer Service & Scoring Center, Academic Nurse Educator Certification Program.

National League for Nursing (NLN) Certification Commission. (2012). *The scope of practice for academic nurse educators.* New York, NY: National League for Nursing.

Nick, J. M., Sharts-Hopko, N. C., & Leners, D. W. (2013). From committee to commission: The history of the NLN's Academic Certified Nurse Educator Program. *Nursing Education Perspectives, 34*(5), 298–302.

Ortelli, T. A. (2006). Defining the professional responsibilities of academic nurse educators: The results of a national practice analysis. *Nursing Education Perspectives*, 27(5), 242–246.

Ortelli, T. (2008). Characteristics of candidates who have taken the Certified Nurse Educator (CNE) examination: A two-year review. *Nursing Education Perspectives*, 29(2), 120–121.

Jan M. Nick

NURSE SCIENTIST

DEFINITION

A nurse scientist is a registered nurse (RN) who investigates issues relevant to the discipline of nursing, including professional practice, education, care delivery, and policy dimensions. A nurse scientist possesses intellectual curiosity and uses the skills of scientific inquiry to design studies that describe phenomena of interest to nurses, create new knowledge, and present that knowledge in a way that it can be applied to nursing practice, education, care delivery, and policy development.

APPLICATION

Nurse scientists are academically prepared at the doctoral level. Nurses with a research doctorate are prepared to design and conduct studies using qualitative and quantitative methods, develop theory, and create and test the usefulness of policy (American Association of Colleges of Nursing [AACN], 2010). It is critical that nurse scientists work with nurses in practice and with interprofessional partners to generate knowledge that is useful for patient care, theory that explains phenomena of interest to nursing, and policy that has an impact on both consumers of health care and professionals who work in the health care arena.

SYNOPSIS

In 1968, the emerging nurse scientist was defined as a nurse who was capable of designing and carrying out research studies and also was knowledgeable in an area that was important to nursing. The goal of these new nurse scientists was to help practicing nurses adapt to a changing health care environment (Kolthoff, 1968). Early doctoral programs to prepare nurse scientists were in other disciplines, such as anthropology, anatomy, and psychology, but evolved to focus on the distinct science of nursing (Gortner, 1991). Nursing research doctoral programs are now numerous, and postdoctoral study is available for additional grounding in a specialty area of nursing research (AACN, 2010). Funding for nursing research is available from many sources, including the National Institute of Nursing Research (NINR & Cantelon, 2010), as well as other governmental and private organizations. Although most funding for nursing research has been directed toward priorities related to patient care, some funding is also now available for research on the science of nursing education. Nursing education research is needed because our curricula and strategies for educating nurses have not changed to reflect the changes in the health care system and in nursing work (Benner, Sutphen, Leonard, & Day, 2010), and national organizations are recognizing the need to develop and test new ways of educating nurses (National League for Nursing [NLN] Board of Governors, 2012). Nurse scientists can now be found working in academic, practice, and industry settings, but most nurse scientists practice in an academic setting (Lewallen & Kohlenberg, 2011). As academic nurse scientists become more numerous, it is more common to find nurse scientists working in smaller academic settings not affiliated with academic medical centers, and often carrying a heavy teaching load that leaves little time for research. In order for nursing science to progress, time for both research and teaching needs to be incorporated into the work life of the nurse scientist in any

N

academic setting (Broome, 2011; Broome, Ironside, & McNelis, 2012). In this way, nursing science will continue to be developed in a variety of settings, and nursing students in all those settings will be mentored by active scientists. If nursing students can see from the beginning of their education that the development and use of nursing science and theories is an accepted and important part of the work of the professional nurse, they will perhaps consider doctoral education for themselves in the future.

RECOMMENDATIONS

With the increasing numbers of doctoral programs in nursing, the number of nurse scientists will continue to grow. The types of science that are investigated by nurses will continue to include topics important to patient care and health policy, as well as building nursing theory. More study is needed to add to the body of knowledge about the science of nursing education, and to better prepare nurses at all levels for the challenges of nursing work in direct patient care, nursing systems, health policy, and other emerging roles. Nursing science can take many forms, and with the development of the doctor of nursing practice degree, more scientific knowledge in the form of evidence-based practice projects with direct application to patient care can be expected.

American Association of Colleges of Nursing (AACN). (2006). *The essentials of doctoral education for advanced nursing practice.* Washington, DC: Author.

American Association of Colleges of Nursing (AACN). (2010). *The research-focused doctoral program in nursing: Pathways to excellence.* Report from the AACN Task Force on the Research-Focused Doctorate in Nursing. Washington, DC: Author.

Benner, P., Sutphen, M., Leonard, V., & Day, L. (2010). *Educating nurses: A call for radical transformation.* San Francisco, CA: Jossey-Bass.

Broome, M. E. (2011). The nurse scientist: A unique contribution to nursing's future. *Nursing Outlook, 59,* 1–3. doi:10.1016/j.outlook.2010.11.008

Broome, M. E., Ironside, P. M., & McNelis, A. M. (2012). Research in nursing education: State of the science. *Journal of Nursing Education, 51*(9), 521–524.

Gortner, S. R. (1991). Historical development of doctoral programs: Shaping our expectations. *Journal of Professional Nursing, 7*(1), 45–53.

Kolthoff, N. J. (1968). Forum: Evolution of the nurse scientist: Emergence and continued development. *Image, 2*(3), 11–12.

Lewallen, L. P., & Kohlenberg, E. (2011). Preparing the nurse scientist for academia and industry. *Nursing Education Perspectives, 32*(1), 22–25.

National Institute of Nursing Research (NINR) & Cantelon, P. L. (2010). *NINR: Bringing science to life* (NIH Publication No. 10–7502). Bethesda, MD: Author.

National League for Nursing (NLN) Board of Governors (2012). *NLN vision: Transforming research in nursing education.* New York, NY: National League for Nursing.

Lynne P. Lewallen

NURSING CARE PLANS

DEFINITION

Nursing care plans (NCPs) provide an organizing framework for the practice of nursing and are "a written reflection of the nursing process" (Ackley & Ladwig, 2014; Gulanick & Myers, 2014, p. 3). The nursing process is a critical thinking approach used to identify and treat problems; it provides guidelines for care to assist clients and their families in reaching self-efficacy goals and optimal health (Ackley & Ladwig, 2014). Nursing process components used to develop NCPs include (a) assessment, (b) diagnosis, (c) planning, (d) implementation, and (e) evaluation.

During assessment, nurses gather subjective and objective data via health interviews, physical examinations, and medical record reviews to plan holistic care. Based on this assessment, nursing diagnoses are identified, which are defined as "a clinical judgment about individual, family, or community experiences/responses to actual or potential health problems/life processes" (Herdman, 2012, p. 515). In planning, client-centered outcomes are decided based on mutual goals and should be "specific, measurable, attainable, realistic, and timed" (Ackley & Ladwig, 2014, p. 7). Interventions are "defined as any treatment based upon clinical judgment and knowledge which a nurse performs to enhance patient/client outcomes" (Bulechek, Butcher, Dochterman, & Wagner, 2013, p. 2). After implementation of planned interventions, nurses evaluate client responses to determine attainment of expected outcomes, and the NCP is revised as needed.

APPLICATION

In education, NCPs are used as a teaching–learning tool to help students understand the dynamic nursing process. Students validate their use of nursing diagnosis by identifying the related factors (contributing) and defining characteristics (signs and symptoms) based on assessment findings. Students select, individualize, prioritize, and implement interventions and evaluate if client outcomes were met to complete the process. NCPs also assist students to integrate classroom learning with clinic experiences by linking cognitive knowledge, including critical thinking and clinical reasoning, with technical skills and attitudes needed for professional nursing practice.

Several models are commonly used to assist nursing students to understand care planning. Gordon's (2010) functional health patterns are helpful to organize assessment data to identify the nursing diagnoses associated with common patterns of client responses. Carpenito's bifocal clinical practice model (Carpenito, 2014) describes how nursing diagnoses, managed with nurse-prescribed (independent) interventions, differ from collaborative problems treated with both independent and interdisciplinary (dependent) interventions. Concept or mind maps, which are visual diagrams of a client's medical and nursing problems, assist students with care planning by illustrating the relationships within the nursing process (Doenges, Moorhouse, & Murr, 2013; Gulanick & Myers, 2014). Clinical (critical) pathways or care maps are another method to provide guidelines for interdisciplinary client care. These tools often incorporate NCPs and are used in practice to evaluate health care outcomes for specific populations, monitor resource utilization, and make comparative judgments (Gulanick & Myers, 2014).

SYNOPSIS

Although the concept of NCPs began to appear in the literature in the 1930s, Henderson (1973) noted, "Since no one can nurse a patient 24 hours a day, 7 days a week, it has always been important to coordinate the efforts of those caring for a sick person through a written plan of some sort" (p. 379). In the 1960s, the "nursing process began to be emphasized as the methodology of clinical care," and the need for a common nursing diagnostic classification system was recognized (Gordon, 1979, p. 487). Since the first National Conference on the Classification of Nursing Diagnoses in 1972, the use of nursing diagnoses has helped to define the profession (Gebbie & Lavin, 1975). Nursing has continued to refine and develop NCPs, adopting standardized taxonomies to provide a common language for documentation and research. These standardized taxonomies include: (a) North American Nursing Diagnoses Association-I nursing diagnoses (Herdman, 2012); (b) Nursing Interventions Classification (NIC; Bulechek et al., 2013); and (c) Nursing Outcomes Classification (NOC; Moorhead, Johnson, Maas, & Swanson, 2013).

Computerized NCPs (CNCPs) are becoming the norm due to the increased use of electronic health records (EHRs). CNCPs and other information systems utilizing distinct taxonomy codes of nursing enable the profession to mine rich databases to measure the unique contributions of nursing to health care. Despite possible advantages, Lee (2005) documented nurses' concerns related to CNCPs, which included inconvenient access, reduced efficiency, inability to individualize care, nursing specialty deficiencies, poor system design, and privacy and legal issues.

RECOMMENDATIONS

As health care is restructured, nurses will play a key role in assisting providers to determine the underlying cause of a problem (root cause thinking) to prevent reoccurrences, prevent readmissions, and promote optimal health (Ackley & Ladwig, 2014). Clients and their families will partner with nurses to navigate increasingly complex health care systems and learn self-management skills needed for health promotion, as well as acute and chronic care (Gulanick & Myers, 2014). To address these health care trends, nursing will need to develop innovative NCPs using new standardized nursing diagnoses, outcomes, and interventions, creating exciting opportunities for nursing education, practice, and research.

Nurses will continue to experience expanded uses of technology to access data, plan care, and facilitate documentation (Ackley & Ladwig, 2014). Faculty will need to ensure nursing students have ample practice using various technologies to develop NCP skills. Further research is needed to assess the effects of technology on the nursing process, especially the use of CNCPs and data mining in nursing education and practice. Regardless of which NCP resource or technology is used, faculty must help students determine the appropriateness of interventions, understand the underlying rationales, tailor the interventions to meet individual client needs, and stress that interventions must be based on current evidence and best practice guidelines to provide high-quality, safe nursing care.

Ackley, B. J., & Ladwig, G. B. (2014). *Nursing diagnosis handbook: An evidence-based guide to planning care* (10th ed.). Maryland Heights, MO: Elsevier Mosby.

Bulechek, G. M., Butcher, H. K., Dochterman, J. M., & Wagner, C. M. (Eds.). (2013). *Nursing interventions classification (NIC)* (6th ed.). St. Louis, MO: Elsevier Mosby.

Carpenito, L. J. (2014). *Nursing care plans: Transitional patient & family centered care* (6th ed.). Philadelphia, PA: Wolters Kluwer/Lippincott Williams & Wilkins.

Doenges, M. E., Moorhouse, M. F., & Murr, A. C. (2013). *Nursing diagnosis manual: Planning, individualizing, and documenting client care* (4th ed.). Philadelphia, PA: F.A. Davis.

Gebbie, K. M., & Lavin, M. A. (Eds.). (1975). Utilization of a classification of nursing diagnoses. In *Classification of nursing diagnoses: Proceedings of the first national conference* (pp. 21–36). St. Louis, MO: Mosby.

Gordon, M. (1979). The concept of nursing diagnosis. *Nursing Clinics of North America, 14*(3), 487–496.

Gordon, M. (2010). *Manual of nursing diagnosis* (12th ed.). Sudbury, MA: Jones & Bartlett.

Gulanick, M., & Myers, J. L. (Eds.). (2014). *Nursing care plans: Diagnoses, interventions, and outcomes* (8th ed.). Philadelphia, PA: Elsevier Mosby.

Henderson, V. (1973). On nursing care plans and their history. *Nursing Outlook, 21*(6), 378–379.

Herdman, T. H. (Ed.). (2012). *NANDA international nursing diagnoses: Definitions and classification, 2012–2014*. Oxford, England: Wiley-Blackwell.

Lee, T. (2005). Nurses' concerns about using information systems: Analysis of comments on a computerized nursing care plan system in Taiwan. *Journal of Clinical Nursing, 14*(3), 344–353. doi:10.1111/j.1365–2702.2004.01060.x

Moorhead, S., Johnson, M., Maas, M. L., & Swanson, E. (Eds.). (2013). *Nursing outcomes classification (NOC): Measurement of health outcomes* (5th ed.). St. Louis, MO: Elsevier Mosby.

Lisa Sue Flood
Rachel Nye

O

ONLINE LEARNING

DEFINITION

Online learning is an instructional method that uses Internet technology, electronic media, and digital innovations to actively engage students and deliver course content in an environment that is potentially rich and diversified. It is expressed in a variety of forms, with varying interpretations among institutions, faculty members, and students (Perry & Pilati, 2011). Technology tools, strategies, and techniques designed to enhance, supplement, and/or replace traditional classroom teaching are generally included in the broad definition of online learning. An online course is defined as one in which at least 80% of the course is online (Allen & Seaman, 2014).

APPLICATION

From the mid-1990s to the present, online learning has steadily gained acceptance and popularity among students and faculty members as an educational practice in nursing education, particularly in registered nurse (RN)–bachelor of science in nursing (BSN) completion and graduate programs (Billings & Halstead, 2012; Perry & Pilati, 2011). Online learning and teaching strategies are used in nursing education for facility orientation, staff development and training, continuing education programs, and tutoring, as well as in formal nursing courses in degree programs. The wide range appeal is attributed to the evolution of the technologically savvy student combined with the need for flexibility, convenience, and accessibility in educational experiences.

Online learning can be engaged synchronously where content is delivered in real time, requiring the student's presence at a designated time, or, more commonly, asynchronously where content is delivered on demand within a course time frame or at the student's own pace (Quinn Griffin & Novotny, 2012). Synchronous learning activities make use of selected technologies such as whiteboards, virtual classrooms, interactive videoconferencing, lecture broadcasts, podcasts, and chat rooms. Asynchronous learning activities may include downloadable PowerPoint presentations, discussion forums, downloadable handouts, electronic textbooks, wikis, blogs, drop boxes, e-mail, and/or electronic office hours. Online learning materials can be instructor-created or commercial software products.

Online learning courses require access to a computer or any device with web browser capability. Online learning programs are typically delivered via a learning management system (LMS) or course management system (CMS) that provides secure, structured, technology-based platforms capable of a multitude of functions such as two-way communication, classroom interactions, simulations, attendance and progress tracking, reporting and storing data, integration with external links, and ways to detect plagiarism (Billings & Halstead, 2012). Current online management systems differ in style, but have similar characteristics in providing opportunity for content-rich and active engagement in student–instructor, student–content, and student–student interactions.

Accrediting agencies for nursing programs have set forth standards for online

O

learning. These standards are used for structuring learning outcomes, delivery of course content, strategies for learning modules, and student evaluation components. Course evaluation tools and national standard rubrics provided by organizations such as Quality Matters (QM) certify excellence in online courses through peer review (Bento & White, 2010).

SYNOPSIS

Researchers have indicated increasing acceptance of online learning among administrators, faculty members, and students (Allen & Seaman, 2014). Online learning tools and methods have transformed nursing education, yet concern remains related to standards, the concern of quality, and effectiveness of this new paradigm. The expectation is that online learning needs to hold to the same standards as in-class face-to-face instruction (Perry & Pilati, 2011). Faculty challenges include the need to rethink teaching roles to become more facilitative, face potential increase in workload, and gain expertise fully using the current technology. Studies have shown that learning through online methods can be the same or superior when compared to face-to-face classes (Hoffmann & Dudjak, 2012); however, not all educators agree (Allen & Seaman, 2014).

Students' access and satisfaction are also considerations in online learning (Picciano, Seaman, & Allen, 2010). Student success in online learning requires basic computer skill, technology self-efficacy, time management skills, and personal motivation. Online learning requires active participation. Studies have shown successful students demonstrate motivation, display self-efficacy with technology, and feel connected to their online classroom (Shen, Cho, Tsai, & Marra, 2013). While students have indicated satisfaction with online learning courses overall, social isolation and retention rates are ongoing concerns.

Overcoming barriers that impede student success and promotion of retention are important issues to address in online learning. Potential barriers to online learning are access to equipment, technology knowledge deficit skill, individual learning styles, faculty teaching styles, motivation, and self-discipline. While recognizing that online learning may not be appropriate for every student or for every faculty member, online learning technology continues to gain wide application in nursing education (Perry & Pilati, 2011).

RECOMMENDATIONS

Active engagement is a key component to student success in online learning (Kang & Im, 2013). Faculty members need to conduct research to determine best practices for promoting active engagement through online communities and to define measures to support student participation in using technology. Further research is needed to expand nursing education's knowledge base of ways to incorporate individual learning styles as well as faculty teaching styles into the online environment (Wuebker, 2013). Adapting the use of emerging instructional design models and existing educational models will help address the issues of quality and effectiveness (Gormley, Colella, & Shell, 2012).

Ongoing faculty development is important and needs to be collaborative with course design experts, faculty work groups, and accrediting bodies (Wang, Shannon, & Ross, 2013). Faculty members need to employ measures to promote academic integrity, improve accessibility, facilitate motivation, and promote self-discipline. The use of technology to its fullest potential will provide a diversified and rich online learning environment for nursing students.

Allen, I. E., & Seaman, J. (2014). *Grade change: Tracking online education in the United States*. Babson Survey Research Group and Quahog Research Group. LLC. Newburyport, MA: Sloan Consortium, Pearson Foundation.

Bento, R., & White, L. (2010). Quality measures that matter. *Issues in Informing Science and Information Technology, 7*, 61–72.

Billings, D. M., & Halstead, J. A. (2012). *Teaching in nursing: A guide for faculty* (4th ed.). St. Louis, MO: Elsevier Saunders.

Gormley, D. K., Colella, C. C., & Shell, D. S. (2012). Motivating online learners using attention, relevance, confidence, satisfaction motivational theory and distributed scaffolding. *Nurse Educator, 37*(4), 177–180.

Hoffmann, R., & Dudjak, L. (2012). From onsite to online: Lessons learned from faculty pioneers. *Journal of Professional Nursing, 28*(4), 255–258.

Kang, M., & Im, T. (2013). Factors of learner-instructor interaction which predict perceived learning outcomes in online learning environment. *Journal of Computer Assisted Learning, 29,* 292–301.

Perry, E., & Pilati, M. (2011). Online learning. *New Directions for Teaching and Learning, 128,* 95–104. doi:2048/10.1002/tl.472

Picciano, A. G., Seaman, J., & Allen, I. (2010). Educational transformation through online learning: To be or not to be. *Journal of Asynchronous Learning Networks, 14*(4), 17–35.

Quinn Griffin, M., & Novotny, J. (2012). *A nuts-and-bolts approach to teaching nursing* (4th ed.). New York, NY: Springer Publishing.

Shen, D., Cho, M., Tsai, C., & Marra, R. (2013). Unpacking online learning experiences: Online learning self-efficacy and learning satisfaction. *Internet and Higher Education, 19,* 10–17.

Wang, C., Shannon, D. M., & Ross, M. E. (2013). Students' characteristics, self-regulated learning, technology self-efficacy, and course outcomes in online learning. *Distance Education, 34*(3), 302–323. doi:10.1080/01587919.2013.835779

Wuebker, M. P. (2013). Adult learners: Improving persistence and performance in online learning environments. *Journal of College Literacy & Learning, 39,* 38–46.

Pamela L. Bonnett
Mary T. Quinn Griffin

ONLINE LEARNING: ASSESSING SOCIAL PRESENCE

O

DEFINITION

There are many definitions of social presence. First defined by Short, Williams, and Christie (1976, p. 65), social presence is the salience or importance of others in a mediated communication setting and the resulting salience of their interpersonal interactions. Similarly, Gunawardena (1995) described social presence as the degree to which an individual is perceived by others to be a "real person" in computer-mediated communication. Tu and McIsaac (2002) refer to social presence as a measure of the feeling of community that individual learners experience in an online classroom. Picciano (2002) defined social presence as the perception a student has of being in and belonging in an online class.

APPLICATION

Over the past decade, distance education has become commonplace within schools of nursing. Both undergraduate and graduate nursing courses, and in many cases entire nursing programs, are now being offered online at many universities. Research has demonstrated that social presence is essential to online learning and has a direct correlation to the degree of satisfaction among students and teachers, as well as the overall effectiveness of the learning experience (Gunawardena & Zittle, 1997; Richardson & Swan, 2003; Tu, 2000). With the loss of the traditional on-campus classroom, one of the greatest challenges for nurse faculty is to create and maintain a sense of social presence without face-to-face interactions. With the absence of eye contact and nonverbal cues such as body language, teachers must find other ways to assess the degree of social presence in the online classroom.

Three categories of indicators to assess social presence in the online classes are emotional expression, open communication, and group cohesion (Garrison, Anderson, & Archer, 2000). Several strategies have been used to enhance these aspects of social presence in online nursing courses. One approach is teacher immediacy, which involves nonverbal behaviors aimed at conveying a feeling of connectedness, closeness, and informality between the student and teacher. Ways to improve teacher immediacy include calling students by their first name, building group cohesiveness by addressing the class as "we" or "us," teacher self-disclosure, using emoticons (e.g., representative symbols to express emotion), and by using humor (Rourke, Anderson, Garrison, & Archer, 2001). A second approach to increasing social presence is through consistent teacher–student interactions or "teaching presence." This may be accomplished through timely responses to e-mails, complimenting students on their work, asking questions, expressing appreciation of student's participation during online classes, and encouraging feedback. Other ideas intended to establish social presence in the online classroom include sending weekly checklists, providing virtual office hours (Baker & Edwards, 2011), and incorporating twitter into the online classroom design (Dunlap & Lowenthal, 2009).

SYNOPSIS

Studies have found that social presence is a significant factor in improving the instructional effectiveness of online classes (Gunawardena, 1995). In an early study by Gunawardena and Zittle (1997), social presence was found to be a strong predictor of student satisfaction in computer-based conferences. Participants in this study who felt a stronger sense of social presence enhanced their experience by using emoticons to express emotion in the absence of face-to-face gesturing. Richardson and Swan (2003) found that students with a high overall perception of social presence also scored higher in terms of perceived learning and perceived satisfaction with the teacher. The level of online interaction is increased with

an improved level of social presence (Tu & McIsaac, 2002). These researchers suggest that social context, online communication, and interactivity are essential elements in establishing a sense of community among online students. Three elements of an educational experience identified in the community of inquiry model (Garrison et al., 2000) are interrelated concepts essential to assessing "presence" in online nursing classes. This model offers a tool by which presence, including social presence, can be assessed. The elements include social presence, cognitive presence (critical thinking process), and teaching presence. Ali, Hodson-Carlton, and Ryan (2004) determined that the major elements of online learning identified by 20 graduate nursing students were congruent with the constructivism theory. An underlying assumption of this theory is that learning is constructed through social interaction among individuals and meaning comes from dialog with others. This study corroborates the importance of creating social presence in online nursing courses. Application of social presence strategies by nursing faculty teaching online courses is essential and has a positive effect on the perceptions of social presence and group interaction among the students (Mayne & Wu, 2011).

RECOMMENDATIONS

With the expansion of advanced technology, there are concerns by nursing faculty that students can experience a sense of disconnect and isolation in the world of web-based education. Because the demand for online nursing programs will most likely only increase in the future, nurse educators must find ways to foster a sense of social presence and community belongingness.

Much of the research on social presence has been conducted by researchers in disciplines other than nursing. Therefore, there is need for nurse researchers to study social presence and its effect on online nursing education. One area where research should focus is on developing best practice teaching strategies that incorporate social presence, cognitive presence, and teaching presence for online nursing education.

Ali, N. S., Hodson-Carlton, K., & Ryan, M. (2004). Student's perceptions of online learning: Implications for teaching. *Nurse Educator, 29*, 111–115.

Baker, C. T., & Edwards, J. T. (2011). A holistic approach for establishing social presence in online courses and programs. *The International HETI Review, 1*. Retrieved from http://www.hetl .org/feature-articles/social-presence-in-online-courses/

Dunlap, J. C., & Lowenthal, P. R. (2009). Tweeting the night away: Using twitter to enhance social presence. *Journal of Information Systems Education, 20*, 129–135.

Garrison, D. R., Anderson, T., & Archer, W. (2000). Critical inquiry in a text-based environment: Computer conferencing in higher education. *The Internet and Higher Education, 2*, 87–105.

Gunawardena, C. N. (1995). Social presence theory and implications for interaction and collaborative learning in computer conferences. *International Journal of Educational Telecommunications, 1*, 147–166.

Gunawardena, C. N., & Zittle, F. J. (1997). Social presence as a predictor of satisfaction within a computer-mediated conferencing environment. *The American Journal of Distance Education, 11*, 8–26.

Mayne, L. A., & Wu, Q. (2011). Creating and measuring social presence in online graduate nursing courses. *Nursing Education Perspectives, 32*(2), 110–114.

Picciano, A. (2002). Beyond student perceptions: Issues of interaction, presence, and performance in an online course. *Journal of Asynchronous Learning Networks, 6*, 21–40.

Richardson, J. C., & Swan, K. (2003). Examining social presence in online courses in relation to students' perceived learning and satisfaction, *Journal of Asynchronous Learning Networks, 7*, 68–88.

Rourke, L., Anderson, T., Garrison, R. D., & Archer, W. (2001). Assessing social presence in asynchronous text-based computer conferencing. *Journal of Distance Education 14*(2), 1–17.

Short, J. A., Williams, E., & Christie, B. (1976). *The social psychology of telecommunications.* London, England: John Wiley.

Tu, C. H. (2000). On-line learning migration: From social learning theory to social presence theory to social presence theory in a CMC environment. *Journal of Network and Computer, 23*, 27–37. doi:10.1006/jnca. 1999–0099

Tu, C. H., & McIsaac, M. (2002). An examination of social presence to increase interaction in online classes. *The American Journal of Distance Education, 16*(3), 131–150.

Teresa D. Ritchie

ONLINE LEARNING: CREATIVITY

DEFINITION

Online learning is a term used to distinguish traditional classroom learning and distance learning in which you are separated by geography (O'Neill, Fisher, Newbold, & Susan, 2008). Creativity is the ability to make new things or think of new ideas.

APPLICATION

Creativity in the online environment is extremely important in order to not make it an isolated experience and instead keep the learner engaged. There are many ways to provide a creative online environment. In fact, the higher the participation in an online course, the higher the satisfaction ratings are with the students (Mitchell, Ryan, Carson, & McCann, 2007). Therefore, there are many ways to engage students through asynchronous and synchronous learning.

Most nursing courses are designed to be asynchronous. Some strategies have

O

been identified to have a creative collaborative learning environment for asynchronous learning. First, the faculty has to become familiar with the course management system to use it to its highest capability. A contract with the students' expectations should be posted, which allows both students and educators to have clear expectations with the particular course. Another way to help the experience not to be so isolated is to have an icebreaker exercise during the first week of class such as having students explain how familiar or comfortable they are with online learning (Vitale, 2010). In addition to the usual PowerPoints with notes, readings, learning objectives, and assignments/quizzes or tests, discussion groups regarding the topics each week are critical. Other ways to engage students is to have a cyberspace office to stay connected to the instructor and class lounge so that students can interact with each other online. A wiki is a collaborative website that can be edited by anyone assigned to it. It works well with group assignments or a whole class final project. It is imperative that the educator gives continuous feedback and interacts with the students in every discussion or assignment.

Synchronous online learning requires a tool such as web-based videoconferencing in order for everyone to interact at the same time from his or her various locations. Synchronous online learning allows for immediate feedback and immediate social support. Learning can be done via audio-, video-, web-based conferencing, or white boarding (Giesbers, Rienties, Tempelaar, & Gijselaers, 2014). Furthermore, instant messaging can be used in communicating between students and virtual office hours for face-to-face time with the nurse educator. Research suggests that adding asynchronous learning to synchronous learning is the most beneficial way to engage learners, but there is limited research (Giesbers et al., 2014).

SYNOPSIS

Online learning is becoming more popular in nursing education. There is overall satisfaction with online courses (Halter, Kleiner, & Hess, 2006; Mitchell et al., 2007). However, there are still some students who prefer the traditional classroom, face-to-face model (Stiffler, 2008). A benchmark study showed that the more active learning and faculty–student interaction, the better the students learned the material (Billings, Connors, & Skiba, 2001). Students become more autonomous and take charge in what and how they learn (Lewis & Price, 2007). Social isolation has been noted in the literature as present and not present. In one study, researchers reported that students felt remote and out of touch (Atack, 2003). Yet, in another study, researchers reported a very social atmosphere for learning (Farrell, Cubit, Bobrowski, & Salmon, 2007). Overall, in order for online learning to be successful, there needs to be a well-developed program with interactive discussions or tutorials to develop the critical thinking and problem-solving skills that nurses need. Also, there needs to be an environment of clear communication and continuous feedback from both the educator and the student (Bonnel, 2008; Bromley, 2010).

RECOMMENDATIONS

The nursing profession has a responsibility to keep up with the constant changes in information technology in order to provide up-to-date evidence-based practice guidelines. In order to do so, educators have to come up with creative ways to keep their students engaged in the online environment. There are many teaching strategies and online teaching platforms that are used to teach.

It is important for the teacher and the students to be familiar with the technology in order to provide creative ways to showcase the learning material. Nurse educators need to integrate online learning activities in order for the students to understand the material but not to lose the importance of communication involved in the nurse–patient relationship. In order for this to be successful, there needs to be tremendous technological support and instructional classes for the faculty (Vitale, 2010).

This area is very much in need of scholarly inquiry. There are very few studies that analyze the nursing students' knowledge, use, and outcomes of the online learning environment and identify which creative ways of teaching have the most positive effects on the learners.

Atack, L. (2003). Becoming a web-based learner: Registered nurses' experiences. *Journal of Advanced Nursing, 44*(3), 289–297.

Billings, D. M., Connors, H. R., & Skiba, D. J. (2001). Benchmarking best practices in web-based nursing courses. *Advances in Nursing Science, 23*(3), 41–52.

Bonnel, W. (2008). Improving feedback to students in online courses. *Nursing Education Perspectives, 29*(5), 290–294.

Bromley, P. (2010). Online learning: Anywhere anytime education for specialist nursing. *Neonatal, Pediatric & Child Health Nursing, 13*(3), 2–6.

Farrell, G. A., Cubit, K. A., Bobrowski, C. L., & Salmon, P. (2007). Using the WWW to teach undergraduate nurses clinical communication. *Nurse Education Today, 27*(5), 427–435.

Giesbers, B., Rienties, D., Tempelaar, D., & Gijselaers, W. (2014). A dynamic analysis of the interplay between asynchronous and synchronous communication in online learning: The impact of motivation. *Journal of Computer Assisted Learning, 30*, 30–50.

Halter, M. J., Kleiner, C., & Hess, R. (2006). The experience of nursing students in an online doctoral program in nursing: A phenomenological study. *International Journal of Nursing Studies, 43,* 99–105.

Lewis, P. A., & Price, S. (2007). Distance education and the integration of E-learning in graduate program. *Journal of Continuing Education in Nursing, 38*(3), 139–143.

Mitchell, E. A., Ryan, A., Carson, O., & McCann, S. (2007). An exploratory study of web-enhanced learning in undergraduate nurse education. *Journal of Clinical Nursing, 16*(2), 2287–2296.

O'Neill, C., Fisher, C., Newbold, C., & Susan, K. (2008). *Developing online learning environments: Best practices for nurse educators.* New York, NY: Springer Publishing.

Stiffler, D. J. (2008). A comparison of web-enhanced vs. traditional classroom teaching in women's health nurse practitioner education. *Topics in Advanced Practice Nursing e-Journal, 8*(3), 1–6.

Vitale, A. (2010). Faculty development and mentorship using selected online asynchronous teaching strategies. *Journal of Continuing Education in Nursing, 41*(12), 549–556.

Jaclyn Conelius

ONLINE LEARNING: MOOC

DEFINITION

An MOOC is a massive open online course available on the Internet for free with unlimited open enrollment to participants globally. Cormier (2008) was the first to use the word MOOC when planning a course offered in Canada.

APPLICATION

What courses for nursing can be offered as MOOCs? In 2012, a health policy course with a focus on the new Affordable Care Act was offered (Kirschner, 2012). This MOOC topic is of interest to a wide audience. There is potential for MOOCs for some nursing courses, but careful selection and content must be considered. Perhaps, MOOCs in nursing could start with courses such as those in the basic sciences, microbiology, or infection control. Such courses could be developed so that the content is relevant to nursing programs globally.

O

Due to the increasing cost of education, it is becoming critical to look at innovative models for teaching and learning. Although the MOOC is not totally new, it is an opportunity for innovation through expansion of the online course format. MOOCs may be the way forward; however, technological support and professional development are critical if faculty members are to develop and deliver innovative and successful MOOCs.

Bellack (2013) questioned if MOOCs posed a threat to faculty and the faculty role, or were a way to ease the faculty shortage. Skiba (2013) stated that with the MOOC, the faculty role is changed from knowledge disseminator to mentor and guide. Faculty members will have to empower and coach students with this new paradigm as students will have to engage and be responsible for their work (Skiba, 2013). The introduction of MOOCs in the present format has implications for school of nursing budgets. MOOCs, although free, may incur expenses that cannot be recouped. Many universities are providing the courses without charge because there is good publicity value and perhaps increase enrollment in the regular programs.

SYNOPSIS

Advanced Learning Interactive Systems Online (ALISON), founded in 2007 in Ireland, developed the first MOOC (Bornstein, 2012). The majority of ALISON learners are in the developing world. ALISON is one of the largest MOOC providers outside the United States and had registered the three-millionth user at the beginning of 2014 (ALISON, 2014). In the United States, the big name MOOC providers are Coursera, Udacity, and EdX. Coursera offers MOOCs and also partners with universities to make MOOCs available. MOOC courses with Coursera are available on mobile devices such as the iPhone and android (Coursera, b, n.d.). Coursera has at least 8.2 million users in 678 courses from 110 institutions (Anderson, 2014). Udacity, founded in 2012, has 1 to 6 million users and offers 36 courses (Udacity, n.d.). EdX, founded in 2012, as of June 23, 2014, had 36 partners.

It offers approximately 200 courses to more than 2.5 million users (EdX, b, n.d.).

MOOC courses are usually at the college or university level. Topics developed for MOOCs are wide ranging and are often broad so that they can attract a diverse audience. Popular topics include the sciences and math, along with topics popular with the public, such as emotional intelligence, social justice, and meditation. Due to the unlimited open enrollment, thousands of students are often enrolled in the same course. Different models have evolved related to the access of course materials and resources. Early MOOC courses provided open access to all resources and materials, while many newer courses provide open access to enrolled students only. MOOCs usually are held for 7 to 9 weeks, with a virtual lecture format and assignments including quizzes. Many have assignments graded by peers (Coursera, a, n.d.). Peer grading is used because it is impossible for faculty to grade thousands of assignments.

The completion rates for MOOCs can range from as low as 13% to as high as 40% or more (Jordan, n.d.). There is also evidence that while many register for an MOOC, many do not watch one course video (Catropa, 2013). Some MOOCs offer completion certificates and a few will offer course credit (EdX, a, n.d.). Coursera reported that students who pay for the company's Signature Track identity verification program, which confirms that they took a course and passed, had some of the highest completion rates. In addition, 70% of those who have signed up for the signature verification option completed the courses (Coursera blog, n.d.). The American Council on Education recognized five MOOC courses for college credit (Kolowich, 2013). All of these courses are run by Coursera and a verified certificate is provided at the end of the course. Perhaps, when MOOCs for undergraduate and graduate nursing students are available, they could be reviewed and approved for college credit by the accrediting bodies and boards of nursing for college credit.

While the video lecture is the usual format for MOOCs, research studies have shown that the more the student is involved in the course, the higher the completion rate (Fowler, 2013). Students involved in discussion board postings with class colleagues showed an increase in final grades (Fowler, 2013). Doing homework also increased the completion rate. Teaching an MOOC can be challenging as there is no student engagement during the class. Some faculty are trying to increase engagement by attaching audio messages to the graded assignments when they are returned (Fowler, 2013). Others are developing discussion board assignments. Some faculty strive to increase course interaction by assigning mentors to the students (Fowler, 2013).

RECOMMENDATIONS

Nursing faculty need to embrace the MOOC and develop course for nursing. Research related to motivation and engagement of students enrolled in the MOOC is needed. Comparison studies on student engagement and course outcomes are also needed. There is a need for the development for innovative assignments and tools to grade and evaluate the student's work securely and accurately when dealing with huge classes. DeSilets (2013) challenges nurses to consider the change in learning and teaching paradigm with the advent of MOOCs and how this will impact continuing professional education. MOOCs are here to stay and they are changing the face of teaching and learning. Nurse educators need to take the lead to ensure MOOCs for nurses to meet the needs of the students and the changing nursing education environment.

ALISON. (2014, February). *World's first MOOC breaks 3 million registered learners worldwide.* Retrieved from http://alison.com/press/World039s-first-MOOC-Breaks-3-Million-Registered-Learners-Worldwide

Anderson, N. (2014, June 23). New Coursera chief stresses the "wow" factor of huge audience for free online courses. *The Washington Post.* Retrieved from http://www.washingtonpost.com/local/education/new-coursera-chief-stresses-the-wow-factor-of-huge-audience-for-free-online-courses/2014/06/23/bf27a1fe-fad4–11e3–8176-f2c941cf35f1_story.html

Bellack, J. P. (2013). MOOCs: The future is here. *Journal of Nursing Education, 52*(1), 3–4. doi:http://dx.doi.org/10.3928/01484834–20121227-10

Bornstein, D. (2012, July 11). Open education for a global economy. *New York Times.* Retrieved from http://opinionator.blogs.nytimes.com/2012/07/11/open-education-for-a-global-economy/

Catropa, D. (2013). Big (MOOC) data. *Inside Higher Ed.* Retrieved from http://www.insidehighered.com/blogs/stratedgy/big-mooc-data#sthash.PmfHXQiD.dpbs

Cormier, D. (2008). *The CCK08 MOOC— Connectivism course, 1/4 way. Dave's Educational Blog.* Retrieved from http://davecormier.com/edblog/2008/10/02/the-cck08-mooc-connectivism-course-14-way/

Coursera, a. (n.d.). *Coursera. Our mission.* Retrieved from https://www.coursera.org/about/

Coursera, b. (n.d.) *Coursera. Take the world's best courses, online for free.* Retrieved from https://www.coursera.org/

Coursera blog. (n.d.). *Congrats to the first students to earn verified course credit with signature track and a chat with the Coursera team.* Retrieved from http://blog.coursera.org/post/48598266910/congrats-to-the-first-students-to-earn-verified

DeSilets, L. (2013). A revolutionary journey into learning/education. *The Journal of Continuing Education in Nursing, 44*(1), 8–9. doi:org/10.3928/00220124–20121227-69

EdX, a (n.d.). *Org.FAQs.* Retrieved from https://www.edx.org/org-faq

EdX, b (n.d.). *Take great online courses at the world's best universities.* Retrieved from https://www.edx.org/

Fowler, G. A. (2013, October 8). An early report card on MOOCs. *Wall Street Journal.* Retrieved from http://online.wsj.com/news/articles/SB10001424052702303759604579093400834738972?mg=reno64-wsj&url=http%3A%2F%2Fonline

.wsj.com%2Farticle%2FSB10001424052702
303759604579093400834738972.html

Jordan, K. (n.d.). *MOOC completion rates: The data*. Retrieved from http://www.katyjordan.com/MOOCproject.html

Kirschner, A. (2012). A pioneer in online education tries a MOOC. *The Chronicle of Higher Education*, November 8, 2014.

Kolowich, S. (2013, February 13). *American Council on Education recommends 5 MOOCs for credit*. Retrieved from http://chronicle.com/article/American-Council-on-Education/137155/

Skiba, D. J. (2013). MOOC's and the future of nursing. *Nursing Education Perspectives, 34*(3), 202–204.

Udacity (n.d.). *Courses*. Retrieved from https://www.udacity.com/courses

Mary T. Quinn Griffin

P

PATIENT SAFETY

DEFINITION

Patient safety is an obligatory component of quality health service planning, delivery, and evaluation. The promotion and preservation of individuals' physiological, psychological, social, cultural, and spiritual integrity as recipients of health services are representative of patient safety. Establishing and maintaining safety for diverse patient populations across multiple health care contexts involves a complex interplay of purposeful individual and collective actions of multiple stakeholders (Benner, Malloch, & Sheets, 2010). Key stakeholders are situated within educational institutions, health care agencies, professional organizations, and regulatory bodies including administrators, decision makers, researchers, educators, clinicians, health care students, patients, and families.

APPLICATION

Patient safety is a foundational underpinning to the education of all nurses regardless of their domain of practice. To optimize patient safety, nursing students and practicing nurses must not only develop but they must also sustain current safety competencies through formalized pre-licensure learning experiences and ongoing continuing education initiatives. Across learning contexts, a number of traditional and technologically mediated educational strategies have been identified as efficacious for the development of patient safety knowledge, skills, and attitudes. Educators, students, and nurses, within a program overtly committed to patient safety, engage in deep learning as they critically examine not only the practice of individual practitioners, but the broader system context in which patient safety is promoted, preserved, and, at times, comprised. In addition to promoting learning, educators are responsible for the detection of circumstances where students' knowledge, skills, or attitudes may jeopardize patient safety. Due diligence, guided by professional and educational standards, necessitates the presence of sound evaluative mechanisms, reporting structures, and policies for remediation or failure. Collectively, stakeholders must be vigilant and communicate individual and system threats on early identification in order to preserve patient safety (World Health Organization, 2011).

SYNOPSIS

Nurse educators' responsibilities for patient safety are guided by an understanding of safety curricula content, teaching and evaluation strategies, and contemporary evidence. Programs have been developed to support practitioners' capacity to fulfill the patient safety mandate. Exemplars of safety curricula include the Multi-Professional Patient Safety Curriculum Guide (World Health Organization, 2011) and the Patient Safety Curriculum (National Patient Safety Foundation, 2014). More specific to the development of nursing students' knowledge, skills, and attitudes for patient safety is the Quality and Safety Education for Nurses Initiative (Quality and Safety Education for Nurses Institute, 2014). Common content within such programs include roles and ethical obligations of individual practitioners; evidence-informed knowledge;

P

patient-centered care; clinical reasoning and health informatics; communication among health care providers; systems theory; and risk detection, management, and recovery.

Content associated with patient safety competencies can be learned through small group activities, case studies, and interactive lectures. Such strategies engage students and explore real-world complexities, which can positively influence patient safety outcomes (Chenot & Daniel, 2010; Forbes & Hickey, 2009). The use of clinical simulations advances opportunities to refine safety competencies within a circumscribed low-risk scenario. Critical reflection during and following a simulated experience allows students to identify their role and the broader system factors that support or threaten patient safety (Benner et al., 2010; Blum & Parcells, 2012). According to Reason, Carthey, & de Leval (2001), there is a heightened risk to patient safety when individual practitioners are blamed for errors, the existence of systemic errors provoking weaknesses are denied, and a patient-centered approach is not present. As such, open discussion about factors contributing to system and practice breakdowns increases awareness of potential threats to patient safety in clinical practice (Palmieri, DeLucia, Peterson, Ott, & Green, 2008).

Nurse educators must not only promote patient safety, but also evaluate the acquisition and application of safety competencies. This necessitates sound and timely evaluative assessments, in compliance with professional practice standards and explicit program expectations (Tanicala, Scheffer, & Roberts, 2011). To this end, tools to measure patient safety knowledge, skills, and attitudes are emerging (Schnall et al., 2008). Educators fulfill a role in supporting patient safety through remediation and mitigation of at-risk situations (Rutkowski, 2007).

The direct measurement of patient safety is potentially elusive and, at present, imprecise. Patient safety is typically measured by the incidence, prevalence, and circumstances surrounding adverse health care events. These include medications errors, nosocomial infections, patient injuries, complaints, and mortality (DiCuccio, 2014). Strategic compilation of findings from discrete databases could contribute to the creation of a historical and contextually informed repository of patient safety violations.

RECOMMENDATIONS

Nurse educators must develop, implement, evaluate, and explicitly communicate the intricacies of evidence-informed safety curricula with their stakeholders. In doing so, the cognitive, moral, ethical, and practice components of patient safety become overt, understood, and expected, regardless of the level of nursing preparation or practice setting. Classroom, laboratory, and clinical nurse educators must be constantly vigilant for threats to patient safety and prepared to intervene.

Nurse educators must ensure the presence of clearly articulated program policies, informed by professional standards, and comply with such policies to mitigate risks to patient safety. Within such a milieu, the emphasis is on risk reduction/prevention, remediation, and correction, as opposed to individual blame and punishment. In addition, it is recommended that nurse educators contribute to the development of a patient safety database that would allow others to learn from emerging patterns of adverse events. Finally, there is a need for further theoretical and empirical understanding of the relationship between patient safety curricula and patient outcomes.

Benner, P. E., Malloch, K., & Sheets, V. (2010). *Nursing pathways for patient safety*. National Council of State Boards of Nursing. St. Louis, MO: Elsevier.

Blum, C. A., & Parcells, D. A. (2012). Relationship between high-fidelity simulation and patient safety in prelicensure nursing education: A comprehensive review. *Journal of Nursing Education, 51*(8), 429–435.

Chenot, T. M., & Daniel, L. G. (2010). Frameworks for patient safety in the nursing curriculum. *Journal of Nursing Education, 49*(10), 559–568.

Dicuccio, M. H. (2014 February 27). The relationship between patient safety culture and patient outcomes: A systematic review. *Journal of Patient Safety.*

Forbes, M. O., & Hickey, M. T. (2009). Curriculum reform in baccalaureate nursing education: Review of the literature. *International Journal of Nursing Education Scholarship, 6*, Article 27.

National Patient Safety Foundation. (2014). *Patient safety curriculum.* Retrieved from http://www.npsf.org/online-learning-center/patient-safety-curriculum-2/

Palmieri, P. A., DeLucia, P. R., Peterson, L. T., Ott, T. E., & Green, A. (2008). The anatomy and physiology of error in adverse health care events. *Advances in Health Care Management, 7,* 33–68.

Quality and Safety Education for Nurses Institute. (2014). *Project overview: The evolution of the quality and safety education for nurses (QSEN) initiative.* Retrieved from qsen.org/about-qsen/project-overview/

Reason, J. T., Carthey, J., & de Leval, M. R. (2001). Diagnosing "Vulnerable system syndrome": An essential prerequisite to effective risk management. *Quality in Health Care, 10*(Suppl. 2), ii21–ii25.

Rutkowski, K. (2007). Failure to fail: Assessing nursing students' competence during practice placements. *Nursing Standard, 22*(13), 35–40.

Schnall, R., Stone, P., Currie, L., Desjardins, K., John, R. M., & Bakken, S. (2008). Development of a self-report instrument to measure patient safety attitudes, skills, and knowledge. *Journal of Nursing Scholarship, 40*(4), 391–394.

Tanicala, M. L., Scheffer, B. K., & Roberts, M. S. (2011). Defining pass/fail nursing student clinical behaviors phase I: Moving toward a culture of safety. *Nursing Education Perspectives, 32*(3), 155–161.

World Health Organization. (2011). *Patient safety curriculum guide: Multi-professional education.* Malta, Greece: WHO.

Sharolyn Mossey

PERSONAL DIGITAL ASSISTANT

DEFINITION

A personal digital assistant (PDA) is a wireless, mobile, electronic device capable of storing, managing, and exchanging information. PDAs are also referred to as mobile computing tools, handheld devices, handheld computers, and smartphones (Johansson, Petersson, & Nilsson, 2013).

APPLICATION

Although the PDA was introduced nearly 20 years ago, its application in nursing education is limited, but it is growing. A PDA enables students or faculty to quickly and conveniently gain access to information while in a clinical or classroom setting; however, no standard for use of these devices has been established in nursing education.

Since first introduced, the technological capability of the PDA has evolved and its use within nursing has subsequently increased (Zurmehly, 2010). PDAs are used as a way to include information technology within nursing education programs (Jenkins, Hewitt, & Bakken, 2006; Koeniger-Donohue, 2008; White et al., 2005). Software applications (APPs) that are compatible with PDAs serve as a resource for student nurses, especially in the area of pharmacology. Nurse practitioners and innovative nurse educators are described as early users of PDAs and APPs (George, Davidson, Serapiglia, Barla, & Thotakura, 2010). Preceptors who use PDAs may influence student use, and may also influence student PDA competency during clinical education through modeling (Cibulka & Crane-Wider, 2011).

The dynamic nature of health care and demand for health-related knowledge necessitates access to a large amount of accurate and reliable information which mobile devices, such as PDAs, can provide (Hudson & Buell, 2011; Johansson et al., 2013; White

P

et al., 2005). PDAs are currently being used by nursing students, in both graduate and undergraduate education, to replace printed resources such as drug reference books, laboratory and diagnostic manuals, and textbooks (Koeniger-Donohue, 2008; Kuiper, 2008; Pattillo, Brewer, & Smith, 2007; Williams & Dittmer, 2009). Faculty utilize PDA technology for organization and student data management during student clinical experiences (White et al., 2005).

SYNOPSIS

The overarching theme of the literature describing PDAs and use in nursing education is the student's ability to manage a PDA and retrieve accurate, reliable, and convenient evidence in the clinical setting with the goal to guide clinical decision making and provide safe care. The Institute of Medicine, National League for Nursing, and The American Association of Colleges of Nursing have recommended increased use of technology in nursing education to meet the growing needs of the health care environment (Koeniger-Donohue, 2008). The PDA can help facilitate the recommendations (Cibulka & Crane-Wider, 2011). There is limited but growing research describing PDA use in nursing education (George et al., 2010; Koeniger-Donohue, 2008; White et al., 2005). Sanchez-Garcia, Lopez-Montesinos, and Fernandez-Aleman (2013) reported that PDAs are the most frequently studied wireless device in nursing education, demonstrating both classroom and clinical application. PDAs have been found to be effective tools in education (Farrell & Rose, 2008; Hudson & Buell, 2011; Johansson et al., 2013; White et al., 2005) by increasing pharmacologic knowledge in the clinical setting (Farrell & Rose, 2008); supporting clinical reasoning (Kuiper, 2008); and connecting nursing theory to clinical application (Hudson & Buell, 2011).

PDAs have a perceived clinical usefulness by nursing students (Cibulka & Crane-Wider, 2011; Hudson & Buell, 2011; Johansson et al., 2013; Pattillo et al., 2007). Student self-reports indicate 21% daily clinical use (Hudson & Buell, 2011), 98% daily use (George et al., 2010), and more frequent use when faculty and preceptors used PDAs as teaching tools (Cibulka & Crane-Wider, 2011).

There are identified benefits and barriers to PDA use in nursing education. Use in the clinical setting is more common than in the classroom; however both have been identified by students as being beneficial to learning (Cibulka & Crane-Wider, 2011; George et al., 2010). Benefits include size, portability, and convenience (Cibulka & Crane-Wider, 2011; White et al., 2005); improved efficiency (George et al., 2010; Johansson et al., 2013); and daily software updates (Pattillo et al., 2007). Barriers are technical problems (Cibulka & Crane-Wider, 2011; George et al., 2010); inconsistent faculty use (White et al., 2005); and costs (Cibulka & Crane-Wider, 2011; Hudson & Buell, 2011).

RECOMMENDATIONS

Textbooks and conventional learning methods may not meet the needs of all students; therefore, educators should become familiar with technology (Williams & Dittmer, 2009). Nursing educators should integrate PDA technology in education (Hudson & Buell, 2011; Johansson et al., 2013; Pattillo et al., 2007). Faculty role modeling is recommended as a method to support student use (Cibulka & Crane-Wider, 2011; Kuiper, 2008).

Because a majority of the literature pertaining to evaluation of PDA use in education is descriptive, using self-report, and is not generalizable, additional study is needed (Zurmehly, 2010). There is a dearth of literature describing student outcomes and standards for use of PDAs in nursing education; thus, educators should take scholarship seriously to evaluate the use of PDAs.

Cibulka, N. J., & Crane-Wider, L. (2011). Introducing personal digital assistants to enhance nursing education in undergraduate and graduate nursing programs. *Journal of Nursing Education, 50*(2), 115–118. doi:10.3928/01484834–20101230-07

Farrell, M. J., & Rose, L. (2008). Use of mobile handheld computers in clinical nursing education. *Journal of Nursing Education, 47*(1), 13–19.

George, L. E., Davidson, L. J., Serapiglia, C. P., Barla, S., & Thotakura, A. (2010). Technology in nursing education: A study of PDA use by students. *Journal of Professional Nursing, 26*(6), 371–376. doi: 10.1016/j.profnurs.2010.08.001

Hudson, K., & Buell, V. (2011). Empowering a safer practice: PDAs are integral tools for nursing and health care. *Journal of Nursing Management, 19*, 400–406. doi: 10.1111/j.1365–2834.2011.01251.x

Jenkins, M. L., Hewitt, C., & Bakken, S. (2006). Women's health nursing in the context of the National Health Information Infrastructure. *Journal of Obstetric, Gynecologic, and Neonatal Nursing, 35*, 141–150. doi:10.1111/J.1552–6909.2006.00009.x

Johansson, P. E., Petersson, G. I., & Nilsson, G. C. (2013). Nursing students' experience of using a personal digital assistant (PDA) in clinical practice—an intervention study. *Nursing Education Today, 33*(10), 1246–1251.

Koeniger-Donohue, R. (2008). Handheld computers in nursing education: A PDA pilot project. *Journal of Nursing Education, 47*(2), 44–77.

Kuiper, R. (2008). Use of personal digital assistants to support clinical reasoning in undergraduate baccalaureate nursing students. *Computers, Informatics, Nursing, 26*(2), 90–98.

Pattillo, R. E., Brewer, M., & Smith, C. M. (2007). Tracking clinical use of personal digital assistant reference resources. *Nurse Educator, 32*(1), 39–42.

Sanchez-Garcia, A. B., Lopez-Montesinos, M. J., & Fernandez-Aleman, J. L. (2013). Wireless devices in nursing education. *Investigación y Educación en Enfermería, 31*(1), 95–106.

White, A., Allen, P., Goodwin, L., Breckinridge, D., Dowell, J., & Garvy, R. (2005). Infusing PDA technology into nursing education. *Nurse Educator, 30*(4), 150–154.

Williams, M. G., & Dittmer, A. (2009). Textbooks on tap: Using electronic books housed in handheld devices in nursing clinical courses. *Nursing Education Perspectives, 30*(4), 220–225.

Zurmehly, J. (2010). Personal digital assistants (PDAs): Review and evaluation. *Nursing Education Perspectives, 31*(3), 179–182.

Carolyn Kollar Tieppo

PHYSICAL ASSESSMENT

DEFINITION

Physical assessment is the detailed examination of the human body using specialized techniques to collect objective data used in clinical decision making (Cole, Hill, & Saunders, 2012; Cox, 2010). Inspection, palpation, percussion, and auscultation are techniques systematically used (Coombs & Moorse, 2002) as well as measuring of vital signs. At the advanced practice level of nursing, the advanced or comprehensive physical assessment follows the completion of a comprehensive health history (Cox, 2010).

APPLICATION

The American Association of Colleges of Nursing (2008) outlined competencies required at the completion of baccalaureate generalist education, which include the integration of knowledge and skills critical to nursing practice. One component of the identified critical skill set is the ability to conduct a physical assessment. As such, most nursing programs in the United States, Canada, and the United Kingdom include instruction on physical assessment in the core curricula (Coombs & Moorse, 2002; Solomon, 1990). The content can be taught as an independent course or integrated throughout the curriculum, with baccalaureate programs more likely to have independent courses than associate degree programs (Giddens & Eddy, 2009).

Physical assessment content is delivered through didactic presentation of

P

techniques, emphasizing body systems, and the identification of normal physiology. Students are then given the opportunity to implement and practice the techniques in a variety of settings and clinical environments. A systems approach from head to toe is generally taught and includes the major systems from the skin, head/neck, to musculoskeletal, and neurologic assessments (Giddens & Eddy, 2009). Both associate degree nursing (ADN) and baccalaureate nursing (BSN) programs commonly teach more than 120 physical assessment skills (Giddens, 2006, 2007; Secrest, Norwood, & DuMont, 2005).

SYNOPSIS

There is a paucity of nursing education literature published in the past 30 years related to physical assessment. Most focus on the depth of physical assessment being taught, the differences between independent versus integrated courses for physical assessment, and whether physical assessment skills learned are beneficial to clinical nursing practice.

Results from a survey of 110 BSN programs confirmed that 98% reported content for physical assessment in their coursework, with nearly two thirds "declaring that assessment is a fundamental part of nursing process basic to all clinical courses" (Solomon, 1990, p. 195). In this sample, 64% of programs reported integrating physical assessment skills into another course, rather than having a stand-alone course. Sixty percent of survey respondents reported placement of physical assessment content in junior-level nursing courses, despite the fact that two thirds of respondents indicated that assessment should be "introduced early in a nursing curriculum" (p. 195). Based on her survey results, Solomon concluded that assessment skills should be incorporated into existing courses rather than adding to an already overloaded program.

Nearly 200 faculty members from ADN and BSN programs were queried regarding curriculum factors, teaching methods,

and content taught related to physical assessment (Giddens & Eddy, 2009). Results showed no statistical difference between educational preparation of the faculty and years of teaching experience in ADN and BSN programs. There was a difference in the method of instruction, with 80% of BSN programs teaching physical assessment as an independent course and allotting more didactic credits to the content. Additionally, more BSN programs than ADN programs reported teaching 15 out of 18 assessment categories (Giddens & Eddy, 2009, p. 27). In an earlier study, Giddens had compared the frequency with which physical assessment skills were employed by associate degree and baccalaureate degree graduates (Giddens, 2006). This study showed no difference between utilization of physical assessment skills based on educational preparation. Giddens suggested that this may reflect the lack of utility of advanced physical assessment commonly taught at the BSN (and not at the ADN) level.

Although many nursing programs teach advanced physical assessment, Zambas (2010) suggested that many skills taught within a systematic physical assessment are rarely used in clinical practice. Evidence for this proposition existed in a late 1990s' survey of baccalaureate students in New Jersey (Barbarito, Carney, & Lynch, 1997). These students reported using only half of the physical assessment skills taught in their formal assessment course in clinical practice, with cardiovascular and respiratory assessments identified as the ones most commonly performed. A survey by Giddens in 2007 supported the findings where she identified an even smaller number of physical assessment skills used in clinical practice (24%) by registered nurses. In this study, most of the utilized core skills were isolated to general observation and inspection, as well as involved cardiovascular and respiratory assessments. Giddens asserted that nursing education should reflect nursing practice, and should focus on teaching content and skills that will be implemented in the practice setting.

RECOMMENDATIONS

As the first step in the nursing process, assessment is critical to successful care delivery and should be integrated throughout nursing preparation. Evidence suggests the heavily laden physical assessment curriculum may not be required or appropriate for the baccalaureate generalist nurse. More research is needed to verify which physical assessment skills are needed by most nurses. This information could be gathered from the clinical sites. Partnerships with health care organizations that employ nurses could offer continuing education for nurses in specialty areas to learn skills that are more specialized. Utilization of technology for teaching physical assessment skills should be further explored as well. Research studies are needed to investigate the effect of using avatars and virtual worlds such as Second Life when teaching clinical skills. Use of the standardized patient when teaching physical assessment needs to be evaluated and compared to real-life situations and simulation scenarios. Researchers have focused on the content taught and the teaching methods used rather than the utilization of skills. No studies were found looking at the competency of nurses to conduct a physical assessment as identified in the *Essentials of Baccalaureate Education for Professional Nursing Practice* (2008). Again, this is an area that warrants further investigation.

American Association of Colleges of Nursing. (2008). *The essentials of baccalaureate education for professional nursing practice*. Retrieved from http://www .aacn.nche.edu/education-resources/ baccessentials08

Barbarito, C., Carney, L., & Lynch, A. (1997). Refining a physical assessment course. *Nurse Educator, 22*(3), 6.

Cole, C., Hill, O., & Saunders, R. (2012). *Pocket companion Jarvis's physical examination and health assessment*. Chatswood, Australia: Elsevier Health Sciences.

Coombs, M. A., & Moorse, S. E. (2002). Physical assessment skills: A developing dimension of clinical nursing practice. *Intensive and Critical Care Nursing, 18,* 200–210.

Cox, C. (Ed.). (2010). *Physical assessment for nurses* (2nd ed.). UK: Wiley-Blackwell.

Giddens, J. (2006). Comparing the frequency of physical examination techniques performed by associate and baccalaureate degree prepared nurses in clinical practice: Does education make a difference? *Journal of Nursing Education, 45*(3), 136–139.

Giddens, J. F. (2007). A survey of physical assessment techniques performed by RNs: Lessons for nursing education. *Journal of Nursing Education, 46*(2), 83–87.

Giddens, J. F., & Eddy, L. (2009). A survey of physical examination skills taught in undergraduate nursing programs: Are we teaching too much? *Journal of Nursing Education, 48*(1), 24–29.

Secrest, J. A., Norwood, B. R., & DuMont, P. M. (2005). Physical assessment skills: A descriptive study of what is taught and what is practiced. *Journal of Professional Nursing, 21*(2), 114–118.

Solomon, J. (1990). Physical assessment skills in undergraduate curricula. *Nursing Outlook, 38*(4), 194–195.

Zambas, S. I. (2010). Purpose of the systematic physical assessment in everyday practice: Critique of a "Sacred Cow." *Journal of Nursing Education, 49*(6), 305–310.

Darlene M. Salas
Mary T. Quinn Griffin

PODCASTING

DEFINITION

Podcasting is defined as the preparation and distribution of digital media containing audio and/or video files. These files are then downloaded to a desktop, laptop, mobile device, or MP3 player (Abate, 2013; Billings & Halstead, 2011; Skiba, 2006). Podcasting was

P

first mentioned in the media in 2004 (Skiba, 2006). Podcasting is derived from the combination of broadcast and the iPod. It is now considered pedagogy and is widely used in nursing and higher education as a component of mobile learning (m-learning), which is viewed as effective, flexible, and innovative. Podcast lectures are distributed to students through iTunes University, known as iTunes U.

APPLICATION

Podcasting is a part of m-learning and is widely accepted and used by students and nurses as part of multitasking, listening, and reading (Schlairet, 2010). Podcasting has been identified as one of the fastest growing technologies in nursing education. Delaney, Pennington, and Blankenship (2010) suggest that current podcast usage is driven by teaching, marketing, service, and technology. In nursing education, podcast use is driven by teaching. The potential of technology to contribute to the improvement in the quality of teaching is what drives the use of podcasting in teaching. Podcasting supports adult learning theory and student self-direction by allowing them to listen to podcast content at their own pace. The use of podcast lectures pre-recorded and assigned to students prior to class allows time for in-class discussion and small group work on case studies applying the content (Billings & Halstead, 2011).

As technology integration has become commonplace, podcasting use has increased. The podcast of live classes assists students in understanding class content by allowing asynchronous review of class material (Billings & Halstead, 2011; Schlairet, 2010). Podcasting allows absent students to listen to the asynchronous podcast to meet the course objectives and be responsible for course content. Furthermore, asynchronous podcasting can be used to provide lecture content when faculty has to cancel class.

Many learning management systems (LMS) used in academia have podcasting capabilities built in the system, allowing faculty members to link podcasts to the online class site. One popular form of podcasting is to capture live classes. An easy way for faculty members to capture lectures for podcasting is with portable flash-memory audio recorders that record directly in the MP3 format. These recordings can be uploaded within minutes of the class to the college server into iTunes U. Faculty members should always identify the date of the class and the topic of the podcast (Billings & Halstead, 2011).

Podcasting supplementary materials are another strategy to enhance learning. Supplementary materials allow students to be engaged and explore topics in greater depth and extend their learning beyond the classroom. Ideas for podcasting include addressing the most common questions from the week, guest lecturers, review of top topics, and creating materials prior to class to allow better preparation (Indiana University, Center for Teaching and Learning, n.d.). A podcast can also allow faculty to deliver quality lecture content and then use face-to-face class time for active learning activities.

SYNOPSIS

Podcasting continues to be an emerging technology (Magg, 2006). It is widely used in nursing and higher education, and accepted by students of the millennial generation who learn via podcasts and other media technology (Abate, 2013). Effective use of podcasting includes quality content that enhances classroom lecture, brief and engaging topics, and material congruent with course objectives. Supplemental podcasting appears to serve as a valuable resource for students who can review content, take notes, and clarify misconception. The supplemental material serves as a foundation for students to apply the content in clinical and classroom activities to enhance critical thinking.

Advantages of podcasting include making content available for additional student review to increase the understanding of difficult concepts and additional note taking (Delaney et al., 2010). Schlairet (2010) reported that students who listen to podcasts and take notes performed higher on examinations than students who do not.

The disadvantage of podcasting a class period is that students may choose not to attend class because the podcast is available (Abate, 2013). It has been suggested that educators introduce additional strategies such as interactive class elements or pop-quizzes to discourage nonattendance (Schlairet, 2010).

RECOMMENDATIONS

Educators can use the podcasted recorded lectures to promote student engagement (Long & Edwards, 2010). Faculty members can record nursing skills for students to review in clinical or in the skills laboratory prior to performing procedures. A podcast should be limited to 10 to 15 minutes in order to reinforce course objectives and enhance content. Faculty can suggest to students that they take notes while listening to the podcast in order to enhance learning. Additional research studies are needed to measure effects of podcasting on student achievement.

Abate, K. S. (2013). The effect of podcast lectures on nursing students' knowledge retention and application. *Nursing Education Perspectives, 34*(3), 182–185.

Billings, D. M., & Halstead, J. A. (2011). *Teaching in nursing: A guide for faculty* (3rd ed.). St. Louis, MO: Elsevier Saunders.

Delaney, E., Pennington, N., & Blankenship, M. B. (2010). The role of podcast lectures in associate degree nursing programs. *Teaching and Learning in Nursing, 5*(2), 54–57. doi:10.1016/j.teln.2009.08.004

Indiana University, Center for Teaching and Learning. (n.d.). *Tips for academic podcasting.* Retrieved from http://ctl.iupui.edu/ common/ uploads/ library/ CTL/ iupui .edu/common/uploads/library/CTL/ CTL34951.pdf

Long, S. R., & Edwards, P., B. (2010). Podcasting: Making waves in millennial education. *Journal for Nurses in Professional Development, 26*(3), 96–101. doi:10.1097/ NND.0b013e3181993a6f

Magg, M. (2006). Podcasting: An emerging technology in nursing education. *Studies in Health Technology and Informatics, 122,* 835–836.

Schlairet, M. (2010). Efficacy of podcasting: Use in undergraduate and graduate programs in a college of nursing. *Journal of Nursing Education, 49*(9), 529–533. doi: 10.3928/01484834–20100524-08

Skiba, D. J. (2006). The 2005 word of the year: Podcast. *Nursing Education Perspectives, 27*(1), 54–55.

Barbara L. Morrison Wilford
Mary T. Quinn Griffin

PORTFOLIO EVALUATION

DEFINITION

A portfolio is a purposeful collection of evidence that may be presented as hard copy or electronically, and is organized to showcase one's efforts, progress, and overall achievements over time in an educational program or professional role.

APPLICATION

A portfolio is regarded as an authentic display of evidence created to highlight the realization of personal, educational, or professional goals; document experiences that contribute to personal and professional development; showcase contributions to the scholarship of a profession; verify attainment of a program's learning outcomes; and/or document the acquisition of specific competencies or behaviors. Development of a portfolio requires careful planning with ongoing critical appraisal of the quality of the evidence, as well as self-reflection and self-evaluation to discover personal strengths, weaknesses, and opportunities for growth that are effectively communicated to others who will judge the significance of the evidence presented. Specific academic and professional applications in nursing include the following: student learning and achievement within a course or program, attainment of curricular outcomes, professional experiences for academic credit and/or program admission, and scholarship for faculty promotion and tenure. Professional applications include documentation for job applications, career ladder promotions, annual performance evaluations, initial and continuing practice certifications, and continued competence for license renewal.

SYNOPSIS

The use of portfolios as a strategy for assessment and evaluation evolved out of a need to identify alternative approaches to traditional objective-item testing in order to better document knowledge and competencies. Over the years, portfolios have become a popular means for judging accomplishments across all grade levels, as well as all professions. Portfolio evaluation in nursing has a strong theoretical foundation that blends Kolb's experiential learning (Kolb, 1984) and Mezirow's transformational learning theories (Mezirow, 2000) with Benner's levels of proficiency in nursing model (Benner, 2001). The creation of a portfolio enables an individual to identify and reflect on experiences that have been a powerful vehicle for learning and have contributed to professional development. Critical thinking to discover meaning in each of the education and practice activities showcased in the portfolio assists the nurse to realize, and others to judge, evolution in the professional role from novice to expert.

Portfolio evaluation in nursing, as in other disciplines, is challenged by three recurring issues. The first issue relates to how much and what sort of evidence is appropriate and necessary to include in a portfolio. The purpose for creating the portfolio will dictate the type of content that should be included. Basic criteria are usually available to guide the selection of portfolio documentation, with specifications for a minimum number of required and optional elements. It is up to the individual developing the portfolio to appraise the quality of his or her documentation, and to select only those items that provide the best evidence to meet the portfolio goals (Clarke, Cortis, & Sowter, 2011).

The second challenge relates to effectively integrating self-reflection and self-evaluation into the portfolio. Meaningful portfolio evaluation relies on the ability of the individual to consciously engage in ongoing reflection to identify strengths and weaknesses, as well as gaps in experiences that point to opportunities for further learning or personal and professional development. This critical review of portfolio documentation enables the individual to recognize and articulate trends in personal and professional development, appreciate the significance of accomplishments, and explain relationships between various experiences and activities. Personal summaries are typically added to a portfolio to allow the individual to explain the importance of a particular experience, or to convey the relationship among a set of documents. Portfolio entries consisting of personal summaries are necessary to prevent erroneous judgments about the significance among portfolio documents to the individual's goals.

The third challenge is how to judge the quality of portfolio evidence in a manner that is valid and reliable. Validity in portfolio evaluation requires empirical evidence that is generated through a process that objectively measures intended constructs. Reliability is established only when multiple raters, including educators, practitioners, and the public, are able to apply the same evaluation criteria and make independent, yet consistent, judgments about the quality and significance of the evidence (Karlowicz, 2010). Efforts to develop sound evaluation methods for portfolio evaluation that demonstrate validity and reliability have been complicated by variability in the content and design of portfolios. Evaluation issues are scoring terminology that is not standardized; rubrics that are too complex for most raters; and lack of agreement by raters regarding characteristics, behaviors, and competencies most valued in nursing education and practice (Garrett, MacPhee, & Jackson, 2013; Hill, 2012; Karlowicz, 2000; McCready, 2007). The difficulties associated with establishing any meaningful process for portfolio evaluation stem from the fact that it is largely a qualitative process while trying to produce quantitative results that can be compared to other objective measures of performance.

RECOMMENDATIONS

Portfolio development is a worthwhile process for the learner and practitioner. The availability of systems to support the creation of e-Portfolios provides an opportunity to enhance the usefulness of the portfolio, as well as advance processes for portfolio evaluation. However, educators and practitioners need to fully consider the benefits and limitations of portfolio evaluation and determine whether this methodology will permit the effective measurement of outcomes and competencies in a way that will yield useful and relevant data to support decisions in education and practice.

Few studies effectively examine the meaning and usefulness of scores derived from portfolio evaluation; and there is no known attempt to determine how portfolio evaluation scores compare with other measures of academic and professional performance. Nursing education programs, accrediting/certification organizations, and others are encouraged to continue identifying ways to integrate portfolios into evaluation plans, to conduct research on the validity and reliability of scoring processes, and to publish experiences with portfolio evaluation.

Benner, P. (2001). *From novice to expert: Excellence and power in clinical nursing practice* (Commemorative ed.). Upper Saddle River, NJ: Prentice Hall Health.

Clarke, D. J., Cortis, J. D., & Sowter, J. (2011). Pilot testing of guidelines to support good practice in the development of professional portfolios. *Nurse Education Today, 31*, e70–e78.

Garrett, B. M., MacPhee, M., & Jackson, C. (2013). Evaluation of an e-Portfolio for the assessment of clinical competence in a baccalaureate nursing program. *Nurse Education Today, 33*, 1207–1213.

Hill, T. L. (2012). The portfolio as a summative assessment for the nursing student. *Teaching and Learning in Nursing, 7*, 140–145

Karlowicz, K. A. (2000). The value of student portfolios to evaluate undergraduate nursing programs. *Nurse Educator, 25*(2), 82–87.

Karlowicz, K. A. (2010). Development and testing of a portfolio evaluation scoring tool. *Journal of Nursing Education, 49*(2), 78–86.

Kolb, D. A. (1984). *Experiential learning.* Englewood Cliffs, NJ: Prentice-Hall, Inc.

McCready, T. (2007). Portfolios and the assessment of competence in nursing: A literature review. *International Journal of Nursing Studies, 44*, 143–151.

Mezirow, J. (2000). Learning to think like an adult: Core concepts of transformation theory. In J. Mezirow (Ed.), *Learning as transformation* (pp. 3–33). San Francisco, CA: Jossey-Bass.

Karen A. Karlowicz

PRECEPTING

DEFINITION

Precepting is modeling, explaining, and sharing the realities of nursing practice to facilitate the development of knowledge and understanding about nursing practice in others. Precepting is enacted by a working nurse, often referred to as a preceptor. The recipient of precepting is a learner: a student in either an undergraduate or graduate program or a new staff member. Precepting is a time-defined relationship with externally defined objectives. Precepting encompasses an introduction to a work environment with a focus on individualized teaching, learning, supporting, and immersing the person being precepted to the realities of nursing practice. Precepting provides the bridge between the conceptual and theoretical learning completed in the classroom and clinical laboratory with the actuality of everyday nursing practice in a health care environment. The goals of precepting are to enhance the learner's knowledge and success, and ultimately to improve the quality of patient care provided.

APPLICATION

In nursing education, precepting is a model in which nursing students are assigned to experienced nurses to learn about nursing practice and the delivery of patient care. Through guidance, supervision, and role modeling, precepting helps to develop knowledge, clinical skills, and professional attitudes in nursing students.

Historically, in undergraduate nursing education, precepting was used in the terminal semester or the capstone experience of the student's curriculum. However, as models of undergraduate nursing education have evolved to include clinical–academic partnerships, immersion learning, and dedicated education units, precepting is becoming more common throughout nursing practice courses in the curriculum (Dean et al., 2013; Jeffries et al., 2013; Raines, 2009). Precepting in these models gives the student insight into the complexities of the nurse's role in the health care setting. Precepting results in a learning experience that extends beyond the nursing care needs of a single patient to fulfilling the needs of a multipatient assignment and the other responsibilities associated with the professional nurse role. It provides the "big picture" of the nurses' responsibilities and accountability beyond the completion of tasks or procedures on a single patient. Precepting is also used in the education of advanced practice nurses because of the opportunity to enhance the development of advanced practice skills as well as socialization to the role of the advanced practice nurse.

A successful precepting experience includes three phases during each encounter: planning, doing, and evaluating. In the planning phase, the preceptor needs to get to know the learner's learning style and prior experiences. This may be facilitated by the faculty member before the student arrives in the clinical setting. Prior to beginning each clinical day, the preceptor needs to review the patient care assignment and identify optimal learning opportunities. The last step of the planning phase involves setting goals and priorities for the student to accomplish and activities to be completed by the end of the clinical day. In the doing phase, the preceptor and learner work together in completing patient care and nursing responsibilities. Allowing the learner to see the nurse in practice and then having the learner perform nursing care activities with the preceptor as a supportive coach is an efficient and effective model of teaching. The last phase involves reflecting on and evaluating the day's accomplishments and providing constructive feedback to the learner.

SYNOPSIS

Precepting is vital to the academic preparation of nursing students (Barker & Pittman, 2010; Carlson, 2013; Omansky, 2010; Raines, 2012). The actions and behaviors of the preceptors influence and shape the meaning and understanding of the practice of nursing for the learner. The relationship between the preceptor and the learner is key to successful functioning and socialization to the role of nurse. Positive characteristics of a good preceptor from the perspective of the learner include being empathetic, respectful, humorous, fair, flexible, and dependable (Stiffler, Arthur, Stephenson, Ray, & Cullen, 2009).

Precepting is a complex and multifactor activity. A good clinical nurse or a good nurse manager is not always good at precepting. Precepting requires strong clinical skills plus an ability to explain complex entities of nursing practice, professional role identity, and strong interpersonal skills. Precepting involves enacting a number of roles simultaneously. Precepting the nurse is acting as a teacher, counselor, role model, coach, protector, socializer, expert, and leader as well as supporting and promoting the growth and development of the learner. In addition, precepting involves open and ongoing communications and feedback with the person being precepted and with the faculty member or program director regarding the learner's progress. For a positive outcome, the nurse precepting, the learner, and the faculty member must work in synchrony. Preceptors do not replace the faculty member in nursing practice education, but extend and complement the role by applying the theoretical knowledge to the complexities and unpredictability of the practice of nursing. Precepting focuses on the development of a learner's clinical competence and socialization to the role of professional nurse.

Quality precepting is preceded by an investment of time and energy in the preparation and education of the nurse preceptor. Learning how to teach others, provide feedback, and balance the dual responsibilities to the student and the patient are critical for successful precepting. Quality preparation for the precepting role results in a more efficient and less stressful experience for everyone.

Many nurses choose to precept because they view it as an enriching and mutually rewarding experience. However, precepting is an added responsibility for the nurses. Recognition of this important role through workload reduction, financial compensation, professional recognition, or other rewards is important.

Precepting is often used interchangeably with mentoring, but they are distinct activities. Precepting has a narrow focus on individualized teaching, learning, and supporting in a clinical setting. Precepting occurs between a nursing student and a registered nurse preceptor or a new staff member and a registered nurse preceptor. Precepting is an educational relationship and takes place in programs that are planned and monitored, are task oriented and focused on the transfer of practical clinical skills, and are time limited. Precepting

is an effective way to bridge the theory–practice gap and a means of transition to the application of knowledge in a clinical setting, whereas mentoring is focused on supporting, inspiring, and nurturing a colleague and is a voluntary relationship often sought out by the people involved (Yonge, Billay, Myrick, & Luhanga, 2007). Mentoring has no specific agenda or goals to accomplish and often evolves into a close relationship with personal and emotional bonds. A mentoring relationship may endure as participants move to different settings, whereas a precepting relationship is assigned and ends with the achievement of the goals or at a predetermined time frame.

RECOMMENDATIONS

Precepting is important to the preparation of the next generation of nurses and for integrating new staff into the work activities and responsibilities. Individuals who are given the privilege of developing the future generation of nurses need to be carefully selected, adequately prepared and supported, and compensated for their contributions to the continuing growth and development of professional nurses. As models of collaborative academic–clinical partnerships continue to grow, evaluation research on the impact of precepting on learning outcomes as well as insight into the professional development of the preceptor are needed.

Barker, E. R., & Pittman, O. (2010). Becoming a super preceptor: A practical guide to preceptorship in today's clinical climate. *Journal of the American Academy of Nurse Practitioners, 22*(3), 144–149.

Carlson, E. (2013). Precepting and symbolic interactionism—a theoretical look at preceptorship during clinical practice. *Journal of Advanced Nursing, 69*(2), 457–464.

Dean, G. E., Reishtein, J. L., McVey, J., Ambrose, M., Burke, S., Haskins, M., & Jones, J. (2013). Implementing a dedicated education unit: A practice partnership with oncology nurses. *Clinical Journal of Oncology Nursing, 17*(2), 208–210.

Jeffries, P. R., Rose, L., Belcher, A. E., Dang, D., Hochuli, J. F., Fleischmann, D., ... Walrath, J. M. (2013). A clinical academic practice partnership: A clinical education redesign. *Journal of Professional Nursing, 29*(3), 128–136.

Omansky, G. L. (2010). Staff nurses' experiences as preceptors and mentors: An integrative review. *Journal of Nursing Management, 18*(6), 697–703.

Raines, D. A. (2009). Competence of accelerated second degree students after studying in a collaborative model of nursing practice education. *International Journal of Nursing Education Scholarship, 6*(1), 1–12.

Raines, D. A. (2012). Nurse preceptors' views of precepting undergraduate nursing students. *Nursing Education Perspectives, 33*(2), 76–79.

Stiffler, D., Arthur, A. J., Stephenson, E., Ray, C., & Cullen, D. L. (2009). A guide for preceptors of advance practice nursing students caring for women and infants. *JOGNN: Journal of Obstetric, Gynecologic & Neonatal Nursing, 38*(5), 624–631.

Yonge, O., Billay, D., Myrick, F., & Luhanga, F. (2007). Preceptorship and mentorship: Not merely a matter of semantics. *International Journal of Nursing Education Scholarship, 4*(1), 1–13. Article 19.

Deborah A. Raines

PREPAREDNESS

DEFINITION

The concept of preparedness is used in many different contexts inclusive of disaster (i.e., emergency, bioterrorism) preparedness and within the psychological literature to explain why certain associations are learned more readily than others. A concept analysis of bioterrorism preparedness (Rebmann, 2006, p. 623) revealed that the antecedents to preparedness are readiness and acceptance to change; the defining attributes comprise gaining knowledge, planning, practicing response behaviors, and evaluating knowledge level, and the consequences of preparedness include recognition of a bioterrorism event and enactment of suitable actions.

APPLICATION

Preparedness of newly qualified health care professionals for the clinical environment has been the topic of debate (Walker et al., 2013). Preparedness can be extrapolated in a multitude of ways including knowing "what you are getting into" (Sedgwick & Yonge, 2007, p. 620) and having the requisite knowledge, skills, and competencies that can be converted into effective clinical practice (Edwards, Smith, Courtney, Finlayson, & Chapman, 2004). Various aspects of how graduates can improve their preparedness for practice have been reviewed and explored (Newton & Cross, 2011; Romyn et al., 2009; Wolff, Regan, Pesut, & Black, 2010). These authors looked at different factors and influences that contribute to the preparedness of graduates for clinical practice, and ultimately their successful transition to a competent health care professional. Graduate-level factors include role preparation (Doody, Tuohy, & Deasy, 2012), role competence (Doody et al., 2012), and personal attributes such as self-confidence in the ability to perform in a role and show interest in the role (Houghton, Casey, Shaw, & Murphy, 2012). Environmental factors influencing graduate preparedness include role clarity, mentorship, and preceptorship programs (Whitehead & Holmes, 2011) and supportive working environments (Wolff et al., 2010).

The role of the graduate nurse within the health care setting varies according to the geographical location, subspecialty, regulatory requirements, and the associated duration of clinical placements within the undergraduate program. Lack of role clarity and varying levels of expectations of graduates can be perceived as a stressor for many newly qualified nurses (Newton & Cross, 2011; Wolff et al., 2010).

Studies focused on assessing the level of competence of graduate nurses highlight the importance of having adequate undergraduate clinical experience (Newton & Cross, 2011). Graduates with previous clinical experience have increased familiarity with ward routine, greater confidence, enhanced ability to communicate with patients and their families, and enhanced sense of belonging (Levett-Jones, Lathlean, Higgins, & McMillan, 2006; Newton & Cross, 2011). Whitehead and Holmes (2011) argue that students were sheltered from the realities of nursing and did not partake in difficult situations, such as dealing with crisis situations and complex patient care needs. Thus, it was suggested from the perspective of stakeholders and nurse leaders that on commencement of employment, graduate nurses lacked sufficient levels of competence in critical aspects of nursing care (Newton & Cross, 2011).

SYNOPSIS

The concept of graduate preparedness within the context of clinical practice is one that is thoroughly debated and challenged. The essence of preparedness within a general context implies that the individual is ready, willing, and able to undertake the duties of a particular role. It also encapsulates the notion that the individual is and will be competent. This mentality toward preparedness for practice is universally acknowledged; however, no single homogeneous definition exists. Furthermore, the educational structures and processes to enable the individual to embody this wider concept of preparedness for clinical practice is something that is constantly challenged, changed, and adjusted to ensure the best possible development and output of graduates; again, this can differ from country to country, resulting in no single coherent model for preparedness for practice. However, the consequences of inadequate preparedness of new graduates for clinical practice can include reality shock, a perception of not being able to adjust to a new role, and competency and skill deficits that have the potential to negatively impact

on the quality and safety of health care provided.

The expectations of clinical staff, nurse leaders, and other key stakeholders vary related to the preparedness of graduate nurses. These varying levels of expectations are a cause for concern as they result in unnecessary stress for graduate nurses. Some researchers have measured the preparedness of graduates to meet the challenges of clinical practice, linking the perception of preparedness to preparedness in relation to terminal program outcomes and program content (Tallentire, Smith, Wylde, & Cameron, 2011). Other researchers have linked preparedness and the measurement of competence in certain domains (Safadi, Jaradeh, Bandak, & Froelicher, 2010). The socialization of nurses to the role of registered nurse is another dimension of preparedness, and requires careful thought and nurturing support systems to ensure that the graduate nurse feels included, valued, respected, and ultimately prepared for practice.

RECOMMENDATIONS

Preparedness in the context of graduates making the transition from a nursing program to practicing as a newly registered nurse is a broad concept. It can be taken to mean that the individual is ready, willing, and able to undertake the duties of a role in clinical practice. However, to ensure a graduate is prepared for the role, adequate role preparation, role competence, self-confidence in the ability to perform in that role, and interest in the role are required. Research is needed to further define preparedness for practice and develop psychometrically tested measures of preparedness for practice.

Doody, O., Tuohy, D., & Deasy, C. (2012). Final-year student nurses' perceptions of role transition. *British Journal of Nursing,* *21*(11), 684–688.

Edwards, H., Smith, S., Courtney, M., Finlayson, K., & Chapman, H. (2004). The impact of clinical placement location on nursing students' competence and preparedness for practice. *Nurse Education Today, 24*, 248–255.

Houghton, C. E., Casey, D., Shaw, D., & Murphy, K. (2012). Students' experience of implementing clinical skills in the real world of practice. *Journal of Clinical Nursing, 22*, 1961–1969.

Levett-Jones, T., Lathlean, J., Higgins, I., & McMillan, M. (2006). The duration of clinical placements: A key influence on nursing students' experience of belongingness. *Australian Journal of Advanced Nursing, 26*(2), 8–16.

Newton, J. M., & Cross, W. M. (2011). Outcomes of a clinical partnership model for undergraduate nursing students. *Contemporary Nurse, 39*(1), 119–127.

Rebmann, T. (2006). Defining bioterrorism preparedness for nurses: Concept analysis. *Journal of Advanced Nursing, 54*(5), 623–632.

Romyn, D. M., Linton, N., Giblin, C., Hendrickson, B., Limacher, L. H., Murray, C., ...Zimmell, C. M. (2009). Successful transition of the new graduate nurse. *International Journal of Education Scholarship, 6*, 1–17.

Safadi, R., Jaradeh, M., Bandak, A., & Froelicher, E. (2010). Competence assessment of nursing graduates of Jordanian universities. *Nursing and Health Sciences, 12*, 147–154.

Sedgwick, M. G., & Yonge, O. (2007). Undergraduate nursing students' preparedness to "go rural." *Nurse Education Today, 28*, 620–626.

Tallentire, V. R., Smith, S. E., Wylde, K., & Cameron, H. S. (2011). Are medical graduates ready to face the challenges of foundation training? *Postgraduate Medical Journal, 87*(1031), 590–595.

Walker, A., Yong, M., Pang, L., Fullarton, C., Costa, B., & Dunning, A. M. T. (2013). Work readiness of graduate health professionals. *Nurse Education Today, 33*(2), 116–122.

Whitehead, B., & Holmes, D. (2011). Are newly qualified nurses prepared for practice? *Nursing Times, 107*(19/20), 20–23.

Wolff, A. C., Regan, S., Pesut, B., & Black, J. (2010). Ready for what? An exploration of the meaning of new graduate nurses' readiness for practice. *International Journal of Nursing Education Scholarship, 7*(1), 1–14. Article 7.

Josephine Hegarty

PROBLEM-BASED LEARNING

DEFINITION

Problem-based learning (PBL) is a strategy for facilitating learning that requires students to think critically, be self-directed, and become proficient at problem solving using real-world scenarios (Schmidt, Rotgans, & Yew, 2011). The strategy is based on adult learning theory principles using student-centered problem-solving approaches.

APPLICATION

PBL principles guide the application of this method in nursing education. This method is student centric in that it empowers the student to take control of the learning process as he or she makes decisions about solving problems in practice-based scenarios. Students are able to obtain their learning goals through the use of facilitation as they discover the gaps in their knowledge necessary for application into clinical practice. Students take more responsibility for their learning, resulting in increased learning skills and job skills (Billings & Halstead, 2011).

Faculty using PBL must act as facilitators of the process, not the subject matter expert. This may be contrary to past teaching philosophies for some faculty and therefore may serve as a block to using PBL in the classroom (Distler, 2008). Students' past experiences are valued and respected as they become more responsible for learning, resulting in the development of critical thinking and problem-solving skills. As a result, students synthesize data, interact with the faculty and students, and use critical thinking to problem solve.

The use of case studies is an integral part of PBL. The case studies are loosely structured by faculty, creating opportunities for students to engage in critical thinking and problem solving (Oermann & Gaberson, 2013). The purpose of the case study is to develop an interactive dialogue among students as they work toward understanding the case study while gathering information and filling knowledge gaps. The loosely structured cases may not have a well-defined answer, providing students the opportunity to explore the problem in more detail. It is this level of exploration and discussion that results in the bridging of the theory–practice gap (Hodges, 2011). This strategy is suitable for adult learners who learn experientially and value the immediate application of information to practice.

SYNOPSIS

PBL began with the education of medical students at McMaster University in 1969 (Distler, 2008). PBL requires the application of adult learning theory, the application of knowledge into practice, and the identification of learning needs of students. Students analyze information that is readily available through various media regarding the problem-based scenario. The traditional method of lecture does not offer opportunities to gather information, process information, and apply the information to practice (Crawford, 2011).

Schmidt et al. (2011) discussed scaffolding in the use of PBL (p. 797). Faculty facilitate meaningful learning during the problem-solving process through the use of scaffolds. Scaffolds are both soft and hard; soft scaffolds are dynamic and based on the action of the faculty to support the learning needs of students, whereas hard scaffolds are static and may include worksheets and other cognitive tools (Schmidt et al., 2011). As students become more comfortable with the PBL process, the scaffolds are removed over time as expertise increases, thereby requiring fewer

resources. This is also referred to as flexible scaffolding.

PBL can be used in face-to-face, hybrid, and fully online nursing education programs. Rounds and Rappaport (2008) found that the use of PBL is time intensive for faculty and students. With face-to-face educational programs, students may work in teams to address the case studies. Teamwork may be more difficult in an asynchronous environment. Faculty who use this method of interactive discussion have found that it fosters a unique closeness between faculty and students.

In their work on the use of PBL with graduate-level nursing, White, Rowland, and Pesis-Katz (2012) looked at a peer-led team-learning model. This model emphasized student interaction using a collaborative approach among students. They found that there was a greater opportunity for students to discuss and apply research findings on current evidence related to the problem-solving case study. Their work was centered on the use of PBL principles including case studies that focused on solving complex real-world problems. Students involved in this model of learning were better able to explore and synthesize knowledge in greater depth.

RECOMMENDATIONS

The implementation of PBL into nursing curricula requires effort and development of faculty (Distler, 2008). All faculty involved in the implementation of PBL in the curricula should be oriented to the principles. In addition, students must also understand the rationale for changing to PBL, how they will be learning, and how they will be evaluated. While this process is time consuming in the early phases, there will be improved student satisfaction and subsequent clinical competence. Faculty may find themselves tempted to revert to traditional methods of learning; however, the rewards for innovation are far reaching (Distler, 2008).

It is important to distinguish between assessment and evaluation when evaluating the results of PBL. Assessment is identifying

P

student learning and evaluation is the outcomes of PBL as a learning strategy (Billings & Halstead, 2011). Faculty need to use both formative and summative evaluation using quantitative and qualitative methods. This will include evidence that students can apply previously acquired knowledge, discuss and debate the case study, and become proficient at critical thinking and problem solving.

Billings, D., & Halstead, J. (2011). *Teaching in nursing: A guide for faculty* (4th ed.). St. Louis, MO: Saunders.

Crawford, T. R. (2011). Using problem-based learning in web-based components of nurse education. *Nurse Education in Practice, 11*(2), 124–130. doi:10.1016/j. nepr.2010.10.010

Distler, J. (2008). Problem-based learning: An innovative approach to teaching physical assessment in advanced practice nursing curriculum. *International Journal of Nursing Education Scholarship, 5*, Article 23. doi:10.2202/1548–923X.1577

Hodges, H. F. (2011). Preparing new nurses with complexity science and problem-based learning. *Journal of Nurse Education, 50*(1), 7–13. doi:10.3928/01484834–20101029-01

Oermann, M. H., & Gaberson, K. B. (2013). *Evaluation and testing in nursing education* (4th ed.). New York, NY: Springer Publishing

Rounds, L. R., & Rappaport, B. A. (2008). The successful use of problem-based learning in an online nurse practitioner course. *Nursing Education Perspectives, 29*(1), 12–16.

Schmidt, H. G., Rotgans, J. I., & Yew, E. H. (2011). The process of problem-based learning: What works and why. *Medical Education, 45*(8), 792–806. doi: 10.1111/j.1365–2923.2011.04035.x

White, P., Rowland, A. B., & Pesis-Katz, I. (2012). Peer-led team learning model in a graduate-level nursing course. *Journal of Nursing Education, 51*(8), 471–475. doi: 10.3928/01484834–20120706-03

John Distler

PROFESSIONAL–COMMUNITY PARTNERSHIP

DEFINITION

Professional–community partnerships are collaborative relationships between a professional/professional group and a community group/agency working in a reciprocal manner to build on strengths and needs of all parties while addressing joint concerns, issues, or problems. These partnerships involve professionals in health care organizations, education, civic, and service organizations. Frequently, these partnerships involve academic institutions and community agencies and may also be known as academic–practice partnerships, academic–service partnerships, education–practice partnerships, academic–community partnerships, or community–campus partnerships. Successful professional–community partnerships involve mutual respect, trust, commitment, open and ongoing communication, shared goals and knowledge, and cooperation. Partners have agreed-upon missions, values, goals, and measurable outcomes; they build upon individual strengths and assets and share resources. These professional–community partnerships expand opportunities for the partners while maximizing partner potential (American Association of Colleges of Nursing and the Association of Nurse Executives, 2010; Beal et al., 2012; Community–Campus Partnerships for Health, 2013).

APPLICATION

Professional–community partnerships can be a useful approach in addressing educational needs and provide rich learning opportunities for students in various programs and across all levels of nursing education. They may lead to improved access to clinical learning opportunities for students, research initiatives, practice sites for faculty, and enhanced recruitment and employment of graduate nursing students by clinical agencies involved in the partnership. Professional–community partnerships can be established with academic nursing programs, professional organizations, and other community health care providers and agencies such as faith communities; schools; community health centers; hospice; shelters; social service agencies; civic, governmental, or health and human service organizations; businesses; or health clinics (Shellenbarger, 2003). As professional–community partnerships develop, participants must be sensitive to potential barriers such as lack of time, lack of resources, lack of knowledge, mistrust, or impaired communication, and work to establish a relationship that builds on strengths and is mutually beneficial to all parties (Beal & Alt-White, 2012).

SYNOPSIS

Partnerships have been in existence in nursing for hundreds of years, starting with health care collaborations with religious communities, followed later by partnerships with physicians, the government, hospitals, and professional organizations (Beal et al., 2012). With recent changes in health care, coupled with the demand for nurses and nursing education, nursing leaders and other health care providers have explored methods of developing approaches to address these issues and partnerships have emerged. More than 15 years ago, a national interest in community partnerships emerged out of the Health Professions Schools in Service to the Nation initiative as the service-learning movement in higher education began to grow. Various health care educators in higher education partnered with communities to address health and social challenges. Leaders in nursing recognized the value of partnerships. In 2010, the American Association of Colleges of Nursing (AACN) and the American Organization of Nurse Executives (AONE) created a joint task force to explore concerns and issues related to academic-practice partnerships. Their work included a review of evidence-based literature, data

collection involving a national survey, focus groups with academic and service leaders, developing a road map for leaders to create and sustain effective partnerships, defining the characteristics of these partnerships, and identifying facilitators and barriers of academic–practice partnerships (Beal et al., 2012). Their work resulted in guiding principles for academic–practice partnerships, which are similar to principles identified in good community–campus partnerships that were developed by the Community–Campus Partnerships for Health (2013). Both groups agree that there are key elements in partnerships that include mutual respect and trust, commitment to the partnership, sharing of knowledge and resources, and the need for evaluation (American Association of Colleges of Nursing and the Association of Nurse Executives, 2012; Community-Campus Partnership for Health, 2013). Additionally, for partnerships to be effective, involved parties must have agreed upon values, goals, and objectives, and use open and clear communication (Beal et al., 2012; Plowfield, Wheeler, & Raymond, 2005).

RECOMMENDATIONS

As professional–community partnerships continue to expand, faculty need further information to ensure successful outcomes of these partnerships. Since much of the literature and research about community partnerships is anecdotal or single site reports, research is needed to understand how to establish, sustain, and evaluate effective partnership activities. Research should use rigorous methods, valid and reliable tools, and sampling approaches with adequate sample sizes that permit generalizability.

A variety of implementation issues should also be considered for faculty interested in pursuing professional–community partnerships. First, faculty need to assess educational and community needs to determine unmet problems and issues that could be best addressed through partnership activities. Then, identification of potential partners is needed. As partnership

P

relationships are developed, time, funding, knowledge, and resources are required to ensure success. Recommended guiding principles concerning partnerships should be followed. Lastly, partners need to plan evaluation activities to determine outcomes of the partnership and impact on key stakeholders. Additional research is needed to ensure that principles of partnerships are effective and used properly. The literature suggests multiple benefits to professional–community partnerships but further research is needed.

American Association of Colleges of Nursing and the Association of Nurse Executives. (2010). *AACN-AONE task force on academic-practice partnerships summary of literature related to academic-service partnerships.* Retrieved from http://www.aacn.nche.edu/leading-initiatives/academic-practice-partnerships

American Association of Colleges of Nursing and the Association of Nurse Executives. (2012). *AACN-AONE task force on academic-practice partnerships guiding principles.* Retrieved from http://www.aacn.nche.edu/leading-initiatives/academic-practice-partnerships

Beal, J. A., & Alt-White, A. C. (2012). *The importance of academic practice partnerships.* Presented at the American Association of Colleges of Nursing Spring 2012 Meeting. Washington, DC: American Association of Colleges of Nursing. Retrieved from www.aacn.nche.edu/leading-initiatives/academic-practice-partnerships

Beal, J. A., Alt-White, A., Erickson, J., Everett, L. Q., Fleshner, I., Karshmer, J.,...Gale, S. (2012). Academic practice partnership: A national dialogue. *Journal of Professional Nursing, 28,* 327–332.

Community-Campus Partnerships for Health. (2013). *Principles of good community-campus partnerships.* Retrieved from http://depts.washington.edu/ccph/principles.html

Plowfield, L. A., Wheeler, E. C., & Raymond, J. E. (2005). Time, tact, talent and trust: Essential ingredients of effective academic-community partnerships. *Nursing Education Perspectives, 26,* 217–220.

Shellenbarger, T. (2003). Professional-community partnerships. In M. H. Oermann & K. T. Heinrich (Eds.), *Annual review of nursing education* (Vol. 1, pp. 43–58). New York: NY: Springer Publishing.

Teresa Shellenbarger

PROFESSIONAL DEVELOPMENT

DEFINITION

Professional development is the process of active participation by nurses in learning activities that assist to develop continuing competence, enhance professional practice, and support achievement of career goals (American Nurses Association [ANA], 2011b, para 3). Development implies a dynamic process that occurs over time. Professional development is the continuing commitment to lifelong learning (Magill-Cuerden, 2007).

APPLICATION

Nurse Practice Acts and the Code of Ethics for Nurses stress the obligation to engage in professional development. Commitment to lifelong learning is a cornerstone of safe nursing practice. In addition, most philosophies of nursing identify professional development as an essential component of nursing practice and education. The ANA Code of Ethics for nurses states that nurses participate in the advancement of the profession through contributions to professional development in practice, education, administration, and knowledge development (ANA, 2001).

Professional development can be as specific as skills training or as broad as enhanced personal development (Cooper, 2009). It begins with basic nursing education and continues in the form of formal degrees, certifications, workshops, journal clubs, continuing education, in-services, and webinars. Nurses choose to develop knowledge through offerings related to specialty areas, or choose to expand upon leadership capabilities through education or mentorship devoted to the development of leadership skills.

Professional development is a requirement for maintaining licensure in many states. In some instances, state boards of nursing mandate continuing development related to specific subject matter, and recertification in many specialties requires knowledge acquisition and proof of continuing education.

To instill the value of lifelong learning in students, it is essential that lifelong learning that leads to professional development is introduced early in the nursing curriculum and maintained as a curricular thread throughout. Initially, baccalaureate students are introduced to professional development through courses and professional organizations; for example, the National Student Nurses Association. Courses in the undergraduate programs where professional development might be included are foundation and leadership courses. Graduate programs include courses in professional development and professional role application. Administrators in schools of nursing foster professional development for faculty by offering opportunities that support participation in professional nursing organizations, attendance at conferences and continuing education events, and by encouraging the attainment of certifications and advanced degrees.

SYNOPSIS

One question posed in the literature is determining whose responsibility it is to monitor professional development. Is it the responsibility of employers, professional organizations, state boards of nursing, or the individual nurse? The ANA (2011a) position statement for professional role competence states that it is not only the responsibility of the nurse to maintain professional competence, but it is also the responsibility of the nursing profession to shape and guide processes

for assuring competence. Furthermore, the employer holds accountability to provide an environment that is conducive to competent practice, and regulatory agencies define minimal standards for regulation of practice to protect the public (ANA, 2011b).

Considering that technological changes and the rate of knowledge acquisition are rapidly increasing in the 21st century, instilling the value of lifelong learning and professional development into students early in education programs is critical. Licensure examinations assure only minimum entry-level competence for professional nurses. Examination contents come from a retrospective model, and the newly licensed nurse has a likelihood of being dated (Huston, 2014). Educators in nursing are responsible for ensuring that students are made aware that knowledge acquisition and identifying one's own learning and development needs are continual expectations of the nursing profession, and that education does not end at graduation.

A culture that values and supports professional development may increase job satisfaction and foster job retention (Cooper, 2009). A national survey of nurses found that a large percentage of nurses who planned to leave nursing positions in the next 3 years responded that they would consider staying if more opportunities for professional development were offered by employers (Ulrich, Buerhaus, Donelan, Norman, & Dittus, 2005). Furthermore, retention is enhanced when professionals are provided with opportunities to expand their knowledge base and skills through preceptorships for students and residencies for graduates (Kearney-Nunnery, 2012). Emphasis in creating a culture in which nurses feel encouraged to grow professionally should be fostered in all health care settings.

Further study is warranted on improving methods of implementing professional development. Cooper (2009) proposes a milestone pathway tool for nurses designed to enhance professional development that is unique to the individual nurse and the specific nursing unit. The tool provides a

P

unit-specific concept map, a milestone pathway template, and a professional development plan. The goal in creating this tool is to avoid a "one size fits all" approach to professional development, and to ultimately affect nurse retention and satisfaction.

RECOMMENDATIONS

Nurses in all career paths need to be empowered to develop professionally. In nursing education, professional development is a concept that needs to be introduced early and continued as a curricular thread throughout the student's academic career. Professional development should be a shared responsibility fostered and promoted by regulatory agencies, organizations, employers, schools of nursing, and the individual nurse. There is a need for further research about the content and quality of nursing professional development, and the creation of better methods to determine how to measure learning and its translation into practice.

> Let us never consider ourselves finished nurses. We must be learning all of our lives.
> —Florence Nightingale

American Nurses Association (ANA). (2001). *Code of ethics for nurses with interpretative statements.* Retrieved from http://www.nursingworld.org/ethics/code/protected_nwcoe303.html

American Nurses Association (ANA). (2011a). *ANA position statement: Professional role competence.* Retrieved from http://gm6.nursingworld.org/MainMenuCategories/Policy-Advocacy/Positions-and Resolutions/ANAPositionStatements/Position-Statements-Alphabetically/Professional-role-Competence.html

American Nurses Association (ANA). (2011b). *Scope and standards of practice for nursing professional development.* Retrieved from http://ananursece.healthstream.com/pages/about.aspx

Cooper, E. (2009). Creating a culture of professional development: A milestone pathway tool for registered nurses. *The Journal of Continuing Education in Nursing, 40*(11), 501–508.

Huston, C. (2014). *Professional issues in nursing: Challenges and opportunities.* Philadelphia, PA: Lippincott Williams & Wilkins.

Kearney-Nunnery, R. (2012). *Advancing your career: Concepts of professional nursing.* Philadelphia, PA: F.A. Davis.

Magill-Cuerden, J. (2007). Leading and managing professional development-improving patient care. *Journal of Nursing Management, 12*(6), 563–566.

Ulrich, B., Buerhaus, P., Donelan, K., Norman, L., & Dittus, R. (2005). How RNs view the work environment: Results of a national survey of registered nurses. *Journal of Nursing Administration, 35*(9), 389–395.

Martha Summers

PROGRESSION TESTING

DEFINITION

Progression testing is the use of standardized tests in designated content areas to assess mastery of essential nursing content as students progress through a nursing curriculum. As a result of progression testing, students gain experience in taking a variety of challenging tests in content areas similar to those addressed by the National Council Licensure Examination for Registered Nurses (NCLEX-RN®). Thus, progression testing complements professor-prepared examinations that also prepare graduates for the NCLEX-RN (Mosser, Williams, & Wood, 2006).

APPLICATION

First-time pass rates on the NCLEX-RN are deemed important determinants of program quality by national accrediting agencies. In addition, graduates of nursing programs may not practice as registered nurses until passing the NCLEX-RN. The NCLEX test plan was revised in 2013 and the passing standard increased as well, reflecting the fact that safe and effective entry-level practice requires a greater level of knowledge, abilities, and skills, due to increased acuity levels of clients (National Council of State Boards of Nursing [NCSBN], 2013). Pressure to pass the NCLEX-RN on the first attempt is important to both nursing programs and graduates, and the NCLEX-RN has become a more challenging exam. Progression testing is one mechanism that can be employed to assist students in mastering and retaining content as they progress through a nursing program, contributing to successful NCLEX-RN pass rates.

The adoption of progression testing within a nursing program is a decision that should be made by the entire faculty, as so many aspects of the program will be affected: how the testing will be used within courses and between levels of the program; policies for the catalog, student handbook, and syllabi of affected courses; and decisions related to fees for testing. Commercially developed standardized assessment programs are available through educational testing and review companies such as Assessment Technologies Institute (ATI) and Elsevier's Health Education Systems, Inc. (HESI testing), with corresponding psychometric parameters for each program. Faculty members are responsible for investigating and selecting the standardized assessment program; determining passing, remediation, and progression policies; and developing an overall progression testing proposal for institutional approval prior to implementation of a progression testing program (Mosser et al., 2006).

SYNOPSIS

Progression testing provides the opportunity for students to test out of each level of a program to progress to the next, and then pass a standardized test to graduate. Utilization of computerized tests that mimic the NCLEX-RN provides additional practice for taking the NCLEX-RN. It is recommended that policies addressing progression testing provide an opportunity for students to review and focus on identified areas of weakness before retesting (Thomas & Baker, 2011). While comprehensive assessments administered at the end of programs are accurate in predicting success, they do not predict failure as well (Harding, 2010). Therefore, early identification of students with low knowledge acquisition is essential in helping them to acquire the necessary content and skills to successfully progress in a program of study (Emory, 2013; Holstein, Zangrilli, & Taboas, 2006).

RECOMMENDATIONS

The pressure for nursing programs to have successful NCLEX-RN pass rates is great, and schools have responded to the challenge in various ways. Morrison, Free, and Newman (2002) reported on seven schools that required a certain score on a designated comprehensive test in order to graduate or take the NCLEX-RN. Nibert, Young, and Britt (2003) examined 45 programs with progression policies and found that progression consequences existed for students who did not pass an end-of-program comprehensive assessment: denial of eligibility for graduation, a failing or incomplete grade in a capstone course, and/or denial of approval to take the NCLEX-RN. Several groups have expressed concern related to using a standardized test to block eligibility to take the NCLEX-RN, with the NLN referring to the practice as "high stakes" testing (Carr, 2011; National League for Nursing [NLN], 2012).

In response to concerns about the use of standardized testing, the NLN (2012) developed fair testing guidelines for faculty and administrators to implement. These guidelines: (a) ensure that tests and decisions based on tests are valid; (b) hold faculty responsible for assessing the abilities of students; (c) use multiple sources of evidence to evaluate basic nursing competence; (d) use tests not only for evaluative measurement, but to support student learning and guide program improvements; and (e) develop comprehensive testing policies that are made readily available to students, informing students as to the

P

purpose of the tests. These guidelines were developed to assist faculty in creating ethical progression policies.

Progression testing provides one mechanism to assist graduates of nursing programs to be successful in passing the NCLEX-RN on the initial attempt. Using progression testing throughout a program provides students with experience in taking NCLEX-RN-based examinations in specific content areas, assisting them to identify their own strengths and weaknesses, and remediating appropriately. Progression testing should not be done in isolation, but accompanied by other intervention strategies to promote students' success: study groups, tutoring, test-taking strategy sessions, and stress reduction techniques (Thomas & Baker, 2011). It is incumbent upon faculty members to regularly review and refine processes used to assess students, in the spirit of continuous quality improvement, and to report results in the literature.

Carr, S. (2011). NCLEX-RN pass rate peril: One school's journey through curriculum revision, standardized testing, and attitudinal change. *Nursing Education Perspectives, 32*(6), 384–388.

Emory, J. (2013). Standardized mastery content assessments for predicting NCLEX-RN outcomes. *Nurse Educator, 38*(2), 66–70.

Harding, M. (2010). Predictability associated with exit examinations: A literature review. *Journal of Nursing Education, 49*(9), 493–497.

Holstein, B., Zangrilli, B., & Taboas, P. (2006). Standardized testing tools to support quality educational outcomes. *Quality Management in Health Care, 15*(4), 300–308.

Morrison, S., Free, K., & Newman, M. (2002). Do progression and remediation policies improve NCLEX-RN pass rates? *Nurse Educator, 27*(2), 94–96.

Mosser, N., Williams, J., & Wood, C. (2006). The use of progression testing throughout nursing programs: How two colleges promote success on the NCLEX-RN. In M. H. Oermann & K. Heinrich (Eds.), *Annual review of nursing education* (Vol. 3, pp. 305–319). New York, NY: Springer Publishing.

National Council of State Boards of Nursing (NCSBN). (2013). *NCSBN board of directors (BOD) voted to raise the passing standard for the NCLEX-RN examination at its meeting on December 17, 2012.* Retrieved from https://www.ncsbn.org/4200.htm

National League for Nursing (NLN). (2012). *The fair testing imperative in nursing education.* New York, NY: Author.

Nibert, A., Young, A., & Britt, R. (2003). The HESI exit exam: Progression benchmark and remediation guide. *Nurse Educator, 28*(3), 141–145.

Thomas, M., & Baker, S. (2011). NCLEX-RN success: Evidence-based strategies. *Nurse Educator, 36*(6), 246–249.

Nancy R. Mosser

PSYCHOMOTOR SKILLS

DEFINITION

Psychomotor skills are movement-oriented activities that involve an overt physical response and mental processes.

APPLICATION

Psychomotor skill development requires understanding the skill and how to perform it, as well as developing the ability to carry out the physical movements accurately, efficiently, and consistently under varying conditions. There are key concepts to understand for teaching psychomotor skills in nursing. First, students should learn the theory and principles underlying the skill prior to practicing it, and assessment of their understanding of those principles should take place outside of the actual performance of the skill. In initial skill learning, students focus on coordinating their movements. If the teacher asks about principles, the focus shifts from the motor component to the cognitive, and this can impede learning. Second, skills require repetitive practice to refine performance, increase consistency, and develop skill automaticity. Considering the need for practice of psychomotor skills, educators should identify the skills that are used frequently in clinical practice, such as intravenous lines maintenance, tracheostomy management, and medication administration. Instruction should focus on those high-use skills and ensure that students have opportunities for repetitive practice of them (Oermann, 2011). This practice is best done in multiple short training sessions, spaced over time, rather than during one long block of time (Spruit, Band, Hamming, & Ridderinkhof, 2013). Third, in skill learning students need specific and informational feedback to guide their movements.

Simulation, as an instructional method, can mimic real experiences with guided experiences (Gaba, 2004). Psychomotor skills can be incorporated into simulation experiences to allow nursing students the opportunity to practice in the context of patient care. From the fundamental practice of sterile gloving to the more complex running of an emergency code, nursing students can learn through repetitive practice in a safe environment. Simulation encourages the deliberate practice of psychomotor skills.

SYNOPSIS

There are three phases of psychomotor skill learning: cognitive, associative, and autonomous (Schmidt & Lee, 2005). Students move through these phases by practicing. The first phase, cognitive, involves understanding the skill or procedure and how to perform it. Feedback to guide performance is critical in the cognitive phase. In the associative phase, students have learned the most effective way of performing the skill and begin to refine performance until it becomes consistent. With continued practice, they move into the autonomous phase where the skill performance is automatic (Schmidt & Lee, 2005).

Students need deliberate practice of skills to move through these phases of psychomotor skill development (Ericsson, Whyte, & Ward, 2007). In deliberate practice, the skill

is practiced repetitively, and students receive specific, informative feedback on their performance (Ericsson et al., 2007; McGaghie, Issenberg, Cohen, Barsuk, & Wayne, 2011). In identifying skills to teach in nursing programs, faculty should consider the need for deliberate practice to retain skills and develop competence. Skills taught early in a nursing program in a foundation or fundamentals course will probably not be retained without practice. A meta-analysis on skill retention found that some skills decay immediately after training and continue to decay over time; if not practiced or used for 1 year, most people perform at less than 92% of their original level (Arthur, Bennett, Stanush, & McNelly, 1998).

There are three domains of learning: cognitive, affective, and psychomotor, and taxonomies have been developed for instruction and assessment in each of these domains. A taxonomy of the psychomotor domain provides a framework for understanding the development of skills and deciding on the expected competency level for each skill. At the lowest level in the taxonomy is imitation learning, in which students observe a demonstration and imitate the performance. With practice, students can follow written instructions rather than having to observe the skill (manipulation level), perform it accurately (precision level) within a reasonable time (articulation level), and finally perform it automatically as a natural part of their patient care (naturalization; Oermann & Gaberson, 2014).

RECOMMENDATIONS

Nurse educators need to understand the phases of psychomotor skill learning and plan for the instruction of these skills, similar to their planning for knowledge acquisition and development of higher-level cognitive skills. Of the three domains of learning, much emphasis has been given in recent years to clinical reasoning, critical thinking, and other cognitive skills. Hagler and Morris (2015) suggested that in some teaching and learning situations, the psychomotor and affective aspects of learning are ignored or expected to develop without planned instruction. Faculty should identify psychomotor skills that are used frequently in clinical practice and for which students must develop their expertise; faculty must also ensure that students have opportunities for deliberate practice of these skills. In a study by Liou, Chang, Tsai, and Cheng (2013), skill reviews enabled nursing students to develop their competence.

An understanding of psychomotor skill development is also important for teachers in order to have appropriate expectations of students in the clinical setting. If students have limited practice after their initial learning, they may perform skills accurately but be slow and inconsistent. More research is needed on how best to teach psychomotor skills in nursing and to identify the most appropriate setting for learning and practicing skills.

Arthur, W., Bennett, W., Stanush, P. L., & McNelly, T. L. (1998). Factors that influence skill decay and retention: A quantitative review and analysis. *Human Performance, 11,* 57–101.

Ericsson, K. A., Whyte, J. IV., & Ward, P. (2007). Expert performance in nursing: Reviewing research on expertise in nursing within the framework of the expert-performance approach. *Advances in Nursing Science, 30*(1), E58–E71.

Gaba, D. M. (2004). The future vision of simulation in health care. *Quality and Safety in Health Care, 13*(Suppl 1), i2–i10.

Hagler, D., & Morris, B. (2015). Teaching methods. In M. H. Oermann (Ed.), *Teaching in nursing and role of the educator: The complete guide to best practice in teaching, evaluation, and curriculum development* (pp. 35–39). New York, NY: Springer Publishing.

Liou, S. R., Chang, C. H., Tsai, H. M., & Cheng, C. Y. (2013). The effects of a deliberate practice program on nursing students' perception of clinical competence. *Nurse Education Today, 33,* 358–363. doi:10.1016/j.nedt.2012.07.007

McGaghie, W. C., Issenberg, S. B., Cohen, M. E. R., Barsuk, J. H., & Wayne, D. B. (2011). Does simulation-based medical education with deliberate practice yield better results than traditional clinical education? A meta-analytic comparative review of the evidence. *Academic Medicine, 86,* 706–711. doi:10.1097/ACM.0b013e318217e119

Oermann, M. H. (2011). Toward evidence-based nursing education: Deliberate practice and motor skill learning. *Journal of Nursing Education, 50,* 63–64. doi:10.3928/01484834–20110120-01

Oermann, M. H., & Gaberson, K. B. (2014). *Evaluation and testing in nursing education* (4th ed.). New York, NY: Springer Publishing.

Schmidt, R. A., & Lee, T. D. (2005). *Motor control and learning: A behavioral emphasis* (4th ed.). Champaign, IL: Human Kinetics.

Spruit, E. N., Band, G. P. H., Hamming, J. F., & Ridderinkhof, K. R. (2013). Optimal training design for procedural motor skills: A review and application to laparoscopic surgery. *Psychological Research* (e-pub ahead of print). doi:10.1007/s00426–013-0525–5

Margory A. Molloy
Jacqueline Vaughn
Marilyn H. Oermann

PUBLIC COMMUNICATION

DEFINITION

Public communication is the process of sharing words or images in a public venue. Traditionally, it has included television, radio, and print media while excluding Internet-based social media. As the use and influence of social media have increased, public communication has evolved to include tools such as blogs, Facebook, and YouTube.

APPLICATION

Public communication is important to nursing education and practice in three major ways: as a process by which students and nurses define and describe the profession of nursing; as a strategy to enhance learning; and as a method for providing population-focused health education. One way that nurses use public communication is to define and describe their responsibilities and duties to the public. Even though providing nursing care is a private undertaking, clients, their families, health care providers, communities, journalists, and politicians are the public. Students should be prepared to describe the critical nature of their work to these individuals and groups.

Public communication strategies can be used to enhance more traditional methods of nursing education. Print media, television, and radio provide opportunities for students to analyze public messages about the profession, create health education campaigns, and examine professional and ethical dilemmas. Social media, including text messaging, blogs, Facebook, and YouTube, enable students to connect with peers, access "real time" information, process their experiences, and work with new concepts outside of the classroom setting. Nurse educators are beginning to integrate these media into the learning experience.

Both traditional and modern public communication strategies can be applied to the process of population-focused information sharing. Students working in community and public health settings can be encouraged to develop public health messages to disseminate via newspaper articles, radio public service announcements, and infographics. Students can be challenged to use social media in public information campaigns to improve health knowledge. By reviewing the scientific literature, students can identify the efficacy of public communication in changing health beliefs or behaviors.

SYNOPSIS

There are three key ideas in understanding public communication. The first is that public communication strategies are not used effectively by nurses to define their work. Buresh and Gordon (2013) described

the absence of nursing's voice and strategies for cultivating an effective public voice (Gordon, 2004). Kazis and Schwendimann (2009) documented a graduate-level elective in which students take on the roles of journalist, radio reporter, news producer, and conference organizer to learn public communication skills. Two public communication campaigns, the American Academy of Nursing's Raise the Voice campaign and the Robert Wood Johnson Foundation's The Future of Nursing Campaign for Action, can be used to increase students' understanding of the importance of communicating the salient elements of professional nursing to the public.

The second key idea is that social media is transforming public communication (Luzon, 2013). The results of this transformation are a blurring of the boundaries between students' public and private lives (Hoflich, 2006; VanDoorn & Eklund, 2013) and the blending of public and private audiences (Luzon, 2013). While the concepts of boundaries, access, and privacy are clear in television, radio, and the print media, they are not as easy to identify and comprehend in Internet-based communication. The National Council of State Boards of Nursing (2011) issued a white paper discussing the key issues of confidentiality and privacy as they related to the use of social media in the practice of nursing. These guidelines should be integrated at all levels of the nursing curriculum.

Use of public communication techniques also enhances nursing education. Traditional public communication strategies used to enhance learning include writing a health promotion newspaper column (McMillan & Raines, 2010); analyzing television shows (Weaver, Salamonson, Koch, & Jackson, 2013); and creating a school-based wellness radio program (Morton, 2008). Social media strategies include using the chat feature of Facebook to facilitate interaction with students (VanDoorn & Eklund, 2013) and using YouTube videos as the basis for NCLEX-style questions to increase learning in the affective domain (May, Wedgeworth, & Bigham, 2013). In addition, Skiba (2008) described

P

uses of Twitter including promoting student collaboration, providing new information, and connecting to the larger world. Roland, Johnson, and Swain (2011) documented that students used blogs to structure newly acquired nursing knowledge and develop a support network.

RECOMMENDATIONS

As the information age continues to develop, nurses will need a well-developed knowledge base that includes multiple public communication strategies. Many students are digital "natives" who have grown up with mass media, technology, and social media but are not aware of the inherent dangers and are inexperienced in the use of these media in a public venue. Nurse educators are obligated to guide students to an understanding of the requirements for responsible use of public communication strategies.

Nurse educators who are not well versed in public communication methodology should engage in professional development activities to build their understanding and expertise. Implementing innovative classroom strategies that use public communication strategies will guide students in their application of these strategies in describing their work and informing consumers. The impact of many of these media has not been widely researched. Future research efforts might include a focus on the efficacy of public communication modalities on the quality of nursing education, the extent of professional advocacy, and change in public health outcomes.

Buresh, B., & Gordon, S. (2013). *From silence to voice: What nurses know and must communicate to the public* (3rd ed.). Ithaca, NY: Cornell University Press.

Gordon, S. (2004). Nurses and public communication: Protecting definitional claims. *Journal of Nursing Management, 12,* 273–278.

Hoflich, J. R. (2006). The mobile phone and the dynamic between private and public communication: Results of an international exploratory study. *Knowledge, Technology & Policy, 19*(2), 58–68.

Kazis, C., & Schwendimann, R. (2009). Bringing nursing to the public. *Journal of Nursing Education, 48*(11), 42–47. doi: 10.3928/01484834–20090828-01

Luzon, M. J. (2013). Public communication of science in blogs: Recontextualizing scientific discourse for a diversified audience. *Written Communication, 30,* 428–457. doi: 10.1177/0741088313493610

May, O., Wedgeworth, M. G., & Bigham, A. B. (2013). Technology in nursing education: YouTube as a teaching strategy. *Journal of Pediatric Nursing, 28,* 408–410. doi: 10/1016/j.pedn.2013.04.004

McMillan, L. R., & Raines, K. (2010). Headed in the "write" direction: Nursing student publication and health promotion in the community. *Journal of Nursing Education, 49,* 418–421. doi: 10.3928/01484834–20100430-05

Morton, J. L. (2008). "I Feel Good!" A weekly wellness radio broadcast for elementary school children. *The Journal of School Nursing, 24*(2), 83–87.

National Council of State Boards of Nursing. (2011). *White paper: A nurse's guide to the use of social media.* Retrieved from https://www.ncsbn.org/Social_Media .pdf

Roland, E. J., Johnson, C., & Swain, D. (2011). Blogging as an educational enhancement tool for improved student performance: A pilot study in undergraduate nursing education. *New Review of Information Networking, 16,* 151–166. doi: 10.1080/13614576.2011.619923

Skiba, D. (2008). Nursing education 2.0: Twitter and tweets. *Nursing Education Perspectives, 29*(2), 110–112.

VanDoorn, G., & Eklund, A. A. (2013). Face to Facebook: Social media and teaching potential of symmetrical, synchronous communication. *Journal of University Teaching & Learning Practice, 10*(1). Retrieved from http://www.ro.uow.edu/ au/jutlp/vol10/iss1/6

Weaver, R., Salamonson, Y., Koch, J., & Jackson, D. (2013). Nursing on television: Student perceptions of television's role in public image, recruitment and education. *Journal of Advanced Nursing, 69,* 2635–2643. doi:10.1111/jan.12148

Susan B. Coyle

PUBLIC POLICY

DEFINITION

Public policy is purposive, goal-directed decisions of official policy makers at local, state, and federal levels that impact the general welfare of the public.

APPLICATION

The topic of public policy, specifically health policy and the role of the nurse as a policy advocate, is no longer in the "nice to know" category for nursing curricula. Developing and strengthening knowledge related to how governments are structured and the processes involved in enacting public policy are now a core competency for students and practicing nurses. Through evidence-based teaching strategies, students are encouraged to develop a voice to respond to public policies that impact health care delivery and the profession of nursing.

There are a number of teaching methods that can be used to engage and connect students with the topic of public policy as it relates to nursing and health care. Two goals, valuing the knowledge and developing a voice to express the knowledge, should guide frameworks for developing learning activities. For example, a framework consisting of presentation of information, learning activities, interpersonal interactions, and evaluation of learning can provide a focus for nurse educators teaching public policy content.

Presentation of information can be done using learning modules that contain behavioral outcomes, reading assignments, web links, slide presentations, videos, and other interactive technology, as well as application learning activities. Learning activities should facilitate students' choices in selecting the activity that best fits their individual learning needs and styles. Student-to-student and student-to-faculty interactions are at the core for meeting learning goals. One example of an interpersonal activity is "Talking Points Memo" whereby students write a memo that succinctly presents information related to a specific example of health policy and the intended and unintended consequences of the policy for health care consumers and/or the profession of nursing. Other students respond to the memo during in class discussions or in virtual classrooms using discussion boards or web and/or screen-casting technology. Faculty comments broaden awareness of the positive and negative impact of public policy on health care delivery and the vital role of nurse as policy advocate. A valuable outcome of this learning activity can be transformation of perspectives related to the policy advocate role.

An example of an experiential learning activity is attendance at state Nurses' Day at the Capitol events that are often sponsored by state nursing associations. These events allow students and practicing nurses the opportunity to practice and hone lobbying strategies. Talking with official policy makers fosters valuing of public policy and helps students gain voices for action.

SYNOPSIS

In the early 1990s, nurse leaders and professional organizations urged educators to include public policy content in nursing curricula. This appeal increased throughout the 2000s (Bowen, Lyons, & Young, 2000; Callahan, 2002; Conger & Johnson, 2000; Faulk & Ternus, 2004, 2006; Reutter & Williamson, 2000). Milio's (2002) visionary statement, "the future of policy-oriented

P

courses will depend on how important professional and academic leaders believe such courses are in preparing nurses to participate in shaping the policies and programs that can improve people's health and health services" (p. 7), has become a reality as today health policy and the role of the nurse as a policy advocate is essential content in baccalaureate and graduate programs.

Evidence to support best practices for integrating public policy information into nursing curriculum is limited and dated. Nurse educators have supported individual courses at baccalaureate and graduate levels (Buerhaus, 1992; Faulk & Ternus, 2006) and incorporation of public policy content into community health and/or leadership courses. There is some evidence to support effectiveness of individual courses in registered nurse (RN) to bachelor of science in nursing (BSN) programs and at graduate levels. Findings from a qualitative study to explore changes in perspectives of RN to BSN students regarding public policy from beginning to end of a public policy in nursing course (Faulk & Ternus, 2006) demonstrated an increased awareness of policy and process, the need for unity as a profession, and the professional role of the nurse including recognition of the need to function as an advocate, educator, and change agent.

Current literature continues to tout the importance of integrating political awareness into nursing programs (Hahn, 2010) and practicing nurses' obligation to enhance political acumen in community and legislative environments (Maryland & Gonzalez, 2012). Best education practices must continue to be explored to help students and practicing nurses value public policy knowledge in order to increase the cadre of politically astute professionals.

RECOMMENDATIONS

All public policy impacts the general welfare of the public. Nurse educators are obligated to health care consumers and to the nursing

profession to move students toward valuing their own role in the public policy process and to help students gain their voice for action. Nurse educators should test and create innovative teaching methods and strategies. The myriad of technology available for teaching in traditional and virtual classrooms must be carefully evaluated to best meet learning needs of diverse student populations and levels of nursing education. As technology considerations are made, educators must stay focused on learning rather than the technology. Seeking input and experiences from colleagues and stakeholders can provide nurse educators with valuable resources. For example, a number of professional nursing organizations at state and national levels have developed educator took kits that serve as guides for teaching public policy to student and practicing nurses.

Research studies are needed that are focused on identifying best methods for incorporating public policy into curricula. As nursing education research expands, educators must seek research initiatives that support evidence-based teaching innovations.

Bowen, M., Lyons, K. J., & Young, B. E. (2000). Nursing and health care reform: Implication for curriculum development. *Journal of Nursing Education, 39*(1), 27–33.

Buerhaus, P. (1992). Teaching health care public policy. *Nursing and Health Care Perspectives, 13*(6), 304–309.

Callahan, S. (2002). Incorporating a political action framework in a BSN program. *Journal of Nursing Education, 39*(1), 34–37.

Conger, C. O., & Johnson, P. (2000). Integrating political involvement and nursing education. *Nurse Educator, 25*(2), 99–103.

Faulk, D., & Ternus, M. (2004). Strategies for teaching public policy in nursing. *Nurse Educator, 29*(3), 99–102.

Faulk, D., & Ternus, M. (2006). Educating public policy advocates: A creative approach. In M. Obermann & K. Heinrich (Eds), *Annual Review of Nursing Education, 4*, 85–100.

Hahn, J. (2010). Integrating professionalism and political awareness into the curriculum. *Nurse Educator, 35*(1), 110–113.

Maryland, M. A., & Gonzalez, R. I. (2012). Patient advocacy in the community and legislative arena. *Online Journal of Issues in Nursing, 17*(1). doi:10.3912/OJIN. Vol117No01Man02

Milio, N. (2002). Building capacity for policy action: Educating today's and tomorrow's nurses. *Journal of Nursing Law, 8*(3), 7–18.

Reutter, L., & Williamson, D. L. (2000). Advocating health public policy: Implication for baccalaureate nursing education. *Journal of Nursing Educator, 39*(1), 21–26.

Debbie Faulk

Q

QUALITY AND SAFETY: QSEN

DEFINITION

Quality and safety are essential outcomes of nursing care. The Quality and Safety Education for Nurses (QSEN), a Robert Wood Johnson Foundation (RWJF), funded grants (2007–2012) and developed competencies (patient-centered care, team work and collaboration, safety, quality improvement, informatics, and evidence-based practice) and resources to accelerate the education of nurses in contemporary quality and safety concepts (QSEN.org). The goal of QSEN, now the QSEN Institute at Case Western Reserve University, is to ensure that all nurses have the knowledge, skills, and attitudes to continuously improve the quality and safety of the health care systems in which they work (Cronenwett et al., 2007, 2009).

APPLICATION

Quality and safety education requires an extension of current nursing education content that focuses on individualized plans of care to include systems of care and systems thinking (Dolansky & Moore, 2013). The QSEN competencies guide this shift, and the knowledge, skills, and attitudes are tailored for undergraduate education (Barton, Armstrong, Preheim, Gelmon, & Andrus, 2009) and graduate education (Pohl et al., 2009). The American Association of Colleges of Nursing (AACN) baccalaureate and doctoral essentials both include quality and safety as key competencies (www.aacn .nche.edu).

The application of quality and safety content occurs in academic and practice settings during the development of overall curricular programming including individual courses, teaching strategies, simulation scenarios, and clinical experiences (Armstrong, Spencer, & Lenburg, 2009). The application of quality and safety education content also occurs in academic clinical partnerships at the institutional (Didion, Kozy, Koffel, & Oneail, 2013), regional, or state levels (Disch, Barnsteiner, & McGuinn, 2013).

Evidence for the use of the QSEN framework is widespread. QSEN competencies are incorporated in nursing textbooks (Ignatavicius & Workman, 2013) and in books regarding quality and safety (Sherwood & Barnsteiner, 2012). Quality and safety competencies are incorporated into the National Council of State Boards of Nursing (NCSBN) nurse residency pilot programs (NCSBN, 2013) and educational programs delivered by professional specialty organizations such as the American Operating Room Nurses. In addition, many nursing models contain the QSEN competencies as an educational competency platform for practicing nurses (www .ohanet.org/wp-content/uploads/2013/03/ QSEN-White-Paper-3.21.13.pdf).

To assist with the integration of quality and safety principles in nursing education, the AACN provided regional Faculty Development Institutes for both baccalaureate and graduate level with the support of the RWJF. These workshops are available without cost and can be accessed from both the AACN and QSEN websites (Barnsteiner et al., 2013; Disch et al., 2013).

Q

SYNOPSIS

Quality and safety competencies can be taught in a variety of settings using many methods. Settings include the classroom, low- and high-fidelity simulation, and clinical setting. The QSEN website contains a database of teaching strategies that can be used in all settings. Teaching strategies are submitted by faculty across the country and peer reviewed. Simulation teaching strategies are available that use single to multiple simulations ranging from pediatrics to the aging adult (Sharpnack & Madigan, 2012). Classroom and clinical teaching strategies are described and evaluated for graduate-level nurses that include and nursing administration (Miltner, Patrician, Dawson, & Jukkala, 2012). In addition, QSEN teaching strategies have been published as root cause analysis (RCA), post-conference quality improvement initiatives, and a safety assessment tool.

A strategy to assist nursing schools to improve academic partnerships and facilitate the competencies of quality and safety is the dedicated education units (DEUs) or educational resource units. These units share the primary objective of developing students' competencies at the individual and organizational levels and emphasize contemporary quality and safety competencies (Didion et al., 2013). Pilot studies published on academic–clinical partnerships have demonstrated promising student outcomes in the facilitation of quality and safety (McKown, McKeon, McKown, & Webb, 2011).

Measurement of nurses' knowledge, skills, and attitudes of quality and safety in nursing education curricula is an important aspect of educational initiatives. Several psychometrically sound instruments have been developed to measure safety (Chenot & Daniel, 2010) and systems thinking (Dolansky & Moore, 2013).

RECOMMENDATIONS

Although progress has been made in quality and safety education in nursing, there are areas needed to accelerate impact. One area is to increase the number of psychometrically valid evaluation tools. This will provide the opportunity to compare data and benchmark progress across academic and clinical sites to determine what works and what does not. Instruments are needed to measure the knowledge, skills, and attitudes in all of the six QSEN competencies. Another area is to identify the essential components of formative and summative evaluation. This includes using research methods to demonstrate efficacy of educational efforts. There is a need to continue faculty development to ensure that all faculty have the capacity to teach quality and safety. Although the QSEN initiative started this work, there continues to be gaps in the capacity for faculty teaching quality improvement. Lastly, to accelerate quality and safety education it is necessary to include an emphasis on quality and safety education in ambulatory care, and long-term care. These additions will contribute to education on improving the patient experience of care, improving health of populations, and reducing per capita cost of health care.

Armstrong, G. E., Spencer, T. S., & Lenburg, C. B. (2009). Using quality and safety education for nurses to enhance competency outcome performance assessment: A synergistic approach that promotes patient safety and quality outcomes. *Journal of Nursing Education, 48*(12), 686–693.

Barnsteiner, J., Disch, J., Johnson, J., McGuinn, K., Chappell, K., & Swartwout, E. (2013). Diffusing QSEN competencies across schools of nursing: The AACN/RWJF Faculty Development Institutes. *Journal of Professional Nursing, 29*(2), 68–74.

Barton, A. J., Armstrong, G., Preheim, G., Gelmon, S. B., & Andrus, L. C. (2009). A national Delphi to determine developmental progression of quality and safety competencies in nursing education. *Nursing Outlook, 57*(6), 313–322.

Chenot, T. M., & Daniel, L. G. (2010). Frameworks for patient safety in the nursing curriculum. *Journal of Nursing Education, 49*(10), 559–568.

Cronenwett, L., Sherwood, G., Barnsteiner, J., Disch, J., Johnson, J., Mitchell, P., ... Warren, J. (2007). Quality and safety education for nurses. *Nursing Outlook, 55*(3), 122–131.

Cronenwett, L., Sherwood, G., Pohl, J., Barnsteiner, J., Moore, S., Sullivan, D. T., ... Warren, J. (2009). Quality and safety education for advanced nursing practice. *Nursing Outlook, 57*(6), 338–348.

Didion, J., Kozy, M. A., Koffel, C., & Oneail, K. (2013). Academic/clinical partnership and collaboration in Quality and Safety Education for Nurses education. *Journal of Professional Nursing, 29*(2), 88–94.

Disch, J., Barnsteiner, J., & McGuinn, K. (2013). Taking a "deep dive" on integrating QSEN content in San Francisco Bay Area Schools of Nursing. *Journal of Professional Nursing, 29*(2), 75–81.

Dolansky, M. A., & Moore, S. M. (2013). Quality and safety in nursing education: The key is systems thinking. *Online Journal of Issues in Nursing, 18*(3).

Ignatavicius, D. D., & Workman, L. M. (2013). *Medical surgical nursing* (7th ed.). Philadelphia, PA: Saunders Elsevier.

McKown, T., McKeon, L., McKown, L., & Webb, S. (2011). Using quality and safety education for nurses to guide clinical teaching on a new dedicated education unit. *Journal of Nursing Education, 50*(12), 706–710.

Miltner, R. S., Patrician, P. A., Dawson, M., & Jukkala, A. (2012). Incorporating quality and safety education into a nursing administration curriculum. *The Journal of Nursing Administration, 42*(10), 478–482.

National Council of State Boards of Nursing. (2013). *Transition to practice model.* Retrieved from http://www.ncsbn.org

Pohl, J. M., Savrin, C., Fiandt, K., Beauchesne, M., Drayton-Brooks, S., Scheibmeir, M., ... Werner, K. E. (2009). Quality and safety in graduate nursing education: Cross-mapping QSEN graduate competencies with NONPF's NP core and practice doctorate competencies. *Nursing Outlook, 57*(6), 349–354.

Sharpnack, P. A., & Madigan, E. A. (2012). Using low-fidelity simulation with sophomore nursing students in a baccalaureate nursing program. *Nursing Education Perspectives, 33*(4), 264–268.

Sherwood, G., & Barnsteiner, J. (Eds.). (2012). *Quality and safety in nursing: A competency approach to improving outcomes.* Hoboken, NJ: John Wiley & Sons, Inc.

Mary A. Dolansky
Dawn McMeekin

R

RECRUITMENT AND RETENTION OF MEN IN NURSING

DEFINITION

Recruitment refers to the process of attracting, screening, and selecting prospective students to a college. Retention is the ability of an institution to retain students through degree completion. Retention rate is the percentage of students who graduate compared to the number of students entering the program.

APPLICATION

Nursing lags behind other health professions in realizing gender parity (American Assembly for Men in Nursing [AAMN], 2013). A more gender inclusive and balanced nursing workforce is important and imperative for our profession. The footings for this begin with changing the perception of the profession of nursing from a female-oriented to a gender-neutral profession, in which men can thrive. Another important step is the review and possible redesign of the curriculum to ensure relevance to both male and female students. Finally, implementing a male-to-male mentorship program and recruiting more men faculty are effective strategies to retain men in nursing (O'Lynn & Tranbarger, 2007). Consequently, the nursing program leadership will need an intentional approach for change documented as a strategic priority with assigned responsibility, accountability, and resources.

Education administrators and faculty will need to make changes to retain men and increase nursing workforce gender diversity. Historically, the ability for nursing education to recruit and retain more men in school has been problematic. The evidence from the literature is clear about this: Nursing education has not made a concerted effort to attract and retain men (MacWilliams, Schmidt, & Bleich, 2013; O'Lynn, 2013; Roth & Coleman, 2008; Villeneuve, 1994). More specifically, attrition of men in nursing school is 15% to 85% and is far greater for men compared to women (Gilchrist & Rector, 2007). One study found that men were six times more likely than women to fail a nursing course (O'Lynn & Tranbarger, 2007).

Accrediting bodies for nursing programs (Accreditation Commission for Education in Nursing; Commission on Collegiate Nursing Education) have focused their attention on diversity in accreditation standards. The AAMN has developed a recognition program, the Excellence in Nursing Education Environments Supportive of Men, which can assist schools with accreditation activities. The AAMN recognition program offers a data-driven evidence-based methodology that nursing schools can implement to foster a gender-inclusive environment and retain male students at rates consistent with female students.

SYNOPSIS

The recruitment of men into nursing school and the retention of those students present major challenges. Several studies have revealed issues that affect recruitment and retention of men in nursing schools, including lack of awareness regarding the opportunities in nursing; nursing as a career choice for men (Bullough, 1994;

Kelly, Shoemaker, & Steele, 1996; LaRocco, 2004); the traditionally feminine imagery of nursing (Evans, 1997; MacPhail, 1996; MacWilliams et al., 2013, Villeneuve, 1994); the image of men nurses as effeminate or homosexuals (MacWilliams et al., 2013; O'Lynn & Tranbarger, 2007); role stress (MacWilliams et al., 2013); questions of male touch (MacWilliams et al., 2013); questions of men as caring, compassionate, and gentle (MacWilliams et al., 2013; Villeneuve, 1994); and the word *nurse* itself (Villeneuve, 1994).

With the launch of the Future of Nursing Campaign for Action, the AAMN established the 20 × 20 Choose Nursing campaign as a national initiative to increase the percent of men in nursing schools across the country to 20% by the year 2020 (AAMN, 2014). Progress in this area is being demonstrated. The enrollment of men in nursing programs has essentially doubled from 6% in 1986 to 11.8% in 2011 (American Association of Colleges of Nursing, 2012). A more recent survey found that men in nursing school enrollment improved slightly to 14% in baccalaureate programs and 15% in both diploma and associate degree programs (National League for Nursing, 2013).

RECOMMENDATIONS

Recruitment and retention of men in the nursing profession is essential. Men add value to patient care and outcomes, provide unique contributions as health care team members, and offer an expanded labor supply. Successful recruitment of men into nursing is dependent on a collaborative effort from the nursing profession, nursing schools, employers, government agencies, and marketers (O'Lynn & Tranbarger, 2007).

Nursing education strategies worthy of consideration are as follows: (a) Make the recruitment and retention of men in the nursing school a strategic priority; (b) develop gender-neutral policies and practices that promote balanced, gender-inclusive educational experiences, textbooks, websites, and nursing-school brochures and advertisement; (c) develop instructional designs that allow for diversity in learning preferences. Male nursing students often express a preference for learning activities that are hands-on, kinesthetic, and task oriented. Other male students may find mildly competitive or peer-directed activities as motivators for learning; (d) increase the number of male nursing faculty including adjuncts, instructors, advisers, and/or mentors; (e) utilize an evidence-based mentoring program for male students as well as providing them the opportunities to work with male nurses in the clinical setting; (f) include in the curriculum a balanced, accurate, historical perspective of the contributions of men to the nursing profession and their care and caring behaviors; (g) Reposition nursing as a gender-neutral profession, which has evolved to include significant clinical responsibilities over the past years; (h) educate middle-school and high-school guidance counselors regarding nursing career opportunities for their male students; and (i) encourage the formation of, or active participation with, local chapters of the AAMN as this is the only organization for students and nurses with a singular purpose of fostering gender diversity through inclusion in nursing schools and the nursing profession.

American Assembly for Men in Nursing (AAMN). (2013). *Excellence in nursing education environments supportive of men.* Retrieved from http://aamn.org/docs/SchoolExcellenceDraft.pdf

American Assembly for Men in Nursing (AAMN). (2014). *20 x 20 choose nursing.* Retrieved from http://aamn.org/choosenursing.shtml

American Association of Colleges of Nursing. (2012). *New AACN data show enrollment surge in baccalaureate and graduate programs amid calls for more highly educated nurses.* Retrieved from http://www.aacn.nche.edu/news/articles/2012/enrollment-data

Bullough, V. L. (1994). Men, women, and nursing history. *Journal of Professional Nursing, 19*(3), 127.

Evans, J. (1997). Men in nursing issues of gender segregation and hidden advantage. *Journal of Advanced Nursing, 26,* 226–231.

Gilchrist, K. L., & Rector, C. (2007). Can you keep them? Strategies to attract and retain nursing students from diverse populations: Best practices in education. *Journal of Transcultural Nursing, 18,* 277–285. Retrieved from http://dx.doi .org/10.1177/1043659607–301305.

Kelly, N. R., Shoemaker, M., & Steele, T. (1996). The experience of being a male student nurse. *Journal of Nursing Education, 35,* 170–174.

LaRocco, S. A. (2004). *Policies and practices that influence recruitment and retention of men in nursing: A grounded theory study of socializing men into nursing.* Unpublished doctoral dissertation, University of Massachusetts, Boston, MA.

MacPhail, J. (1996). Men in nursing. In J. R. Kerr & J. MacPhail (Eds.), *Canadian nursing: Issues and perspectives* (pp. 74–81, 3rd ed.). St. Louis, MO: Mosby-Yearbook.

MacWilliams, B. R., Schmidt, B., & Bleich, M. R. (2013). Men in nursing: Understanding the challenges men face working in this predominantly female profession. *American Journal of Nursing, 113,* 38–44. Retrieved from http://journals.lww.com/ ajnonline/Fulltext/2013/01000/Men_in_ Nursing.26.aspx.

National League for Nursing. (2013). *Annual survey of schools of nursing, Fall 2012.* Retrieved from http//www.nln.org/ research/slides/index.htm

O'Lynn, C. E. (2013). *A man's guide to a career in nursing.* New York, NY: Springer Publishing Company.

O'Lynn, C. E., & Tranbarger, R. (2007). *Men in nursing: History, challenges, and opportunities.* New York, NY: Springer Publishing Company.

Roth, J. E., & Coleman, C. L. (2008). Perceived and real barriers for men entering nursing: Implications for gender diversity. *Journal of Cultural Diversity, 15,* 148–152.

Villeneuve, M. J. (1994). Recruiting and retaining men in nursing: A review of the literature. *Journal of Professional Nursing, 10,* 217–228.

Reynaldo R. Rivera
William T. Lecher

REFLECTIVE WRITING

DEFINITION

Reflective writing is an assignment that involves the deliberate and recursive contemplation of thoughts, feelings, and interactions about significant clinical experiences that results in self-awareness and improved practice (Asselin, Schwartz-Barcott, & Osterman, 2013; Kennison & Misselwitz, 2002). As such, reflective writing proffers a unique and complex mode of thinking.

APPLICATION

Faculty can encourage students' critical thinking skills, as well as their metacognition—thinking about thinking—through the use of reflective writing as a pedagogical strategy. Although similarities exist among academic writing, narrative pedagogy, and writing programs (writing across the curriculum, writing in the disciplines, and writing to learn), there are distinct differences. For instance, narrative pedagogy entails openly sharing practice experiences, whereas reflective writing about practice experiences is intended to be a confidential dialogue among trusted teachers or mentors. Students may be asked, but not required, to share their reflective writing. In initiating reflective writing as pedagogy, it is important for faculty to clarify the purpose of the assignment, describe the reflective process, and ensure confidentiality of submitted work.

Most experts purport that the process of reflection, the starting point for reflective writing, incorporates three dynamic stages: awareness of unsettling or surprising thoughts and feelings, critical analysis of the situation, and development of a new perspective (Freshwater, 2008; Regmi & Naidoo, 2013). For instance, in the first stage, a medication error may prompt the student to worry about the patient's response and anxiety or guilt about making the mistake. Following along in stage two, the student analyzes the

R

sequence of steps leading to the error and interactions during that time, trying to figure out how the error happened. In stage three, the student learns what practice change will prevent a recurrence of the mistake.

There are several models of varying complexity that systematically guide students' reflection and reflective writing through steps, cycles, or cue questions. Baker's (1996) semi-structured four-step model works well with students who are new to the reflective writing process (Kennison, 2012). A more challenging model is Johns's (2004) Structured Reflective Cycle (SRC) that provides cue questions pertaining to Carper's (1978) four patterns of knowing: ethical, personal, aesthetic, and empirical. A fifth pattern, reflectivity, has been added. A more recent model (Kim, LauzonClabo, Burbank, Leveillee, & Martins, 2010), Critical Reflective Inquiry (CRI), uses cue questions to guide students through three distinct interrelated phases, processes, and outcomes. In so doing, the CRI model shows three progressive depths of thinking: descriptive, reflective, and critical. While one model of reflection has not been found to be more effective than another, reflective models to guide faculty-developed cue questions may structure the writing and, therefore, facilitate learning.

SYNOPSIS

Reflecting on, and writing about, significant practice experiences helps students connect theory with practice (Langley & Brown, 2010), articulate everyday ethical comportment, and learn from successes and mistakes (Benner, Sutphen, Leonard, & Day, 2010). Students report that reflective writing makes them think, analyze, and improve their practice; offers a record of practice experiences; and provides a platform for expression (Hong & Chew, 2008). Reflecting on practice is fostered when students have one or two patient assignments as opposed to larger patient assignments (Benner et al., 2010). Over time and with practice, students achieve higher levels of reflection (Ip et al., 2012; Langley

& Brown, 2010) with the goal of continually improving practice.

While reflective writing is recognized as effective pedagogy, there is a dearth of research on learning outcomes on reflective writing. A recent experimental study (Naber & Wyatt, 2014) used a pretest–posttest design to compare the effects of a reflective writing intervention on the critical thinking skills and dispositions of baccalaureate nursing students. After a 6-week reflective writing intervention, the experimental group's posttest scores showed a significant increase in the truth-seeking subscale of critical thinking dispositions when compared to the control group. In an earlier descriptive study, Kennison (2006) found a positive correlation between teacher ratings of baccalaureate students' reflective writings and the students' critical thinking scores.

Taylor-Haslip (2010) found that students' levels of reflection evidenced in their writing correlated with clinical performance and examination scores. In a related study, researchers used a 4-week reflective writing strategy to determine whether the level of reflection improved (Ip et al., 2012). Results indicated a significant difference in frequency and percentage of higher levels of reflection between baseline and posttests (Ip et al., 2012). In a 3-week continuing education program using reflective writing of clinical situations, participants demonstrated a significant increase in self-reflection scores (Asselin & Fain, 2013).

In a recent study, faculty and graduate students agreed that reflective journal writing in an online graduate course enabled self-awareness of attitudes, strengths/weaknesses, personal meaning, and understanding of problems from others' perspectives (Langley & Brown, 2010). Survey results support previous findings that lack of time for students to reflect and for faculty to grade the reflection were common barriers. Designating time for students to reflectively write during their scheduled clinical experience is recommended to lessen this concern (Hong & Chew, 2008) and facilitate direct teacher feedback for students' questions.

Barriers to effective reflective writing have been noted in the literature. Students may write what they believe the teacher wants to hear, deliberately omitting errors and problematic behavior for fear of lower grades. However, students need a safe haven to reflect about their own and others' practice mistakes (Benner et al., 2010; Kennison, 2012) without fear of negative grading consequences. Experts recommend that reflective writing not be used as a means of assessing students' clinical performance. Faculty identified grading reflective writing as problematic and a barrier to using the strategy (Langley & Brown, 2010). Rather than assigning a grade, the reflective writing may be evaluated for *process* and level of reflection (Kennison, 2012). Time constraints remain a common problem for students (Ip et al., 2012; Kennison, 2012; Langley & Brown, 2010) who prefer shorter writing assignments. Knowing that reflective writing about complex clinical experiences takes time and practice, the teacher may be at odds trying to satisfy students with short writing assignments insufficient for developing depth of thinking. However, shorter writing assignments at the onset of reflective writing across a nursing program may well be appropriate for students new to the writing process. Additionally, graduate students in an online course identified lack of trust in those reading their reflective writing as a detriment (Langley & Brown, 2010).

Reflective writing may conjure anxiety and vulnerability as students open themselves to expressing their deepest feelings about emotionally laden practice experiences. The teacher or facilitator needs to openly support students in a nonjudgmental way. Developing reflective writing as effective pedagogy depends on faculty development on how to use the strategy, clearly delineated purpose and expectations, dialogical feedback focusing on process, and confidentiality in a trusting supportive environment (Kennison, 2012).

RECOMMENDATIONS

While there is widespread use of reflective writing and the literature supports its value as a pedagogical strategy, there is a paucity of research on resultant outcomes, specifically on practice changes. Additionally, there is little empirical evidence that any one model or method is most effective in facilitating reflective writing (Asselin & Fain, 2013). Finally, best practices in facilitating and evaluating reflective writing added to the nurse educator's repertoire of teaching skills.

Asselin, M. E., & Fain, J. A. (2013). Effect of reflective practice education on self-reflection, insight, and reflective thinking among experienced nurses. *Journal for Nurses in Professional Development, 29*, 111–119.

Asselin, M. E., Schwartz-Barcott, D., & Osterman, P. A. (2013). Exploring reflection as a process embedded in experienced nurses' practice: A qualitative study. *Journal of Advanced Nursing, 69*(4), 905–914.

Baker, C. R. (1996). Reflective learning: A teaching strategy for critical thinking. *Journal of Nursing Education, 35*, 19–22.

Benner, P., Sutphen, M., Leonard, V., & Day, L. (2010). *Educating nurses: A call for radical transformation.* San Francisco, CA: Jossey-Bass.

Carper, B. A. (1978). Fundamental patterns of knowing in nursing. *Advances in Nursing Science, 1*(1), 13–24.

Freshwater, D. (2008). Reflective practice: The state of the art. In D. Freshwater, B. J. Taylor, & G. Sherwood (Eds.), *International textbook of reflective practice in nursing* (pp. 1–18). West Sussex, UK: Wiley-Blackwell.

Hong, L. P., & Chew, L. (2008). Reflective practice from the perspective of the bachelor of nursing students in International Medical University (IMU). *Singapore Nursing Journal, 35*(3), 5–15.

Ip, W. Y., Lui, M. H., Chien, W. T., Lee, I. F., Lam, L. W., & Lee, D. T. (2012). Promoting self-reflection in clinical practice among Chinese nursing undergraduates in Hong Kong. *Contemporary Nurse, 41*(2), 253–262.

Johns, C. (2004). *Becoming a reflective practitioner* (2nd ed.). Oxford, UK: Blackwell.

Kennison, M. (2006). The evaluation of students' reflective writing for evidence of critical thinking. *Nursing Education Perspectives, 27*, 269–273.

Kennison, M. (2012). Developing reflective writing as effective pedagogy. *Nursing Education Perspectives, 33,* 306–311.

Kennison, M., & Misselwitz, S. (2002). Evaluating reflective writing for appropriateness, fairness and consistency. *Nursing Education Perspectives, 23,* 238–242.

Kim, H. S., LauzonClabo, L. M., Burbank, P., Leveillee, M., & Martins, D. (2010). Application of critical reflective inquiry in nursing education. In N. Lyons (Ed.), *Handbook of reflective inquiry: Mapping a way of knowing for professional reflective inquiry* (pp. 159–172). New York, NY: Springer.

Langley, M. E., & Brown, S. T. (2010). Perceptions of the use of reflective learning journals in online graduate nursing education. *Nursing Education Perspectives, 3,* 12–17.

Naber, J., & Wyatt, T. H. (2014). The effect of reflective writing interventions on the critical thinking skills and dispositions of baccalaureate nursing students. *Nurse Education Today, 34,* 67–72.

Regmi, K., & Naidoo, J. (2013). Understanding the processes of writing papers reflectively. *Nurse Researcher, 20*(6), 33–39.

Taylor-Haslip, V. (2010). Guided reflective journals depict a correlation to the academic success of nursing students. *Teaching and Learning in Nursing, 5,* 68–72.

Monica Metrick Kennison

REMEDIATION

DEFINITION

Remediation is the act or process of correcting a fault or deficiency (*American Heritage Dictionary*, 2009). Remediation in nursing education is the process by which review and reinforcement of the material covered during instructing can be performed in such a way so as to improve the learners' understanding and application of the information (Reinhardt, Keller, Ochart Summers, & Schultz, 2012).

APPLICATION

Remediation in nursing education can take a number of forms. As an avenue for review of content covered in a didactic setting, the remediation can be an additional lecture, a question-and-answer review, a practice test and multiple questions, an oral presentation to peers, or a paper presented to the instructor.

To review and correct a clinical practice situation, the skills learning laboratory is an apt place for remediation, thus keeping patients safe until the skill is mastered. Practice is a form of remediation when the skill is witnessed and corrected by an instructor, practitioner, or peer. In essence, remediation in nursing education is the reteaching or review of content previously given in course instruction. Student concerns during remediation activities are an excellent opportunity to clarify content and expand the learner's understanding of the topic.

SYNOPSIS

The use of remediation has been a solid tool used during instruction activities since the inception of nursing education. Content and skills are taught, demonstrated, return demonstrated, corrected, and retaught. The skills check-off is in essence the final step in instruction and is a document that verifies remediation.

Of recent concern is the efficacy of remediation in preparation of nursing students for standardized progression, exit examinations, and National Council Licensure Examination-Registered Nurse (NCLEX-RN®) licensing examination. Research demonstrates that progression and exit examinations can predict NCLEX-RN success. There are numerous reports in nursing education literature describing remediation programs developed to assist students with success on the NCLEX-RN (Bonis, Taft, & Wendler, 2007; Frith, Sewell, & Clark, 2005; Heroff, 2009; McGann & Thompson, 2008; Mills, Wilson, & Bar, 2001; Morrison, Free, & Newman, 2008; Sifford & McDaniel, 2007). A set of best practices for remediation can be synthesized from this literature. Common to these reports was a structured approach to remediation delivered through a faculty-facilitated specialized course. Using best practices as described in the nursing literature, individualized remediation plans are created and address the barriers to success for each student. A systemic review by Pennington and Spurlock (2010) offers an empiric model of evaluation as the gold standard for the development and evaluation of a remediation course. Also, common in these reports is the need to address individualized student needs. To accomplish this, each student is asked to identify strengths and weaknesses and develop a personal plan of study for remediation. Test-taking strategies, measures to alleviate test anxiety and improve self-confidence, and learning to read and answer NCLEX-style questions are also a part of many of these programs.

The effect of low self-esteem can complicate remediation and plays a critical role in the remediation process. The faculty member must be able to provide both mentorship and motivation to students who are quite likely suffering from a lack of self-esteem and confidence. At the same time, the faculty must also encourage students to take control of their own learning to meet their identified learning goals. In a situation where each individual represents a unique combination of strengths and needs, a remediation approach has to be tailored to serve the interests of the individual student (Reinhardt et al., 2012).

RECOMMENDATIONS

While content review for specific areas of nursing knowledge is included in most remediation programs, this is not the sole focus of remediation activities. Test-taking strategies, measures to alleviate test anxiety and improve self-confidence, and learning to read and answer NCLEX-style questions are also a part of many of these programs. Using best practices as described in the literature, a faculty-facilitated remediation course can

be established with the goal of assisting students to determine their own learning goals, create individualized remediation plans, and address barriers to success (Reinhardt et al., 2012).

American Heritage Dictionary. (2009). *The American Heritage® Dictionary of the English Language* (4th ed.). (2009). Boston, MA: Houghton Mifflin Company.

Bonis, S., Taft, L., & Wendler, M. C. (2007). Strategies to promote success on the NCLEX-RN: An evidence-based approach using the ACE Star Model of Knowledge Transformation. *Nursing Education Perspectives, 28*(2), 82–87.

Frith, K. H., Sewell, J. P., & Clark, D. J. (2005). Best practices in NCLEX-RN readiness preparation for baccalaureate student success. *Computers, Informatics, Nursing, 23*(6), 322–329.

Heroff, K. (2009). Guidelines for a progression and remediation policy using standardized tests to prepare associate degree nursing students for the NCLEX-RN at a rural community college. National Council Licensure Examination-Registered Nurse. *Teaching & Learning in Nursing, 4*(3), 79–86.

McGann, E., & Thompson, J. M. (2008). Factors related to academic success in at-risk senior nursing students. *International Journal of Nursing Education Scholarship, 5,* Article 19.

Mills, L. W., Wilson, C. B., & Bar, B. B. (2001). A holistic approach to promoting success on NCLEX-RN. *Journal of Holistic Nursing, 19*(4), 360–374.

Morrison, S., Free, K. W., & Newman, M. (2008). Do progression and remediation policies improve NCLEX-RN pass rates? Reprinted with permission from *Nurse Educator, 31*(3), 54s–56s.

Pennington, T. D., & Spurlock, D. (2010). A systematic review of the effectiveness of remediation interventions to improve NCLEX-RN pass rates. *Journal of Nursing Education, 49*(9), 485–492.

Reinhardt, A. C., Keller, T., Ochart Summers, L., & Schultz, P. (2012). Strategies for

R

success: Crisis management model for remediation of at-risk students. *Journal of Nursing Education, 51*(6), 305–311.

Sifford, S., & McDaniel, D. M. (2007). Results of a remediation program for students at risk for failure on the NCLEX exam. *Nursing Education Perspectives, 28*(1), 34–36.

Anita C. Reinhardt

RESEARCH COURSE

DEFINITION

Research is a scientific process of systematic inquiry or study to validate and refine existing knowledge and to develop new knowledge in a discipline (Polit & Beck, 2012). Research constitutes the empirical and scientific body of nursing science.

APPLICATION

Research is a challenging course to teach. The complexity of teaching a research course is related to creating methods to actively engage students. Furthermore, incorporating three major sciences—ethics, statistics, and nursing theory—adds to the complexity. The evidence-based practice (EBP) and translational research movements in health sciences have emphasized the role of research in education and practice and guided the course structure and teaching methods.

The nursing program should be structured to ensure that students at all levels attain different research competencies (American Association of Colleges of Nursing [AACN], 2006). For example, undergraduate students should be taught to analyze and apply evidence. In teaching research with graduate students, emphasis should be on critical appraisal and synthesis of the research finding to identify best practices for specific patient populations.

This means all students will be critical consumers of research. Critical consumers determine credibility and applicability to practice. The AACN *Position Statement on Nursing Research* identified the competencies for different levels of nursing programs (AACN, 2006).

It is important to clarify the difference between the skills taught in a research course and those skills needed for EBP. The ultimate goal of EBP is to integrate the best available evidence into practice. Models are available to guide incorporation of evidence into nursing practice (Newhouse, Dearholt, Poe, Pugh, & White, 2007; Titler et al., 2001).

SYNOPSIS

Different experiential learning techniques have been used to teach research in nursing and health sciences (Sowan & Jenkins, 2013; Stern, 2005; Tsai, Cheng, Chang, & Liou, 2014). These include developing research questions for different research designs using the PICOT format; writing an integrative literature review; engaging students in the research process through conducting interviews and data collection; analyzing data collected from or by students; critically appraising of quantitative and qualitative studies; writing a research proposal; interacting with expert researchers who are invited as guest speakers; and presenting posters.

In addition, educators have taught the research course using EBP projects as a successive multipart assignment built on identifying a practice problem and ending with writing a recommendation for practice (Sowan & Jenkins, 2013). Other effective trends in teaching the research course include collaboration with an academic librarian to teach information literacy skills, group-focused collaborative learning activities, service-learning projects, participating in journal clubs, and joint assignments with a corequisite clinical course (August-Brady & Adamshick, 2013; McCurry & Martins, 2010; Sowan & Jenkins, 2013).

RECOMMENDATIONS

It is recommended that consideration be given to teaching research as an interdisciplinary course. In an interdisciplinary course, groups of health professionals can focus on creating evidence for a particular patient population, thus enhancing interprofessional collaboration. Strategies for creatively engaging students in the research course should be created, used, and evaluated, thus promoting active learning. Research should be taught within the framework of lifelong learning and be integrated throughout the nursing curriculum.

American Association of Colleges of Nursing (AACN). (2006). *AACN position statement on nursing research*. Retrieved from http://www.aacn.nche.edu/publications/position/NsgResearch.pdf

August-Brady, M., & Adamshick, P. (2013). Oh, the things you will learn: Taking undergraduate research to the homeless shelter. *Journal of Nursing Education, 52*(6), 342–345.

McCurry, M. K., & Martins, D. C. (2010). Teaching undergraduate nursing research: A comparison of traditional and innovative approaches for success with millennial learners. *Journal of Nursing Education, 49*(5), 276–279.

Newhouse, R. P., Dearholt, S., Poe, S., Pugh, L. C., & White, K. (2007). *Johns Hopkins nursing evidence-based practice model and guidelines*. Indianapolis, IN: Sigma Theta Tau International.

Polit, D., & Beck, C. T. (2012). *Nursing research: Generation and assessing evidence for nursing practice* (9th ed.). Philadelphia, PA: Lippincott Williams & Wilkins.

Sowan, A. K., & Jenkins, L. (2013). Use of the seven principles of effective teaching to design and deliver an interactive hybrid nursing research course. *Nursing Education Perspectives, 34*(5), 31–38.

Stern, P. (2005). A holistic approach to teaching evidence-based practice. *American Journal of Occupational Therapy, 59*(2), 157–164.

Titler, M. G., Kleiber, C., Steelman, V. J., Rakel, B. A., Budreau, G., Everett, L. Q.,...Goode, C. J. (2001). The Iowa model of evidence-based practice to promote quality care. *Critical Care Nursing Clinics of North America, 13*(4), 497–509.

Tsai, H., Cheng, C., Chang, C., & Liou, S. (2014). Preparing the future nurses for nursing research: A creative teaching strategy for RN-to-BSN students. *International Journal of Nursing Practice, 20*(1), 25–31.

Azizeh Sowan

RESEARCH ETHICS

DEFINITION

Research ethics is the application of fundamental ethical principles to ensure that research is conducted in a morally acceptable and responsible manner. Ethical issues can arise at any time during the research process from the initial design of the study to data collection, analysis, and publication (Aita & Richer, 2005).

APPLICATION

All health care workers practicing in a modern evidence-based culture should have an appreciation of the ethics that underpin rigorous research (Bowater & Wilkinson, 2012). An understanding of research ethics is imperative for all practicing nurses and therefore should be explicitly included in modern nursing curricula. Students need to learn the background, theory, and skills associated with ethically acceptable research. Case studies and role-play are recommended teaching strategies for helping students actively participate in discussions based on applying ethics to complex human situations (Bowater & Wilkinson, 2012; Eisen & Berry, 2002).

R

SYNOPSIS

Violations of human rights by research in the 20th century emphasized the need for ethical standards that should be adhered to when conducting research (Aita & Richer, 2005). The Nuremberg Code (1947) highlighted issues of informed consent, freedom from coercion, and the assurance that there is an appropriate risk–benefit ratio for the participant. The Declaration of Helsinki (1964), and its subsequent amendments, was developed to address the ethical principles for medical research and included the issue of children and individuals who could not give voluntary consent. The Belmont Report (1974) addressed the three fundamental principles underlying the acceptable conduct of research involving human participants: respect for persons, beneficence, and justice. In present-day research, the main ethical procedures that need to be adhered to in conducting research are informed consent, risk–benefit assessments, confidentiality, anonymity, and data protection.

Informed consent involves ensuring that participants are given adequate, clearly understandable information about the research and risk–benefits involved in participation. Participants must also be given the choice to consent voluntarily to participate in the research or decline participation without any consequences (Polit & Beck, 2006). The five elements of informed consent are competence, disclosure, understanding, voluntariness, and consent (Beauchamp & Childress, 2001). In nursing research, there are challenges to this process in terms of protecting vulnerable groups. Examples of vulnerable groups include children, the elderly, and people with cognitive impairment. Research involving vulnerable participants must be conducted in a sensitive, ethical manner with full awareness of the participants' capacity and consent.

Furthermore, when nursing research uses qualitative methodologies, there are implications for consent arising primarily from the problem and population being studied (Houghton, Casey, Shaw, & Murphy, 2010). Researchers may not be able to accurately predict the course of the research process from the outset, and may be required to negotiate and revise the research protocol for the duration of the study (Munhall, 1988).

To adhere to the principle of beneficence, the risk–benefit ratio of participating in the research must be explicated. The researcher is responsible to make it clear to the subject what potential harm may occur as a result of participation, as well as the potential benefits for the subject. Furthermore, the language of the risk–benefit ratio to the participant must be written at a level that can be understood. For nurses engaging in research, they must consider the relationship they may have with participants (Orb, Eisenhauer, & Wynaden, 2001), and also their dual role as both nurse and researcher (Casey, 2004; Houghton et al., 2010).

Issues of confidentiality and data protection are of utmost importance in research ethics. In quantitative research, assurance of anonymity should be made, whereby even the researcher is not able to identify the participants in the study (Polit & Beck, 2006). In qualitative research, even though the researcher knows the participant, anonymity is completely preserved. Data protection refers to the storage, safekeeping, retention, destruction, or reuse of personal data in research. There are international and country-specific guidelines on how data should be stored securely and for how long. It is imperative that researchers comply with these guidelines to safeguard the privacy of participants.

RECOMMENDATIONS

Educators in nursing need to ensure that students and qualified nurses are equipped to recognize and understand the ethical implications for health care. Nurse researchers need to be cognizant of the principles that guide ethical decisions in the research process. Understanding the specific implications for research with human participants, particularly vulnerable populations, and the differences between qualitative and quantitative research are essential. Practicing nurses need to know how to ensure that patients are being treated in an ethical and respectful manner by researchers entering the clinical setting. Case studies and role-play have been recognized as a potential strategy for developing ethical knowledge and skills. Furthermore, encouraging students to read and critique research reports could be considered as a valuable means for assessing their understanding of ethics in nursing research.

Aita, M., & Richer, M. C. (2005). Essentials of research ethics for healthcare professionals. *Nursing & Health Sciences, 7*(2), 119–125.

Beauchamp, T. L., & Childress, J. F. (2001). *Principles of biomedical ethics* (5th ed.). New York, NY: Oxford University Press.

The Belmont Report. (1974). *Ethical principles and guidelines for the protection of human subjects of research.* Retrieved from http://www.hhs.gov/ohrp/humansubjects/guidance/belmont.html

Bowater, L., & Wilkinson, M. (2012). Twelve tips to teaching (legal and ethical aspects of) research ethics/responsible conduct of research. *Medical Teacher, 34*(2), 108–115.

Casey, D. (2004). Challenges of collecting data in the clinical setting. *Nursing Times Research, 9*(2), 131–141.

Declaration of Helsinki. (1964). *Ethical principles for medical research involving human subjects.* Retrieved from http://www.wma.net/en/30publications/10policies/b3/

Eisen, A., & Berry, R. M. (2002). The absent professor: Why we don't teach research ethics and what to do about it. *The American Journal of Bioethics: AJOB, 2*(4), 38–49.

Houghton, C. E., Casey, D., Shaw, D., & Murphy, K. (2010). Ethical challenges in qualitative research: Examples from practice. *Nurse Researcher, 18*(1), 15–25.

Munhall, P. L. (1988). Ethical considerations in qualitative research. *Western Journal of Nursing Research, 10*(2), 150–162.

The Nuremberg Code. (1947). Retrieved from http://www.hhs.gov/ohrp/archive/nurcode.html

Orb, A., Eisenhauer, L., & Wynaden, D. (2001). Ethics in qualitative research. *Journal of Nursing Scholarship, 33*(1), 93–96.

Polit, D. F., & Beck, C. T. (2006). *Essentials of nursing research: Methods, appraisal, and utilization* (6th ed.). Philadelphia, PA: Lippincott, Williams and Wilkins.

Catherine Houghton

RESEARCH LITERACY

DEFINITION

Research literacy is an essential competency for evidence-based nursing practice in this age of rapid technology and knowledge generation. Specifically, research literacy is the ability to locate, understand, and critically evaluate evidence for application in practice (Nolan & Behi, 1996). This topic is distinct from research *capacity*, which is the ability to *conduct* research (Fitchett, Tartaglia, Dodd-McCue, & Murphy, 2012; Wayne et al., 2008).

APPLICATION

Research literacy is considered a component of research mindedness that includes comprehension of the significance and relationship of research to practice; abilities to draw on research to inform practice; awareness of various research approaches and strategies; appreciation of the strengths and limitations of different research methods; and critical and open-minded appraisal of research findings and literature (Maidment, Chilvers, Crichton-Hill, & Meadows-Taurua, 2011). Skills instrumental to research literacy are formulating researchable questions; accessing information from multiple sources including electronic sources; differentiating which information to consider as evidence; critically evaluating and synthesizing evidence; interpreting evidence to make clinical judgments; incorporating research findings into

R

communications with colleagues, patients, and community groups; maintaining ethical, responsible, and compassionate standards of practice; routine reflection on practice from multiple perspectives; and participation in the culture of research (Kreitzer, Sierpina, & Fleishman, 2010).

Several approaches to teaching research literacy have been explored in nursing and other health disciplines. Promotion of critical thought is considered foundational for teaching and learning research literacy. Broad curricular strategies include curricular integration (Halcomb & Peters, 2009; Peckover & Winterburn, 2003). For example, integration could take place following a core research course with skills practice, and by enabling students to apply earlier acquired research skills (Lasater et al., 2009). Approaches that have been explored include collaborating with librarians for searching and e-literacy skills (Genoni, Merrick, & Willson, 2006; Hossain, Perrin, & Cumming, 2012; Janke, Pesut, & Erbacker, 2012; Phelps, 2013); direct clinical practice for application of research findings (Gray, 2010; Jakubec & Astle, 2013); and mentoring with experienced researchers (Leung, Verhoef, & Dryden, 2005; Maidment et al., 2011).

SYNOPSIS

Skills of research literacy include formulating researchable questions, accessing information, analyzing research findings for evidence, critically evaluating and synthesizing research findings, interpreting evidence to make clinical judgments, referencing research in communications, and maintaining ethical standards in all practices. It is recommended to use teaching and learning activities that engage students in the critical appraisal of evidence in ways that draw out practice relevancies and direct everyday practice (Jakubec & Astle, 2013; Lasater et al., 2009). Collaboration among nursing students, faculty, librarians, clinical practitioners, and managers has been found to be an effective teaching–learning strategy for enhancing research literacy. Underpinning

all strategies is faculty engagement in critical appraisal of research literature that is essential for teaching and learning success (Wayne et al., 2008).

RECOMMENDATIONS

Expanded technology and knowledge generation have put an increased pressure on the education of research-literate nurses. Nursing students must receive the necessary foundational skill preparation in their professional education to competently link research literacy to their everyday practice. Critical thinking, searching, appraisal, communication, and application skills are central competencies of the research-literate nurse. Achieving these competencies is a complex and collaborative activity that is constantly evolving.

As technology advances, it is important for nurse educators to understand how to guide students in the critical appraisal of research finding. Nursing educators must demonstrate research literacy in every course in which they teach. Finally, there is a current need for scholarship on research literacy for nursing practice and education, particularly in relation to the essential components of research literacy, effective teaching approaches, and evaluation strategies.

Fitchett, G., Tartaglia, A., Dodd-McCue, D., & Murphy, P. (2012). Educating chaplains for research literacy: Results of a national survey of clinical pastoral education residency programs. *The Journal of Pastoral Care & Counseling, 66*(1), 3.

Genoni, P., Merrick, H., & Willson, M. A. (2006). Scholarly communities, e-research literacy and the academic librarian. *The Electronic Library, 24*(6), 734–746.

Gray, M. T. (2010). Research odyssey: The evolution of a research partnership between baccalaureate nursing students and practicing nurses. *Nurse Education Today, 30*(4), 376–382.

Halcomb, E. J., & Peters, K. (2009). Nursing student feedback on undergraduate research education: Implications for teaching and learning. *Contemporary Nurse, 33*(1), 59–68.

Hossain, H., Perrin, C., & Cumming, K. (2012). Information literacy and its application in nursing education. *International Journal of Modern Education and Computer Science, 4*(10), 1–8.

Jakubec, S. L., & Astle, B. J. (2013). Students connecting critical appraisal to evidence-based practice: A teaching-learning activity for research literacy. *Journal of Nursing Education, 52*(1), 56–58.

Janke, R., Pesut, B., & Erbacker, L. (2012). Promoting information literacy through collaborative service learning in an undergraduate research course. *Nurse Education Today, 32*(8), 920–923.

Kreitzer, M. J., Sierpina, V., & Fleishman, S. (2010). Teaching research literacy: A model faculty development program at Oregon College of Oriental Medicine. *Explore, 6*(2), 112–114.

Lasater, K., Salanti, S., Fleishman, S., Coletto, J., Jin, H., Lore, R., & Hammerschlag, R. (2009). Learning activities to enhance research literacy in a CAM college curriculum. *Alternative Therapies in Health and Medicine, 15*(4), 46–54.

Leung, B., Verhoef, M. J., & Dryden, T. (2005). Mentorship programs within a network to build research literacy & capacity in complementary & alternative medicine (CAM) practitioners. *Journal of Complementary and Integrative Medicine, 2*(1), 9.

Maidment, J., Chilvers, D., Crichton-Hill, Y., & Meadows-Taurua, K. (2011). Promoting research literacy during the social work practicum. *Aotearoa New Zealand Social Work, 23*(4), 3.

Nolan, M., & Behi, R. (1996). From methodology to method: The building blocks of research literacy. *British Journal of Nursing, 5*(1), 54–57.

Peckover, S., & Winterburn, S. (2003). Teaching research to undergraduate community nursing students: Reflections upon curriculum design. *Nurse Education in Practice, 3*(2), 104–111.

Phelps, S. F. (2013). Designing the information literacy competency standards for nursing. *Medical Reference Services Quarterly, 32*(1), 111–118.

Wayne, P. M., Buring, J. E., Davis, R. B., Andrews, S. M., John, M. S., Kerr, C. E.,…Schachter, S. C. (2008). Increasing research capacity at the New England School of Acupuncture through faculty and student research training initiatives. *Alternative Therapies in Health and Medicine, 14*(2), 52–58.

Sonya L. Jakubec

RESEARCH PRACTICUM

DEFINITION

A research practicum (RP) can be defined as a course of study that involves the supervised practical application of previously acquired knowledge, skills, and theories of research (Mount Holyoke College, 2014). The term *research* means a systematic investigation designed to develop or contribute to generalizable knowledge (Research, 2013). The word *practicum* (Plural: practica) was first used in 1904, originated from the German word *Praktikum* (Latin *practicum*), and is synonymous with externship, internship, apprenticeship, and training (Practicum, n.d.; Practicum, 2014). A practicum can be a school or college course in a specialized field of study that is designed to give students supervised practical application of previously studied theory. The title practicum generally refers to on-the-job training. It is a common graduation requirement in a number of majors including graduate and undergraduate nursing programs. In nursing, the practicum can be in education, clinical practice, research, management, or administration.

APPLICATION

RP is an effective teaching method that facilitates a hands-on or immersion experience for students. As a unique opportunity designed for highly motivated students, eligibility requirements may be stipulated by the university or department, and entry into this course may be through a strict filtering process. Objectives of RP may include to provide practical and guided experience that demonstrates aspects of the collaborative research process, apply knowledge of research methods in the research setting, obtain a positive experience on research, gain valuable professional development training, prepare students for graduate school, and assist students in choosing a career path (Emory University Rollins School of Public Health, 2014). The practicum exposes the students to the delights and frustrations involved in research as well.

The credits for an RP can be based on course duration, and can be determined by the faculty and the student based on the curriculum. The RP can be faculty, preceptor, or mentor directed, and be done at an external agency. If the RP is with an external agency, identifying a competent research mentor and maintaining ongoing open communication between the student, mentor, and the faculty is important for successful completion. The roles, responsibilities, and timeline must be clearly identified.

Based on the level of involvement, the students may have to complete the human subjects' protection training required by the university and external agency. The tasks assigned to the students may include data collection, data entry, literature review, questionnaire design, institutional review board (IRB) application, technique validation, and data analysis (Miller & Rinetelmann, 2007). For active involvement such as data collection, the students must be listed in the IRB application. Otherwise, the students can only work with de-identified data. The student may be responsible for maintaining a codebook, data analysis, and reporting in a timely fashion. While not the focus of an RP, the student may present the study along with the faculty or research mentor, or be coauthor on the work. The student may be required to complete a final RP report evaluating the experience. This will help faculty validate

the course in meeting the learning objectives and make the needed changes in the RP for future students.

SYNOPSIS

The RP can be facilitated in two ways: faculty-mentored research and collaborative research at a local, national, or international facility. The RP and faculty mentoring have been found to provide a positive experience and confidence in research (Howard, Beauchesne, Shea, & Meservey, 1996; Ravert, Boyer, Harmon, & Scoffield, 2004). Challenges for successful implementation of RP may consist of providing resources, matching schedules, choosing venue for dissemination of results, finding knowledgeable and motivated mentors, planning, and paying attention to detail (Ravert et al., 2004). Academic partnership with other universities, service institutions, or public health and community-based settings can also offer opportunities for students to participate in research activities (Frank, 2008).

While clinical and leadership practica are well grounded in the current nursing practice, RP is just emerging. With only 1% of nurses conducting research at present, hands-on-training to students may generate and maintain the passion for research (Deatrick & Given, 2011). It is essential to ensure adequate student preparation to avoid feelings of frustrations and lack of confidence.

RECOMMENDATIONS

It is recommended that careful structuring and preparation of students could offer opportunities for original research (Kirkpatrick, Tweedell, & Semogas, 2011). Furthermore, journaling about the RP experience may help catch those moments to guide students in planning the RP.

Early exposure to hands-on research to foster interest and prepare future researchers is recommended. Generating interest early in the RP moves with highs and lows, and is a work in progress. A zealous research mentor can ignite the passion in the students to enjoy research and provide new understanding. Faculty should view mentoring as an opportunity to guide students in the RP that may expand the marketability of the students for diverse job opportunities.

Deatrick, J. A., & Given, B. (2011). Creating a pipeline for tomorrow's nurse researchers (Editorial). *Research in Nursing & Health, 34,* 171–175.

Emory University Rollins School of Public Health. (2014). *Examples of practicum objectives.* Retrieved from http://www.sph .emory.edu/current_students/career_services/currentstudents/practicum_objectives.html

Frank, B. (2008). Enhancing nursing education through effective academic-service partnerships (Chap. 2). In M. H. Oermann (Ed.), *Annual review of nursing education* (Vol. 6 , pp. 25–43). New York, NY: Springer Publishing.

Howard, E. P., Beauchesne, M. A., Shea, C. A., & Meservey, P. M. (1996). Research practicum: Linking education to practice. *Nurse Educator, 21*(6), 33–37.

Kirkpatrick, H., Tweedell, D., & Semogas, D. (2011). Transformative learning through a research practicum for undergraduate nursing students. *Journal of Nursing Education, 50*(10), 595–598.

Miller, S. M., & Rinetelmann, K. (2007). Research practicum in rehabilitation counselor education: Learning research through hands-on experience. *Rehabilitation Education, 21*(1), 27–32.

Mount Holyoke College. (2014). *Student projects: Research practicum vs research project.* Retrieved from https://www.mtholyoke .edu/irb/practicum

Practicum. (n.d.) *Random House Kernerman Webster's college dictionary* (2010). Retrieved from http://www.thefreedictionary.com/ practicum

Practicum. (2014). *Merriam-Webster's online dictionary.* Retrieved from http://www .merriam-webster.com/dictionary/ practicum

Ravert, P., Boyer, B., Harmon, K., & Scoffield, H. (2004). Learning nursing research through faculty-mentored projects. *Nurse Educator, 29*(4), 170–174.

Research. (2013). *The American Heritage® dictionary of the English language, fourth edition.* Retrieved from http://www.thefreedictionary.com/research

Rachel Joseph

RESILIENCE IN NURSING EDUCATION

DEFINITION

Resilience in nursing education is the relationship between risk and protective factors causing an individual to bounce back and even thrive in the face of adversity. Human resilience is a dynamic interaction among personal characteristics, adversity, and the environment (McAlister & McKinnon, 2009). Personal characteristics such as inner strengths or capabilities are enhanced by contextual support, thus altering protective factors that enable resilient individuals to adapt and thrive in the face of significant adversity or stressors (Ahern, 2006; Stephens, 2013; Taylor & Reyes, 2012) and to achieve a positive outcome (Haas, 2004). Windle (2011) asserts that the experience of resilience changes as an individual develops, and that adaptation is mediated through bidirectional relationships that create the multiple layers of life contexts.

APPLICATION

Fostering resilience is essential in educating nurses to care and engage with human beings in creating therapeutic connections. Stressors, including the intimate nature of nursing care and turbulent health care environments, require nursing students to be resilient (Chesser-Smyth, 2005). Work-related adversities have accumulative negative effects on nursing students' health and psychological well-being, exposing them to physical and emotional jeopardy (Stephens, 2012). Nursing students are very quickly catapulted into working in high-stress and high-risk environments where stress, adversity, and risk are all antecedents of resilience. Resilience enables the student to rebound and is a required quality for success in nursing (Jackson, Firtko, & Edenborough, 2007; Taylor & Reyes, 2012). Nursing education can foster and support nurses to be resilient.

Hunter (2012) studied perceptions, satisfaction, and risks in the therapeutic bond within the context of a therapeutic engagement. Resilience is vicarious, acting as a counterbalance in reducing the possibility of traumatization for nurses and patients. Resilience supports reframing of negative events and enhances coping skills (Hernandez, Gangsei, & Engstrom, 2007).

Protective factors are attributes of resilience and modify how a nursing student copes with risk and stress. Such factors include rebounding, determination, self-efficacy, self-esteem, social support, personal control, flexibility, and a sense of humor. The consequences of resilience mean that a nursing student can recover, adjust, personally grow, and thrive in a high-risk environment (Mealer et al., 2012).

SYNOPSIS

Nurse educators can prepare nursing students to be resilient in recovering from adversity to develop personal growth. Taylor and Reyes (2012) identified that successfully negotiating nursing studies enhances resilience. Nursing students' perceptions of their ability to solve difficult problems were higher at the beginning of the semester than at the end, thus questioning the efficacy of resilience development.

McAlister and McKinnon (2009) describe resilience as a process of adjusting to adversity that can be learned and supported. Hodges, Keeley, and Grier (2005) call for teaching and learning strategies that elicit discovery of personal meaning and affective learning in developing professional resilience among nursing students. Engagement

and connection, cocreated learning experiences, and freedom to experiment in creating shared professional meaning and values that are essential to resilient professional nurses are encouraged as teaching and learning strategies.

Experiential learning, creative self-expression, explorations of original thinking, increased assertiveness, enhanced communication, and greater collaboration are key in promoting resilience in nursing (McDonald, Jackson, Wilkes, & Vickers, 2013). Resilience education should focus on the undergraduate program where nursing students learn to build identities and coping strategies, as well as discern and build strengths. Clinical supervisors and facilitators who engage in open genuine dialogue support development of resilience in practice.

RECOMMENDATIONS

In supporting resilience, nurse educators must be resilient themselves. Having a healthy work-life balance and looking after one's physical, emotional, and spiritual health will create resilience. It is recommended that the resilient behaviors of nurses be identified in order to develop a repertoire of recognizable resilient skills (Hodges, Keeley, & Troya, 2008). This repertoire of resilient skills can serve as a model of resilient behaviors that may create a greater self-awareness of resilience among nursing students. In addition, resilience can be incorporated into professional development processes so that nursing students can develop resilient behaviors early in their nursing career. Encouraging nursing students to use humor and to participate in social activities that are health focused, such as a running group or hosting fun-based team-building opportunities, strengthens resilience and fosters the capacity to rebound when faced by adversity.

Ahern, N. R. (2006). Adolescent resilience: An evolutionary concept analysis. *Journal of Pediatric Nursing, 21*(3), 175–185.

Chesser-Smyth, P. A. (2005). The lived experience of general student nurses on their first clinical placement: A phenomeno-logical study. *Nurse Education in Practice, 5,* 320–327.

Haas, J. (2004). Resilience. In S. Peterson & T. Bredow (Eds.), *Middle range theories: Application to nursing research* (pp. 341–367). Philadelphia, PA: Lippincott.

Hernandez, P., Gangsei, D., & Engstrom, D. (2007). Vicarious resilience: A new concept in work with those who survive trauma. *Family Processes, 46*(2), 229–241.

Hodges, H., Keeley, A., & Grier, E. C. (2005). Professional resilience, practice longevity, and Parse's theory for baccalaureate education. *Journal of Nursing Education, 44*(12), 548–554.

Hodges, H., Keeley, A. C., & Troya, P. J. (2008). Professional resilience in baccalaurate-prepared acute care nurses: First steps. *Nursing Education Perspectives, 29*(2), 80–89.

Hunter, S. (2012). Walking in sacred spaces in the therapeutic bond: Therapists' experiences of compassion satisfaction coupled with the potential for vicarious traumatization. *Family Processes, 51,* 179–192.

Jackson, D., Firtko, A., & Edenborough, M. (2007). Personal resilience as a strategy for surviving and thriving in the face of workplace adversity: A literature review. *Journal of Advanced Nursing, 60*(1), 1–9.

McAlister, M., & McKinnon, J. (2009). The importance of teaching and learning resilience in the health disciplines: A critical review of the literature. *Nurse Education Today, 29,* 371–379.

McDonald, G., Jackson, D., Wilkes, L., & Vickers, M. (2013). Personal resilience in nurses and midwives: Effects of a work-based educational intervention. *Contemporary Nurse, 45*(1), 134–143.

Mealer, M., Jones, J., Newman, J., McFann, K. K., Rothbaum, B., & Moss, M. (2012). The presence of resilience is associated with a healthier psychological profile in intensive care unit (ICU) nurses: Results of a national survey. *International Journal of Nursing Studies, 49,* 292–299.

Stephens, T. M. (2012). *Increasing resilience in adolescent nursing students.* PhD Dissertation University of Tennessee, Knoxville, TN.

Stephens, T. M. (2013). Nursing student resilience: A concept clarification. *Nursing Forum, 48*(2), 125–133.

Taylor, H., & Reyes, H. (2012). Self-efficacy and resilience in baccalaureate nursing studies. *International Journal of Nursing Education Scholarship, 9*(1), 1–13.

Windle, G. (2011). What is resilience? A review and concept analysis. *Reviews in Clinical Gerontology, 21,* 152–169.

Gerardina Harnett

RETENTION: NONTRADITIONAL STUDENTS

DEFINITION

Retention of nontraditional students in nursing refers to the rate at which students successfully stay in a program of study. Jeffreys (2003) describes program retention as the enrollment in a program, either part or full time, and taking the required courses; this may include repeating courses for which there has been withdrawal and/or failure.

Jeffreys (2003) describes nontraditional students as having any of the following characteristics: 25 years or older, commuter, individuals with children, representatives of minority racial and/or ethnic groups, males, General Equivalency Diploma (GED) graduates, English as a second language students, and those who require remedial classes. Ross-Gordon (2011) also includes those who are single parents, financially independent, and working full-time or attending part-time. Nontraditional students include adults returning to earn their first degree, postbaccalaureate students switching careers, and/or individuals returning to earn a second degree, often in an online or accelerated format.

R

APPLICATION

By 2022, more than 526,800 nurses will be needed in the United States (Bureau of Labor Statistics, 2014). The National Center for Education Statistics (2013) reported that from 2000 to 2011, enrollment of students aged 25 and older increased 41% in degree-granting institutions. Further, the Center predicts a rise of 14% in nontraditional student enrollments from 2011 to 2020. Recruiting increased numbers of nontraditional students, including men and those of diverse ethnic backgrounds, will help reduce health disparities currently existing among underserved populations (American Association of Colleges of Nursing [AACN], 2014). Thus, it is critical that nurse educators create an environment that is supportive and encouraging for these unique students who do not take the traditional path to their nursing degree.

Nontraditional students have been one group of individuals who have an increased risk for attrition (Harris & O'Rourke, 2014). Normally older and more ethnically diverse, these students often have multiple stressors, including financial strain, employment constraints, and family and community responsibilities (Harris & O'Rourke, 2014). Ethnically diverse students are at increased risk for attrition due to additional barriers, including lack of awareness of their cultural needs by nursing programs, feelings of isolation, lack of faculty support, and language barriers (Harris & O'Rourke, 2014). Some need to juggle schedules of children and aging parents as they try to negotiate time for class, clinical, labs, and studying. These conflicting priorities may lead to guilt, anxiety, and frustration as they make sacrifices to provide balance in their lives.

SYNOPSIS

Due to the uniqueness of nontraditional learners, a variety of teaching strategies may be used to capture participants' learning needs. Visual, auditory, and kinesthetic styles are recognized by most nurse educators. Even though adults learn by a variety of methods, 80% are predominately visual learners. The ways in which adults learn have an enormous effect on their ability to acquire and apply knowledge, seek learning experiences, and enjoy participating in the education process (Blevins, 2014).

Knowles's theory of andragogy may be the best known theoretical approach for adult learners. According to this framework, adults prefer self-direction in learning; bring a vast reservoir of experience; exhibit a readiness to learn based on a need to know or do; prefer problem-centered learning; and exhibit a relatively high degree of internal motivation (Ross-Gordon, 2011). Faculty can serve as change agents in creating supportive learning environments by incorporating adult learning theory and research into the classroom, and by advocating for adult-oriented programs and services. The design and delivery of programs are critical to successful experiences for nontraditional students (Ross-Gordon, 2011).

Building on life experiences can create an environment that connects new knowledge to past expertise. Inviting students to share pertinent experiences enriches class discussion and can be a successful strategy for adult learners. Engagement provides an environment that makes material relevant, and real-life stories build on adult learner experiences in the classroom (Day, Lovato, Tull, & Ross-Gordon, 2011).

One explanation for attrition of nontraditional second-degree students is a mismatch between student expectations from prior career learning experiences and the reality of nursing curricula (Sedgewick, 2013). The literature pertaining to second-degree nursing students suggests that these students often consider nursing to be a practical, meaningful profession that will allow them to help others, as well as provide secure, well-paying careers (Sedgewick, 2013).

RECOMMENDATIONS

Nontraditional students often meet rigorous admission criteria, yet attrition rates remain high (Rouse & Rooda, 2010). With the development of effective interventions, schools of nursing can decrease attrition rates. The following interventions can assist in this endeavor: providing a thorough orientation that emphasizes the pace and intensity of the program; inviting alumni of the program to provide firsthand testimony regarding methods of handling the demands of a fast-paced program; offering student assistance in preparing a personal budget and identifying additional sources of financial support; and offering students opportunities for counseling and stress relief (Rouse & Rooda, 2010).

It is incumbent on administrators of nursing programs to make admission decisions that result in the highest possible retention rates of prepared students for the profession. Rosenberg, Perraud, and Willis (2007) found that inadequate screening of potential applicants was a concern. Many health science programs assess noncognitive factors in an attempt to identify applicants who understand the commitment they are making. In addition, the essential characteristics of compassion, integrity, altruism, motivation, interpersonal skills, and respect are requisite for success (Rosenberg et al., 2007).

In developing educational programs, faculty must understand the principles of adult learning, generational influences, and learning styles. The learning process is improved when education is presented with teaching methods that are coordinated with students' preferred learning styles. When learning needs are met, there is enhanced understanding and retention of information that ultimately impacts patient care (Blevins, 2014).

Focus group sessions are effective methods for providing data on program evaluation, outcomes, and needs that can support retention. Robert, Pomarico, and Nolan (2011) used focus groups in nursing courses to identify students' learning needs, expectations for faculty, and preferred teaching methods. Faculty received feedback at various points in the program to build on qualities the students would bring to the program, and to adapt teaching strategies (Robert et al., 2011).

Learning communities, where students share strengths and collaborate on specific projects, can be ideal for this population. In designing programs, educators need to acknowledge student goals and the unique strengths they bring to the study and practice of nursing (Raines, 2011). Clear expectations and structure are important to nontraditional learners who expect that professors are well organized and content is clear and concise (Day et al., 2011).

Clinical instructors can be instrumental in working with nontraditional students. Cangelosi (2007) presents examples of how a clinical instructor made all the difference. These faculty members used pedagogical skills and clinical competence to show students how to integrate classroom learning in the clinical setting. Successful instructors were described as being there and taking extra time (Cangelosi, 2007). Clinical instructors who made a difference for students used themselves as bridges in facilitating student learning and encouraged students to create bridges of their own (Cangelosi, 2010).

Nontraditional students need to be provided with opportunities to engage in partnerships with nurses in the clinical setting to foster self-confidence (Sedgewick, 2013). Fewer placements of longer duration would facilitate a sense of connection and give more time to develop supportive relationships (Sedgewick, 2013).

Although nontraditional students may present themselves as self-assured, confident, and mature, they often seek reassurance that they have made the right career choice. Consequently, transitioning into the nursing program can be difficult, with students reporting feelings of being overwhelmed in response to the fast pace and heavy workload (Sedgewick, 2013).

Combining rigorous admission screening with a thorough assessment of student goals can provide a foundation for strong support systems needed by nontraditional students throughout the nursing program. Providing clear expectations, incorporating adult-learning principles, and creating learning communities that support partnerships

R

in the clinical area are critical to success. As we strive to make the health care workforce look more like the patient population, retaining these nontraditional students will help decrease disparities in health care as we educate the next generation of nurses.

American Association of Colleges of Nursing (AACN). (2014). *Enhancing diversity in the workforce.* Washington, DC: American Association of Colleges of Nursing. Retrieved from http://www.aacn .nche.edu/media-relations/fact-sheets/ enhancing-diversity

Blevins, S. (2014). Understanding learning styles. *MedSurg Nursing, 23*(1), 59–60.

Bureau of Labor Statistics. (2014). *Quick facts: Registered nurses.* Occupational Outlook Handbook (2014–2015 Ed.). Washington, DC: U.S. Department of Labor. Retrieved from http://www.bls.gov/ooh/health-care/registered-nurses.htm

Cangelosi, P. R. (2007). Accelerated second-degree baccalaureate nursing programs: What is the significance of clinical instructors? *Journal of Nursing Education, 46*(9), 400–405.

Cangelosi, P. R. (2010). Voices of faculty of second-degree baccalaureate nursing students. *Journal of Nursing Education, 49*(3), 137–142.

Day, B. W., Lovato, S., Tull, C., & Ross-Gordon, J. (2011). Faculty perceptions of adult learners in college classrooms. *The Journal of Continuing Higher Education, 59*(2), 77–84.

Harris, R. C., & O'Rourke, M. E. G. (2014). Addressing the challenges of nursing student attrition. *Journal of Nursing Education, 53*(1), 31–37.

Jeffreys, M. R. (2003). Nontraditional undergraduate nursing student retention and success. In M. H. Oermann & K. T. Heinrich (Eds.), *Annual review of nursing education* (Vol. 2, pp. 61–90). New York, NY: Springer.

National Center for Education Statistics. (2013). *Digest of education statistics, 2012 (NCES 2014–2015).* Washington, DC: U.S. Department of Education. Retrieved from http://nces.ed.gov/fastfacts/display .asp?id=98

Raines, D. A. (2011). What attracts second degree students to a career in nursing? *Online Journal of Issues in Nursing, 16*(1), 1.

Robert, T. E., Pomarico, C. A., & Nolan, M. (2011). Assessing faculty integration of adult learning needs in second-degree nursing education. *Nursing Education Perspectives, 32*(1), 14–17.

Rosenberg, L., Perraud, S., & Willis, L. (2007). The value of admission interviews in selecting accelerated second-degree baccalaureate nursing students. *Journal of Nursing Education, 46*(9), 413–416.

Ross-Gordon, J. M. (2011). Research on adult learners: Supporting the needs of a student population that is no longer nontraditional. *Peer Review, 13*(1), 26–29.

Rouse, S. M., & Rooda, L. A. (2010). Factors for attrition in an accelerated baccalaureate nursing program. *Journal of Nursing Education, 49*(6), 359–361.

Sedgewick, M. (2013). Comparison of second-degree and traditional undergraduate nursing students' sense of belonging during clinical placements. *Journal of Nursing Education, 52*(11), 657–661.

Theresa Tavella Quell
Carole A. Pomarico

RISK ASSESSMENT

DEFINITION

Risk assessment is defined as the threatened ability of nursing students at all levels of education to gain access, progress in a nursing program, graduate, and pass licensing examinations for pre-licensure; and certification examinations for advanced practice nurses. Factors identified for at-risk students include speaking English as a second language (ESL); first generation attending college; retaking prerequisite science courses to obtain at least a C; not having completed or within 5 years taken prerequisite college or college preparatory courses (algebra, biology, chemistry); not scoring within the average range or higher of a pre-entrance standardized test; less than a 3.0 science and overall grade point average (GPA); work hours increase: greater than or equal to 20 hours part-time or greater than or equal to 40 hours full-time to finance undergraduate and graduate education, and those with family responsibilities, especially those with a lack of a family/support system.

APPLICATION

The importance of at-risk students' characteristics for passing the National Council Licensure Examination-Registered Nurse (NCLEX-RN®) as an outcome measure of prelicensure nursing programs is evidenced by the plethora of research studies conducted by nurse educators for more than 20 years. Breckenridge's Risk Assessment Profile, Strategies for Success (RAPSS) instrument development has evolved for more than two decades with risk indicator additions based on evidence. RAPSS consists of 13 items used to assess at-risk students for admission and progression through nursing programs to determine strategies to enhance student success, as well as to predict students' graduation rates, licensure, and certification examination pass rates (Breckenridge, 2006, 2010; Breckenridge, Wolf, & Roszkowski, 2012). The RAPSS score assists directors, faculty, and advisors to identify students during the admissions process, prospectively, who benefit from a remediation program aimed at improving the potential for academic success. The application of the RAPSS is a central component in the Students at Risk, Strategies for Success (SRSS) and Nursing Workforce Diversity (NWD) program (Breckenridge, 2013), whereby the purpose is to assist underserved, underrepresented, and diverse nursing students to achieve success by completing a bachelor of science in nursing (BSN) degree and pass the NCLEX-RN as first-time candidates. This program is intended to close the gap of poverty, educational disparities, and preparation for at-risk students and increase the number of diverse underserved registered nurses (RNs) joining the workforce. A structured learning, risk-reduction approach increases the retention of currently enrolled students and provides financial support through stipends or scholarships. Programs for the recruitment and remediation of disadvantaged and ethnically diverse baccalaureate nursing students continue to be developed, especially through the NWD Program of Health Resources and Services Administration (HRSA). Condon et al. (2013) developed the Success in Learning Individualized Pathways Program (SLIPP) at a private west coast baccalaureate school of nursing implemented to promote academic success for nursing students who were at a higher risk for attrition than traditional nursing students.

SYNOPSIS

Several studies have identified risk factors targeted to develop interventions for student success for more than 20 years. Billings and Halstead (2012), found that ESL students experienced several barriers that put the students at risk for academic achievement. These included lack of self-confidence; reading, writing, and learning difficulties; isolation prejudice; and lack of family and financial support. Scheele, Pruitt, Johnson, and Xu (2010) identified that Asian students struggle with English language difficulties around gender and tense; in spoken Asian languages, gender and tense are not differentiated. Several studies have outlined barriers for Hispanic students. Bond et al. (2008) reported that problems Hispanic students face are lack of financial support, emotional and moral support, mentoring, professional socialization, academic advising, and technical support. Moceri (2010) identified nonflexible or nonculturally appropriate curricula and language barriers as detrimental obstacles for Hispanic students. Mount Carmel's Learning Trail student success program, developed in 2003, assists Hispanic students to be successful by providing mentoring, tutoring, counseling and follow-up (Billings & Halstead, 2012).

R

The risk of failing the NCLEX-RN increases with the number of C or lower grades students receive in nursing courses. In addition to academic performance, variables of test anxiety and student-predicted NCLEX-RN scores need to be considered regarding students at risk. Hopkins (2008) developed a model of student support utilizing specified academic predictors including the SAT or ACT; cumulative GPA; math and reading scores; and nonacademic variables: age, race, and gender. After at-risk students are identified, a mechanism for referring the student to support systems should be implemented. For example, McGahee, Gramling, and Reid (2010) proposed limiting admission to nursing programs to students with no more than one science course failure.

RECOMMENDATIONS

Benner, Sutphen, Leonard, and Day (2010) noted that there are schools and health care organizations that offer outreach and pipeline programs for high school students, and encouraged that these types of programs be strengthened through financial support, recruitment, and retention infrastructures. Jeffreys (2012) recommended to avoid predicting retention of students based only on demographic characteristics. The environmental factors regarding living arrangements, financial status, family financial support for school, family responsibilities, family emotional support, transportation arrangements, and financial aid and/or scholarships were more influential for retention than other factors. Jeffreys (2012) noted that retrospective studies have been the norm to determine nursing student performance outcomes, but recommends prospective assessment of risk and early intervention to maximize retention of at-risk students. Consistent with this assertion, RAPSS is criterion based, incorporating both demographic and academic risk indicators for student applicants at the time of the admission process. This measure determines if students are in need of additional remediation to prospectively meet the admission requirements and progress in a nursing program. If students are at risk and in need of support services, Breckenridge (2013) recommends that remediation begins in the pre-entry phase of an SSR.

Benner, P., Sutphen, M., Leonard, V., & Day, L. (Eds.). (2010). *Educating nurses: A call for radical transformation*. San Francisco, CA: Jossey-Bass.

Billings, D., & Halstead, J. (Eds.). (2012). *Teaching in nursing: A guide for faculty* (4th ed.). St. Louis, MO: Saunders.

Bond, M. L., Gray, J., Baxley, S., Cason, C., Denke, L., & Moon, M. (2008). Voices of Hispanic students in baccalaureate nursing programs: Are we listening? *Nursing Education Perspectives*, 136–142.

Breckenridge, D. M. (2006). Hospital diversity initiative for new access students: NETS, career ladder program. *Pennsylvania Nurse, 61*(4), 22–23.

Breckenridge, D. M. (2010). A time to give back. In J. Fitzpatrick, C. Shultz, & T. Aiken (Eds.), *Giving through teaching: How nurse educators are changing the world* (pp. 379–381). New York, NY: Springer.

Breckenridge, D. M. (2013). Project Director, Grant Award: D19HP24300–01-00. *Students at risk, strategies for success*, Nursing Workforce Diversity (NWD) program funded by U.S. Department of Health Resources and Services Administration (HRSA).

Breckenridge, D. M., Wolf, Z., & Roszkowski, M. (2012). Risk assessment profile and strategies for success instrument: Determining prelicensure nursing students' risk for academic success. *Journal of Nursing Education, 51*(3), 160–166.

Condon, V., Morgan, C., Miller, E., Mamier, I., Zimmerman, G., & Mazhar, W. (2013). A program to enhance recruitment and retention of disadvantaged and ethnically diverse baccalaureate nursing students. *Journal of Transcultural Nursing, 24*(4), 397–407. doi:10.1177/1043659613493437

Hopkins, T. H. (2008). Early indication of at-risk nursing students: A student support model. *Journal of Nursing Education, 47*(6), 254–259.

R

Jeffreys, M. (2012). *Nursing students retention: Understating the process and making difference.* New York, NY: Springer.

McGahee, T., Gramling, L., & Reid, T. (2010). NCLEX-RN success: Are there predictors. *Southern Online Journal of Nursing Research,* 10(4). Retrieved from www.snrs.org.

Moceri, J. (2010). Being Cabezona: Success strategies of Hispanic nursing students. *International Journal of Nursing Education,* 7(1), 1–15.

Scheele, T., Pruitt, R., Johnson, A., & Xu, Y. (2010). What do we know about educating Asian ESL nursing students? A literature review. *Nursing Education Perspectives,* 32(4), 244–249.

Diane M. Breckenridge

RISK FOR FAILURE

DEFINITION

Students are at risk for failure when they do not meet course objectives or fulfill course requirements. If course objectives are not met and requirements are not fulfilled, the result is course failure. When successful completion of a course is required in order to progress in a program of study, failure may delay future coursework until the course is successfully repeated. Students may be at risk for failure at any time and in any type of educational program.

APPLICATION

"Risk for failure" has implications for students enrolled in nursing programs both in their satisfactorily meeting course requirements and progressing through to complete a nursing program, as well as in their passing the National Council Licensure Examination (NCLEX) at the completion of the program. Desirable outcomes are that students be retained in the program to complete all coursework satisfactorily, to progress through

their program to completion in a timely manner, and finally to pass the NCLEX, preferably on the first attempt. Undesirable outcomes include student attrition, delayed program completion, and lack of success on the NCLEX. Voluntary attrition occurs when students elect to drop out of the program for personal reasons or because they are unsure about nursing as a career choice. Involuntary attrition occurs when students are dismissed from the program due to failure in nursing coursework. Failure in the NCLEX on the first attempt requires additional testing and delays employment as a nurse. For students, the consequences of failure either in coursework or in the NCLEX can include disappointment, frustration, lack of confidence in their ability to be successful on subsequent NCLEX attempts, and a sense of having wasted financial resources, time, and energy completing coursework (O'Donnell, 2009). The nursing program is affected by student attrition with empty program seats and lost tuition revenue. Furthermore, if a student does not pass the NCLEX, a decreased pass rate occurs, which may impact the program's reputation and accreditation (Hadenfeldt, 2012).

Intrinsic and extrinsic variables such as students' age and ethnicity, educational background, goal determination, family responsibilities, external support sources, and financial resources may influence the student's chances of success or put them at risk for failure (Hadenfeldt, 2012; Jeffreys, 2004; Shelton, 2003). Younger or traditional students (defined as 24 years of age or younger) may better be able to focus on educational pursuits with fewer interruptions due to family and employment responsibilities, and they may have retained study skills developed in high school. Nontraditional students, on the other hand, may draw from a wealth of life experiences to overcome obstacles and they may be highly motivated to accomplish the tasks needed to be successful (Jeffreys, 2004; Shelton, 2003). Ethnically diverse students may face unique family, language, and cultural barriers. Because these students are often first-generation college students,

R

family members may not understand the need to provide relief from or assistance with responsibilities so that students have time to study (Gardner, 2005). Knowledge and confidence acquired through success in previous educational coursework, and determination to achieve educational goals, may positively impact persistence through difficult nursing coursework (Jeffreys, 2004). Family responsibilities and external support affect students' ability to be successful (Gardner, 2005; Jeffreys, 2004). When coursework is added to household and employment responsibilities, students may feel overwhelmed. An unanticipated family crisis (i.e., illness, death, divorce) can impact attendance and student academic achievement (Hadenfeldt, 2012; Jeffreys, 2004). Lack of financial resources can influence student success as students are responsible for educational and household expenses and may be required by employers to maintain a minimum number of employment hours to retain jobs and health insurance. Poor high school coursework achievement, college prerequisite science course failures, low science course grade point average, nursing coursework failure, and lack of success in pre-entrance and nursing program assessment testing are variables that suggest students might be at risk for failure for nursing program completion and NCLEX success (Fraher, Belsky, Carpenter, & Gaul, 2008; Seago, Keane, Chen, Spetz, & Grumbach, 2012).

Nursing program characteristics can increase or decrease risk for failure. Admission policies must assure that students who are admitted to the program have demonstrated the ability to be successful in scholarly work and that these abilities can be applied to nursing coursework and ultimately to the NCLEX. If students are deficient in English composition, math, or other academic skills, preparatory coursework should be completed prior to beginning nursing coursework. Lack of preparation will put the student at risk for failure. Once in the program, faculty knowledge regarding necessary course content, strategies to promote critical thinking, and the latest NCLEX test

plan is essential. Faculty support including demonstrating interest in the student, providing counsel, and assisting the student in activating support resources can make a difference in success (Shelton, 2003). Academic and social support such as tutoring and peer study groups may make a difference in the student's ability to be successful.

Strategies to assist students who are at "risk for failure" can be implemented when lack of success is identified early in the semester. In a study by Hadenfeldt (2012), performance improvement plans were utilized with students in a community college nursing program who were not meeting academic, behavioral, or attendance requirements in a course. The plans outlined which specific course objectives were not being met and provided instructor recommendations regarding resources to promote success. Students were required to develop a brief personal strategy for success. The plans increased success, especially with traditional students. In addition, most of these students passed the NCLEX on the first attempt (Hadenfeldt, 2012). In an intervention trialed by Harris, Rosenberg, and O'Rourke (2014) in an associate degree nursing program in a historically Black college, students at risk for failure were identified early and recruited into voluntary participation in the Student Success Program (SSP). The SSP consisted of group meetings, individual mentoring with the program director, and completion of eight learning modules, which included identification of available resources. Faculty were also provided with workshops regarding various learning styles and strategies for maintaining a culturally sensitive classroom. Although not all desired outcomes were achieved, the faculty reported ongoing success in the use of the learning strategies, and the study resulted in a positive change in the admission requirements for the program (Harris et al., 2014).

SYNOPSIS

There are student and nursing education program characteristics that put a student at risk for failure in a nursing education program that may result in program attrition or failure on the NCLEX examination. Program completion and passing of the NCLEX are necessary achievements toward nursing licensure. Early identification of students at risk for failure provides an opportunity to intervene with educational and support systems.

Strategies to improve student success on the NCLEX include the use of learning assessment tools, engaging all faculty in the process of preparation by promoting critical thinking in students, providing additional support for students who have been unsuccessful on previous coursework, and intensive remediation activities for those at risk for failure on comprehensive testing during the final semester of the program (Reinhardt, Keller, Summers, & Schultz, 2012).

RECOMMENDATIONS

Future research is needed regarding interventions to promote student success and effectiveness to complete the program and achieve success on the first attempt on the NCLEX.

Fraher, E. P., Belsky, D. W., Carpenter, J. M., & Gaul, K. (2008). *A study of associate degree nursing program success.* A final report compiled by the University of North Carolina at Chapel Hill. Retrieved from http://www.shepscenter.unc.edu/hp/publicaitons/NCCCS_ADN_Report.pdf

Gardner, J. (2005). Barriers influencing the success of racial and ethnic minority students in nursing programs. *Journal of Transcultural Nursing, 16,* 155–162. doi: 10.1177/1043659604273546

Hadenfeldt, C. J. (2012). Effects of an intervention plan on nursing student success. *Journal of Nursing Education, 51*(2), 89–94.

Harris, R. C., Rosenberg, L., & O'Rourke, M. E. G. (2014). Addressing the challenges of nursing student attrition. *Journal of Nursing Education, 53*(1), 31–37.

Jeffreys, M. R. (2004). *Nursing student retention: Understanding the process and making a difference.* New York, NY: Springer Publishing.

O'Donnell, H. (2009). The emotional impact of nursing student attrition rates. *British Journal of Nursing, 18*(12), 745–754.

Reinhardt, A. C., Keller, T., Summers, L. O., & Schultz, P. (2012). Strategies for success: Crisis management model for remediation of at-risk students. *Journal of Nursing Education, 51*(6), 305–311.

Seago, J. A., Keane, D., Chen, E., Spetz, J., & Grumbach, K. (2012). Predictors of students' success in community college nursing programs. *Journal of Nursing Education, 51*(9), 489–495.

Shelton, E. N. (2003). Faculty support and student retention. *Journal of Nursing Education, 42*(2), 68–76.

Cynthia Hadenfeldt

R

SCHOLARSHIP

DEFINITION

The American Association of Colleges of Nursing (AACN) defines nursing scholarship as, "...those activities that systematically advance the teaching, research, and practice of nursing through rigorous inquiry that (a) is significant to the profession, (b) is creative, (c) can be documented, (d) can be replicated or elaborated, and (e) can be peer-reviewed through various methods" (AACN, 1999b, p. 1).

APPLICATION

Scholarship is the necessary ingredient for expanding the field of nursing education and improving nursing practice (AACN, 2006). In order for nursing to meet the current challenges of health care delivery, scholarship in nursing must be a salient part of all nursing practice. Boyer's (1990) model of scholarship has been frequently cited in the literature as a guide for understanding scholarship in nursing. This model includes four main aspects of scholarship: discovery—the generation of new knowledge; teaching—teachers and students cross the bridge to understand and achieve a better learning environment; application—the use of knowledge for development and change; and integration—interprofessional collaboration leading to improved understanding of responsibilities and roles. Furthermore, the AACN (1999b) position is that scholarship in nursing does not exist unless the knowledge is made public for further testing and debate.

Nurse educators are responsible for deriving a variety of creative teaching–learning activities to facilitate the principles of scholarship throughout all levels of nursing curricula and health care systems. Scholarship within nursing education must focus on classroom research, evidence-based practice (EBP), and providing the structure that nurses need to give the most efficient instruction to patients (Robert & Pape, 2011).

SYNOPSIS

Scholarship in nursing education became known in the early 1960s after Bixler and Bixler (1959) publicly questioned the validity of nursing as a true profession. Their major concern was the lack of scientific merit to nursing traditions and practices. Nursing scholars of that era took on the challenge of developing the science of nursing through establishing nursing theory that could direct scientific research specifically to nursing practices (Meleis, 1987). In the beginning, scholarship in nursing focused on formulating theories that provided new knowledge to guide and explain the science of nursing. Scholarship activity was generally kept within academia, and was viewed as a path to career advancement with emphasis on research and publication. Nursing scholarship within the clinical workplace was given much less prominence and importance.

The changes in world health care and delivery have influenced nursing leaders to reconceptualize the notion of scholarship in nursing. The report from the Carnegie Foundation for the Advancement of Teaching introduced a new model of scholarship (Boyer, 1990), which included the integration, application, teaching, and discovery of knowledge. Building on this model, the AACN's (1999b) position paper outlined guidelines for nursing education to meet the challenges of health care reform and delivery of care. More emphasis was placed on scholarship in nursing education that promoted the discovery of new knowledge through clinical research and EBP (AACN, 1999a, 2006). Different forms of scholarship have become the acceptable way of advancing nursing knowledge and growing the profession. Today, scholarship in nursing includes the discovery, integration, application, and teaching of new knowledge within both research-focused academic settings and non-research-focused clinical settings. In keeping with this trend, nursing education programs have established the doctor of nursing practice (DNP) with the aim of preparing practicing nurses to be leaders in EBP. Scholarship is focused on the translation of nursing research into practice and the integration of new knowledge to improve clinical decision making (Terry, 2012). The nursing profession has progressed through not only the discovery of new knowledge in the discipline but also the integration and application of this knowledge through EBP (AACN, 2006).

RECOMMENDATIONS

Social and political influences have created significant challenges for the nursing profession in this decade and will continue to do so in the future. Nursing scholarship will continue to grow in importance as EBP becomes more widely established, and the expectation for better patient outcomes becomes the norm (Brown, 2014). Nursing education must prepare nurses to become involved in nursing scholarship activities to create their own EBP and collaborate with other professions to improve patient care. Educators must be committed to teaching students about the importance of nursing scholarship in practice in order to influence health care decisions and advance the profession. Students must understand that practice includes identifying clinical problems, using technology to retrieve evidence, reading and analyzing research, weighing evidence, and implementing change (Schmidt & Brown, 2012). Nurse scholars must continue to develop midrange and practice theories that are more useful in clinical settings and lead practice nurses in basing their patient care on evidence.

American Association of Colleges of Nursing (AACN). (1999a). *Hallmarks of scholarly nursing practice.* Washington, DC: Author.

American Association of Colleges of Nursing (AACN). (1999b). *Position statement on defining scholarship for the discipline of nursing.* Retrieved from http://www.aacn.nche.edu/publications/positions/scholar.htm

American Association of Colleges of Nursing (AACN). (2006). *Position statement on defining scholarship for the discipline of nursing.* Retrieved from *http://www.aacn.nche.edu/publications/position/defining-scholarship*

Bixler, G. K., & Bixler, R. W. (1959). The professional status of nursing. *The American Journal of Nursing, 59*(8), 1142–1147.

Boyer, E. L. (1990). *Scholarship reconsidered: Priorities of the professoriate.* Princeton, NJ: Carnegie Foundation for the Advancement of Teaching.

Brown, S. J. (2014). *Evidence-based nursing: The research-practice connection.* Burlington, MA: Jones & Bartlett.

Meleis, A. I. (1987). ReVisions in knowledge development: A passion for substance. *Scholarly Inquiry for Nursing Practice, 1*(1), 5–19.

Robert, R. R., & Pape, T. M. (2011). Scholarship in nursing: Not an isolated concept. *MEDSURG Nursing, 20*(1), 41–44.

Schmidt, N. A., & Brown, J. M. (2012). *Evidence-based practice for nurses: Appraisal and application of research.* Sudbury, MA: Jones & Bartlett.

Terry, A. J. (2012). *Clinical research for the doctor of nursing practice.* Sudbury, MA: Jones & Bartlett.

Cheryl Riley-Doucet

SELF-DIRECTED LEARNING

DEFINITION

Conceptualized almost five decades ago, self-directed learning (SDL) was developed by educational learning expert Rogers (1981) and subsequently revised by Tough (1971) and Knowles (1975). Rogers initially described the concept of self-direction, which was then refined by Tough who noted that adult learners are self-directed in their own personal learning needs and are motivated to seek out and gain the knowledge and skills required to meet those needs (O'Shea, 2003). Knowles further defined the core principles required for SDL as being individually driven, formulated, conducted, and evaluated either with or without the support of others (Knowles, 1975). Criticized in the literature for differing interpretations, primary elements led to years of debate and additional modifications. Today SDL, in contrast to teacher-led instruction, identifies the core principle of SDL as learning, which is intrinsically and extrinsically derived, articulated, and executed by the individual. SDL has been embraced in higher education and health care in direct response to societal and technological changes. These changes have accelerated and accentuated the critical need to develop survival skills to adapt in these complex environments. O'Shea (2003) considers SDL as an essential component in nursing today.

APPLICATION

SDL is a process that empowers the learner to take personal responsibility for learning by establishing learning goals, identifying and accessing resources, adopting activities to facilitate learning, and evaluating learning performance. The use of SDL in nursing can guide learners and educators to facilitate and develop skills and confidence for independent lifelong learning. In nursing education,

it is no longer acceptable to prepare the learner by merely transferring knowledge; educators must facilitate the student's ability to independently acquire new skills both today and in the future as current practices are likely to become obsolete.

Benefits of SDL in nursing literature include developing skills of inquiry and attaining new knowledge through increased learner confidence, adaptability in new situations, and personal autonomy. SDL minimizes the notion of curriculum hypertrophy created by the exponential growth of knowledge (Abrahamson, 1978). Students learn a process to define and analyze problems effectively to respond to whatever the future brings.

Use of SDL compared to teacher-directed learning has not always been successfully implemented in nursing education (White, 2006). Assessing student and educator readiness along with appropriate and adequate preparation is critical for success. Students need to operate as self-directed learners and learn how to control what they want to learn; learn how to question; access resources; and motivate self. This process is often foreign to undergraduate students and can easily frustrate the learner, creating anxiety and distress (Hewitt-Taylor, 2001; Lunyk-Child, 2005). Educators of SDL are charged with creating a learning environment that can facilitate learning with mutual respect, maintain rigor, and support the development of knowledge, skills, and attitude (Kim, Olfman, Ryan, & Eryilmaz, 2014; O'Shea, 2003; Pryce-Miller, 2010). Multiple forms of SDL have been successfully used in nursing education including reflections, independent study, informal discussion or group work, distance or online learning modules, and teleconferencing (O'Shea, 2003).

The purported benefits of SDL can be optimized by assessing readiness for SDL, preparing the learners and educators, and identifying learning styles. Furthermore, the student's motivation, learning style, and specific learning situations must be taken into account (Candy, 1991).

SYNOPSIS

There are three main factors required for understanding SDL. These are understanding of the different perspectives and frameworks on SDL, shifting from traditional teaching to a more facilitated process, and assessing readiness of the individual learner. Historically, two main perspectives on implementation of SDL in education have existed. One perspective is that SDL is a process that takes into account the level of the learner and the organizational processes required to facilitate SDL. The second perspective identifies SDL as a personal attribute where the academic institution develops learners who possess intellectual autonomy (Candy, 1991). Recent works by Vonderwell and Turner (2005) support the blending of the two perspectives by identifying key personal characteristics that can be used to leverage the SDL process. Key characteristics of self-directed learners are varied but generally include ability to work independently, ability to self-manage, a desire for learning, and a skill in problem solving (Candy, 1991; Knowles, 1975). Ultimately, the goal is to produce a self-directed learner for life.

Teaching methods for SDL are different from traditional teacher-directed instructions (White, 2006). Faculty development that supports educators to learn and maintain the competency in facilitating SDL is essential. Brown and Libberton (2007) discussed the need for educators to identify the learning needs of students and use a variety of teaching methodologies to support SDL. In addition, the school needs to embrace a culture of mutual respect and shared responsibility in which teachers facilitate SDL in the curriculum. Learning contracts and reflections have been ideal methods of teaching SDL (Hewitt-Taylor, 2001). Problem-based learning has also assisted students to learn the skills required to identify measures to solve the problem.

Readiness for SDL for the student is individualized and exists on a continuum. If student readiness is low when completing an SDL assignment, the result may be high anxiety. In contrast, if the student with high readiness is given a very structured assignment with numerous teacher instructions, his or her anxiety may also be high (Fisher, King, & Tague, 2001). Several scales to assess readiness for SDL have been developed. One of the most recent scales was developed by Fisher and King (2010).

RECOMMENDATIONS

SDL is important in nursing. Guiding students to inquire about and acquire new knowledge is necessary to meet the challenges in the complex, rapidly changing health care environment. SDL enables individuals to take initiative and responsibility for learning. There is a need for current research with SDL at all levels of nursing education.

Abrahamson, S. (1978). Disease of the curriculum. *Journal of Medical Education, 53*(12), 951–957.

Brown, J., & Libberton, P. (2007). *Principles of professional studies in nursing.* Baskingstoke, England: Palgrave.

Candy, P. (1991). *Self-direction for lifelong learning: A comprehensive guide to theory and practice.* San Francisco, CA: Jossey-Bass.

Fisher, M., & King, J. (2010). The self directed learning readiness scale for nursing education revisited. *Nurse Education Today, 30*(1), 44–48.

Fisher, M. K., King, J., & Tague, G. (2001). Development of self-directed learning readiness scale for nursing education. *Nurse Education Today, 21,* 516–525.

Hewitt-Taylor, J. (2001). Self directed learning: Views of teachers and students. *Journal of Advanced Nursing, 36*(4), 496–504.

Kim, R., Olfman, L., Ryan, T., & Eryilmaz, E. (2014). Leveraging a personalized system to improve self-directed learning in online educational environments. *Computers & Education, 70*(1), 150–160.

Knowles, M. (1975). *Self-directed learning.* New York, NY: Associated Press.

Lunyk-Child, O. C. (2005). Self directed learning: Faculty and student perspectives.

Journal of Nursing Education, 40(3), 116–123.

O'Shea, E. (2003). Self directed learning in nurse education: A review of the literature. *Issues and Innovations in Nursing Education,* 43(1), 62–70.

Pryce-Miller, M. (2010, November 20). *Are first year undergraduate student nurses prepared for self-directed learning?* Retrieved from www.nursingtimes.net

Roger, C. (1981). Education, a personal activity. *Educational Change and Development,* 3(3), 1–12.

Tough, A. (1971). *The adult's learning project: A fresh approach to theory and practice in adult learning.* Toronto, Canada: Institute for Studies in Education.

Vonderwell, S., & Turner, S. (2005). Active learning and preservice teachers' experience in an online course: A case study. *Journal of Technology and Teacher Education,* 13(1), 65–84.

White, C. (2006). Smoothing out transitions: How pedagogy influences medical students' achievements of self regulated goals. *Advances in Health Science Education Theory and Practices,* 12(3), 279–297.

Kari Gali

SELF-EVALUATION

DEFINITION

Self-evaluation is a process in which a person engages in a subjective appraisal of self. This process may be structured by self-enhancement, self-verification, self-assessment, and self-improvement (Sedikides & Strobe, 1995).

APPLICATION

Self-evaluation in the nurse coach literature is part of the self-development process and applies to both the client and coach (Dossey, Luck, & Schaub, 2014). It is an integral process of self-development, self-assessment, self-reflection, and self-care. Self-evaluation may occur as a reflective process with or without the use of a tool or a specific goal. Reflection has the potential to help one transform on a personal, organizational, or social level (Fleming, 2007). The process aids one in determining if, how, and why the desired outcomes have been achieved. Self-evaluation may be sparked or enhanced through interpersonal relationships or events. When one performs an evaluation, assessing both merit and worth, the evaluator's own values may enter the process.

Evaluation occurs regularly in nursing and is supported by recommendations throughout nursing literature in scope of practices, processes, and standards of care. The American Nurses Association (ANA) Standard of Nursing Practice #14 is "Professional Practice Evaluation," stating that the "registered nurse evaluates his or her own practice in relation to professional practice standards and guidelines, relevant statutes and regulation" (ANA, 2010).

As one evaluates programs, student outcomes, and patient interactions, the role of self cannot be forgotten. Throughout professional nursing practice, organizations and institutions' formal yearly evaluations occur. In best practice models, self-evaluation occurs prior to a discussion with an administrator. In the self-evaluation process, the nurse uses self-reflection to self-assess, identify, and delight in areas of accomplishment as well as identify potential opportunities for growth. Self-evaluation is further enhanced through dialogue with the administrator, leading to new goals and enhanced self-development.

As with any evaluation, self-evaluation may be focused on either process or outcomes. Process refers to the content of the self-evaluation and outcome refers to the actual results of the self-evaluation (Pender, Murdaugh, & Parsons, 2006). When self-evaluation is focused on outcomes, it may include the completion of projects, student teaching, or certain achievements such as publishing, certifications, presentations, and completion of

S

research. Self-evaluation concerning process may include reflection on factors that hindered or facilitated goal achievement; it may include teaching or leadership style, interpersonal relationships, time management, or team cohesiveness. Self-evaluation is enhanced through feedback from others as different perspectives may be offered, providing further opportunities for growth and development.

Students, practitioners, and faculty have opportunities to use simulation, video recording, and standardized patients as content for self-evaluation. For example, reviewing a videotape of a standardized patient encounter assessing verbal and nonverbal communication in a safe, structured environment can be an approach to self-evaluation. Self-evaluation may be overly critical; thus, the use of group feedback and reflection may help nurses learn from peers and view self with compassion and honesty.

SYNOPSIS

Self-evaluation has value in personal, clinical, and educational interactions in facilitating personal growth. Self-evaluation has a place in both formative and summative evaluations, to enable participants to derive meaning from the evaluations and view them as growth producing. Viewing self-evaluation as a process integral to professional and personal growth increases and expands the process beyond a yearly activity. Both formal and informal processes exist to assist with self-evaluation; it may be sparked by self-reflection, somatic responses, or interactions with others. Application of self-evaluation to our personal wellness can assist us in feeling whole and inspired about life, as our self- image may be enhanced.

RECOMMENDATIONS

As nurses and nurse educators assist clients and students with self-evaluation, self-evaluation of the nurse and educator is vital. In addition, the process should be ongoing and not dependent upon a yearly workplace evaluation. Thus, self-evaluation should be the target of nursing research initiatives,

to assess benefits, identify processes, and address both formal and informal methods of self-evaluation. Reflection, a key component to the self-evaluation process, needs to become a daily practice, supported by workplace–institution initiatives. Additional tools and processes need to be developed for quantitative and qualitative studies to be conducted on self-evaluation. Educational offerings can offer insights to change perspective of self-evaluations, increase dialogue, and identify benefits, so personal growth and meaning for all nurses are enhanced.

American Nurses Association (ANA). (2010). *Nursing: Scope and standards of nursing practice* (2nd ed). Silver Spring, MD: Nursebooks.org

Dossey, B. M., Luck, S., & Schaub, B. G. (2014). *Nurse coaching: Integrative approaches for health and wellbeing.* North Miami, FL: International Nurse Coach Association.

Fleming, P. (2007). Reflection a neglected art in health promotion. *Health Education Research, 22*(5), 658–664.

Pender, N., Murdaugh, C., & Parsons, M. (2006). *Health promotion in nursing practice* (5th ed.). Upper Saddle River, NJ: Pearson Prentice Hall.

Sedikides, C., & Strobe, M. (1995). The multiply motivated self. *Personality and Social Psychology Bulletin, 21*, 1330–1335. doi:10.1177/01461672952112010

St. Leger, A. S., & Walsworth-Bell, J. P. (1999). *Change promoting research for health services.* Buckingham, England: Open University Press.

Deborah McElligott

SELF-EVALUATION: MEASUREMENT

DEFINITION

Self-evaluation is a process and a skill by which individuals judge their level of clinical knowledge and skill performance measured against external standards, with the goal of self-improvement (Tyser, McCrea, & Knupfer, 2012).

APPLICATION

Ubiquitous to health care organizations are performance-evaluation processes. A critical aspect of regulating performance and clinical competence includes the evaluation of self. In nursing education, self-evaluation can be used to enhance other evaluative methods in providing a complete picture of student performance. Moreover, the use of self-evaluation during nursing education can be a means to develop this critical skill. Self-evaluation, when utilized accurately, has the potential to promote self-awareness and self-directed learning that can continue beyond nursing school.

There are several instruments, and various methods, for self-evaluation that have been employed in clinical education. An exploratory study conducted by Abbott, Carswell, McGuire, and Best (1988) indicated that self-evaluation was positively perceived as a method for providing direction for learning. One of the earliest instruments used was the Nurse Competence Scale (NCS), which was developed for practicing nurses. The scale assesses the competence of students in topics such as therapeutic interventions and ensuring quality. It also includes competence-related factors, such as age, gender, and supervision. It was determined that self-assessment provided a basis for competence development and should be used systematically during education (Kajander-Unkuri et al., 2014). Methods have included a video-recorded benchmark. In this instance, students were videotaped performing a task and asked to assess their performance using global rating scales. Self-evaluation was repeated after viewing the benchmark video. It was concluded that the utilization of a benchmark may improve accuracy of self-evaluations (Hawkins, Osborne, Schofield, Pournaras, & Chester, 2012). It was also observed that the utilization

of video benchmarks, versus written evaluation guidelines, improved the accuracy of self-evaluation and clinical competence in nursing students performing Foley catheterization skills (Yoo, Yoo, & Lee, 2010).

SYNOPSIS

While self-directed learning and self-regulation are desired outcomes in the practice environment, the accuracy of self-evaluation to promote those outcomes is frequently unreliable. Students' self-evaluations are often inversely related to their actual performance; thus, crucial to the accuracy of self-evaluation is the specific, timely, and constructive feedback, offered in a safe environment, by credible and trusted supervisors (Baxter & Norman, 2011; Dolmans, 2013; Sargeant et al., 2010; Yoo et al., 2010). Furthermore, accurate, informed self-evaluation requires consideration of internal and external sources such as the learning–practice climate, credibility of information processes, personal attributes, and relationships with others. Tensions that arise between internal and external sources, and overall self-evaluation, such as the idea that one is a good person, versus momentary self-evaluation in a given context, such as clinical performance, can further lead to inaccuracies with the self-assessment (Sargeant et al., 2010).

Informing the learner about strengths and weaknesses in order to identify learning needs has been utilized widely. Other external methods, such as high-quality positive and negative feedback, should be employed in order to enhance the accuracy of the students' self-evaluations (Plakht, Shiyovich, Nusbaum, & Raizer, 2013). Instructors should also take into consideration the role that motivation plays in the positivity of self-evaluations. Evidence suggests that self-evaluation inflation correlates with promotion concerns (Scholer, Ozaki, & Higgins, 2014).

RECOMMENDATIONS

Applications of self-assessment are known to increase self-awareness of learning. For

S

learners, in order to become competent in evaluating their abilities, they should be guided toward self-assessment (Kurt, 2014). Caution should be utilized when considering the use of self-evaluation scales as a teaching–learning tool, or to assess nursing students' competencies. Specific guidelines for evaluation must be clearly expressed to the student, and the consideration of benchmark demonstrations should be addressed. Further, it is important to consider self-evaluation in combination with expert feedback in nursing, because of the general tendencies for students to under-evaluate or over-evaluate their performance.

There is a need for current evidence regarding the effectiveness of requiring student self-evaluations in nursing education. Specifically, research should be done to validate self-evaluation tools, and to determine the correlations with self-evaluation and goal setting, performance improvement, and self-efficacy.

Abbott, S. D., Carswell, R., McGuire, M., & Best, M. (1988). Self-evaluation and its relationship to clinical evaluation. *Journal of Nursing Education, 27*(5), 219–224.

Baxter, P., & Norman, G. (2011). Self-assessment or self deception? A lack of association between nursing students' self-assessment and performance. *Journal of Advanced Nursing, 67*(11), 2406–2413.

Dolmans, D. H. (2013). Self-assessment and dialogue: Can it improve learning? *Advances in Health Sciences Education: Theory and Practice, 18*(2), 193–195.

Hawkins, S. C., Osborne, A., Schofield, S. J., Pournaras, D. J., & Chester, J. F. (2012). Improving the accuracy of self-assessment of practical clinical skills using video feedback—The importance of including benchmarks. *Medical Teacher, 34*(4), 279–284.

Kajander-Unkuri, S., Meretoja, R., Katajisto, J., Saarikoski, M., Salminen, L., Suhonen, R., & Leino-Kilpi, H. (2014). Self-assessed level of competence of graduating nursing students and factors related to it. *Nurse Education Today, 34*(5), 795–801.

Kurt, M. (2014). Collaborative assessment: Fostering ownership in assessment. *Education, 134*(3), 332–339.

Plakht, Y., Shiyovich, A., Nusbaum, L., & Raizer, H. (2013). The association of positive and negative feedback with clinical performance, self-evaluation and practice contribution of nursing students. *Nurse Education Today, 33*(10), 1264–1268.

Sargeant, J., Armson, H., Chesluk, B., Dornan, T., Eva, K., Holmboe, E.,...van der Vleuten, C. (2010). The processes and dimensions of informed self-assessment: A conceptual model. *Academic Medicine, 85*(7), 1212–1220.

Scholer, A., Ozaki, Y., & Higgins, T. (2014). Inflating and deflating the self: Sustaining motivational concerns through self-evaluation. *Journal of Experimental Social Psychology, 51*, 60–73.

Tyser, M. P., McCrea, S. M., & Knupfer, M. (2012). Pursuing perfection or pursuing protection? Self-evaluation motives moderate the behavioral consequences of counterfactual thoughts. *European Journal of Social Psychology, 42*, 372–382.

Yoo, M. S., Yoo, Y., & Lee, H. (2010). Nursing students' self-evaluation using a video recording of Foley catheterization: Effects on students' competence, communication skills, and learning motivation. *Journal of Nursing Education, 49*(7), 402–405.

Remylin S. Bruder
Reynaldo R. Rivera

SERVICE LEARNING

DEFINITION

Service learning is a "teaching and learning method that connects meaningful community service experiences with academic learning, personal growth, and civic responsibility" (National Dropout Prevention Center Network, 2014, p. 1).

APPLICATION

The goal of service learning is to prepare students to become civic-minded with the ability to use critical-thinking skills for solving real-life problems and to see themselves as change agents as a result of their community-learning experiences (Cress, 2014). Service learning promotes greater social awareness, increased cultural competency, increased empathy, improved communication skills, and a continued commitment to service in the future (Amerson, 2010, 2012; Kelleher, 2013; Murray, 2013; Wehling, 2008). Students commonly see the experience as "eye-opening" to the challenges that vulnerable or disenfranchised populations face in their daily lives and the privileges students may take for granted (Amerson, 2012; Hunt & Swiggum, 2007).

SYNOPSIS

The pedagogy of service learning requires that service activities are linked directly with the academic objectives; students must be active participants engaged in the planning and development of the service; reciprocity must exist between the student and the community–client; and reflection must be incorporated into the experience (Amerson, 2014). The students must first be introduced to service-learning concepts and be prepared to engage in collaborative work with the community. Preparation should include the process of engaging in meaningful reflection, information about the country or community, cultural practices of the local community, and preparation for the cultural shock that may occur.

The core principles of global service learning are cultural competence, compassion, curiosity, courage, collaboration, creativity, and capacity building (McKinnon & Fealy, 2011). Students must engage in active, experiential learning opportunities during community-based activities where they work with community members in reciprocal learning partnerships. Curiosity, compassion, and courage are needed to step outside the student's comfort zone to engage in collaboration and capacity building with diverse communities using creative approaches to solve everyday problems. These actions facilitate development of critical-thinking skills. Students frequently indicate that service-learning projects or immersion programs are more effective teaching strategies than the traditional classroom lecture or videos.

Numerous nurse researchers have demonstrated the value of international service learning as an effective strategy for the development of cultural competency in nursing students (Amerson, 2010, 2012; Bentley & Ellison, 2007; Curtin, Martins, Schwartz-Barcott, DiMaria, & Soler Ogando, 2013; Green, Comer, Elliott, & Neubrander, 2011; Hunt & Swiggum, 2007; Larson, Ott, & Miles, 2010). Faculty should consider the following recommendations when planning a service-learning project with nursing students: match the economic status of the intended community with the goals of the curriculum; plan a time frame for work in the host country that will be manageable; provide opportunities for students to work outside their comfort zone; encourage visits to homes within the community; require students to provide direct care and teaching; and use a variety of methods of reflection, including journaling, discussion, and photography (Amerson, 2014). Language skills play a critical role in engaging with communities in international settings. Therefore, students should participate in language classes prior to the service-learning experience. Socioeconomic issues and the current health care environment of the host country are often a part of the prerequisite learning in preparation for working internationally. Debriefing is important upon return to the United States to help students understand the ambiguous feelings of privilege and guilt that may occur after working in poverty-stricken countries. Although these recommendations are suggested primarily for use with international service learning, the principles may be adapted for use with service learning in local communities as well.

S

RECOMMENDATIONS

Nurse educators have demonstrated effective outcomes in the area of transcultural self-efficacy for nursing students following service learning in a variety of settings and with diverse vulnerable populations. It is recommended that evaluation of the student's perception of the service-learning experience, and the client's perception of the cultural competency displayed by the student, be evaluated. Future studies should focus on client satisfaction and the efficacy of health education or interventions being delivered during the service-learning project.

Amerson, R. (2010). The impact of service-learning on cultural competence. *Nursing Education Perspectives, 31*(1), 18–22.

Amerson, R. (2012). The influence of international service-learning on transcultural self-efficacy in baccalaureate nursing graduates and their subsequent practice. *International Journal of Teaching and Learning in Higher Education, 1*(1), 6–15.

Amerson, R. (2014). Research-based recommendations for implementing international service-learning. *Journal of Professional Nursing, 30*(2), 175–179.

Bentley, R., & Ellison, K. J. (2007). Increasing cultural competence in nursing through international service-learning experiences. *Nurse Educator, 32*(5), 207–211.

Cress, C. (2014). *Defining a service-learning pedagogy of access and success. Campus Compact.* Retrieved from http://www.compact .org/resources/future-of-campus-engagement/defining-a-service-learning-pedagogy-of-access-and-success/4229/

Curtin, A. J., Martins, D. C., Schwartz-Barcott, D., DiMaria, L., & Soler Ogando, B. M. (2013). Development and evaluation of an international service learning program for nursing students. *Public Health Nursing, 30*(6), 548–556.

Green, S. S., Comer, L., Elliott, L., & Neubrander, J. (2011). Exploring the value of an international service-learning experience in Honduras. *Nursing Education Perspectives, 32*(5), 302–307.

Hunt, R. J., & Swiggum, P. (2007). Being in another world: Transcultural student experiences using service learning with families who are homeless. *Journal of Transcultural Nursing, 18*(2), 167–174.

Kelleher, S. (2013). Perceived benefits of study abroad programs for nursing students: An integrative review. *Journal of Nursing Education, 52*(12), 690–695.

Larson, K. L., Ott, M., & Miles, J. M. (2010). International cultural immersion: En vivo reflections in cultural competence. *Journal of Cultural Diversity, 17*(2), 44–50.

McKinnon, T. H., & Fealy, G. (2011). Core principles for developing global service-learning programs in nursing. *Nursing Education Perspectives, 32*(2), 95–101.

Murray, B. S. (2013). Service-learning in baccalaureate nursing education: A literature review. *Journal of Nursing Education, 52*(11), 621–626.

National Dropout Prevention Center/Network. (2014). *Service-learning overview.* Retrieved from http://www.dropoutprevention.org/effective-strategies/service-learning

Wehling, S. (2008). Cross-cultural competency through service-learning. *Journal of Community Practice, 16*(3), 293–315.

Roxanne Amerson

SERVICE LEARNING: COMMUNITY HEALTH IMPROVEMENT

DEFINITION

Service learning is a teaching method that integrates formal learning with student activities designed to better a community. Ideally, the learning and the service are shared mutually among all participants: students, instructor, and community partners. Since both the learning and the service in service learning are highly variable, they generally resist reductive theoretical descriptions (Cruz & Giles, 2000; Moore, 2013). While service learning has become popular in numerous disciplines, it is particularly suited to community health nursing education.

APPLICATION

The term *service learning* has been used to designate a type of pedagogy since the late 20th century. Service learning principles have been incorporated in nursing education since its earliest recorded beginnings. Nurses and nursing students historically have learned and practiced in schools, places of business, places of worship, homes, communities, and wherever people gather to live, work, and worship. Community health nursing clinical practice can be called service learning provided that the criteria of community partnership and mutual gain are met.

Integrating concepts of social determinants of health, social justice, cross-cultural nursing, family nursing, and vulnerability into learning goals are basic to the practice of service learning (Gillis & MacLellan, 2010; Groh, Stallwood, & Daniels, 2011). Other important goals in service learning are increased critical self-awareness, growth in empathy, and acquisition of insight into the complexity of chronic health conditions. Learning goals are typically documented by thematic analysis of data from student reflective journaling or postexperience debriefing. The data support claims that students acquire skills in cross-cultural interaction and problem solving in resource-challenged environments (Amerson, 2012; Green, Comer, Elliott, & Neubrander, 2011).

Service learning projects in nursing education have focused on a wide variety of populations in various sites: older adults (Ross, 2012; Tsai, 2013), families with a mentally ill member (du Plessis, Koen, & Bester, 2013), children in school programs (Bassi, 2011; Eymard, Breaux, & Dozar, 2013), and international projects (Amerson, 2012; Green et al., 2011). Pijl-Zieber and Kalischuk (2011) describe a shift in nursing education based on two factors. One factor is the increasing shortage of traditional clinical placements. The second factor is that in order to achieve healthier populations, nurses need to practice the principles of primary health care where people actually live, work, play, and worship.

Service outcomes will naturally depend upon the nature of the service delivered. Sometimes this is specific and easily measurable within a short time frame (Belcher et al., 2012). In other cases, the service has an open-ended future. Assessing the health impact of such nursing interventions requires longitudinal data collection and analysis. In addition, health outcomes are likely to be the result of multiple factors.

Nursing service learning can begin with a needs assessment of a particular population such as school children (Eymard et al., 2013), older adults (Ross, 2012; Tsai, 2013), and international communities (Amerson, 2012; Green et al., 2011). In some cases, identifying the needs and making appropriate referrals by advocating for change could be an outcome of the service. Nursing service learning, as with service learning in other disciplines, has tended to focus on learning outcomes rather than service outcomes because of the complexity of measuring service outcomes (Cruz & Giles, 2000).

SYNOPSIS

Service learning is natural to nursing with its commitment to the health and healing of people across the life span. Nurse educators and nursing students engage in mutually beneficial learning and service activities in partnership with populations. Service learning is particularly suited to help nursing students learn the social determinants of health and disease, cross-cultural nursing, and social justice. Student nurses can acquire skills in complex assessments, communication, advocacy, teaching, referral, and problem solving.

RECOMMENDATIONS

While learning outcomes are well documented in nursing service learning studies, the service outcomes are discussed less. As nursing moves through the 21st century toward greater investment in population health with prevention as a priority, measuring the health impact of nursing service learning is likely to gain more importance.

Amerson, R. (2012). The influence of international service-learning on transcultural self-efficacy in baccalaureate nursing graduates and their subsequent practice. *International Journal of Teaching and Learning in Higher Education, 24,* 6–15.

Bassi, S. (2011). Undergraduate nursing students' perceptions of service-learning through a school-based community project. *Nursing Education Perspectives, 32*(3), 162–167.

Belcher, A., Conner, L., Anderson, J. M., Branham, J., Levett, M., Paddock, G.,...Zonca, M. (2012). Education-service partnership to promote best practices in a latent tuberculosis infection program. *Public Health Nursing, 29*(1), 62–70.

Cruz, N., & Giles, D. (2000). Where's the community in service-learning research? *Michigan Journal of Community Service Learning, Special Issue,* 28–34.

du Plessis, E., Koen, M. P., & Bester, P. (2013). Exploring home visits in a faith community as a service-learning opportunity. *Nurse Education Today, 33*(8), 766–771.

Eymard, A., Breaux, P., & Dozar, K. (2013). Transformative learning in nursing students through a service learning project with a vulnerable community. *Journal of Nursing Education and Practice, 3,* 35–43. doi:10.5430/jnep.v3n3p35

Gillis, A., & MacLellan, M. (2010). Service learning with vulnerable populations: Review of the literature. *International Journal of Nursing Education Scholarship, 7*(1), Article 41. doi:10.2202/1548–923X2041

Green, S. S., Comer, L., Elliott, L., & Neubrander, J. (2011). Exploring the value of an international service-learning experience in Honduras. *Nursing Education Perspectives, 32*(5), 302–307.

Groh, C. J., Stallwood, L. G., & Daniels, J. J. (2011). Service-learning in nursing education: Its impact on leadership and social justice. *Nursing Education Perspectives, 32*(6), 400–405.

Moore, D. T. (2013). *Engaged learning in the academy: Challenges and possibilities.* New York, NY: Palgrave Macmillan.

Pijl-Zieber, E., & Kalischuk, R. (2011). Community health nursing practice education: Preparing the next generation. *International Journal of Nursing Education Scholarship, 8*(1), 1–13. doi:10.2202/1548–923X.2250

Ross, M. E. (2012). Linking classroom learning to the community through service learning. *Journal of Community Health Nursing, 29*(1), 53–60. doi:10.1080/0737001 6.2012.645746

Tsai, C. -H. (2013). To accept the elderly and learn from them: Senior citizen care center. *Tzu Chi Nursing Journal, 7,* 32–35.

Ruby K. Dunlap

SIMULATION: CLINICAL REASONING

DEFINITION

Clinical reasoning is the cognitive and metacognitive process used for analyzing knowledge as it relates to individual patients and distinct clinical situations (Banning, 2008). Clinical reasoning is a process of making professional judgments, evaluating evidence to solve problems, and making diagnostic and patient management decisions (Higgs, Burn, & Jones, 2001). It is a deliberate process of weighing alternatives against evidence and choosing the most appropriate intervention for the patient (Tanner, 2006). The terms *critical thinking, decision making,* and *clinical judgment* are often used interchangeably with clinical reasoning (Simmons, 2010). The terms are interrelated concepts; however, they are not the same and their differences, although subtle, are important to recognize (Victor-Chmil, 2013).

APPLICATION

Developing clinical reasoning skills is essential to the development of competent, high-functioning clinical nurses. Developing clinical reasoning is a challenge that nursing educators have struggled with for decades. Traditional teaching methods may be insufficient to develop clinical reasoning skills when an adult learner is involved. Recently, the suggestion of using human patient simulation (HPS), also known as high-fidelity patient simulation (HFPS), training has been considered as a learning strategy to assist in the development of clinical reasoning and teamwork skills for nurses as well as other clinical disciplines (Baldwin, 2007; Bremner, Aduddel, Bennett, & VanGeest, 2006; Gierach & Evenson, 2010; Lasater, 2007). Typically, HPS actively engages the learner, incorporating the use of both clinical reasoning and teamwork skills (Fanning & Gaba, 2007). The simulation culminates in a debrief that affords the learner the opportunity to reflect on the simulation encounter and learn experientially (Fanning & Gaba, 2007). Experiential learning is a tenet of adult learning strategy described by Kolb (1984). According to Benner, Stannard, and Hooper (1996), the purpose of the thinking-in-action approach is to allow students to simulate clinical reasoning through patient circumstances as they occur. The thinking-in-action approach encourages educators to recreate scenarios using HPS as a connection between didactic education and experiential learning where students can use problem solving and clinical skills to provide patient care in a safe environment (Vyas, Ottis, & Caligiuri, 2011). Simulation effectiveness has been positively associated with improvement of critical thinking and clinical reasoning in complex patient care situations and assists in improving student confidence (Lewis, Strachan, & Smith, 2012).

SYNOPSIS

The demands of patient safety standards, the implementation of the Affordable Care Act, and the increased use of HPS technology has provoked nurse educators to reevaluate educational methods. The paucity of clinical educational sites has made HPS a viable nursing educational option. Integrating HPS into nursing curricula may provide nurses with improved learning and development of clinical judgment (Lasater, 2007). The use of simulation-based learning includes an adult learner who is actively engaged, both cognitively and emotionally (Fanning & Gaba, 2007). Fanning describes the simulation encounter and the subsequent nonjudgmental debrief process as being tailored to the objectives and needs of the participant and team. When used correctly, the results of a well-developed and executed simulation can impact not only the acquisition of skills but positively affect clinical judgment and decision making (Fanning & Gaba, 2007). Clinical simulation is being used as a tool in the development of clinical reasoning in nursing education with promising results. Clinical simulation therefore fulfills Tanner's (2006) description of a clinical reasoning skill set as the ability to sort information, prioritize, reflect, and create conclusions.

The review on clinical reasoning is concentrated on the nursing student. It can be hypothesized that nursing students are novices at clinical reasoning and therefore the most suitable subjects. Simulation has been found to provide a safe environment to practice decision making and prioritization when used as part of a nursing curriculum (Gierach & Evenson, 2010). Gierach used a mass casualty simulation to test the clinical knowledge of nursing students and their ability to hone their clinical reasoning skills. Results indicated that the debriefing process assists the nursing student with incorporation of nursing principles and concepts, and with reflecting on their strengths and areas for improvement (Gierach & Evenson, 2010).

Baldwin (2007) used emergency department clinical scenarios developed for nursing students to enhance clinical reasoning skills. The author concluded that the simulation experience provided a safe venue for students to practice their clinical reasoning skills both individually and as a group (Baldwin, 2007).

Another reported finding was that the reflective debriefing sessions were instrumental in solidifying clinical reasoning concepts while allowing the students to evaluate their own progress (Baldwin, 2007).

RECOMMENDATIONS

Nurse educators have a substantial responsibility of educating future nurses; therefore, the integration of innovative teaching modalities is crucial for the development of sound clinical reasoning. One of the modalities that has emerged in recent years is HPS. Clinical reasoning is the process of applying nursing knowledge to a clinical situation in order to initiate an appropriate patient intervention. The literature over the past decade substantiates the investment in innovative teaching methods such as HPS to develop and improve clinical reasoning skills in nurses.

HPS requires scenario-specific objectives and meticulous planning to achieve the desired effects. The simulated scenarios are therefore able to be replicated on demand until the desired outcome is reached. This can be seen as an effective educational strategy, not only for improving clinical reasoning but because HPS may be used to address the growing ethical dilemma of practicing on human patients (Bremner et al., 2006). This eliminates the need for finding a human patient with the desired disease state in order to practice a particular skill or to develop clinical reasoning.

Further nursing research is needed to study the effect of simulation and structured debriefing on clinical reasoning, including replicating studies, which have demonstrated students' improved critical reasoning in complex patient care simulations. HPS is being integrated in nursing school curricula; therefore, a longitudinal study on the clinical reasoning skills of nursing students who have used HPS would be valuable. Additionally, future research would benefit from larger sample sizes and studying clinical reasoning in diverse nursing populations for improved generalizability.

Baldwin, K. B. (2007). Friday night in the pediatric emergency department: A simulated exercise to promote clinical reasoning in the classroom. *Nurse Educator, 32*(1), 24–29.

Banning, M. (2008). Clinical reasoning and its application to nursing: Concepts and research studies. *Nurse Education in Practice, 8*(3), 177–183.

Benner, P., Stannard, D., & Hooper, P. L. (1996). A "thinking-in-action" approach to teaching clinical judgment: A classroom innovation for acute care advanced practice nurses. *Advanced Practice Nursing Quarterly, 1*(4), 70–77.

Bremner, M. N., Aduddell, K., Bennett, D. N., & VanGeest, J. B. (2006). The use of human patient simulators: Best practices with novice nursing students. *Nurse Educator, 31*(4), 170–174.

Fanning, R. M., & Gaba, D. M. (2007). The role of debriefing in simulation-based learning. *Simulation in Healthcare, 2*(2), 115–125.

Gierach, M., & Evenson, C. (2010). Clinical reasoning in the classroom: A triage simulation. *Nurse Educator, 35*(6), 228–230.

Higgs, J., Burn, A., & Jones, M. (2001). Integrating clinical reasoning and evidence-based practice. *AACN Clinical Issues, 12*(4), 482–490.

Kolb, D. (1984). *Experiential learning; experience as a source of learning and development.* Englewood Cliffs, NJ: Prentice Hall.

Lasater, K. (2007). High-fidelity simulation and the development of clinical judgment: Students' experiences. *Journal of Nursing Education, 46*(6), 269–276.

Lewis, R., Strachan, A., & Smith, M. M. (2012). Is high fidelity simulation the most effective method for the development of nontechnical skills in nursing? A review of the current evidence. *The Open Nursing Journal, 6*, 82–89.

Simmons, B. (2010). Clinical reasoning: Concept analysis. *Journal of Advanced Nursing, 66*(5), 1151–1158.

Tanner, C. A. (2006). Thinking like a nurse: A research-based model of clinical judgment in nursing. *Journal of*

Nursing Education, 45(6), 204–211. doi: 10.1111/j.1365–2648.2010.05262.x

Victor-Chmil, J. (2013). Critical thinking versus clinical reasoning versus clinical judgment: Differential diagnosis. *Nurse Educator, 38*(1), 34–36.

Vyas, D., Ottis, E. J., & Caligiuri, F. J. (2011). Teaching clinical reasoning and problem-solving skills using human patient simulation. *American Journal of Pharmaceutical Education, 75*(9), 189. doi:10.5688/ajpe759189

M. Isabel Friedman
Barbara DeVoe

SIMULATION: ETHICS

DEFINITION

Simulation ethics is a framework used by educators and students who participate in simulated clinical experiences to define the correctness or incorrectness of their activities. The domains of this framework are beneficence and autonomy.

APPLICATION

Simulation has become a growing component in nursing education both in schools and health care facilities. It is a constructivist pedagogy, which has arisen out of a growth in technology, a decrease in clinical opportunities, and a shortage of nursing faculty. When the framework of ethics is applied to simulation, it raises issues related to patients, students, and the simulationist.

Beneficence and autonomy as applied to simulation imply that patients should not be exposed to undue risk and should be permitted to determine who will care for them and what care they will receive. The majority of academic health care is delivered in large urban academic medical centers that care for a large portion of underserved patients. The underserved do not have many options for great care and are therefore in a place of limited choice. The presence of large numbers of students seeking clinical experience in academic medical centers means that patients are at higher risk of receiving care from less than fully-qualified practitioners. These risks include multiple attempts at a procedure, increased discomfort, and unnecessary errors. The use of simulation for training reduces the number of experiences needed in the real-world clinical settings and provides more accomplished and experienced students to the clinical area.

Beneficence is an important reason for the use of simulation in critical, high-risk, low-volume clinical situations. By preparing students and practitioners to deal effectively with each other in high-risk/low-volume occurrences, the likelihood of success and positive patient outcomes is enhanced. Also, the use of simulation permits the identification of errors and strategies used for error recovery. Many real-world errors go undiscovered, whereas simulation-based errors and recoveries are easily identified during debriefing and incident review. Thus, simulation permits educators to develop strategies to identify and prevent errors.

As a constructive pedagogy, simulation must be conducted in a transparent and reflective way. The debriefing process is a key component, which adds to learning. Learning from mistakes and identification of opportunities enhances the learning and self-efficacy of the student. Constructivist learning occurs when the student and teacher interact in a way that internalizes learning of external facts.

The ethics of the simulation instructor is an important element. This person develops valid and appropriate scenarios. In addition, he or she conducts appropriate debriefing and assessment, which will provide the student with insight and learning. The instructor treats students with respect and confidentiality. Thus, learning is a positive experience.

Students have ethical requirements as well. They must maintain confidentiality of the scenario to assure the learning of others and be willing to suspend disbelief of the scenario as being authentic. Acceptance of the situation as reality is essential to the learning process. This places the burden on simulation creators to use authentic situations and responses presented in a realistic and engaging scenario.

SYNOPSIS

Simulation "provides students with an opportunity to learn and practice in a controlled environment that closely mirrors the realities and complexities of practice without the risk of causing harm to patients" (Ironside, Jefferies, & Martin, 2009, p. 333). Patient autonomy and social justice rights are often violated in the pursuit of practitioner education. Simulation provides a beneficent outcome for the many underserved patients who are often the recipients of student care in large academic medical centers. Simulation brings improvements to the safety of patient care. Using simulation can help identify errors and how practitioners recover from errors. This knowledge leads to changes in practice and process. These improved processes enhance patient safety.

Simulation is often used to assist interprofessional practitioners to learn to communicate in a more effective manner. This improved communication increases patient safety and outcomes. By engaging in interprofessional communication in both high- and low-risk simulations, and then reflecting on communication styles and effectiveness, practitioners learn new skills. Real-world experiences do not always allow for this joint reflection on communication.

RECOMMENDATIONS

This pedagogy is evaluated in view of the needs of students and the effectiveness of the methodology. It is valuable in evaluating competency in procedures, decision making, and critical thinking by using methods such as role-playing, videos, and manikins (Jeffries, 2005; Piper & Czekanski, 2012).

Ricketts (2011) believes that the primary goal of any simulation is to improve the safety of care and to help the learner achieve competence by applying theoretical knowledge to clinical practice. "The use of simulation

wherever feasible conveys a critical educational and ethical message to all: patients are to be protected whenever possible and they are not commodities to be used as conveniences of training" (Ziv, Wolpe, Small, & Glick, 2003, p. 783).

The question of what is appropriate for learning in simulation versus real clinical practice is still being debated. There is agreement that using simulation is appropriate in high-risk, low-volume situations and in situations where learners can practice basic skills without causing patient harm or discomfort. The question of how much simulation is appropriate and what is lost through simulation is still being determined. This is a question of beneficence by providing the greatest good to the greatest number.

Simulation does not provide the student with the variety of human encounters and human responses that are available in the real world. Students do not enhance their ability to interpret the subtle clues conveyed by real-life experiences. These subtle movements, facial expressions, and voice tones are not easily replicated. The ability to interpret such signals is an important portion of competence in decision making and assessment (Watson et al., 2012). Therefore, the ethic of beneficence requires that careful monitoring of the use of simulation as a substitute for clinical experience is in place.

Ironside, P. M., Jeffries, P. R., & Martin, A. (2009). Fostering patient safety competencies using multiple-patient simulation experiences. *Nursing Outlook, 57*(6), 332–337.

Jeffries, P. R. (2005). A framework for designing, implementing, and evaluating simulations used as teaching strategies in nursing. *Nursing Education Perspectives, 26*(2), 96–103.

Piper, L., & Czekanski, K. (2012). Use of a simulated administrative decision-making exercise in an online master's nursing administration course. *Journal of Nursing Education, 51*(6), 343–344.

Ricketts, B. (2011). The role of simulation for learning within pre-registration nursing education—A literature review. *Nurse Education Today, 31*(7), 650–654.

Watson, K., Wright, A., Morris, N., McMeeken, J., Rivett, D., Blackstock, F.,...Jull, G. (2012). Can simulation replace part of clinical time? Two parallel randomised controlled trials. *Medical Education, 46*(7), 657–667.

Ziv, A., Wolpe, P. R., Small, S. D., & Glick, S. (2003). Simulation-based medical education: An ethical imperative. *Academic Medicine, 78*(8), 783–788.

Letty R. Piper

SIMULATION: FACULTY DEVELOPMENT

DEFINITION

Faculty development is described as a tool for improving educational competencies necessary for teachers to promote academic excellence (Wilkerson & Irby, 1998). The goal of faculty development is to empower teachers to stand out in their role as educators and encourage lifelong learning for both themselves and their students. Faculty development for nurse educators using high-fidelity patient simulation (HFPS) as a teaching technique is essential.

APPLICATION

A paradigm shift in nursing education has evolved from teacher centric to student centric (Cannon-Diehl, 2009; Drummond-Young et al., 2010). Over the past 10 years, nursing academicians have responded to this paradigm change by embracing new evolving technologies. HFPS is one of those technologies. Patient simulators are being purchased with the hope that nursing educators will embrace the new technology; however, many are not prepared to utilize this teaching strategy for instruction. This presents a challenge since there is no standard curriculum

for teaching with this innovative pedagogy (Jeffries, 2008).

With the introduction and expansion of the learner-centric methodology of simulation in the academic and clinical arenas, nurse educators need to acquire the knowledge and skills to teach with simulation in order to deliver robust experiential education (Jeanette, Parker, Nadeau, Pelayo, & Cook, 2012; Jeffries, 2005; Shellenbarger & Edwards, 2012). It is important to remember that an educator who has expertise in his or her respective field becomes a novice when he or she commences using HFPS as a teaching strategy (Gaba, 2007).

Benner's novice to expert theory (Benner, 1984) was the framework used by the California Simulation Alliance (www.californiasimulationalliance.org) to develop a simulation collaborative for faculty enhancement using an apprenticeship program. In this model, each level of competency has a specific methodology focusing on learning objectives that move nurse educators through the various stages of Benner's theory. This program has produced many nursing faculty with the expertise to teach with simulation and has been replicated throughout the nursing simulation community (Waxman & Telles, 2009). In addition, Jeffries (2008) proposed the Simulations Take Educator Preparation (STEP) plan to help educators realize the important aspects of teaching with simulation: standardized materials, train the trainer, encourage the development of a simulation design team, and plan to coordinate and implement simulation activities.

As a result of the growing importance of simulation in nursing education, a multicenter, multimodal study to investigate the use of simulation was conducted by a partnership between the National League for Nursing (NLN) and the Laerdal® Corporation. The resulting publication, *Simulation in Nursing Education: From Conceptualization to Evaluation*, is an excellent resource that outlines the criteria for nurse educators to produce high-quality educational experiences for students using simulation (Jeffries,

2007). A virtual Simulation Innovation and Resource Center (SIRC) offers web-based courses in scenario design, debriefing and guided reflection, teaching and learning strategies, technology, curriculum integration, and simulation center design (Bentley & Seaback, 2011). Both the book and website provide standardized resources for nurse educators teaching with simulation. The Society of Simulation in Healthcare (2012) developed a curriculum and assessment for simulation educators to attain a Certification as a Healthcare Simulation Educator (CHSE). In addition, attendance at local, regional, national, and international simulation conferences and workshops, as well as learning from colleagues with collaborative one-on-one educational sessions, are useful strategies for educators to increase their knowledge base for teaching with simulation (Shellenbarger & Edwards, 2012).

SYNOPSIS

The central tenet of clinical simulation is the ability to create a safe, realistic learning environment where students have the opportunity to apply their acquired knowledge; practice nursing, teamwork, and communication skills; and apply clinical decision making under the guidance of well-trained simulation educators (Jeffries, 2008; Nehring, Wexler, Hughes, & Greenwell, 2013). The aforementioned educational methods discussed provide opportunities to enhance the educational expertise for nurse educators using simulation. However, competencies for simulation educators, a universal language, and a standardized curriculum are required as simulation is integrated into nursing curricula. The learning curve to become proficient in simulation is individual and must be constantly honed (Jeffries, 2008). In order for nursing faculty to embrace this innovative pedagogy, faculty development must be ongoing and supported.

RECOMMENDATIONS

Collaboration with interprofessional partners in the clinical setting and academia is essential for the future direction of simulation-based learning activities. There is a paucity of literature describing the competencies necessary for health care educators and most notably a lack of research for the competencies for simulation-based nursing educators. There is a need for evidence-based research that focuses on faculty development needs as well as curriculum development and evaluation of this pedagogy (Jeffries, 2008). It would be optimal for nursing and other health care educators to lead this initiative.

Benner, P. (1984). *From novice to expert: Excellence and power in clinical nursing practice.* Menlo Park, CA: Addison-Wesley.

Bentley, R., & Seaback, C. (2011). A faculty development collaborative in interprofessional simulation. *Journal of Professional Nursing, 27*(6), e1–e7.

Cannon-Diehl, M. R. (2009). Simulation in healthcare and nursing: State of the science. *Critical Care Nursing Quarterly, 32*(2), 128–136.

Drummond-Young, M., Brown, B., Noesgaard, C., Lunyk-Child, O., Maich, N. M., Mines, C., & Linton, J. (2010). A comprehensive faculty development model for nursing education. *Journal of Professional Nursing, 26*(3), 152–161.

Gaba, G. M. (2007). The future vision of simulation in healthcare. *Simulation in Healthcare, 2,* 126–135.

Jeanette, M., Parker, R. A., Nadeau, J., Pelayo, L. W., & Cook, J. (2012). Developing nurse educator competency in the pedagogy of simulation. *Journal of Nursing Education, 51*(12), 685–691. doi: 10.3928/01484834–20121030-01

Jeffries, P. R. (2005). A framework for designing, implementing, and evaluating simulations used as teaching strategies in nursing. *Nursing Education Perspectives, 26*(2), 96–103.

Jeffries, P. R. (Ed.). (2007). *Simulation in nursing education: From conceptualization to evaluation.* New York, NY: National League for Nursing.

Jeffries, P. R. (2008). Getting in S.T.E.P. with simulations: Simulations take educator

S

preparation. *Nursing Education Perspectives, 29*(2), 70–73.

Nehring, W. M., Wexler, T., Hughes, F., & Greenwell, A. (2013). Faculty development for the use of high-fidelity patient simulation: A systematic review. *International Journal of Health Sciences Education, 1.* Retrieved from http://dc.etsu.edu/ijhse/vol1/iss1/4

Shellenbarger, T., & Edwards, T. (2012). Nurse educator simulation: Preparing faculty for clinical nurse educator roles. *Clinical Simulation in Nursing, 8*(6), e249–e255. doi: 10.1016/j.ecns.2010.12.006

Society of Simulation in Healthcare. (2012). *Certification standards and elements.* Retrieved from https://ssih.org/uploads/static_pages/PDF's/Certification/CHSE%20Standards.pdf

Waxman, K. T., & Telles, C. L. (2009). The use of Benner's framework in high-fidelity simulation faculty development: The bay area simulation collaborative model. *Clinical Simulation in Nursing, 5*(6), e231–e235. doi: 10.1016/j.ecns.2009.06.001

Wilkerson, L., & Irby, D. M. (1998). Strategies for improving teaching practices: A comprehensive approach to faculty development. *Academic Medicine, 73*(4), 387–396.

Barbara DeVoe
M. Isabel Friedman

SIMULATION: GENERAL

DEFINITION

Simulation is an active learning strategy that uses devices or techniques to develop an environment that closely represents a clinical setting, as well as provides educators safe, hands-on approaches to teaching and assessing psychomotor, communication, and critical-thinking skills (Blevins, 2014). Simulation is "a dynamic process involving the creation of a hypothetical opportunity that incorporates an authentic representation of reality, facilitates active student engagement, and integrates the complexities of practical and theoretical learning with opportunity for repetition, feedback, evaluation, and reflection" (Bland, Topping, & Wood, 2011, p. 668).

APPLICATION

A variety of simulator types can be used from the very simplistic to very high tech. Simulator types include part-task simulators that focus on a specific part of the body (e.g., mannequins used in cardiopulmonary resuscitation training); simulated patients who are trained to act like patients; screen-based computer simulators that use web or computer-assisted programs; and integrated simulators that are capable of producing physiological responses (e.g., full-sized adult, pediatric, or obstetrical simulators; Durham & Alden, 2008).

Jeffries' (2005) simulation in the nursing education framework has been widely used in nursing education. The model has six specific areas that must be addressed when designing simulations: objectives, planning, fidelity, complexity, cues, and debriefing. Objectives describe what the students should know or be able to do at the end of the simulation. Planning activities address each objective and identify needed information related to role expectations, mental and physical comorbid conditions, timelines, expected outcomes, props, and equipment.

Fidelity or realism focuses on the need for the experience to reflect clinical reality. Cues are provided by the faculty who act as facilitators and provide learner support and debriefing. Debriefing allows students an opportunity to engage in reflective learning and to link theory, research, and practice into effective interventions in complex situations (Jeffries, 2005).

SYNOPSIS

The beneficial outcomes of including simulation throughout an undergraduate nursing program are reduced levels of anxiety in students, increased knowledge retention, and development of psychomotor, communication, and critical-thinking skills within a safe environment (Stroup, 2014). Kelly, Hager, and Gallagher (2014) asked 102 nursing students to rank 11 components of simulation in terms of making a contribution to enhancing clinical judgment. Facilitated debriefing, post-simulation reflection, and guidance by the educator were ranked as most beneficial. Reviewing the audio-taped simulation and patient case notes was ranked as least beneficial.

Jeffries et al. (2011) implemented a simulation-based cardiovascular assessment program in four universities using a full-sized adult mannequin. Thirty-six advanced practice nursing students participated and reported significant improvements in their self-confidence to perform cardiovascular assessment, and were extremely satisfied with the simulation methods as an effective teaching strategy. Sixty second-year associate degree nursing students participated in an obstetrical simulation experience and audio-taped their reflections of the experience. Qualitative analysis revealed three themes: the nonthreatening environment, enhancement of learning, and feeling more prepared to practice (Partin, Payne, & Slemmons, 2011). Three hundred third-year nursing students reported high-fidelity simulation using three differing scenarios to be enjoyable, challenging, and matched well with course content (Wotton, Davis, Button, & Kelton, 2010). Students also found debriefing to be important for clarification and providing a rationale for practice. Students did, however, report having short episodes of feeling confused when the simulated patient's clinical condition changed. Kaplan and Ura (2010) developed a simulation-based learning experience to increase senior nursing students' confidence, as well as their ability to safely and effectively prioritize, delegate, and implement care. Ninety-seven students rated that they agreed or strongly agreed that the simulation experience was well organized, realistic, and increased their understanding of prioritization and delegation.

Over three quarters of the participants also reported having more confidence in their leadership abilities. Brewer (2011) conducted an integrated review of the literature and summarized that students and faculty view simulation positively, yet most of the studies are qualitative with the need for more quantitative research.

The use of simulation has been found to be an effective, interactive teaching strategy. Nursing students have reported simulation experiences provide safe, informative opportunities to practice communication and technical skills. Outcomes of simulation experiences that have been reported include increased self-confidence levels, enhanced leadership skills, and feeling more prepared for real-time clinical experiences.

RECOMMENDATIONS

The need to provide undergraduate nursing students with clinical experiences that will foster competencies in acute and chronic illness management, clinical reasoning, assessment, diagnosis, and intervention is paramount. Challenges of finding clinical placements for students have made it difficult for nurse educators to provide necessary experiences. One solution to address clinical placement shortage is the use of simulation.

According to Bland, Topping, and Tobbell (2014), nurse educators should also be aware of the limitations of using simulation in terms of authenticity. Although high-fidelity simulators are designed to be realistic with heart rates, breath sounds, moaning, and crying, some students may still find these experiences lacking authenticity. Further research is needed to better understand the relationships between fidelity, authenticity, and learning to improve the effectiveness of simulation in nursing education.

Bland, A. J., Topping, A., & Tobbell, J. (2014). Time to unravel the conceptual confusion of authenticity and fidelity and their contribution to learning within simulation-based nurse education. A discussion paper. *Nurse Education Today, 34*(7), 1112–1118.

Bland, A. J., Topping, A., & Wood, B. (2011). A concept analysis of simulation as a learning strategy in the education of undergraduate nursing students. *Nurse Education Today, 31*(7), 664–670.

Blevins, S. (2014). The impact of simulation on patient care. *MEDSURG Nursing, 23*(2), 120–121.

Brewer, E. P. (2011). Successful techniques for using human patient simulation in nursing education. *Journal of Nursing Scholarship, 43*(3), 311–317.

Durham, C. F., & Alden, K. R. (2008). Enhancing patient safety in nursing education through patient simulation. In R. G. Hughes (Ed.), *Patient safety and quality: An evidenced-based handbook for nurses* (pp. 221–260). Rockville, MD: Agency for Healthcare Research and Quality.

Jeffries, P. R. (2005). A framework for designing, implementing, and evaluating simulations used as teaching strategies in nursing. *Nursing Education Perspectives, 26*(2), 96–103.

Jeffries, P. R., Beach, M., Decker, S. I., Dlugasch, L., Groom, J., Settles, J., & O'Donnell, J. M. (2011). Multi-center development and testing of a simulation-based cardiovascular assessment curriculum for advanced practice nurses. *Nursing Education Perspectives, 32*(5), 316–322.

Kaplan, B., & Ura, D. (2010). Use of multiple patient simulators to enhance prioritizing and delegating skills for senior nursing students. *Journal of Nursing Education, 49*(7), 371–377.

Kelly, M. A., Hager, P., & Gallagher, R. (2014). What matters most? Students' rankings of simulation components that contribute to clinical judgment. *Journal of Nursing Education, 53*(2), 97–101.

Partin, J. L., Payne, T. A., & Slemmons, M. F. (2011). Students' perceptions of their learning experiences using high-fidelity simulation to teach concepts relative to obstetrics. *Nursing Education Perspectives, 32*(3), 186–188.

Stroup, C. (2014). Simulation usage in nursing fundamentals: Integrative literature review. *Clinical Simulation in Nursing, 10,* e155–e164.

Wotton, K., Davis, J., Button, D., & Kelton, M. (2010). Third-year undergraduate nursing students' perceptions of high-fidelity simulation. *Journal of Nursing Education, 49*(11), 632–639.

Karen S. Dunn

SIMULATION: HUMAN PATIENT

DEFINITION

Simulation is a pedagogy method used to improve, promote, and actively engage students in a realistic clinical situation using a human patient, or a computerized patient simulator to mimic real-life clinical situations (Jeffries, 2005). Human patient simulations are a forum for actively engaging nursing students in critical thinking and application of knowledge.

APPLICATION

Simulation has taken on many forms over the numerous years it has been used in nursing education (Nehring & Lashley, 2009). Human patient simulation and the use of high-fidelty technology have added a broader dimension to simulation use in nursing education. The long history of simulation in nursing education has included the use of anatomical models such as jointed skeletons; task trainers such as models of arms and legs used to practice injections and first aid; and low-fidelity patient simulators. Fidelity denotes the extent to which the entity imitates reality (Nehring & Lashley, 2009).

Jeffries (2008) suggests that high-fidelity patient simulations (HFPSs) can be used as innovative approaches to nursing education at a time when the world has a shortage of nurse educators, by allowing students clinical opportunities to learn without compromising a patient's safety. She suggests more research should be completed with reliable methods to test skill acquisition and learning outcomes assessment, so as to increase the evidence used to support its use as a learning strategy. Benner, Sutphen, Leonard, and Day (2010) found that by engaging students in active learning, they are more readily able to recall and apply knowledge when it is needed later.

The most appropriate theoretical framework for this type of educational intervention is the Nursing Education Simulation Framework (NESF) developed by the National League for Nursing (NLN). The conceptual framework allows one to design, implement, and evaluate teaching strategies using simulations within the nurse educational setting (Jeffries, 2005). It is made up of five components that are as follows: best practices in education, student factors, teacher factors, simulation design, and outcome measurements. By including best practices in education, faculty focus on how students learn and provide the means that optimizes learning and critical-thinking skills. Student factors include the importance of being responsible for learning, being self-directed, and being motivated. Teacher factors include providing faculty with the training and technological support they need in order to design and implement the new learning strategies. Simulation design should support course goals, learning outcomes, and skill competencies. Faculty should also consider the complexity, fidelity, cues, and debriefing that will be implemented within the learning exercise. Outcome measures are focused on student critical-thinking skills gained from the simulation experience and the translation of theoretical concepts.

SYNOPSIS

Simulation in human patients provides for a safe method of actively engaging students in clinical scenarios using HFPS as innovative approaches to nursing education. Opportunities for students to develop and advance their clinical knowledge and skills are critical. HFPS provides innovative approaches to nursing education (Jeffries, 2008). Simulation provides a valuable intermediate step to preparing nursing students to care for patients in a clinical setting. Oliver, Ambrose, and Wynn (2011) integrated a mental health problem of depression with suicidal ideations with management of an adult health postoperative surgical patient simulation. The HFPS was beneficial in identifying students' unwillingness to explore feelings they were uncomfortable with and therefore allowed faculty to assist students in improving communication while managing a depressed obese patient on a medical–surgical floor (Oliver, Ambrose, & Wynn, 2011). The use of human patient simulation has become an integral part of nursing education. Simulation is useful in both undergraduate and graduate education.

RECOMMENDATIONS

Human patient simulations serve as a valuable and practical method to assist students in learning to work as a team and problem solve through consensus building. Faculty should be provided with the needed training and technological support in order to successfully design and implement learning strategies using human patient simulation. Faculty development should include continuing education on design and development of scenarios that mimic clinical situations to improve critical-thinking skills. Faculty should be accountable for priming students on what to expect and how to prepare for the simulation experience; however, students need to be self-directed and motivated to learn. Objectives should be determined and communicated in advance in regard to how simulation will be used for learning and for evaluation. Simulation is a positive and effective pedagogy to help students understand critical content and develop communication skills in nursing education. There is a need to continue research and add to the evidence to support student outcomes gained from the use of simulation in undergraduate and graduate nursing education.

Benner, P., Sutphen, M., Leonard, V., & Day, L. (2010). *Educating nurses: A call for radical transformation*. San Francisco, CA: Jossey-Bass.

Jeffries, P. R. (2005). A framework for designing, implementing, and evaluating simulations used as teaching strategies in nursing. *Nursing Education Perspectives, 26*(2), 96–103.

Jeffries, P. R. (2008). Getting in S.T.E.P. with simulations: Simulations take educator preparation. *Nursing Education Perspectives, 29*(2), 70–71. Retrieved from http://search .ebscohost.com

Nehring, W. M., & Lashley, F. R. (2009). Nursing simulation: A review of the past 40 years. *Simulation & Gaming, 40*(4), 528–552. Retrieved from http://search.ebsco-host.com

Oliver, J. S., Ambrose, S. M., & Wynn, S. D. (2011). Using simulation innovation to facilitate learning nursing concepts: Medical and mental health. *Journal of Nursing Education, 50*(2), 120. doi: 10.3928/01484834–20110120-02

JoAnn S. Oliver

SIMULATION: INTERPROFESSIONAL

DEFINITION

Interprofessional simulation (IPS) includes both educators and learners from two or more professions who join to create interactive and collaborative learning activities that replicate real-world situations (Gaba, 2007; Zhang, Thompson, & Miller, 2011). Simulation activities can occur in a wide array of settings, including simulation centers, in situ, and virtual settings such as Second Life®. Various health care simulation formats include immersive simulations, human patient simulators, standardized patients, and serious games. The goal of IPS is to further develop knowledge, communication, and clinical skills, and enhance respectful attitudes that yield competent team performance (Gaba, 2007; Institute of Medicine [IOM], 2003).

APPLICATION

Regardless of setting and format, simulation is increasingly being viewed as a facilitating technology that transcends traditional educational boundaries and allows students in pre-licensure and postgraduate health care programs to acquire the competencies needed for interprofessional practice (Zhang et al., 2011). The necessity of numerous roles in a simulation scenario naturally lends itself to interprofessional collaboration. Nursing and medicine are the two professions included most frequently in IPS (Zhang et al., 2011).

Although each profession must educate students in preparation for their future roles, it is considered essential that team members understand the roles of each of the other team members. Simulation of health care practice allows participants to question their perceptions of these roles brought from previous exposure, culture, and media (National League for Nursing [NLN], 2012). Considerable efforts in standardization of structure and process for successful interprofessional health care simulation are underway.

The Society for Simulation in Healthcare (SSH) is a multiprofession organization that promotes excellence in interprofessional health care education, practice, advocacy, and research through a variety of simulation modalities (SSH, 2011). SSH has had a rigorous accreditation program for simulation centers since 2008 (SSH, 2011). The SSH has developed both beginning and advanced levels of certification for educators using simulation. Both the levels of certification criteria include elements of interprofessional collaboration. Certification is open to all health care professionals (SSH, 2014).

In nursing, six competencies of Quality and Safety Education for Nurses (QSEN) have been defined as patient-centered care, teamwork and collaboration, evidence-based practice, quality improvement, safety, and informatics (Cronenwett et al., 2007). IPS is essential to the integration of these patient safety competencies in education and practice, particularly the competencies of teamwork and collaboration and quality improvement.

Although there are natural and structural inclinations for interprofessional collaboration in simulation, significant barriers remain in implementation. Scheduling participants from different programs or professions who have varied schedules is a continual challenge. Perhaps the most-cited obstacle to IPS is limited resources. This broad category includes the costs of simulation and how that should be shared among the professions, as well as a lack of recognition by administration of the workload necessary to execute IPS (Gough, Hellaby, Jones, & MacKinnon, 2012; NLN, 2012). Other barriers include faculty and administration resistance to change and proximity to other health care programs (NLN, 2012).

Health care educators in academe and practice are finding ways around the obstacles of IPS. Two highly successful IPS programs focused on medical and nursing students (Liaw et al., 2014; Paige et al., 2014). Paige et al. (2014) implemented a high-fidelity, interprofessional simulated operating room (OR) experience with undergraduate nursing students, nurse anesthesia students, and medical students. This quasi-experimental study looked at self-efficacy and teamwork before and after simulation experiences. Overall, students tended to overestimate their practice of team-based behaviors. Statistically significant improvement in self-efficacy and team performance after IPS intervention were reported (Paige et al., 2014). The authors concluded that high-fidelity IPS of the OR improves students' team-based attitudes and performance.

Liaw et al. (2014) developed a program of IPS (Sim-IPE) aimed to improve communication between nursing and medical students. In their Sim-IPE program, communication strategies, such as Situation, Background, Assessment, Recommendation (SBAR) and Check-Back, were implemented in handover reporting of a deteriorating patient (Liaw

et al., 2014). Self-confidence, perception of interprofessional learning, and satisfaction with the simulation were measured. Statistically significant increases in confidence and perception for both medical and nursing students along with overall satisfaction in the simulation program were reported (Liaw et al., 2014).

SYNOPSIS

The SSH promotes IPS and offers accreditation to organizations that implement simulation (SSH, 2011) as well as certification for simulation educators of all health care professions (SSH, 2014). Inadequate resources, primarily costs, and educator workload remain sufficient obstacles to many institutions that desire the implementation of IPS.

Implications to health care are obvious. IPS offers academic health care educators an early opportunity to develop students' self-efficacy, team performance (Paige et al., 2014), self-confidence, communication skills, and appreciation for interprofessional teamwork (Liaw et al., 2014). Health care educators in the practice setting are implementing IPS opportunities to foster competence and excellence in health care teams. It is believed that this systematization of IPS will revolutionize professional practice and lead to marked advancements in patient safety (Liaw et al., 2014).

RECOMMENDATIONS

The IOM (2010) urges a further increase in the use of simulation as a training tool for teaching health care clinicians, especially in the areas of team training. While the anecdotal and empirical evidence supports this shift in education and training of health care providers, several cautions should be noted. First, Milton (2013) advises that nurse educators have an obligation to carefully incorporate nursing theoretical-based curricula with IPS and never compromise theoretical core beliefs of nursing. Second, while some mention the challenge of finding appropriate places in nursing curriculum to insert IPE opportunities (NLN, 2012), it is a transformation in thinking and planning that will integrate IPE simulation into nursing curriculum as naturally as it occurs in professional practice. Third, the NLN (2012) recommends careful attention to matching student levels across the various programs in order to maximize success of IPS.

Simultaneously, educators in practice and academe are building a body of knowledge regarding IPS. Initially, the use of an evaluation framework to define outcomes and a quality improvement model to structure designing and testing could provide the scientific foundation for systematically measuring the effectiveness of IPS (Zhang et al., 2011). Further, multisite longitudinal research studies are required to provide evidence of the transferability of skills developed during IPS to patient care, as well as the overall impact on both education and health care (Gough et al., 2012). With the current state of IPS knowledge, high-quality mixed and multimethod approaches should be encouraged to provide a richer picture and more robust analyses of IPS interventions and outcomes (Gough et al., 2012).

The ultimate goal of IPS is excellence in team performance. Health care educators in academic and practice realms must focus efforts on developing IPS for larger units of participants such as teams, units, and entire health care organization (Gaba, 2007).

Cronenwett, L., Sherwood, G., Barnsteiner, J., Disch, J., Johnson, J., Mitchell, P., . . . Warren, J. (2007). Quality and safety education for nurses. *Nursing Outlook, 55*(3), 122–131.

Gaba, D. M. (2007). The future vision of simulation in healthcare. *Simulation in Healthcare, 2*(2), 126–135.

Gough, S., Hellaby, M., Jones, N., & MacKinnon, R. (2012). A review of undergraduate interprofessional simulation-based education (IPSE). *Collegian, 19*(3), 153–170. doi:org/10.1016/j.colegn.2012.04.004

Institute of Medicine (IOM). (2003). *Health professions education: A bridge to quality.* Washington, DC: National Academies Press.

Institute of Medicine of the Natural Academies. (2010). *The future of nursing: Leading change, advancing health.* Washington, DC: National Academies Press.

Liaw, S. Y., Koh, Y., Dawood, R., Kowitlawakul, Y., Zhou, W., & Lau, S. T. (2014). Easing student transition to graduate nurse: A SIMulated Professional Learning Environment (SIMPLE) for final year student nurses. *Nurse Education Today, 34*(3), 349–355.

Milton, C. L. (2013). Ethical issues surrounding interprofessional collaboration. *Nursing Science Quarterly, 26*(4), 316–318. doi:10.1177/0894318413500314

National League for Nursing (NLN). (2012). *A nursing perspective on simulation and interprofessional education (IPE): A report from the National League for Nursing's think tank on using simulation as an enabling strategy for IPE.* Retrieved from http://www.nln .org/facultyprograms/facultyresources/ pdf/nursing_perspective_sim_education .pdf

Paige, J. T., Garbee, D. D., Kozmenko, V., Yu, Q., Kozmenko, L., Yang, T., . . . Swartz, W. (2014). Getting a head start: High-fidelity, simulation-based operating room team training of interprofessional students. *Journal of the American College of Surgeons, 218*(1), 140–149. doi:10.1016/j. jamcollsurg.2013.09.006

Society for Simulation in Healthcare (SSH). (2011). SSH accreditation process 9.10: Informational guide for the accreditation process from the SSH Council for accreditation of healthcare simulation programs. *Society for Simulation in Healthcare.*

Society for Simulation in Healthcare (SSH). (2014, March 4). *CHSE-A certified healthcare simulation educator-advanced [certification process].* Retrieved from http://ssih.org/ chse-a

Zhang, C., Thompson, S., & Miller, C. (2011). A review of simulation-based interprofessional education. *Clinical Simulation in Nursing, 7*, e117–e126. doi:10.1016/j. ecns.2010.02.008

Margaret A. Harris

SIMULATION: MEDICATION SAFETY

DEFINITION

Nursing educators can use simulation to train students in the intricacies of medication administration, rather than practicing these high-risk skills solely on patients. Simulation is a controllable strategy that puts genuine equipment in the hands of students so that they can practice complex skills such as reconstitution from powder to intravenous solution, dilution to recommended concentration, and rate of infusion. Within a simulated environment, educators can allow performance error so that there is subsequent "learn by doing" that is not feasible on acute care units.

APPLICATION

Faculty bear the responsibility of keeping patients safe while simultaneously offering nursing students the opportunity to experience authentic patient care situations. However, students are often not given the opportunity to administer complex medications during routine clinical rotations, and especially during critical events when accuracy is vital within the context of a high-stress situation. So rather than relying so heavily on random opportunity in clinical to practice this set of skills, virtual environments can be created that model actual medication requirements. In simulation, students are presented with real medication orders, which may even include prescribing error, so that both critical thinking and technical skill can be assessed.

Scholars well entrenched in medication safety research have postulated that in order to improve the numeracy, calculation competence, and technical acumen needed for safe medication administration, there must exist a culture of education that is adaptive to both evolving clinical environments and our the 21st century nursing students (Weeks, Sabin, Pontin, & Woolley, 2013). It is time to move away from the model that includes classic didactic instruction followed by an assessment of numeracy via a conventional medication calculation exam. Evidence suggests that abstract word-based assessments that are void of contextual features present in clinical practice are not reliable indicators of student medication calculation ability (Wright, 2012). Poor performance on a written examination may be due to inability to visualize the problem, compounded by limited opportunity to handle the equipment and supplies (Sabin, 2013).

While nursing faculty may be able to teach formulas in classroom settings, simulation allows time and space for the student to see the problem in context. Building a mental image of the calculation through hands-on practice allows the student to envision the problem in a concrete fashion. In using simulation, faculty can colocate the demands for conceptual calculation and technical requirements within authentic learning and assessment environments. Such review of calculation plus hands-on administration using equipment may help to reinforce error-reducing practices.

Educators have found that using simulation to practice medication administration is not only convenient, but successful in improving student ability to perform calculations (Costello, 2011; Pauly-O'Neill & Prion, 2013). Analysis of a systematic literature search regarding the use of simulation to improve medication calculation skill revealed that using simulated scenarios that include real-life medication calculation examples allowed students to better develop critical-thinking skills as well as decrease their anxiety (Zahara-Such, 2013).

SYNOPSIS

Nonadherence to the "Rights Method" causes medication error. However, according to the Institute of Medicine's landmark report *To Err Is Human: Building a Safer Health Care System* (IOM, 1999), an error can be further defined as the wrong plan to achieve an aim. In other words, a registered nurse (RN) or nursing student may correctly identify the patient, drug, dose, route, and time, but fail to displace air bubbles from a syringe; hence, underdosing can occur. Setting traditional pumps incorrectly or overriding smart pump technology (those devices programmed with drug-specific safety software) may result in delivering a medication too rapidly.

In a study of smart pump technology and medication administration, authors report that success rates on secondary infusions were low (55.6%) regardless of the type of infusion pump used (Trbovich, Pinkney, Cafazzo, & Easty, 2010). Medication left in the dead space of infusion tubing is another pitfall in medication administration that is related to an inability to set the rate and volume correctly (Broselow, Luten, & Schuman, 2008). Sears, Goldsworthy, and Goodman (2010) reports the results of a randomized controlled study showing that students made fewer errors in clinical rotations after exposure to simulation-based experiences than those without. Research that illustrates a significant relationship between authentic learning environments and success in medication calculation helps support the notion that this exposure is a vital step in the construction of knowledge (Weeks, Clochesy, Hutton, & Moseley, 2013).

Participating in drug administration within a simulated environment puts the emphasis on application and demonstration within a wider context that cannot be ensured during a clinical rotation (Sabin et al., 2013). Added benefits include the opportunity to model expert performance, scaffold learning, reflect on performance with support, and enculturate students to the essential features of safe practice (Macdonald, Weeks, & Moseley, 2013).

RECOMMENDATIONS

Traditional didactic strategies based on word problems divorced from real-world context may be too abstract for many learners. Research has supported the use of more adaptive pedagogy including the use of simulation to capture expert practices and recreate them in a virtual setting, providing tangible materials that can be manipulated rather than formulas on a page. Syringes, infusion pumps, intravenous bags, labeled drug vials, and medication sheets can all be made available as the student extracts the important information from the medical orders and ultimately delivers a medication safely.

Broselow, J., Luten, R., & Schuman, A. (2008). Preventing death by decimal point. *Contemporary Pediatrics, 25*, 35–44.

Costello, M. (2011). The use of simulation in medication calculation instruction: A pilot study. *Nurse Educator, 36*(5), 181–182.

Institute of Medicine (IOM). (1999). *To err is human: Building a safer health care system.* Washington, DC: National Academy Press.

Macdonald, K., Weeks, K. W., & Moseley, L. (2013). Safety in numbers 6: Tracking pre-registration nursing students' cognitive and functional competence development in medication dosage calculation problem-solving: The role of authentic learning and diagnostic assessment environments. *Nurse Education in Practice, 13*(2), e66–e77.

Pauly-O'Neill, S., & Prion, S. (2013). Using integrated simulation in a nursing program to improve medication administration skills in the pediatric population. *Nursing Education Perspectives, 34*(3), 148–153.

Sabin, M. (2013). Write and wrong: authenticity and medication dosage calculation. *Nurse Education in Practice, 13*(2), e2–e3.

Sabin, M., Weeks, K. W., Rowe, D. A., Hutton, B. M., Coben, D., Hall, C., & Woolley, N. (2013). Safety in numbers 5: Evaluation of computer-based authentic assessment and high fidelity simulated OSCE environments as a framework for articulating a point of registration medication dosage calculation benchmark. *Nurse Education in Practice, 13*(2), e55–e65.

Sears, K., Goldsworthy, S., & Goodman, W. M. (2010). The relationship between simulation in nursing education and medication safety. *Journal of Nursing Education, 49*(1), 52–55.

S

S

Trbovich, P. L., Pinkney, S., Cafazzo, J. A., & Easty, A. C. (2010). The impact of traditional and smart pump infusion technology on nurse medication administration performance in a simulated inpatient unit. *Quality & Safety in Health Care, 19*(5), 430–434.

Weeks, K. W., Clochesy, J. M., Hutton, B. M., & Moseley, L. (2013). Safety in numbers 4: The relationship between exposure to authentic and didactic environments and nursing students' learning of medication dosage calculation problem solving knowledge and skills. *Nurse Education in Practice, 13*(2), 43–54.

Weeks, K. W., Sabin, M., Pontin, D., & Woolley, N. (2013). Safety in numbers: An introduction to the nurse education in practice series. *Nurse Education in Practice, 13*(2), e4–e10.

Wright, K. (2012). The assessment of drug calculation skills–time to rethink the whole process. *Nurse Education Today, 32*(4), 341–344.

Zahara-Such, R. (2013). Improving medication calculations of nursing students through simulation: An integrative review. *Clinical Simulation in Nursing, 9*, e379–e383.

Susan Pauly-O'Neill

SIMULATION: PATIENT SAFETY

DEFINITION

Simulation is the technique of imitating real experiences with guided experiences that replicate significant aspects of the real world in a fully interactive manner (Gaba & DeAnda, 1987). It is performed primarily for the purpose of study or training. Simulation has roots in aviation; like the aviation industry, simulation in health care is aimed at safety of the consumer, or, more specifically, the patient.

APPLICATION

Nursing has generated many useful structures and standards for the implementation of simulation toward patient safety. In an annual message, the president of the International Nursing Association for Clinical Simulation and Learning (INACSL) recently affirmed that patient safety is the primary focus of health care simulation (Durham, 2014). INACSL has been a leader in the promotion and dissemination of evidence-based practice standards for clinical simulation methodologies, research, and education. INACSL updated the standards for best practice in simulation, which consist of terminology, professional integrity of participants, participant objectives, facilitation, facilitator, the debriefing process, and participant assessment and evaluation (Clinical Simulation in Nursing, 2013).

Through collaborative work with the National League for Nursing, Jeffries created the Jeffries' simulation model (Jeffries, 2005). The model was developed from the theoretical and empirical literature related to simulation and identifies essential aspects of simulation design that bolster student outcomes. The factors of model include teacher factors, student factors, educational practices, design of specific simulation experiences, and student outcomes (Jeffries, 2005).

During the same time period, a group of nurse researchers developed a comprehensive approach to ensure patient safety competencies were being addressed in nursing education. The six competencies of quality and safety education for nurses (QSEN) are patient-centered care, teamwork and collaboration, evidence-based practice, quality improvement, safety, and informatics (Cronenwett et al., 2007). It has been stipulated that these competencies cannot be mastered through a didactic approach (Cronenwett et al., 2007). Simulation is essential to the integration of patient safety competencies in nursing education and their sustainment in nursing practice.

Nursing literature specific to simulation and patient safety includes the evaluation of patient safety competencies (Henneman et al., 2010), improvement of patient safety behaviors (Gantt & Webb-Corbett, 2010), and improvement in medication administration performance (Harris, Pittiglio, Newton, & Moore, 2014; Sears, Goldsworthy, & Goodman, 2010). Henneman et al. (2010)

examined the types of errors that occurred or were recognized and corrected in a simulated clinical environment. The authors reported that all students committed an error and thus concluded that greater emphasis is needed on effective educational interventions to teach patient safety (Henneman et al., 2010). These findings endorse simulation as an effective method to evaluate patient safety competencies.

Looking to influence patient safety behaviors in student nurses, Gantt and Webb-Corbett (2010) reported improved patient safety behaviors with simulation as an educational intervention. The authors found that simulation provides an opportunity to teach patient safety with well-defined standards for performance of many QSEN competencies. These findings support the use of simulation to incorporate QSEN competencies. Simulation methods should be reconceptualized by nursing faculty as not only teaching tools for clinical situations, but as tools that can be used by greater numbers of students at various levels of nursing to integrate patient safety competencies (Harris et al., 2014).

Nursing research has also focused on medication safety using simulation as an educational intervention (Harris et al., 2014; Sears et al., 2010). Harris, Pittiglio, Newton, and Moore (2014) examined the effects of simulation on safe medication preparation in junior-level nursing students and reported significantly higher performance in students who experienced simulation. Sears, Goldsworthy, and Goodman (2010) used a quasi-experimental design to examine whether the use of simulation could help reduce medication errors and reported study results that demonstrate a positive effect of simulation on the reduction of medication administration errors. Although samples in both studies were small, findings suggest that simulation education may contribute to a reduction in medication errors involving student nurses. Both studies contribute to knowledge in the area of simulation in nursing education and patient safety specific to medication administration; replication and expansion in this area are recommended (Harris et al., 2014; Sears et al., 2010).

It is noteworthy that most research in the area of simulation and patient safety has been performed in adult patient simulation with little focus on the pediatric population (Zhang, Thompson, & Miller, 2011). Simulations may be of particular interest to pediatric patient safety because of children's size and the nature of physiologic reserves, as well as the added stress to health care providers that parents at the bedside can bring (Gaba, 2007; Harris, 2011). Simulation intervention in pediatric nursing education has shown significant increases in student clinical scores and anecdotal reports of increased confidence in the clinical setting (Harris, 2011).

SYNOPSIS

Simulation in nursing education has shown to be useful in evaluation of patient safety competencies and improving those competencies, specifically in the area of medication administration safety. From an integrative review of patient safety and simulation in nursing education, Berndt (2014) reported simulation to be more effective than traditional didactic methods. Furthermore, it was concluded that existing evidence supports the efficacy of simulation in teaching patient safety competencies. Future research needs to include more rigorous design with larger samples from multiple sites.

Simulation helps reduce medical errors and encourages patient safety. Although the up-front costs of establishing simulation centers may be high, the long-term cost will be recovered from the consequent decrease in medical errors and subsequent increase in patient safety (Abraham, Wade, O'Connell, Desharnais, & Jacoby, 2011). The key drivers to further simulation efforts to improve patient safety include public interest, liability insurers, professional organizations, accrediting bodies, and government regulatory organizations (Gaba, 2007).

RECOMMENDATIONS

In many health systems currently, emphasis is placed on basic science education, individual knowledge and skill, and an apprenticeship model of training. Simulation needs to play a principal role in the education, training, and clinical care sustainment of health care providers. Simulation provides both structure and standardization of basic education, training, and continued education of practitioners to achieve excellence in patient safety. A transformation of the entire education, training, and continued education of health care providers is called for in the literature (Gaba, 2007; Zhang et al., 2011). Simulation will be an important bottom-up tool for creating and maintaining a culture of safety and for fostering changes in work procedures and communication systems (Gaba, 2007).

Abraham, J., Wade, D. M., O'Connell, K. A., Desharnais, S., & Jacoby, R. (2011). The use of simulation training in teaching health care quality and safety: An annotated bibliography. *American Journal of Medical Quality, 26*(3), 229–238. doi: 10.1177/1062860610384716

Berndt, J. (2014). Patient safety and simulation in prelicensure nursing education: An integrative review. *Teaching and Learning in Nursing, 9*, 16–22. doi:org/10.1016/j.teln.2013.09.001

Cronenwett, L., Sherwood, G., Barnsteiner, J., Disch, J., Johnson, J., Mitchell, P., . . . Warren, J. (2007). Quality and safety education for nurses. *Nursing Outlook, 55*(3), 122–131. doi:10.1016/j.outlook.2007.02.006

Durham, C. (2014). President's message: Patient safety the focus of healthcare simulation. *Clinical Simulation in Nursing, 10*, e1–e2. doi:org/10.1016/j.ecns.2013.12.001

Gaba, D. M. (2007). Out of this nettle, danger, we pluck this flower, safety; healthcare vs. aviation and other high-hazard industries. *Simulation in Healthcare, 2*(4), 213–217.

Gaba, D., & DeAnda, A. (1987). A comprehensive anesthesia simulation environment: Recreating the operating room for research and training. *Anesthesiology, 69*, 387–394.

Gantt, L. T., & Webb-Corbett, R. (2010). Using simulation to teach patient safety behaviors in undergraduate nursing education. *Journal of Nursing Education, 49*(1), 48–51. doi:10.3928/01484834–20090918-10

Harris, M. A. (2011). Simulation-enhanced pediatric clinical orientation. *Journal of Nursing Education, 50*(8), 461–465. doi: 10.3928/01484834–20110429-05

Harris, M. A., Pittiglio, L., Newton, S. E., & Moore, G. (2014). Using simulation to improve the medication administration skills of undergraduate nursing students. *Nursing Education Perspectives, 35*(1), 26–29. doi:10.5480/11–552.1

Jeffries, P. R. (2005). A framework for designing, implementing, and evaluating simulations used as teaching strategies in nursing. *Nursing Education Perspectives, 26*(2), 96–103.

Henneman, E. A., Roche, J. P., Fisher, D. L., Cunningham, H., Reilly, C. A., Nathanson, B. H., & Henneman, P. L. (2010). Error identification and recovery by student nurses using human patient simulation: Opportunity to improve patient safety. *Applied Nursing Research, 23*(1), 11–21.

Sears, K., Goldsworthy, S., & Goodman, W. M. (2010). The relationship between simulation in nursing education and medication safety. *Journal of Nursing Education, 49*, 52–55. Retrieved from http://dx.doi.org/10.3928/01484834–20090918

Zhang, C., Thompson, S., & Miller, C. (2011). A review of simulation-based interprofessional education. *Clinical Simulation in Nursing, 7*(4), e117–e126. doi:10.1016/j.ecns.2010.02.008

Margaret A. Harris

SIMULATION: PROGRAM EVALUATION

DEFINITION

The use of high-fidelity simulation (HFS) in nursing education has been described as simulation that incorporates a computerized full-body manikin that can be programmed to provide a realistic physiological response to student actions (Cant & Cooper, 2010, p. 4). Program evaluation of simulation is a methodological data collection and review process intended to inform decisions and improve program efficacy.

APPLICATION

Integration of simulation across the curriculum represents one of the several "best practices in simulation pedagogy" (McGaghie, Issenberg, Petrusa, & Scalese, 2010). The absence of a consistent framework to measure and evaluate simulation-associated outcomes is a major challenge to incorporating simulation into nursing curricula (Onello & Regan, 2013).

Historically, evaluation of simulation in education has emphasized the measurement of outcomes (i.e., knowledge gain and skill acquisition) and comparisons of simulation with standard teaching methods (Kable, Arthur, Levett-Jones, & Reid-Searl, 2013). Specific reports of curricular or program-level evaluation of simulation are extremely limited (Arthur, Levett-Jones, & Kable, 2013; Kable et al., 2013; Schiavenato, 2009). Exploration to design and develop standardized methods of simulation outcome measurement has been called for at national and international levels (Cant & Cooper, 2010).

SYNOPSIS

Although a gold standard for evaluation of simulation has not appeared in the literature (Kardong-Edgren, Adamson, & Fitzgerald, 2010), researchers are studying systematic assessment methods and developing standardized tools for evaluating simulation (Elfrink Cordi, Leighton, Ryan-Wenger, Doyle, & Ravert, 2012).

The nursing education simulation framework (NESF) was developed through a partnership with the National League for Nursing and the Laerdal Corporation. Jeffries (2005) published the framework for designing, implementing, and evaluating simulations in nursing education. Constructs of the framework include teacher–student factors, educational practices, student outcomes, and design characteristics. Wide variance in the volume and strength of evidence in support of the constructs and subcomponents was found in a recent review of the literature (Groom, Henderson, & Sittner, 2013).

Sportsman, Schumacker, and Hamilton (2011) used the perception of clinical competence model as a framework to study the impact of simulation in an undergraduate nursing curriculum using students' sense of clinical competence and other metrics of success. A five-variable model with input (student–faculty characteristics) and process variables (learning strategies and clinical learning environment) explained BSN students' perceptions of their clinical competence. Sportsman et al. used this model and three instruments to collect, explore, and interpret data from BSN and AD students participating in a series of courses using simulation experiences. Acceptable reliability coefficients were reported for the three instruments (Sportsman, Schumacker, & Hamilton, 2011).

Simulation allows for evaluation of student behaviors in the affective, cognitive, and psychomotor learning domains, and assessment should address learning in these domains (Sando et al., 2013). Reviewing extant literature, Kardong-Edgren, Adamson, and Fitzgerald (2010) identified 22 simulation evaluation tools and acknowledged four tools most closely addressing the three learning domains simultaneously.

Davis and Kimble (2011) identified six rubrics for use in measurement of simulation-related objectives and appraised how well these quantified students meet curricular outcomes expected of baccalaureate nursing programs as articulated in *The Essentials of Baccalaureate Education for Professional Nursing Practice* (American Association of Colleges of Nursing [AACN]). Stating that although rubrics "structured around meeting the essentials have the ability to provide evidence of positive student learning outcomes via HPS outcomes evaluation" (Davis & Kimble, 2011, p. 609), the authors acknowledge none of the evaluated rubrics; however, addressed the three domains of learning and measured all nine AACN essentials. A majority was in pilot form and required additional psychometric development.

The Program for Nursing Curriculum Integration (PNCI), developed by Medical Education Technologies Inc. (METI, Sarasota, FL), is a comprehensive educational package incorporating the use of simulation designed to help educators integrate simulation broadly throughout nursing curricula. The program requires the iSTAN® simulator and uses an evaluation instrument (Simulation Effectiveness Tool [SET]), which measures simulation effectiveness via student self-report of confidence and learning. Although Schiavenato (2009) states "an important step in the evaluation of simulation in nursing education is divorcing it from any particular product" (p. 390), the SET has been psychometrically tested in a multisite national study and found to be a reliable instrument (Elfrink Cordi et al., 2012).

Arthur, Levett-Jones, and Kable (2013) leveraged international consensus among simulation experts and developed 15 evidence-based quality indicator statements to guide evaluation of simulation implementation within nursing curricula (Arthur et al., 2013, p. 1361). To evaluate simulation quality in undergraduate nursing curriculum, Kable, Arthur, Levett-Jones, and Reid-Searl (2013) constructed a set of tools from the quality indicators. One tool, the Student Evaluation Instrument, has been described as applicable across simulation practices, program levels, and curricula and holds promise for use in interdisciplinary simulation evaluation settings (Kable et al., 2013). Testing of the other instruments has been undertaken to expedite refinement of the quality indicators for evaluation of simulation experiences (Arthur et al., 2013).

In 2011, the International Nursing Association for Clinical Simulation and Learning (INACSL) published seven standards of best practice in simulation. One of these performance standards specifically addresses outcome evaluation and assessment of simulation-based experiences (Sando

et al., 2013). The evaluation standard includes detailed guidelines for formative, summative, and high-stakes evaluation of simulation experiences. The standard identifies priority areas for development of an evaluation framework across the gamut of use to address inconsistent outcome definitions, nonreporting of instrument psychometric properties, and lack of methodological rigor noted in the simulation literature (Onello & Regan, 2013).

RECOMMENDATIONS

As this discussion suggests, simulation evaluation instruments are indeed evolving, but have not assessed all elements concomitant with the quality implementation of simulation across nursing curricula (Kable et al., 2013). A gold standard for evaluation of simulation remains elusive, and simulation-related outcome measurement issues persist as one of today's greatest pedagogical challenges (McGaghie et al., 2010).

As simulation gains wider use in nursing education, evaluation efforts must focus on the instruments that currently show the most promise for further refinement and development (Kardong-Edgren et al., 2010), so that a standardized or universal method of outcome measurement for quality implementation in curricular integration of simulation can emerge.

The Simulation Evaluation Instrument, developed by Todd, Manz, Hawkins, Parsons, and Hercinger (2008) and briefly presented here in work by Davis and Kimble (2011) and Kardong-Edgren et al. (2010), may be positioned for further development in that the tool currently evaluates simulated learning across three learning domains, quantifies meeting of curricular outcomes as articulated in AACN *Essentials,* and possesses robust psychometric properties. Recognizing that evaluation methods must be guided by a broader reconceptualization of simulation encompassing varied methods used throughout nursing curricula, the NESF (Jeffries, 2005) hold promise for further development. The framework and its essential constructs and sub-constructs have been suggested to provide a foundation and serve as a fundamental guide for evaluation of the evolving methodology of simulation-based education (Groom et al., 2013).

American Association of Colleges of Nursing. (2008). *The essentials of baccalaureate education for professional nursing practice.* Retrieved from http://www.aacn.nche.edu/education-resources/Bacc Essential08.pdf.

Arthur, C., Levett-Jones, T., & Kable, A. (2013). Quality indicators for the design and implementation of simulation experiences: A Delphi study. *Nurse Education Today, 33*(11), 1357–1361.

Cant, R. P., & Cooper, S. J. (2010). Simulation-based learning in nurse education: Systematic review. *Journal of Advanced Nursing, 66*(1), 3–15.

Davis, A. H., & Kimble, L. P. (2011). Human patient simulation evaluation rubrics for nursing education: Measuring the essentials of baccalaureate education for professional nursing practice. *Journal of Nursing Education, 50*(11), 605–611.

Elfrink Cordi, W. L., Leighton, K., Ryan-Wenger, N., Doyle, T. J., & Ravert, P. (2012). History and development of the simulation effectiveness tool [SET]. *Clinical Simulation in Nursing, 8*(6), e199–e210.

Groom, J. A., Henderson, D., & Sittner, B. J. (2013). National League for Nursing—Jeffries simulation framework state of the science project: Simulation design characteristics. *Clinical Simulation in Nursing, 10*(7), 337–344. doi: org/10.1016/j.ecns.2013.02.004

Jeffries, P. R. (2005). A framework for designing, implementing, and evaluating simulations used as teaching strategies in nursing. *Nursing Education Perspectives, 26*(2), 96–103.

Kable, A. K., Arthur, C., Levett-Jones, T., & Reid-Searl, K. (2013). Student evaluation of simulation in undergraduate nursing programs in Australia using quality indicators. *Nursing and Health Sciences, 15,* 235–243.

Kardong-Edgren, S., Adamson, K. A., & Fitzgerald, C. (2010). A review of currently published evaluation instruments for human patient simulation. *Clinical Simulation in Nursing, 6,* e25–e35.

McGaghie, W. C., Issenberg, S. B., Petrusa, E. R., & Scalese, R. J. (2010). A critical review of simulation-based medical education research: 2003–2009. *Medical Education, 44*(1), 50–63.

Onello, R., & Regan, R. (2013). Challenges in high fidelity simulation: Risk sensitization and outcome measurement. *The Online Journal of Issues in Nursing, 18*(3). doi:10.3912/OJIN.Vol18No03PPT01

Sando, C. R., Coggins, R. M., Meakim, C., Franklin, A. E., Gloe, D., Boese, T.,…Borum, J. C. (2013). Standards of best practice: Simulation standard VII: Participant assessment and evaluation. *Clinical Simulation in Nursing, 9,* e30–e32.

Schiavenato, M. (2009). Reevaluating simulation in nursing education: Beyond the human patient simulator. *Journal of Nursing Education, 48*(7), 388–394.

Sportsman, S., Schumacker, R. E., & Hamilton, P. (2011). Evaluating the impact of scenario-based high-fidelity patient simulation on academic metrics of student success. *Nursing Education Perspectives, 32*(4), 259–265.

Todd, M., Manz, J. A., Hawkins, K. S., Parsons, M. E., & Hercinger, M. (2008). The development of a quantitative evaluation tool for simulations in nursing education. *International Journal of Nursing Education Scholarship, 5,* Article 41.

Maura C. Schlairet

SIMULATION: SCENARIO CREATION

DEFINITION

Scenario creation is the process of designing, testing, implementing, and evaluating course lessons that can be taught by using creative teaching strategies. Scenarios for

S

use in simulation mimic the reality of a clinical environment and are designed to demonstrate procedures, decision making, and critical thinking through techniques such as role-playing, case studies, and the use of interactive videos or mannequins (Jefferies, 2005).

APPLICATION

The National League for Nursing designed a framework to assist nursing educators in scenario creation. This model guides the educator based on the findings obtained from an empirically supported tool. The components found in this model are based on the concepts of information, problem solving, student support, fidelity, and debriefing (Billings & Halstead, 2011).

The first step in this model is to outline the objectives. The objectives should relate to problem-solving skills needed to provide care, and be appropriate to the level of student. The focus of the simulation should be based on problems students typically encounter in clinical practice.

When planning the time schedule, one should plan not only the time limit for the scenario, but the debriefing period that follows the simulation. When a specific period of time has been identified for the scenario, the educator needs to end the scenario on time. The educator should be aware that each student or group of students will perform at different paces and levels; therefore, scenarios should be designed to challenge the skills and cognitive stages of the different learners.

Scenario creation includes the assignment of roles for students to assume during the simulation. The roles of nurse, physician, other health care professionals, and family members are a few of the roles that may be assigned to the scenario. Assigning roles during a scenario allows students the opportunity to gain a better understanding of group process. The students gain experience in group process and development of therapeutic communication skills (Clapper, 2010).

Reflection questions need to be designed for use during the debriefing period that follows completion of the scenario. These reflection questions provide the students with guided opportunities to think back on the situation in which they participated. The debriefing period at the end of the scenario is crucial as it allows time for the learner to evaluate the session under the guidance of an instructor.

SYNOPSIS

The use of scenarios in nursing education offers the opportunity for students to be actively involved in an experience shared by all of the students in the group (Fuszard, 2001).

A well-designed scenario using simulation can reach all types of learners because it encompasses the cognitive, psychomotor, and affective domains of learning. The visual learner would have the opportunity to observe the skills, the auditory learner would learn from listening to the class talk about the simulation experience, and the kinesthetic learner could benefit from the hands-on use of equipment and demonstration (Billings & Halstead, 2011). Therefore, scenario creation promoting active learning and using real-life clinical situations with varied learning experiences are critical for creation of scenarios.

Students are continually engaged in the learning process through interactive learning and faculty can encourage students to make connections between key concepts (Jefferies, 2005). Scenarios should be based on evidence-based references, as well as quality and safety patient care standards that drive nursing practice. It has also been suggested that scenarios be validated through peer review and pilot testing and reviewed annually for currency (Waxman, 2010).

RECOMMENDATIONS

Health care is becoming more complex due to all of the advances in science and technology. The nurse of today must be able to critically think in this increasingly complex environment. Education techniques using scenarios based on realistic, complex situations provide an efficient way to structure learning activities needed to practice. Nurses in practice and in academia need to work together to create suitable scenarios to meet the changing health care needs. Research studies comparing student learning outcomes between traditional clinical models and simulation with tailored scenarios need to be explored. Faculty development should be aimed at providing the knowledge and skills required to create interesting real-life scenarios that match the learning objectives of the student.

Billings, D. M., & Halstead, J. A. (2011). *Teaching in nursing: A guide for faculty* (4th ed.). St. Louis, MO: Elsevier Saunders.

Clapper, T. C. (2010). Beyond Knowles: What those conducting simulation need to know about adult learning theory. *Clinical Simulation in Nursing,* 6(1), e7–e14. doi:10.1016/j.ecns.2009.07.003

Fuszard, B. (2001). *Innovative teaching strategies in nursing* (3rd ed.). Gaithersburg, MD: Aspen.

Jefferies, P. R. (2005). A framework for designing, implementing and evaluating simulations used as a teaching strategy in nursing. *Nursing Education Perspectives, 26,* 96–103.

Waxman, K. T. (2010). The development of evidence-based clinical simulation scenarios: Guidelines for nurse educators. *Journal of Nursing Education, 49*(1), 29–35.

Mary Grady
Mary T. Quinn Griffin

SIMULATION: TRANSFORMATIVE LEARNING

DEFINITION

Simulation involves the use of human-like manikins, or human patient simulators (HPSs), ranging from low fidelity to high fidelity. High fidelity refers to the most technologically advanced versions, which mimic many human physiological reactions to trauma, illness, and interventions. The manikin is designed to look human and to respond in a human-like manner. The responses are controlled by an instructor or facilitator via a computer, which enables the direction of scenarios that mimic illness and trauma. Nursing students are able to practice nursing interventions, such as medication administration, after assessing alterations in health in the HPS. The facilitator can then replicate physiological changes in health status and acuity in response to the student's interventions as required for the clinical scenario. Often the HPS is placed in a room designed to mimic a clinical environment to realistically simulate a nursing practice experience.

APPLICATION

Depending on the desired learning outcomes and pedagogical structures that underpin a simulation-based clinical curriculum, dominant learning theories must be considered to facilitate high-fidelity simulated learning sessions. Depending on whether the goal is the rote learning of factual knowledge and psychomotor skills or, conversely, the enhancement of problem solving, nurse educators should consider the application of theory in designing HPS-based clinical scenarios. Guidelines for behaviorist-based simulation include the incorporation of low levels of acuity and complexity to avoid overwhelming adult learners, the repetition of learning experiences, theory supplementation, and the incorporation of modular learning. Guidelines for constructivist-based simulation include access to a variety of information resources in the simulation laboratory; the negotiation of learning objectives between the instructor and the students; and the creation of scenarios that involve uncertainty, increased acuity, and amplified environmental noise. To guide the educator on which form of pedagogy to apply, it is pertinent also to consider the role that social discourse and transformative learning theory play in a simulation-based learning environment.

HPS-based clinical scenarios are in reality social endeavors that lead to the collaborative creation of knowledge (Parker & Myrick, 2012). Therefore, social discourse and perspective transformation in Mezirow's (1994, 1995) transformative learning theory should come to the forefront. HPS-based clinical scenarios, with the use of group process, peer filtering of knowledge, and critical reflection, are well suited for contributing to transformation of the student's meaning schemes and perspectives. HPS-based clinical scenarios are also useful in delivering disorienting dilemmas that upset learners' knowledge and understanding of health care and skill application. Upsetting perceived knowledge, values, and beliefs about clinical practice through exposure to high-fidelity simulation helps students learn to reinterpret a dilemma and ultimately incorporate new meanings into their cognitive schema. Similarly to constructivist pedagogy, transformative learning theory empowers students to define goals, make choices, and problem solve. Furthermore, the instructor can model experiential engagement and encourage regular, noncompetitive feedback (Mezirow, 1991).

Other strategies specific to HPS that might be considered include repeating HPS scenario sessions, increasing students' exposure to HPS to foster the development of trusting relationships, and using video playback to promote critical reflexivity. Nurse educators should also consider using incremental disorientating dilemmas for more junior learners instead of exposing them to emotionally charged experiences to avoid overwhelming and hindering their ability to cognitively process the scenario. For many students, especially more novice learners, there appears to be a significant potential for self-esteem and confidence in their clinical knowledge and skills to be threatened in a high-fidelity simulated clinical session. Further recommendations to counter these potential threats include gradually increasing peer observation, assessing the overuse of signal and noise, increasing or decreasing the simulation facilitator's direct interjection of support during a clinical scenario, leveling acuity and interpersonal conflict to the level of the student, maintaining role authenticity, and providing students with the tools necessary to become orientated to the simulation environment.

SYNOPSIS

The current body of research has shown evidence from students and educators of perceived efficacy in simulation (Mould, White, & Gallagher, 2011; Smith-Stoner & Hand, 2008); perceived confidence building (Fisher & King, 2013); and moderate evidence of improved skill performance and/or retention (Cant & Cooper, 2010; Levett-Jones, Lapkin, Hoffman, Arthur, & Roche, 2011). Unfortunately, the current state of knowledge has specific limitations, including an overemphasis on the simple description of a phenomenon (Rourke, Schmidt, & Garga, 2010). However, external validity is lacking as a result of informal evaluation methods and problems with rigor (Harder, 2010). Although the external validity may be questionable, the current body of research broadly endorses simulation as a valid educational practice.

More specific endorsement of HPS-based nursing education can be seen in relation to the application of transformative learning theory. In particular, HPS enhances social dialogue and, subsequently, peer-validated socially derived knowledge (Leigh & Hurst, 2008; Parker & Myrick, 2010). Although HPS-based clinical scenarios have the potential to transform students' meaning schemes with regard to clinical practice and knowledge, they also have the potential to overwhelm the cognitive capacity and cause feelings of anxiety, stress, fear, and disengagement (Parker & Myrick, 2012). To this end, Dunnington (2014) recommended avoiding simple instrumental utilization of high-fidelity HPS, considering context and engaging learners in clinical scenarios.

RECOMMENDATIONS

The proliferation of HPSs in undergraduate nursing education raises questions about the application of well-informed pedagogical practices. Despite a growing body of research into this technology-based learning tool, there is insufficient evidence on which to base decisions on best practice to both structure simulation-based curriculum and facilitate HPS-based clinical scenarios that meet the learning needs of the modern adult learner (Cant & Cooper, 2010; Rourke et al., 2010). Although HPS-based clinical scenarios facilitate group process and social construction of knowledge (Leigh & Hurst, 2008; Parker & Myrick, 2010), there has been limited research into these social processes. Fisher and King (2013) noted that further research is needed in the areas of simulation and interprofessional collaboration as it relates to health care education.

Ultimately, there is a need to move beyond the hypothetico-deductive approach and build a theoretical framework based on the processes that occur in high-fidelity simulation. This movement will also foster future research that more accurately reflects the complex social processes that those who participate in HPS-based clinical scenarios experience. Uncovering the social processes that occur with the HPS-based simulated clinical learning environment will assist nursing educators in developing simulation-based curricula that are truly transformative learning for the modern adult learner.

Cant, R. P., & Cooper, S. J. (2010). Simulation-based learning in nurse education: Systematic review. *Journal of Advanced Nursing, 66*(1), 3–15.

Dunnington, R. M. (2014). The nature of reality represented in high fidelity human patient simulation: Philosophical perspectives and implications for nursing education. *Nursing Philosophy, 15*(1), 14–22.

Fisher, D., & King, L. (2013). An integrative literature review on preparing nursing students through simulation to recognize and respond to the deteriorating patient. *Journal of Advanced Nursing, 69*(11), 2375–2388.

Harder, B. N. (2010). Use of simulation in teaching and learning in health sciences: A systematic review. *Journal of Nursing Education, 49*(1), 23–28.

Leigh, G., & Hurst, H. (2008). We have a high-fidelity simulator, now what? Making the most of simulators. *International Journal of Nursing Education Scholarship, 5*(1), 1–9.

Levett-Jones, T., Lapkin, S., Hoffman, K., Arthur, C., & Roche, J. (2011). Examining the impact of high and medium fidelity simulation experiences on nursing students' knowledge acquisition. *Nurse Education in Practice, 11*(6), 380–383.

Mezirow, J. (1991). *Transformative dimensions of adult learning.* San Francisco, CA: Jossey-Bass.

Mezirow, J. (1994). Understanding transformative theory. *Adult Education Quarterly, 44*(4), 222–232.

Mezirow, J. (1995). Transformation theory of adult learning. In M. R. Welton (Ed.), *In defense of the lifeworld* (pp. 39–70). New York, NY: SUNY Press.

Mould, J., White, H., & Gallagher, R. (2011). Evaluation of a critical care simulation series for undergraduate nursing students. *Contemporary Nurse, 38*(1–2), 180–190.

Parker, B., & Myrick, F. (2010). Transformative learning as a context for human patient simulation. *Journal of Nursing Education, 49*(6), 326–332.

Parker, B. C., & Myrick, F. (2012). The pedagogical ebb and flow of human patient simulation: Empowering through a process of fading support. *Journal of Nursing Education, 51*(7), 365–372.

Rourke, L., Schmidt, M., & Garga, N. (2010). Theory-based research of high fidelity simulation use in nursing education: A review of the literature. *International Journal of Nursing Education Scholarship, 7,* Article 11.

Smith-Stoner, M., & Hand, M. W. (2008). A criminal trial simulation: Pathway to transformative learning. *Nurse Educator, 33*(3), 118–121.

Brian Parker

S

SOCIAL PRESENCE

DEFINITION

Social presence is the ability of learners and instructors in a community of learning to project their personal characteristics into the community, presenting themselves as real people through the use of emotional expression, open communication, and various means to establish group cohesion (Garrison, Anderson, & Archer, 2000). Social presence plays a pivotal role in both setting the educational climate and as a support for scholarly discourse.

APPLICATION

Social presence has importance in the education of nurses due to the emergence of entire programs of nursing being delivered in an online environment. A computer-mediated platform for education has very few affective cues on which participants can base interactions. There are no opportunities for eye contact, or observation of body language or facial expressions. The community of inquiry model (COI) developed by Garrison, Anderson, and Archer (2000) demonstrates the role of social presence as one of the major elements of the learning experience, along with cognitive presence and teaching presence in creating a learning community or community of inquiry. Creating this sense of community predisposes participants to enhanced interaction, is beneficial to student engagement, increases motivation and satisfaction with the learning environment, and increases perception of learning in online classes (Rovai, 2002).

For nursing instructors, the challenge is to create an online community with a climate of social presence, incorporating and understanding the experiences of learners, and integrating affective and cognitive aspects into course design. While all members of an online learning community have shared responsibility for establishing a social discourse and dialog, it is the instructor who most likely influences establishment and maintenance of the social presence as well as a teaching presence within an online course.

Strategies for creating a climate of trust and social presence include weaving affective aspects into all learning experiences using techniques such as welcoming messages, instructor self-disclosure, instructor expressions of emotion, the use of inclusive pronouns, and expressing concern and appreciation for student efforts. Strategies used to maintain the engagement of student-to-student and student-to-instructor interactions and communication include structuring collaborative learning activities, positive and timely feedback, answering questions with demonstrated enthusiasm for the subject, continuing a thread in a student discussion, referencing prior to student's posts in discussions, asking questions, and demonstrating an instructor presence in the course of the instruction.

SYNOPSIS

The definition of social presence started as a way to explain the effects that a communication medium can have on how people communicate (Short, Williams, & Christie, 1976). With the emergence of online education, researchers began to apply the definition to computer-mediated educational models and to further refine the definition (Garrison et al., 2000). Currently there is not one agreed upon definition of social presence and it continues to evolve in the education literature.

There is also little agreement on how to measure social presence. Research on social presence has focused on surveys, coding schemes, observing behaviors of social presence, and perceptions of students about computer-mediated learning formats (Gunnawardena & Zittle, 1997; Richardson & Swan, 2003; Tu, 2002). Both Gunnawardena and Zittle (1997) and Richardson and Swan (2003) demonstrated a relationship between social presence and satisfaction with online learning, as well as perceived learning.

A study among registered nurses (RN)–bachelor of science in nursing (BSN) students examined social presence and its relationship to satisfaction and perceived learning (Cobb, 2011). Findings supported the research by Gunnawardena and Zittle (1997) regarding the relationship between social presence and satisfaction with online learning, further supported the reliability and validity instrument, and also corroborates Richardson and Swan's (2003) finding of social presence positively correlated with perceived learning. Likewise, a pilot study by Mayne and Wu (2011) reported that the inclusion of specific social presence techniques had a positive impact on group interaction as well as online learning expectations.

The focus of current research on social presence has shifted from socioemotional support to an understanding of how it supports the educational objectives and outcomes of the learning community. While effective communication is important, it cannot be separated from the academic and purposeful nature of education, including cognitive and teaching presence (Garrison, Anderson, & Archer, 2010). Research findings have demonstrated the interdependence of learning and emotion and suggest that the role each plays is more complex than previously thought. Social presence is a concept that taps into the affective or emotional aspects of learning models, based on an assumption that social presence has a positive effect on learning outcomes.

On the other hand, recent studies of social presence and the COI theoretical model have challenged the idea that social presence is a major influence in learning. While students view it as a means to share, express their views, and collaborate (Akyol et al., 2009), the concept of teaching presence, specifically the instructor-to-student interaction and the course design, exerts a major influence on student learning and indicates that teaching and social presence are highly correlated (Bangert, 2008).

RECOMMENDATIONS

Continued studies need to be conducted to further define social presence and the role it plays in both blended and online learning. This would necessitate research to determine the effect on learners in various settings, the influence of group-based social presence on the learning process, and the outcomes of learning using this model. While social presence and sustained communication are necessary components of meaningful learning, the challenge is to both conceptualize and measure meaningful learning. Continued studies on social presence and teaching presence need to be designed in order to define the constructs in a way that they can inform the teaching and learning process (Annand, 2011).

Akyol, Z., Arbaugh, J., Cleveland-Innes, M., Garrison, D. R., Ice, P., Richardson, J., & Swan, K. (2009). A response to the review of the community of inquiry framework. *Journal of Distance Education, 23*(2), 123–136.

Annand, D. (2011). Social presence within the community of inquiry framework. *The International Review of Research in Open and Distance Learning, 12*(5). Retrieved from http://www.irrodl.org/index.php/irrodl/rt/printerFriendly/924/1855

Bangert, A. (2008). The influence of social presence and teaching presence in the quality of online critical inquiry. *Journal of Computing in Higher Education, 20*(1), 34–61.

Cobb, S. C. (2011). Social presence, satisfaction, and perceived learning of RN-to-BSN students in web-based nursing courses. *Nursing Education Perspectives, 32*(2), 115–119.

Garrison, D. R., Anderson, T., & Archer, W. (2010). The first decade of the community of inquiry framework: A retrospective. *The Internet and Higher Education, 13*(1–20), 5–9.

Garrison, D. R., Anderson, T., & Archer, W. (2000). Critical inquiry in a text-based environment: Computer conferencing in higher education. *The Internet and Higher Education, 2*(2–3), 87–105.

Gunnawardena, C. N., & Zittle, F. J. (1997). Social presence as a predictor of

S

satisfaction with a computer-mediated conferencing environment. *American Journal of Distance Education, 11*(8), 26.

Mayne, L. A., & Wu, Q. (2011). Creating and measuring social presence in online graduate nursing courses. *Nursing Education Perspectives, 32*(2), 110–114.

Richardson, J. C., & Swan, K. (2003). Examining social presence in online courses in relation to students' perceived learning satisfaction. *Journal of Asynchronous Learning Networks, 7*(1), 68–88.

Rovai, A. (2002). A preliminary look at the structural differences of higher education classroom communities in traditional and ALN courses. *Journal of Asynchronous Learning Networks, 6*(1), 41–56.

Short, J., Williams, E., & Christie, B. (1976). *The social psychology of telecommunications.* London: John Wiley.

Tu, C. H. (2002). The measurement of social presence in an online learning environment. *International Journal on E-Learning, 1*(2), 34–45.

Linda Mayne

Standardized Patient

DEFINITION

Inception of the standardized patient was introduced by Dr. Howard Barrows in 1963. Originally called a programmed patient and then a simulated patient, the name was later changed to underline the major advantage and strongest feature of this type of simulation—to provide a standardized patient problem that will not vary in presentation from student to student. According to Barrows (1993), the term *standardized patient* is "the umbrella term for both a simulated patient (a well person trained to simulate a patient's illness in a standardized way) and an actual patient (who is trained to present his or her own illness in a standardized way)" (p. 443). The Association of Standardized Patient Educators (2013) calls a standardized patient an individual who, portraying the role of a patient, is trained to consistently teach, assess, and evaluate students in physical presentation and health history.

APPLICATION

The use of simulation in nursing education has increased over the last decade. Decreased clinical sites, concerns for patient safety, rapid and constant technological innovations, and the push for interprofessional education are necessitating the need for more use of simulation in nursing education. Standardized patients play an important role in simulation. Standardized patients provide students in academia with additional training outside a textbook by putting them face to face with patients who can provide the physical, psychological, and emotional aspects of clinical practice.

Standardized patients allow the instructor control of the teaching methodology and environment (Barrows, 1993; Cantrell & Deloney, 2007). Standardized patients can be present when real patients are not, and they can be brought into environments (classrooms, for example) when and where it is not feasible or practical to have a real patient. Faculty can control the learning objectives and integrate psychosocial issues into the case scenarios with standardized patients. Furthermore, cases or portrayals can be homogenous and accurately reproduced for other students so that all students are exposed to the same case study.

The use of standardized patients can alleviate problems associated with evaluation. As opposed to preceptor input and instructor observation, which can incur unreliability and bias (Ebbert & Connors, 2004), standardized patients allow for careful evaluation of the student's clinical ability, interstudent comparison, and teaching methodology (Barrows, 1968). Because standardized patients can provide a reliable means for teaching and evaluating, they are often used to provide an outcome measure of students' clinical competence, to access faculty effectiveness in teaching, and to assess clinical decision making. The reliability of standardized patient evaluations of student performance has been shown to be moderate to substantial when compared to a second rater team trained in the same manner (Bolstad, Xu, Shen, Covelli, & Torpey, 2012).

SYNOPSIS

The use of standardized patients to teach communication skills is frequently reported in the literature. Students and instructors can speak freely about the disease process without fear of upsetting a real patient, and learners can receive immediate and constructive feedback. Conversations that students may rarely encounter in academic clinical practice, such as end-of-life discussions and communicating bad news, can be practiced in a safe, nonthreatening environment. Communication skills are enhanced by the use of standardized patients. Recent studies have shown that, when compared to alternate teaching methods for teaching communication skills, students preferred training that included standardized patients (Lagan et al., 2012). In addition, communication skills were significantly superior ($p < .0001$) when standardized patients were used (Schlegel, Woermann, Shaha, Rethans, & van der Vleuten, 2011), and knowledge and self-efficacy increased with students trained with standardized patients.

The use of standardized patients to teach health examination skills has been found to be an effective educational technique (Grice, Wenger, Brooks, & Berry, 2013). Students can practice physical assessment skills in a safe environment without the concern of tiring, hurting, or inconveniencing a patient. Furthermore, the student does not aggravate the patient's disease. Physical examination skills can be practiced over and over until the student and/or instructor are satisfied that the technique is correct (Barrows, 1968, 1993; Cantrell & Deloney, 2007). The use of standardized patients in health assessment can alleviate problems related to unreliable feedback and inconsistent physical presentations, which are often encountered when students

use peers to hone examination skills in the laboratory setting. Feedback can come not only from the instructor but from the standardized patient as well, who many times has been trained to give valid and reliable feedback to students (van Zanten, Boulet, & McKinley, 2007).

Providing nursing students with practical experiences related to psychosocial and mental health illnesses can be challenging to nurse educators due to shortened clinical time and a lack of experienced psychiatric faculty (Hermanns, Lilly, & Crawley, 2011). Simulations that incorporate standardized patients are able to not only provide students with educational experiences involving these patient encounters and diagnoses but also the opportunity to practice therapeutic communication skills that are essential in psychiatric and mental health nursing (Lang & Hahn, 2013). In recent studies, standardized patients have allowed students the opportunity to screen for adolescent depression and suicide (Fallucco, Conlon, Gale, Constantino, & Glowinski, 2012) as well as alcohol and substance abuse (Satterfield et al., 2012). Authors in both studies reported that knowledge and confidence increased for students who participated in the simulations.

RECOMMENDATIONS

Many standardized patient programs are associated with schools of medicine, limiting the access some schools of nursing have to this type of simulation. Additionally, the cost of recruiting, training, and managing a pool of standardized patients excludes some nurse education programs from enjoying the benefits of standardized patients. While the feedback standardized by patients provided to students has been shown to be beneficial to learning, there is no standardized approach for how to train standardized patients to give effective feedback to students nor are there established guidelines for providing feedback to standardized patients (Bokken, Linssen, Scherpbier, van der Vleuten, & Rethans, 2009). To strengthen the benefits that standardized patients bring to simulation, future

S

development in these areas is recommended in nursing education.

Association of Standardized Patient Educators. (2013). *About ASPE*. Retrieved from http://www.aspeducators.org/

Barrows, H. S. (1968). Simulated patients in medical teaching. *Canadian Medical Association Journal, 98*(14), 674–676.

Barrows, H. S. (1993). An overview of the uses of standardized patients for teaching and evaluating clinical skills. *AAMC. Academic Medicine, 68*(6), 443–451; discussion 451.

Bokken, L., Linssen, T., Scherpbier, A., van der Vleuten, C., & Rethans, J. J. (2009). Feedback by simulated patients in undergraduate medical education: A systematic review of the literature. *Medical Education, 43*(3), 202–210.

Bolstad, A. L., Xu, Y., Shen, J. J., Covelli, M., & Torpey, M. (2012). Reliability of standardized patients used in a communication study on international nurses in the United States of America. *Nursing & Health Sciences, 14*(1), 67–73.

Cantrell, M. J., & Deloney, L. A. (2007). Integration of standardized patients into simulation. *Anesthesiology Clinics, 25*(2), 377–383.

Ebbert, D. W., & Connors, H. (2004). Standardized patient experiences: Evaluation of clinical performance and nurse practitioner student satisfaction. *Nursing Education Perspectives, 25*(1), 12–15.

Fallucco, E. M., Conlon, M. K., Gale, G., Constantino, J. N., & Glowinski, A. L. (2012). Use of a standardized patient paradigm to enhance proficiency in risk assessment for adolescent depression and suicide. *The Journal of Adolescent Health, 51*(1), 66–72.

Grice, G. R., Wenger, P., Brooks, N., & Berry, T. M. (2013). Comparison of patient simulation methods used in a physical assessment course. *American Journal of Pharmaceutical Education, 77*(4), 1–5.

Hermanns, M., Lilly, M. L., & Crawley, B. (2011). Using clinical simulation to enhance psychiatric nursing training of baccalaureate students. *Clinical Simulation in Nursing, 7*(2), e41–e46. doi:10.1016/j.ecns.2010.05.001

Lagan, C., Wehbe-Janek, H., Waldo, K., Fox, A., Jo, C., & Rahm, M. (2012). Evaluation of an interprofessional clinician-patient communication workshop utilizing standardized patient methodology. *Journal of Surgical Education, 70*(1), 95–103.

Lang, C. S., & Hahn, J. A. (2013). BLAST model: An innovative approach to prepare second-degree accelerated BSN students for inpatient psychiatric clinical experiences. *Journal of Psychosocial Nursing, 51*(3), 38–45.

Satterfield, J. M., O'Sullivan, P. O., Satre, D. D., Tsoh, J. Y., Batki, S. L., Julian, K.,...Wamsley, M. (2012). Using standardized patients to evaluate screening, brief intervention, and referral to treatment (SBIRT) knowledge and skills acquisition for internal medicine residents. *Substance Abuse, 33*, 303–307.

Schlegel, C., Woermann, U., Shaha, M., Rethans, J. J., & van der Vleuten, C. (2011). Effects of communication training on real practice performance: A role-play module versus a standardized patient module. *Journal of Nursing Education, 51*(1), 16–22.

van Zanten, M., Boulet, J. R., & McKinley, D. (2007). Using standardized patients to assess the interpersonal skills of physicians: Six years' experience with a high-stakes certification examination. *Health Communication, 22*(3), 195–205.

Tonya Rutherford-Hemming

STORY THEORY

DEFINITION

Story is an inner human resource for meaning making (Smith & Liehr, 2014). The purpose of this middle-range story theory is to describe and explain story as the context for a nurse-to-person health-promoting process. Fundamental concepts of story theory include intentional dialogue, connecting with self in relation, and creating ease. Story is connecting with self in relation through intentional dialogue to create ease (Smith & Liehr, 2014).

APPLICATION

Prioritizing the holistic aspects of care in nursing education can be challenging for educators (McMahon & Christopher, 2011). This middle-range theory is particularly applicable in nursing education because it focuses on the true work of the nurse, which is caring. The theory is based on the premise that telling a story to a nurse who is truly present to really hear the person's concerns about what matters most is a caring process that has the power to create a nurse-person process that leads to healing.

Using story theory to plan nursing care begins with a focus on the person's response to a complicating health challenge. This approach is consistent with the American Nurses Association (ANA) definition of nursing: "The protection, promotion, and optimization of health and abilities, prevention of illness and injury, alleviation of suffering through the diagnosis and treatment of the human health response, and advocacy in the care of individuals, families, communities, and populations" (ANA, 2003). The human response is multidimensional, assessed through story, and addresses the physical and psychosocial needs of patients, thus creating a holistic assessment.

Integrating story theory into an existing course is based on the belief that students must first understand the concepts of the theory before they can apply them in practice (Flanagan & McCausland, 2007). Story theory concepts are intentional dialogue, connecting with self in relation, and creating ease. Because of the abstract nature of these concepts, faculty guidance is essential in understanding and applying the concepts. Intentional dialogue is the purposeful engagement with another to gather the story of a health challenge. Intentional dialogue centers on true presence by focusing on the story teller, and querying emergence is clarifying what is not understood as the person is telling the story. Connecting with self in relation is an awareness of self in the present moment. Creating ease is an energizing release that comes from telling the story to a person who is truly present to listen and to hear what matters most to the person about his or her health situation (Smith & Liehr, 2014).

If the student is expected to apply story theory in practice, then the student needs to be shown how to use it. Students begin by reading the literature to gain an understanding of the concepts of the theory, and how the theory can be used to provide care. Faculty guidance is critical through discussions of the theory, as well as during role modeling use of the theory in the clinical setting. Sharing story theory applications in the clinical group in post-conferences offers students further understanding of the theory as it can be applied to practice. This approach to applying story theory in practice takes place over an entire semester so that students can develop deep meaning of the theory.

SYNOPSIS

Story theory has been applied in an honors program (Carpenter, 2010). The following objectives were developed for the honors student based on two goals: (a) The student will use the theory to plan the care for a person experiencing a complicating health challenge and (b) the student will facilitate clinical group interaction and dialogue to assist other students in the clinical group to relate story theory concepts to clinical practice.

The student gathered a story about what mattered most, that is, what was most important to the patient. The story served as data to clarify the human response to illness that was made manifest by the patient. To put the theory into practice, the student was instructed to gather two perspectives— the acute care perspective and the patient perspective. The acute care perspective was the usual care information that all students

S

gather, and includes subjective and objective data from the patient grouped into nursing diagnostic categories for the planning of care. The patient perspective was the story about what mattered most to the patient. This was gathered through intentional dialogue, which requires being truly present in a quiet and undisturbed manner.

Students were asked to describe insights about nursing care that came from the postconference discussions (Carpenter, 2010). Comments made by students include a noted difference between the acute care perspective and the patient's perspective; for example what is important to the patient may not be his or her dressings or medication. The patient's concern about living from one day to the next is understandable, given the situation. When asked to describe the most important learning experienced in this situation, student comments included: developed a sense of importance in listening to the patient, developed an increased understanding of the big picture that we often lose in regular clinical, pulled together information we get from all of our classes, and tied the priorities of patients into the plan of care. The honors student evaluation of the experience was positive. She indicated she developed insight into holistic care through learning that health care providers have different priorities than those of patients, that the experience had a huge impact on her nursing practice, and led to an interest in continuing work with a future independent study. Incorporating story theory into the clinical course was effective in expanding the existing curriculum and raising the quality of the clinical experience.

RECOMMENDATIONS

The following implications can be drawn for applying the middle-range theory of story with students in the clinical practice experience. This approach takes student learning beyond the emphasis on disease to the complicating health challenge as experienced by the patient, and thus raises the level of student learning in clinical courses. Story theory provides a theory-guided method to teach caring. It is generally noted that caring can be a difficult concept to teach. Framing caring as intentional dialogue to be truly present with the person to gather the story shows students a way to engage in a caring relationship, which is the essence of nursing. Therefore, students come to get a sense of the difference between a medical perspective and a nursing perspective, focused on the patient's experience of the complicating health challenge.

Story theory can be applied to any clinical course when there is the intention to put theory into action. Middle-range theory is at a level of abstraction that can be readily applied to the practice situation. The use of a particular theory in practice requires a value for educating students to come to know the unique perspective of nursing, which is caring about the human response. This means that the faculty member values the nursing perspective, and holds a commitment to integrate this perspective in the education of students. And lastly, application of story theory enriches the faculty and student experience by focusing on the true work of nursing—caring about the person's experience of the complicating health challenge.

American Nurses Association (ANA). (2003). *Nursing: A social policy statement* (2nd ed.). Silver Springs, MD: author.

Carpenter, R. (2010). Using story theory to create an innovative honors level nursing course. *Nursing Education Perspectives, 31*(1), 28–32.

Flanagan, N. A., & McCausland, L. (2007). Teaching around the cycle: Strategies for teaching theory to undergraduate nursing students. *Nursing Education Perspectives, 28*(6), 310–314.

McMahon, M. A., & Christopher, K. A. (2011). Toward a mid-range theory of nursing presence. *Nursing Forum, 46*(2), 71–82.

Smith, M., & Liehr, P. (2014). Story theory. In *Middle range theory for nursing* (3rd ed.). New York, NY: Springer Publishing.

Roger D. Carpenter

STUDENT ADVISING

DEFINITION

Student advising in nursing can constitute varied components and involve a variety of approaches. Academic advising involves the interaction with students in a formal pre-set meeting such as in a classroom or office (Jefferys, 2012). Student advising also occurs in less formal ways such as casual conversations, interactions in workplaces, professional activities, and in varied correspondence.

APPLICATION

Student advising in nursing education is manifested by encouraging educational and career goals, promoting feelings of self-worth, believing in the student's ability to succeed, listening to problems and concerns, showing interest in academic progress, presenting a realistic outlook, and offering assistance (Jefferys, 2012). This process can start with high school students and run through the spectrum of educational levels in nursing. Advising is especially important in choosing nursing as a career and navigating the many options for continued education after entry to practice.

SYNOPSIS

Nursing as a profession is rich with career and educational opportunities. Workforce predictions indicate a growing need for nurses and a highly educated nursing workforce. There has been a steady increase in the number of individuals entering nursing and returning for continued academic education. The desire to pursue a career in nursing can range from early adolescence to later life. For some, the vocational call starts in childhood, and for some, nursing represents a viable employment option as the health care industry continues to grow. Some enter nursing after completing degrees in other fields.

At any phase in nursing, student advising can be beneficial. Nursing has a variety of options for entry to practice and it can be especially valuable for students to discuss these options with advisors. Education in a licensed practical nurse (LPN) program, diploma program, associate degree, program and bachelor's degree program are all options for entry to practice. Supporting students to make the best choice involves academic abilities, financial resources, educational resources, understanding long-term goals, and demands of the job market. For example, a high school student considering an LPN program, because it is the least expensive and of shortest duration, needs to know the limits this nondegree program will have on job opportunities. Changes in health care and the U.S. economy have a major impact on health care careers; therefore, choosing the most appropriate program that will afford the greatest long-term career options is preferable.

Once individuals have entered the nursing workforce, advising continues to play a major role in career direction. The *Future of Nursing* report (Institute of Medicine [IOM], 2011) and other powerful forces in the profession have sparked nurses to return to the academic setting. Intentional advising, workplace support, and increasing collaboration among academic organizations can support the attainment of an educated workforce; this is a major initiative for health care quality (IOM, 2011).

Increased options for graduate degrees in nursing can prompt experienced nurses to seek the advice of experienced professionals, academic advisors, and others for support. Nurses struggle with decisions around graduate education, such as the decision to pursue a doctorate of nursing practice (DNP), preparation as a nurse practitioner or nurse educator, and other emerging roles for nurses. Practical advice from peers, health care leaders, and mentors can support appropriate choices.

Once students enter a program of study, advising can be a key to student retention and socialization. Attitudes and approaches to advising can be varied, and students may perceive advising from extremely valuable to overly authoritative. The quality of advising

S

can be varied by the faculty's knowledge, attitudes, and experience. Often colleges and universities have minimal requirements for advising that focus on course selection. Beyond minimum requirements, formal and informal advising activities can strongly support the student–faculty relationship. When the relationship is positive, it can foster development of the students' professional identity, support success in learning, and encourage professional choices in academic paths of higher education (August-Brady, 2008). However, poor advising can have unfortunate repercussions to a student's academic experience. Advising and supportive resources are especially critical to minorities and underrepresented student groups who face unique challenges. A positive advising relationship has the capacity to help students achieve and to integrate students into the nursing profession (Jeffreys, 2012).

Approaches to how students seek out and receive advising are open to many options. Emerging technology has made an impact on communication. In the era of Facebook Instant Messenger, Live Journal Blogger, Web Shots, and campus blogs, current and prospective students have countless opportunities for nontraditional communication that can assist in advising (Aleman & Wartman, 2009). How these and future communication tools will influence career choices, professional relationship development, networking, and informed decision making remains to be seen. Those professionals with formal advising responsibilities need to investigate and experiment with technological opportunities.

RECOMMENDATIONS

Advising in the field of nursing can take on a variety of dimensions. Pre-career counseling, continuing education choices, career options, and personal growth are all areas in which advising is valuable. Practice organizations and academic institutions value advising as an integral component of success and the continued development of nurses.

Formal and informal advising can shape careers, support positive professional relationships, and ensure a high-quality nursing workforce. Academic organizations have policies to support advising for students and encourage positive attitudes regarding this pivotal relationship. Emerging technologies can offer new options for communication as a component of advising in a fast-changing world.

Aiken, L., Sloane, D., Bruyneel, L., Van den Heede, L., Griffiths, P., Busse,…Sermeus, W. (2014). Nurse staffing and education and hospital mortality in nine European countries: A retrospective observational study. *Lancet*. Retrieved from http://dx.doi.org/10.1016/S0140–6736(13)62631–8

Aleman, A., & Wartman, K. (2009). *Online social networking on campus. Understanding what matters in student culture*. New York, NY: Routledge.

August-Brady, M. (2008). *Nursing as a career*. In B. Moyer & R. Wittmann-Price (Eds.), *Nursing education. Foundations for practice excellence* (pp. 55–62). Philadelphia, PA: F. A. Davis.

Institute of Medicine. (2011). Th*e future of nursing: Leading change, advancing health*. Washington, DC: The National Academies Press.

Jeffreys, M. (2012). *Nursing student retention. Understanding the process and making a difference* (2nd ed.). New York, NY: Springer.

Sally O. Gerard

STUDENT-CENTERED LEARNING

DEFINITION

Student-centered learning shifts the focus of action from the teacher to the learners. These methods include active learning, in which students work together to solve problems, answer questions, formulate questions of their own, discuss, explain, debate, or brainstorm during class. The student-centered learning experience is not a passive one, as it is based on the premise that active learning helps students to learn independently (MacHemer & Crawford, 2007). Student-centered learning is grounded in constructivist learning theories. Constructivism evolved from a number of learning theories, each contributing valuable ideas that have shaped our present understanding. The learner is central and must be actively engaged in seeking and constructing learning (Attard, Di Ioio, Geven, & Santa, 2010).

APPLICATION

In the traditional approach, most class time is spent with the professor lecturing and the students watching and listening. The students tend to work individually on assignments, and cooperation may not be encouraged. On the other hand, student-centered learning is authentic learning. Guidelines include providing an authentic context that reflects the way the knowledge is applied in real life, access to expert performance and modeling, multiple roles and perspectives, and collaborative construction of knowledge. Application of student-centered learning is a reflective process. Reflection is an intersubjective process that promotes deeper learning; it involves consciously thinking about and analyzing what one has done or is doing. Reflection provides a method for professionals to promote lifelong learning.

Student-centered learning is a collaborative endeavor that involves groups of learners working together to solve a problem, complete a task, or create a product. It is based on the idea that learning is a natural social process. Learning occurs though active engagement among peers, in either face-to-face or online forums.

Furthermore, Semple (2000) believes that learning is a collaborative process in which multiple perspectives are considered. This type of learning, where students work in teams to collaborate on problems and projects with clear assignments, can assure positive interdependence and individual accountability.

SYNOPSIS

The literature shows that student-centered methods are superior to the traditional teacher-centered approach in enhancing: short-term mastery, long-term retention, depth of understanding, acquisition of critical thinking or creative problem-solving skills, formation of positive attitudes toward the subject, and level of confidence in knowledge or skills (Attard et al., 2010).

Student-centered learning emerged as a concept within the field of educational pedagogy and has been a topic of discussion in higher education and within national policy making for the past few decades. While the concept of student-centered learning is relatively new, the idea of looking at the way in which teaching is conducted and how learning processes work has spanned over almost two centuries. Student-centered learning first focused on changes to pedagogical approaches and making educational processes more flexible to increase student participation in learning. When constructivism theory gained popularity, reflection on successful approaches led to new or modified concepts, contributing to the body of knowledge of student-centered learning. Constructivism is based on the idea that learners must construct and reconstruct knowledge in order to learn effectively. Thus, from a constructivist perspective, it was accepted that knowledge is not passively received from the world, from others, or from authoritative sources. Rather, all knowledge is created as individuals and groups adapt to and make sense of their experiential worlds (MacLellan & Soden, 2004, 2007).

RECOMMENDATIONS

Student-centered learning was designed to develop cutting-edge professional skills, such as problem solving, group process, and group facilitation. Lifelong learning skills are viewed by nurse educators as essential for professional nursing practice (Young & Paterson, 2007).

Student-centered learning takes place in diverse settings including the classroom, hospital, and community. It is recommended that student-centered learning be applied across the curriculum so that students acquire the skills and knowledge for professional nursing practice, which often includes highly scientific, technological, and political environments.

Attard, A., Di Ioio, E., Geven, K., & Santa, R. (2010). Student-centered learning: An insight into theory and practice. *International Journal for the Scholarship of Teaching & Learning, 1*(1), 1–18.

MacHemer, P. L., & Crawford, P. (2007). Student perceptions of active learning in a large cross-disciplinary classroom. *Active Learning in Higher Education, 8*(1), 9–30.

MacLellan, E., & Soden, R. (2004). The importance of epistemic cognition in student-centered learning. *Instructional Science, 32*(3), 253–268.

MacLellan, E., & Soden, R. (2007). The significance of knowledge in learning: A psychologically informed analysis of higher education students' perceptions. *The International Journal Scholarship of Teaching and Learning, 1*(1), 1–18.

Semple, A. (2000). Learning theories and their influence on the development and use of educational technologies. *Australian Science Teachers Journal, 46*(3), 21.

Young, L. E. (Ed.) & Paterson, B. L. (2007). *Teaching nursing: Developing a student-centered learning environment* (pp. 5–19). New York, NY: Lippincott Williams & Wilkins.

Irena L. Kenneley

STUDENT CHEATING

DEFINITION

Cheating is to break a rule or law, usually to gain an advantage at something or to elude through fraud or trickery (Merriam-Webster, 2014). In nursing education, cheating regards some level of fraud surrounding academic assessment, performance, or completion of a required component of a degree.

APPLICATION

The concept of cheating has been a long-standing issue in the academic setting. Despite being a most trusted profession, nursing shares the broad issues of cheating at all levels of academic preparation. Few institutions formally collect information on cheating, and even fewer make it public so as to not be perceived by the outside world as having a problem (Bi, 2013). However, student cheating does provide a continuous source of challenge for many academic organizations. Advancing technology and competition in nursing programs further escalate issues of dishonesty.

SYNOPSIS

Cheating is described under the broader spectrum of academic integrity. The specific types of cheating can include unauthorized collaboration, using unauthorized resources, plagiarism, falsification of documents, and exam security (Morgan & Hart, 2013). New and unexpected ways to achieve fraud in the academic and clinical setting continue to evolve and poses great concern for institutions and the profession. Cheating has been associated with workplace dishonesty (Harper, 2006).

Various forms of cheating are quite numerous and can range from wandering eyes during an exam to highly sophisticated, technology-based deceit. The utilization of technology can help deter cheating; however, at the same time, it creates opportunities for cheating via technological devices. The Harvard Cheating Scandal involved the use of social media as students communicated on Facebook to complete an assignment (Schlozman, 2013). In an age where technology is so ingrained into the fabric of young adults, the source for the standard of knowing is technology, rather than the ability to articulate knowing in depth and in breadth. This situation creates ambiguity in what constitutes cheating. Faculty are challenged to have a specific discussion of what constitutes cheating, as well as what is acceptable and unacceptable. In addition, students who witness or suspect cheating should have a safe mechanism for reporting.

In the age of technology, new ways of cheating are present and always evolving. For example, exams and content can be stolen, photographed with phones, posted online, tweeted, or copied. Furthermore, students can obtain course papers and other course content from existing websites that are either free or come with a charge. To complicate the matter, some faculty who are not from the digital generation can be unaware of the ways students can cheat using technology (Schlozman, 2013). Many institutions and nursing programs have instituted academic integrity policies that are included in the student handbook and the course syllabus.

RECOMMENDATIONS

To address the concerns of cheating in a high-tech world, faculty need to assess teaching learning strategies. Writing assignments should require students to integrate information that is not readily available from online sources (Marcoux, 2010). Traditional on-site programs should develop interactive learning activities that demonstrate the students' knowledge of content. Technology should be incorporated into all learning settings with frank conversations of appropriate student use.

Faculty will need to learn new technologies and strategies based on the setting in which they teach and model ethics and values for using information in a manner that reflects integrity (Marcoux, 2010). Specific content regarding plagiarism, use of online information, and reliable resources are crucial to a generation that has instantaneous access to information. Policies and documents regarding academic integrity should be incorporated at all levels of academia.

Bi, F. (2013). Better data can help colleges fight cheating. *The Chronicle of Higher Education, 60*(2), 12–13.

Harper, M. (2006). High tech cheating. *Nurse Education Today, 26*(8), 672–679.

Marcoux, B. (2010). Student cheating with technology. *Teacher Librarian, 38*(1), 70.

Merriam-Webster Online. (2014). Retrieved from http://www.meriam-webster.com/dictionary/cheating

Morgan, L., & Hart, L. (2013). Promoting academic integrity in an online RN-BSN program. *Nursing Education Perspectives, 34*(4), 240–243.

Schlozman, S. (2013). Cheating in the age of Facebook. *Psychology Today, 46*(2), 47–48.

Sally O. Gerard

STUDENT COMPUTER COMPETENCY

DEFINITION

The health care environment for the 21st century involves nurses who are directly engaged with clinical information systems and technology to improve the quality and safety of patient care. Being proficient in the use of computers and applications extends beyond computer literacy and involves informatics competency. Competency is the capacity to perform at a particular task, including the understanding of knowledge, clinical, technical, and communication skills, and the ability to problem solve through the use of clinical judgment (Schroeter, 2008). Computer literacy is defined as an understanding of the concepts, terminology, and operations that relate to general computer use. Nurse informatics (NI) are the skills required by the registered nurse to integrate nursing science, computer science, and information science to manage and communicate data, information, and knowledge in nursing practice (Conrick, Hovenga, Cook, Laracuente, & Morgan, 2004). Nurses must have informatics competency, which includes the knowledge and skills necessary to use computers and information technology in nursing practice in order to have a meaningful and effective role in a wired and connected health care delivery system.

APPLICATION

Technology Informatics Guiding Education Reform (TIGER, 2009) is an initiative formed by a group of nurse leaders in 2004 to create a vision with specific actions and strategies to improve nursing education, practice, and patient care through the use of health information technology (The TIGER Initiative, 2007). The American Association of Colleges of Nursing (AACN) in 2008 suggested introductory-level nursing informatics competencies for the bachelor of science in nursing (BSN) curriculum. The TIGER Initiative (2007) developed recommendations for competencies for nurses and nursing students: basic computer competencies, information literacy, and information management. Basic computer competencies include basic computer operation; word processing skills; use of spreadsheet and database programs; Internet skills, including e-mail and the use of search engines; library databases; and computer simulations as part of the learning experience (Elder & Koehn, 2009). Exposing students to nursing-specific software such as computerized medication administration, point-of-care technology, patient charting using an electronic medical record (EMR), barcoding, and mobile applications can increase students' abilities to distinguish the need for information; advance their critical abilities to process information; and foster a positive appreciation for information literacy in delivering safe patient care (Flood, Gasiewicz, & Delpier, 2010). Computer and information literacy provide the foundation for informatics competencies, including critical-thinking skills, the ability to use technology to solve information problems, knowledge of standardized languages and classifications, and promotion of evidence-based practice (Hebda & Calderone, 2010).

Teaching students to discriminate and assess the relevance, validity, and accuracy of information acquired from consumer information websites as opposed to research-based journal articles through posttest and modules are techniques that faculty can utilize to integrate library system and electronic database system usage (Edwards & O'Connor, 2011).

SYNOPSIS

The TIGER education and faculty aim is for all practicing nurses and students to have the necessary skills to practice nursing in the high-tech environment (Hebda & Calderone, 2010). Graduating students from nursing programs must possess informatics competency in order to recognize the need for information, know how to obtain it, understand its use, and be able to evaluate the information (Edwards & O'Connor, 2011). Curriculum development should include strategies that can assess a nursing student's competency for both undergraduate and graduate levels on informatics knowledge and competency skills, especially in the areas of computer skills in data access, use of decision support systems, and health information management. As the health care environment continues to adopt and implement new emerging technologies, future nurses entering the workforce need to be armed with the computer and informatics skills necessary to be competent in the nursing profession.

RECOMMENDATIONS

TIGER calls for informatics competencies at all levels of nursing and has defined specific skills for all nurses, both beginning nurses and experienced nurses (Hebda & Calderone, 2010). Nursing faculty's lack of familiarity with computerized systems such as electronic health records (EHRs) and informatics competencies contribute to the limited informatics content in nursing curriculum (Ornes & Gassert, 2007). The goal of the TIGER initiative is twofold: first, to enable informatics tools, principles, and practices to be used by nurses to make health care safer, effective, efficient, patient centered, timely, and equitable; and secondly, to integrate these technologies into nursing education and practice (The TIGER Initiative, 2007; Walker, 2010). The action plan includes making changes in nursing education by integrating informatics competencies into the nursing curriculum; taking an active role in the design of informatics tools that are user-friendly and evidence based; working with nursing organizations to communicate the vision to their members; and integrating industry standards for health information technology interoperability (The TIGER Initiative, 2007; Walker, 2010). The rapid advances in computer information technology have important workplace implications and educational/training opportunities for both nursing students and educators worldwide.

American Association of Colleges of Nursing (AACN). (2008). *The essentials of baccalaureate education for professional nursing practice.* Retrieved from http://www.aacn.nche.edu/Education/baccessentials08.pdf

Conrick, M., Hovenga, E., Cook, R., Laracuente, T., & Morgan, T. (2004). *A framework for nursing informatics in Australia; a strategic paper* (p. 34). Brisbane, Australia: Australian Government Department of Health and Ageing.

Edwards, J., & O'Connor, P. A. (2011). Improving technology competency in nursing students: The Passport Project. *The Journal of Educators Online, 8*(20), 1–20.

Elder, B. L., & Koehn, M. L. (2009). Assessment tool for nursing student computer competencies. *Nursing Education Perspectives, 30*(3), 148–152.

Flood, L., Gasiewicz, N., & Delpier, T. (2010). Integrating information literacy across a BSN curriculum. *Journal of Nursing Education, 49,* 101–104.

Hebda, T., & Calderone, T. (2010). What nurse educators need to know about the TIGER initiative. *Nurse Educator, 35,* 56–60. doi: 10.1097/NNE.0b013e3181ced83d

Ornes, L., & Gassert, C. (2007). Computer competencies in a BSN program. *Journal of Nursing Education, 46,* 75–78.

Schroeter, K. (2008). *Competence literature review.* Denver, CO: Competency and Credentialing Institute.

Technology Informatics Guiding Education Reform (TIGER). (2009). *TIGER Informatics Competencies Collaborative (TICC) final report.* Retrieved from www.tigersummit.com

The TIGER Initiative. (2007). *Evidence and informatics transforming nursing: 3-Year action steps toward a 10-year vision.* Retrieved from www.tigersummit.com

Walker, P. (2010). The TIGER initiative: A call to accept and pass the baton. *Nursing Economics, 28,* 352–355. Retrieved from http://proquest.umi.com/pqdlink-did=2173757041&sid=2&Fmt=3-&clientId=9269&RQT=309&VName=PQD

Mary Joy Garcia-Dia
Amy Reiterman

STUDENT DISABILITY

DEFINITION

Disability is defined by the Americans with Disabilities Act (ADA) as "a physical or mental impairment that substantially limits one or more of the major life activities, a record of such impairment, or being regarded as having such an impairment" (ADA, 2008). Such physical and mental disabilities may result from birth, acute or chronic disease, or trauma. One in five people in the United States report having a disability (U.S. Census Bureau, 2012). The term *disabled student* is sometimes thought of as inappropriate, as it implies that this is the person's most important feature. In its place, many have adopted the term *student with a disability* (Hutcheon & Wolbring, 2012). In nursing education, a student with a disability is a qualified individual with a documented disability who

S

needs accommodations to have equal access to instruction, class, or programs.

APPLICATION

Nursing educators have the responsibility to support students with disabilities. In addition, they have access to resources to support students with disabilities. As in all of higher education, nursing schools are required to provide suitable academic adjustments to guarantee discrimination does not occur on the basis of a disability (Ed.gov, n.d.). Academic adjustments may include auxiliary aides and services or modifications to academic requirements. Reduced academic loads, course substitutions, note takers, recording devices, sign language interpreters, and extended test-taking time are other examples of modifications (Ed.gov, n.d.). An example of an auxiliary aide for faculty is the DO IT Faculty Room, from the University of Washington, which provides strategies to create classroom environments that maximize learning for all students.

As more classes are delivered on the web, it is critical that students have access to online materials such as closed captioned video lectures for hearing impaired students and voice-activated software to enable automated text typing for students unable to use a keyboard. Although not specific for educators, guidelines and assistance for web accessibility can be found in Section 508 of the Rehabilitation Act, as well as at WebAIM.

Nursing educators can support students with disabilities by helping them build self-determination skills. Allowing students to engage in the setup of their services, or encouraging them to explore various technologies and learning strategies, can increase their sense of ownership. Students with disabilities may need encouragement to persist in applying to multiple nursing programs, since individual nursing school admission requirements vary according to the Nurse Practice Act in each state and according to technical or core performance standards in each program (Maheady & Fleming, 2005). Students with disabilities may also need

reassurance or help in locating appropriate adaptive devices to succeed in clinical courses. A wide range of adaptive technologies are available, such as clear surgical masks that enable lip reading; amplified or pressure-sensitive stethoscopes for nursing students with hearing loss; thermometers with audio temperature readings for visually impaired nursing students; and sphygmomanometers that can be operated with one hand for students with physical disabilities (Maheady & Fleming, 2005; Shaw, Madaus, & Banerjee, 2009).

SYNOPSIS

Students in preschool through 12th grade are entitled to a free, appropriate public education to be provided in the least restrictive environment. Once these students enter the postsecondary environment, such as nursing school, they bear the responsibility to self-identify, request, and document the need for services, which is one of the main barriers to nursing education (Helms, 2006, p. 195; Peterson, VanDycke, Roberson, & Sedaghat, 2013). Students are no longer automatically entitled to services. The Office of Civil Rights (OCR) provides a pamphlet outlining the rights and responsibilities of students with disabilities preparing for higher education, based on Section 504 of the Rehabilitation Act of 1973 and Title II of the ADA of 1990. Both acts prohibit discrimination on the basis of disability (Ed.gov, n.d.).

On the other hand, nursing schools are "not required to lower or substantially modify essential requirements," nor do they need to "make adjustments that would fundamentally alter the nature of a service, program or activity or that would result in an undue financial or administrative burden" (Ed.gov, n.d.). In addition, nursing schools do not need to "provide personal attendants, individually prescribed devices, readers for personal use or study or other devices or services of a personal nature" (Ed.gov, n.d.), but do need to ensure equal access. Nursing schools are also responsible for keeping any information related to student disability confidential (Peterson et al., 2013).

RECOMMENDATIONS

Nurse educators have the responsibility to ensure all students have equal access in education, which includes physical access to the face-to-face or online classroom and clinical practicum sites, along with programmatic access to all course materials. Students with disabilities must follow the institutional policies and procedures for obtaining accommodations, and that information should be identified in every course syllabus. Accommodations are determined on a case-by-case basis, must be reasonable, and must not alter the essential functions of the class. Not only does the classroom need to be accessible, but nursing educators need to keep abreast of adaptive technology options for students with disabilities to enable clinical practicum success and nursing technical skill mastery.

The National Organization of Nurses with Disabilities (NOND) encourages best practices in nursing education and employment. The Job Accommodation Network serves as a clearing house with specific information for employers accommodating nurses with disabilities.

Role models are needed for all nurses and nursing students. Students with disabilities often report feelings of isolation and vulnerability. University and nursing school settings do not typically allow students with disabilities "media of expression, social outlets, or opportunities to embrace their identities" (Hutcheon & Wolbring, 2012). The NOND and ExceptionalNurse.com websites offer profiles and videos of successful nurses with disabilities at all levels of education and practice. More research is needed on how students with disabilities perceive nursing education (Ashkroft et al., 2008).

Nursing educators need to learn more about accommodations and universal design principles for students with disabilities. Ashkroft et al. (2008) address the need for nursing educators to further their own understanding in several domains related to students with disabilities: accommodations in the clinical setting; personal attitudes and biases; legal requirements, professional obligations and university policies that impact admission, accommodation, and evaluation; internal nursing school processes for accommodations; and the stigma students may face accessing nursing as a profession. Nursing faculty who embrace opportunities for gaining knowledge in these areas and who utilize the available resources will not only enhance their own perspectives but also enhance the experience and success for nursing students with disabilities, which will ultimately increase the diversity and quality of the future nursing workforce.

Americans with Disabilities Act of 1990, as Amended, 42 U.S.C.A. § 12101 et seq. (2008). Retrieved from http://www.ada.gov/pubs/adastatute08.htm

Ashkroft, T., Chernomas, W., Davis, P., Dean, R., Seguire, M., Shappiro, C., & Swiderski, L. (2008). Nursing students with disabilities: One faculty's journey. *International Journal of Education Scholarship, 5*(1). Retrieved from http://www.exceptionalnurse.com/NursingStudentsWithDisabilities2008.pdf

Ed.gov. (n.d.). *Students with disabilities preparing for postsecondary education: Know your rights and responsibilities.* Retrieved from http://www2.ed.gov/print/about/offices/list/ocr/transition.html

Helms, L. (2006). Disability law and nursing education: An update. *Journal of Professional Nursing, 22*(3), 190–196.

Hutcheon, E. J., & Wolbring, G. (2012). Voices of "disabled" post-secondary students: Examining higher education "disability" policy using an ableism lens. *Journal of Diversity in Higher Education, 5*(1), 39–49. doi:10.1037/a0027002

Maheady, D. C., & Fleming, S. E. (2005). "Homework" for future nursing students with disabilities. *Minority Nurse.* Retrieved from http://www.minoritynurse.com/article/%E2%80%9Chomework%E2%80%9D-future-nursing-students-disabilities

S

Peterson, L. Y., VanDycke, J. L., Roberson, R. L., & Sedaghat, J. M. (2013). Promoting student transition from entitlement services to eligibility resources. *Intervention in School and Clinic, 49*(2), 99–107. doi:10.1177/1053451213493173

Shaw, S. F., Madaus, J. W., & Banerjee, M. (2009). Enhance access to postsecondary education for students with disabilities. *Intervention in School and Clinic, 44*(3), 185–190. doi:10.1177/1053451208326047

U.S. Census Bureau. (2012). Retrieved from https://www.census.gov/newsroom/releases/archives/miscellaneous/cb12–134.html

Janet Resop Reilly

STUDY ABROAD PROGRAMS

DEFINITION

Study abroad programs are educational activities completed in a country outside that of a student's home institution. Such programs are focused on educational experiences that provide course credit for general education or credit toward a major. Study abroad programs include but are not limited to classroom courses and experiential activities (McKinnon & McNelis, 2013).

APPLICATION

Study abroad programs in nursing are educational in focus and contribute toward the completion of nursing or non-nursing course credit in a host country. Most study abroad programs in U.S. Schools of Nursing are offered as general education or special sessions, not as credit toward a major (McKinnon & McNelis, 2013). Participants in study abroad programs may complete courses individually or as a group. Students may participate in study abroad programs independently or accompanied by faculty from the home institution, as in faculty-led programs. Study abroad programs vary in duration according to the individual courses, objectives, and activities to be completed.

Increased demand for study abroad programs in nursing education stems from a pressing need to develop students as global citizens prepared to navigate the challenges and opportunities of a diverse patient population and an increasingly interconnected world. In addition to course and core degree objectives, study abroad programs are conducted with an emphasis on the development of global citizenship, civic engagement, and cultural sensitivity (Frenk et al., 2010; Kelley, Connor, Kun, & Salmon, 2008; Reising et al., 2008). Participation in study abroad programs as students or faculty promotes professional growth, develops expertise in global health, and enhances nurses' role as locally responsive and globally connected members of a global health system (Frenk et al., 2010).

SYNOPSIS

Though primarily cognitive and educational in focus, participation in study abroad programs also promotes growth in the intrapersonal and interpersonal domains of human development (Braskamp, Braskamp, & Merrill, 2009). When challenged to adapt to unfamiliar surroundings, languages, transport systems, and cultures, students develop a sense of self-efficacy, a concept defined by Bandura (1997) as "an individual's confidence in his/her ability to negotiate the challenges inherent in the larger social world" (Gardner, Steglitz, & Gross, 2009, p. 20). In addition to self-efficacy, students attain a sense of awareness and respect for the culture and global perspectives (Braskamp et al., 2009).

By interacting with others in a host country, students may develop interpersonally into culturally sensitive individuals who are better able to view the world as one in which we function as members of an interdependent global society (Bosworth et al., 2006; Braskamp et al., 2009). This perspective fosters a longer-term outcome of a "broader view of health care, comparisons with other health care systems, and advocacy" (Bosworth et al., 2006, p. 37) in addition to the development of professional and civic responsibility (Reising et al., 2008).

The interpersonal and intrapersonal growth resulting from study abroad program participation contributes to the development of global citizens who are better able to assess and approach the challenges they will meet as nurses working with diverse populations (Frenk et al., 2010; Reising et al., 2008). The achievement of such growth is dependent upon students' ability to reflect on their experiences abroad. Reflection on their experiences encourages students' awareness and ability to better articulate the outcomes of their experiences (Gardner et al., 2009; Lewin, 2009).

RECOMMENDATIONS

Despite growing interest in study abroad programs in nursing education, continued development of such programs is restricted by a lack of clarity regarding the issue of credit toward a major in schools of nursing. Such ambiguity has led schools of nursing to establish study abroad programs as extra courses available to students who are able to pay additional fees (McKinnon & McNelis, 2013). Examination and definition of regulations surrounding credit toward a major for study abroad programs are needed to encourage growth in student participation and program development. Further development in study abroad programs should also address the possibility of reciprocity for coursework completed abroad to students' home institution. Examination into reciprocity of course credit in addition to credit toward a major in nursing education may encourage continued growth in study abroad programs by preventing delay in coursework or graduation as a result of participation. As study abroad programs continue to develop, it is also ethically imperative to promote further studies examining the effects of programs on host communities.

Bandura, A. (1997). *Self-efficacy: The exercise of control.* New York, NY: W. H. Freeman.

Bosworth, T. L., Haloburdo, E. P., Hetrick, C., Patchett, K., Thompson, M. A., & Welch, M. (2006). International partnerships to promote quality care: Faculty groundwork, student projects, and outcomes. *Journal of Continuing Education in Nursing, 37*(1), 32–38.

Braskamp, L. A., Braskamp, D. C., & Merrill, K. C. (2009). Assessing progress in global learning and development of students with education abroad experiences. *Frontiers: The Interdisciplinary Journal of Study Abroad, 18,* 101–118.

Frenk, J., Chen, L., Bhutta, Z. A., Cohen, J., Crisp, N., Evans, T.,…Zurayk, H. (2010). Health professionals for a new century: Transforming education to strengthen health systems in an interdependent world. *Lancet, 376*(9756), 1923–1958.

Gardner, P., Steglitz, I., & Gross, L. (2009). Translating study abroad experiences for workplace competencies. *Peer Review, 11*(4), 19–22.

Kelley, M. A., Connor, A., Kun, K. E., & Salmon, M. E. (2008). Social responsibility: Conceptualization and embodiment in a school of nursing. *International Journal of Nursing Education Scholarship, 5*(1), Article 28.

Lewin, R. (2009). Transforming the study abroad experience into a collective priority. *Peer Review, 11*(4), 8–11.

McKinnon, T. H., & McNelis, A. M. (2013). International programs in United States schools of nursing: Driving forces, obstacles, and opportunities. *Nursing Education Perspectives, 34*(5), 323–328.

Reising, D. L., Shea, R. A., Allen, P. N., Laux, M. M., Hensel, D., & Watts, P. A. (2008). Using service-learning to develop health promotion and research skills in nursing students. *International Journal of Nursing Education Scholarship, 5*(1), Article 29.

Kathleen de Leon

S

SUBSTANCE ABUSE

DEFINITION

Substance abuse is defined as a disorder comprised of a collection of symptoms including behavioral, cognitive, and physiological components (American Psychiatric Association [APA], 2013). A person with substance abuse continues using the substance or substances despite significant problems with role responsibilities, legal issues, and relational conflicts.

The diagnosis of a substance use disorder (APA, 2013) is determined by an array of behaviors over a calendar year, leading to a substantial impairment in functioning, including an inability to complete key family responsibilities, education, or work obligations, and placing self or others in dangerous situations and legal problems. Relapse and drug craving are common in those persons with a long-term history of substance abuse when exposed to drug-related stimuli.

The National Survey on Drug Use and Health (NSDUH) is a survey which documents substance abuse prevalence in the United States. Research findings revealed that substance use and dependency is a threat, which occurs in approximately 6% of the U.S. population (U.S. Department of Health and Human Services [DHHS], 2013). The age groups that are most affected by illicit drug use are among young adults (18–25 years) and middle-aged adults (50–59 years), which link to the typical ages of traditional nursing students and the nursing workforce. The most commonly abused substances are marijuana, pain relievers for non-medicinal use, and cocaine. The documented number of persons who admitted heroin use has almost doubled since 2007 (373,000 to 620,000). Men and persons affected with mental health comorbidities are at greater risk for chemical dependency.

APPLICATION

Student nurses must be educated on the pathology of addiction, risk and protective factors, the signs and symptoms of substance use, addiction and withdrawal, treatment options, potential for recovery, nursing interventions, therapeutic responses, and anticipatory guidance to educate and support families of those affected by substance abuse. Sullivan (1995) documented that substance abuse content typically includes 1 to 5 hours over the entirety of the nursing program. Topics may be embedded into lectures tied to pathology of disease and elective courses.

Nurses may not recognize substance abuse and be unprepared to manage abuse issues. Some nurses hold negative attitudes toward patients with substance abuse issues and recovery and often prefer not caring for them (Beckstead, 2002, 2005; Happell, Carta, & Pinikahana, 2002; Kornegay Bugle, Jackson, & Rives, 2004). Students must be prepared to recognize and report peers with suspected impairment. Health care providers who are suspected of substance misuse are commonly not confronted by their peers utilizing the *Don't Ask Don't Tell* attitude (Monroe & Kenaga, 2011).

SYNOPSIS

The relevant review of literature on substance use and abuse as it relates to the discipline of nursing includes prevalence; risk factors for misuse; knowledge and attitudes of student nurses, nurses, and other health care professionals regarding patients or colleagues who misuse substances; management concerns such as disciplinary efforts or alternatives to discipline and reentry into practice policies; and nursing curricula related to substance abuse. Studies directly linking nursing students, nurses, and nursing faculty with substance abuse or dependency are limited. Often, terms used for substance abuse are used interchangeably and include chemical use, abuse or misuse, dependency or impairment, addiction, and withdrawal.

RECOMMENDATIONS

Students should understand the risk and protective factors for alcohol and drug use.

Nurse educators need to be aware of the most common risk factors for alcohol and drug use. These are parental approval of drug and alcohol use, parental monitoring, parental or older siblings with drug and alcohol use, development of antisocial behavior, associating with peers with problem behavior, risk-taking behavior, poor school performance, and easy access to alcohol or drugs (Haber, 2001; DHHS, 2013; West, 2003). Students need a solid understanding of the nurse practice act and their legal obligation to report substance abuse.

American Psychiatric Association (APA). (2013). *Diagnostic and statistical manual of mental disorders*, 5th ed. Washington, DC: Author.

Beckstead, J. W. (2002). Modeling attitudinal antecedents of nurses' decisions to report impaired colleagues. *Western Journal of Nursing Research, 24*(5), 537–551.

Beckstead, J. W. (2005). Reporting peer wrongdoing in the healthcare profession: The role of incompetence and substance abuse information. *International Journal of Nursing Studies, 42*(3), 325–331.

Haber, J. (2001). Management of substance abuse and dependence problems within families. In M. A. Naegle & C. E. D'Avanzo (Eds.), *Addictions and substance abuse: Strategies for advanced practice nursing* (pp. 305–331). Upper Saddle River, NJ: Prentice Hall.

Happell, B., Carta, B., & Pinikahana, J. (2002). Nurses' knowledge, attitudes and beliefs regarding substance use: A questionnaire survey. *Nursing & Health Sciences, 4*(4), 193–200.

Kornegay, K., Bugle, L., Jackson, E., & Rives, K. (2004). Facing a problem of great concern: Nursing faculty's lived experience of encounters with chemically dependent nursing students. *Journal of Addictions Nursing, 15*(3), 125–132.

Monroe, T., & Kenaga, H. (2011). Don't ask don't tell: Substance abuse and addiction among nurses. *Journal of Clinical Nursing, 20*(3–4), 504–509.

Sullivan, E. (1995). *Nursing care of clients with substance abuse*. St. Louis, MO: Mosby.

U.S. Department of Health and Human Services (DHHS). (2013). *Substance abuse and mental health services administration*. National Outcome Measures. Retrieved from http://www.nationaloutcomemeasures.samhsa.gov/./index.asp

West, M. (2003). A kaleidoscopic review of literature about substance abuse impairment in nursing: Progress toward identification of early risk indicators? *Journal of Addictions Nursing, 14*(3), 139–144.

Cheryl D. Schlamb

Teaching Assistants

DEFINITION

Teaching assistants (TAs) provide support to faculty and students in course-related tasks or in the simulation or laboratory resource center. Undergraduate TAs (UTAs) are appointed or employed based on satisfactory completion of the course, meeting a minimum grade point average (GPA), and successful faculty-to-student matches. The use of UTA is a newly emerging practice in nursing education and may prove valuable, especially in light of current and future increases in student enrollments and shortages of nursing faculty.

APPLICATION

UTAs have been used successfully in many disciplines to lead discussion sessions, grade assignments, tutor other students, conduct office hours, and enter grades (Goff & Lahme, 2003; Herrman & Waterhouse, 2010; Reges, 2003). UTAs may assist in programs of nursing by supporting faculty, providing additional academic resources to students, and increasing the UTA skills in peer leadership and course material mastery while exposing undergraduate students to the faculty role as a potential career choice (Chandler, 2005; Goldsmith, Stewart, & Ferguson, 2006; Herrman & Waterhouse, 2010).

SYNOPSIS

TAs and faculty mentors may benefit greatly from the TA role. UTAs learn to connect with students on a mentoring level and assist them with strategies to enable learning and thriving in the academic environment. UTAs develop skills in leadership, project management, and communication. Furthermore, they may begin to appreciate the role of the nurse educator and see it as part of their career trajectory. Faculty benefit by being able to focus on higher-level demands of teaching, including developing classes, incorporating creative strategies into teaching methods, conducting classroom assessment and higher-level evaluation measures, and other faculty tasks. Faculty also glean benefits from the close relationships developed with UTAs and are able to provide valuable mentoring while being relieved of selected administrative and clerical roles. Students are perhaps the most fortunate beneficiaries of the UTA programs. They have the opportunity to learn from fellow students, to develop mentoring relationships with peers, and to have increased resources for development.

The role of UTAs may vary based on the needs of the students, the teaching formats of the educational program, and the individual wishes of faculty. Authors have identified the potential tasks of the UTA to include proctoring examinations, taking examinations to the testing center or running examinations, providing review sessions for students on a weekly basis or in preparation for examinations, tutoring students who are struggling with class content, checking the American Psychological Association (APA) format in student assignments, maintaining course records for mandatory assignments, commenting on field experience assignments, grading short assignments or those easily analyzed via established rubrics, entering student scores into grade programs or online grade books, grading quizzes, leading discussion groups, providing peer education in the laboratory setting, and stocking or preparing the lab (Chandler, 2005; Goldsmith et al., 2006; Herrman & Waterhouse, 2010).

In addition, faculty play an important role in ensuring the success of the UTA program. Ongoing communication, clear delineation of expectations, and supervision of tasks are critical. UTAs should not be asked to handle difficult student situations or to take on responsibilities outside their level, skill, and expertise. Faculty who delegate by clearly explaining the UTA's tasks and details find that UTAs are of significant assistance in their educational workload. Without such delegation, UTAs may appear to add to the faculty burden. It is important to maintain a close working relationship with UTAs and ensure that the experience is positive in their course of study.

Other disciplines allow TAs, usually at the graduate level, to teach didactic classes, develop examinations, and evaluate higher-level assignments. In nursing, they are used more in undergraduate clinical nursing education. Graduate student TAs may be helpful, but their personal course work and requirements, family demands, and short-term needs may limit their value as TAs.

A shortage of nursing faculty and pressure to increase student enrollment is leading schools to reconfigure the nursing curriculum. Strategies to increase enrollment in nursing education programs include increasing numbers of faculty and supplementary staff to support clinical and classroom teaching. One component of this redesign could be to develop a TA program for undergraduate students (Herrman & Waterhouse, 2010). In an example UTA program, students apply and register for a pass–fail course. They work 28 hours with a faculty member or provide support in the simulation resource center. In addition, the UTAs sign a contract delineating behavior and the obligations of the UTA role and participate in a group orientation highlighting confidentiality, working with students, and role expectations. This program demonstrated success in allowing faculty to ensure time spent on class lectures and other teaching methods, assisted students in receiving extra support for their learning, and provided UTAs with valuable experiences. Participants report satisfaction with the program (Herrman & Waterhouse, 2010).

Chandler (2005) described a UTA program in which undergraduate students are paired with graduate TAs and faculty to support a large freshmen class of nursing students. Evaluation of this program revealed positive outcomes including increased mentoring of students, development of UTA leadership qualities, and faculty perceptions of an ease in workload. Goldsmith, Stewart, and Ferguson (2006) employed third-year nursing students to assist more novice students to learn skills in the lab setting, leading to positive outcomes in learning and course implementation.

RECOMMENDATIONS

As with any new teaching method or innovative program, the use of TAs in nursing education demands ongoing and rigorous evaluation. Each nursing program must assess needs and the possibility for UTAs to fill critical gaps in educational practices. The relatively intangible outcomes of UTAs, benefit to TAs, and impact on faculty workload necessitate evaluation using both quantitative and qualitative methods.

The need for clear delineation of the UTA role and ongoing evaluation of student and faculty outcomes is imperative. Collins and Simco (2006) describe the use of reflection and reflective journaling to ensure that UTAs incorporate principles of teaching and learning rather than simply completing tasks to support faculty and students.

Future analysis may explore how UTA programs cultivate interest in careers as nurse researchers and faculty members, support faculty mentoring, and accommodate additional numbers. Because the teaching role and the teaching–learning process are inherent to the education of students, TAs are logical additions to the provision of undergraduate education and may prove useful in a variety of academic settings.

Chandler, G. E. (2005). Growing nurse leaders: An undergraduate teaching assistant program. *Journal of Nursing Education, 44*(12), 569–572.

Collins, J., & Simco, N. (2006). Teaching assistants reflect: The way forward? *Reflective Practice: International and Multidisciplinary Perspectives, 7*(2), 197–214.

Goff, C., & Lahme, B. (2003). Benefits of a comprehensive undergraduate teaching assistant program. *PRIMUS: Problems, Resources, and Issues in Mathematics Undergraduate Studies, 13*(1), 75–84.

Goldsmith, M., Stewart, L., & Ferguson, L. (2006). Peer learning partnership: An innovative strategy to enhance skill acquisition in nursing students. *Nurse Education Today, 26*(2), 123–130.

Herrman, J. W., & Waterhouse, J. K. (2010). Benefits of using undergraduate teaching assistants throughout a baccalaureate nursing curriculum. *Journal of Nursing Education, 49*(2), 72–77.

Reges, S. (2003). Using undergraduate students as teaching assistants in a state university. *ACM SIGSCE Bulletin, 25*(2), 103–107.

Judith W. Herrman

TEXT MESSAGING

DEFINITION

Text messaging (a.k.a. texting) is the use of portable networked devices such as mobile phones to share short electronic messages comprised of alphanumeric characters and symbols.

APPLICATION

Text messaging provides a convenient method of short communication that is easily accessible in today's digitally connected world. According to Pew Internet Research (Brenner, 2013), which conducted interviews on 6,010 adults aged 18+ years, 91% of Americans have cell phones, and 88% of these individuals use their cell phones to send or receive text messages. Given the ubiquitous usage of text messaging for social communication, this tool may be employed for more specific purposes in clinical education and health care. Text messaging may be used at various levels in the overall health care setting; it may be used as a supplement to the education of health care professionals, communication among health care professionals in practice, and contact with patients throughout their health care regime.

SYNOPSIS

The literature regarding text messaging highlights a variety of uses for this brief form of communication. Text messaging has been used to enhance instructions in the basic sciences for nursing students. According to Richardson, Littrell, Challman, and Stein (2011), text messaging is used to encourage first-year nursing students to preview their anatomy notes for upcoming lectures or to review their notes shortly following lecture. Short one-sentence questions were texted or e-mailed to the students to prompt further discussion of the basic anatomy content.

Text messaging has also been used to enhance communication between health care providers. According to Howard, Fox, and Coyer (2014), text messaging aids communication between coordinating academics and off-campus clinical nursing administrators. Descriptive findings from this study indicated that the text messaging efforts improved cohesiveness between these academic units, as well as increased approachability and feelings of collaboration between the administrators and professors.

Text messaging has enhanced communication with patients and improved health outcomes. In such cases, text message reminders resulted in changes in the patient's behavior. Free et al. (2011)

implemented a text messaging smoking cessation program (txt2stop) to support patients in their abstinence from a detrimental habit. Short motivational messages encouraged patients to keep to their program; this approach worked, as patients who received the reminders were biochemically verified to have abstained from smoking at 6 months. In a 2009 systematic review of 25 studies involving cell phone and text-messaging intervention (Krishna, Boren, & Balas, 2009), with a total of 38,060 participants in 12 clinical areas and 13 countries, 19 studies assessed patient outcome care. The number of texts sent to patients varied throughout the studies (1–5 texts/week), yet there were significant improvements regarding patient compliance with medications, stress level, smoking quit rates, and self-efficacy. In addition, Gurol-Urganci, de Jongh, Vodopivec-Jamsek, Atun, and Car (2013) reported evidence from seven studies involving 5,841 participants that mobile text-message reminders improved the rate of attendance of health care appointments compared to no reminders. These results were similar to phone call reminders, yet cheaper. Further evidence for text messaging and behavior modification is presented in the article by Park, Howie-Esquivel, Chung, and Dracup (2014) as messaging increased adherence to antiplatelet therapy as evidenced by Medication Event Monitoring Systems (MEMS) and text message response rates. These articles suggest that text messaging may provide a doorway to patient care that closely mimics the encouragement individuals receive through social connections. Lua and Neni (2012) showed that patients had favorable opinions toward using short message service (SMS), a text-messaging service component of mobile phones, for epilepsy education, drug-taking reminders, and clinic appointment reminders. A follow-up study (Lua & Leni, 2013) showed that patients who received text messages exhibited significantly improved medication adherence and clinical attendance compared to the control group.

RECOMMENDATIONS

Current literature supports the use of text messaging to enhance patient outcomes with respect to medication compliance and encouragement to be persistent in healthy choices (e.g., quit smoking). Weaver, Lindsay, and Gitelman (2012) reinforce that text messaging between the patient and health care provider allows for convenient, direct, and immediate communication, as recipients are more likely to read and respond to the message right away. However, in regard to communication between health care professionals, there is room for improvement. In contrast to Howard et al. (2014), a recent publication (Wu et al., 2014) suggests that text messaging may not be entirely beneficial in the health care realm due to increased tendencies to misinterpret the intended message, since text messages provide short instructions with minimal context. In addition, text messages minimized the face-to-face time needed between health care providers, leading to a sense of depersonalization and negative impact on work relationships. These findings provide incentive for improving the use of text messaging in the education of health care professionals. Future efforts to clarify brief messages of notification and inquiries of patient care are warranted. Education may be needed to emphasize components that must always be included in a brief message, for example, in order to provide appropriate context to the topic and to minimize misunderstanding.

In regard to nursing education, perhaps training for text message correspondence may begin early when basic science courses are taught and first correlated with clinical outcomes. In addition, text messaging may also be used to promote discussion in early coursework when students may be less confident to ask questions during lecture (Richardson, Littrell, Challman, & Stein, 2011). Short messages may be sent to the instructor to inquire further about the topic being discussed. As text messaging is sure to maintain popularity in the near future, educators may take advantage of this tool to promote discussion instead of depersonalizing correspondences.

Brenner, J. (2013). *Pew Internet: Mobile. Pew Internet & American Life Project.* Retrieved from http://pewinternet.org/Reports/2013/Cell-Activities.aspx

Free, C., Knight, R., Robertson, S., Whittaker, R., Edwards, P., Zhou, W.,...Roberts, I. (2011). Smoking cessation support delivered via mobile phone text messaging (txt2stop): A single-blind, randomised trial. *Lancet, 378*(9785), 49–55.

Gurol-Urganci, I., de Jongh, T., Vodopivec-Jamsek, V., Atun, R., & Car, J. (2013). Mobile phone messaging reminders for attendance at healthcare appointments. *The Cochrane Database of Systematic Reviews, 12,* CD007458.

Howard, C., Fox, A. R., & Coyer, F. (2014). Text messaging to support off-campus clinical nursing facilitators: A descriptive survey. *Nursing Education Today, 34*(6), e32–e36.

Krishna, S., Boren, S. A., & Balas, E. A. (2009). Healthcare via cell phones: A systematic review. *Telemedicine Journal and E-Health, 15*(3), 231–240.

Lua, P. L., & Neni, W. S. (2012). Feasibility and acceptability of mobile epilepsy educational system (MEES) for people with epilepsy in Malaysia. *Telemedicine Journal and E-Health, 18*(10), 777–784.

Lua, P. L., & Neni, W. S. (2013). A randomised controlled trial of an SMS-based mobile epilepsy education system. *Journal of Telemedicine and Telecare, 19*(1), 23–28.

Park, L. G., Howie-Esquivel, J., Chung, M. L., & Dracup, K. (2014). A text messaging intervention to promote medication adherence for patients with coronary heart disease: A randomized controlled trial. *Patient Education and Counseling, 94*(2), 261–268.

Richardson, A., Littrell, O. M., Challman, S., & Stein, P. (2011). Using text messaging in an undergraduate nursing course. *Journal of Nursing Education, 50*(2), 99–104.

Weaver, B., Lindsay, B., & Gitelman, B. (2012). Communication technology and social media: Opportunities and implications for healthcare systems. *Online Journal of Issues in Nursing, 17*(3), 3.

Wu, R., Appel, L., Morra, D., Lo, V., Kitto, S., & Quan, S. (2014). Short message service or disService: Issues with text messaging in a complex medical environment. *International Journal of Medical Informatics, 83*(4), 278–284. doi:10.1016/j.ijmedinf.2014.01.003

April Richardson Hatcher

THEORETICAL THINKING

DEFINITION

Theoretical thinking is the application of direct experience, correspondence with what is known, and an understanding of the logic of the relationships among the elements of the theory. It includes an understanding of nursing phenomena, differentiating between relevant and irrelevant phenomena, and deciding how theory applies to nursing practice and research (Meleis, 2012).

APPLICATION

In the process of learning, students put theory into practice throughout the educational program (Kuhn, 1970; Tomey & Alligood, 2006). In this way, students incrementally build their understanding of theories that inform practice. Carper (1978) highlights the importance of paying critical attention to the question of what knowledge is of most value in the discipline of nursing. She holds that knowing in nursing is a combination of the patterns of empiric, aesthetics, personal, and ethical.

SYNOPSIS

A major goal put forth by nursing leaders in the 20th century was the development of nursing knowledge on which to base practice,

T

improve quality of care, and inform nursing research (Scott, Matthews, & Kirwan, 2014). Alligood (Tomey & Alligood, 2006) contends that nursing theoretical works are vital to the future of both the discipline and the profession of nursing. She believes that research alone produces isolated information, whereas research and theory together produce nursing science. The science of nursing includes theoretical frameworks that are learned and applied in practice and research. Guiding students to value theoretical thinking in nursing is of utmost importance. This means that faculty model theoretical thinking as they lay the foundation for the courses in which they teach.

RECOMMENDATIONS

Theoretical thinking is necessary for excellent nursing practice and therefore is essential. Current thinking encourages the achievement of a therapeutic relationship with the patient that is theory based. Necessary to achieve this is self-awareness (Carper, 1978; Musker, 2011) coupled with a full understanding of the benefit of a therapeutic relationship for the patient. This requires knowledge of the theoretical framework in nursing that ties directly to caring as an essential element of a therapeutic relationship. To achieve this, careful reading and faithful interpretation of nursing theory are required.

Carper, B. A. (1978). Fundamental patterns of knowing in nursing. *Advances in Nursing Science, 1*(1), 13–23.

Hussey, T. B. (2004). Intellectual seductions. *Nursing Philosophy, 5*, 104–111.

Kuhn, T. S. (1970). *The structure of scientific revolutions*. Chicago, IL: University of Chicago Press.

Meleis, A. I. (2012). *Theoretical thinking: Development and progress*. Philadelphia, PA: Wolters Kluwer Health/Lippincott Williams and Wilkins.

Musker, K. (2011). Nursing theory-based independent practice: A personal experience of closing the theory practice gap. *Advances in Nursing Science, 34*(1), 67–77.

Scott, P. A., Matthews, A., & Kirwan, M. (2014). What is nursing in the 21st century and what does the 21st century health system require of nursing? *Nursing Philosophy, 15*, 23–34.

Tomey, A. M., & Alligood, M. R. (2006). *Nursing theorists and their work*. St. Louis, MO: Mosby.

Aoife Lane

THEORY–PRACTICE INTEGRATION

DEFINITION

Theory–practice integration is the use of nursing ideas, values, and science to guide purposeful implementation of highly skilled actions that go beyond routine technical skills to prevent or resolve patient care problems (Schon, 1983; Thompson, 2000). Theory–practice integration is cyclical in that each informs and builds on the other. New practice problems identify gaps in knowledge, which drive theory revision, generation, and new scientific study. Theory–practice integration overlaps with the concepts of critical thinking, evidence-based practice, and clinical decision making.

APPLICATION

The goal of nursing education is to prepare students to enter practice as competent, autonomous, and accountable professional nurses. Theory–practice integration in education begins with teaching basic physical and social science principles, leading to psychomotor and interview skills in controlled laboratory settings, culminating in clinical experiences with real patients. As the knowledge base grows, students integrate theory and practice in solving patient care problems. Benner, Tanner, and Chesla (2009) describe developmental stages toward expert practice. Novice students learn theory and psychomotor skills that are context free, concrete, and rule driven. Educators then design clinical experiences where students use skills and rules in real situations to move students to the advanced beginner stage. By graduation, students become competent in theory–practice integration as they reflect on what they are doing in unique, uncertain situations as they are practicing (Schon, 1987).

Educators design curricula and clinical experiences to enhance student ability to move from novice, to advanced beginner, to competent practitioner (Benner, Tanner, & Chesla, 2009). To do this, educators must design courses and educational methods that integrate theoretical knowledge (or knowing that), and practical knowledge (or knowing how) (Benner, 1984). Professional knowledge is the blending of theoretical and experiential knowledge, enabling the nurse to solve unique practice problems. Schon (1983) called this reflection in action, grounded in the use of theory in the here and now, where practitioners are problem solvers using metacognitive processes as the situation unfolds. Students must learn how to use metacognitive processes to gather patient data, analyze data to identify patterns, develop a potential nursing diagnosis based on theoretical knowledge, plan interventions, implement the plan, and evaluate outcomes (Thompson, 2000). While theory is based on research that attempts to control known variables, practice situations involve uncontrolled and initially chaotic variables that need quick clinical decisions. Educators need to help students identify a framework to guide them through the problem-solving process.

Students in clinical practice can be frightened by the need to accept risk and responsibility for decisions and action in practice (Benner et al., 2009). Educators must be attuned to this and assist students to work through this uncomfortable process. If the student resists accepting responsibility for actions, then stagnation, boredom, or withdrawal from learning can occur. As students gain experience, integration of theory into practice becomes more intuitive and less emotional.

SYNOPSIS

Nursing has evolved from a technical practice that uses trial and error to a professional practice that uses theory-based scientific evidence, clinical reasoning, and critical thinking to guide actions. Thompson (2000) identified the fallacy that professional practice is theory-less. Failure to draw on theoretical knowledge leads to inappropriate interventions that are inefficient and fail to solve patient problems (Meleis, 1997; Thompson, 2000). Theory helps direct care away from ineffective interventions and assists to prioritize actions in unique individual patient situations. Therefore, nursing education must move students from simple memorization of facts and procedural skills to reflection in action; thus, using metacognitive processes as professional practice is based on thought and reflection rather than routine assumptions (Thompson, 2000). This can be difficult as students use memorization in beginning courses of basic physical and social sciences and then move to theory–practice integration. When students become competent in theory–practice integration, they become skilled, autonomous, and accountable for their practice.

RECOMMENDATIONS

Curriculum design and teaching methods emphasize coaching and learning by doing enhanced theory–practice integration (Schon, 1987). Coaching in the art of reflection and clinical practicum courses where dialogue between student and teacher includes advice, criticism, explanations, and descriptions regarding patient care enhance theory–practice integration. High-fidelity simulation and debriefing methods used commonly in nursing education also support reflection in action.

Nursing education must teach students to become information literate. To use scientific evidence, students need to know how to access it, analyze it, and apply it to practice problems (Cannon & Boswell, 2012). While students grow up using personal information sources such as Google, Yahoo, Wikipedia, and other nonprofessional Internet search engines to find information, educators need to move them to professional information sources. It is essential to teach students how to use computerized search engines to find evidence for practice. Educators need to direct students to use professional peer-reviewed sources such as Cochrane Reviews, CINAHL, PubMed, and government and professional practice websites for practice recommendations, research, and practice standards. Requiring the use of professional resources supports thinking and decision making using theory–practice integration. Investigation of how to support student transition from the use of personal information resources to professional resources is needed.

Further development of teaching strategies that improve student rational learning and critical thinking is needed (Cannon & Boswell, 2012). Formative evaluation implements a constructionist model of learning where the teacher coaches the student into reframing problems that are goal oriented for both patient and student (Schon, 1987). Formative evaluation provides feedback on incorrect thinking, redirects problem solving, and can provide opportunities for modeling clinical decision making and coaching reflection in action (Oermann & Gaberson, 2013). The Socratic method of asking students to examine the logic behind selected tasks and judgments can support rational learning. Syntactical learning methods support understanding of the relationships and patterns in patient care. Faculty should talk students through their decision-making process and clarify the intuitive process that meshes theory with practice. Inquiry learning methods that engage students in questioning, exploring, and categorizing challenges in nursing care help to close the loop in theory–practice integration and further advance nursing science, theory, and practice (Ironside, 2007).

Benner, P. (1984). *From novice to expert: Excellence and power in clinical nursing practice*. Menlo Park, CA: Addison-Wesley.

Benner, P., Tanner, C., & Chesla, C. (2009). *Expertise in nursing practice: Caring, clinical judgment, and ethics* (2nd ed.). New York, NY: Springer Publishing.

Cannon, S., & Boswell, C. (2012). *Evidence-based teaching in nursing: A foundation for educators*. Sudbury, MA: Jones & Bartlett.

Ironside, P. (Ed.). (2007). *On revolutions and revolutionaries: 25 years of reform and innovation in nursing education*. New York, NY: National League of Nursing.

Meleis, A. I. (1997). *Theoretical nursing: Development and progress* (3rd ed.). Philadelphia, PA: Lippincott.

Oermann, M. H., & Gaberson, K. B. (2013). *Evaluation and testing in nursing education* (4th ed.). New York, NY: Springer Publishing.

Schon, D. A. (1983). *The reflective practitioner*. New York, NY: Basic Books.

Schon, D. A. (1987). *Educating the reflective practitioner: Toward a new design for teaching and learning in the professions*. San Francisco, CA: Jossey-Bass.

Thompson, N. (2000). *Theory and practice in human services*. Philadelphia, PA: Open University Press.

Christine M. Thomas

TRANSFORMATIVE LEARNING

DEFINITION

Transformative learning (TL) is the process of effecting change in a frame of reference (Mezirow, 1997). This means that there is a question of one's assumptions about what is known, thus leading to a transformed view of the situation.

APPLICATION

TL is an adult learning theory, and can be an effective approach to assist the student in the clinical setting to become an autonomous thinker (Parker & Myrick, 2010). Guiding the student to reflect on assumptions and beliefs that come with caring for persons from different cultures and life experiences can be an effective teaching approach to facilitate TL. Students may experience being challenged when facing life views that are different from their own, thus creating an opportunity for critical appraisal. This transforming approach can assist students to reach short-term goals and objectives, which may ultimately lead to becoming an autonomous thinker (Mezirow, 1997).

SYNOPSIS

TL is a learning theory formulated first by Paulo Freire in 1970. He found that adult learners, when posed with a problem, need to question assumptions, pose questions, and conceptualize the problem within the context of the social, political, and economic influences in their lives (Derix, 1998). He indicated that the frame of reference is the lens by which one views the world. Therefore, the context is the frame of reference.

The 10-step process leads the nurse to become an autonomous thinker. The educator's role in the steps is to gently ask questions that provoke thought and insight. The goal is to change the lens the nurse is looking through (McAlister, Tower, & Walker, 2007; Mezirow, 1997).

Adult learners tend to realize how and why they perceive their current world, and take action to come to a different view of the world (Mezirow, 1997). This can be achieved by multiple exposures to new problems requiring the student to assess his or her own feelings and perceptions about the problem, including limitations in knowledge, requiring the student to assess assumptions and perceptions about the problem. The student must be given time to process the problem while discovering underlying assumptions, either positive or negative. After the underlying assumptions have been identified, the student completes a critical self-reflection uncovering the foundation of the underlying assumptions. Once the source is identified, the student participates in critical discourse, where the

information is shared in a group and the group assists in problem solving. Finally, the student acknowledges the change in the frame of reference, thus culminating in a new perspective (Mathew-Maich, Plog, Jack, & Dobbins, 2010; McGonigal, 2007).

RECOMMENDATIONS

In order to implement TL in nursing education, instructors must create the environment. This environment must be nonthreatening and supportive. This environment promotes trust between student and instructor, which is paramount to the discourse required in transformational learning. Instructors need to create objectives that foster critical thinking, self-examination, and critical appraisal that encourage autonomy and, ultimately, TL.

The instructor must take time to get to know the students by inquiring about thoughts and feelings (McAlister et al., 2007). This strategy will foster trust in the classroom. An exercise to meet this strategy might be short journal entries throughout the semester. Short introduction with a brief history may help to make the students feel they are heard and valued. It is also important to know there are others in the class like them.

Transformational learning is a teaching approach that promotes critical autonomous thinking. The changing work environment and fast pace of technology require the new worker to be an autonomous free thinker, able to adapt to multiple situations. The nurse educator will play a key role in the development of the student who is an autonomous thinker undergoing constant transformation in thinking (Parker & Myrick, 2010).

Derix, J. (1998). Transformative learning in the practice of adult education: An overview. *PAACE Journal of Lifelong Learning,* 7, 1–14.

Mathew-Maich, N., Plog, J., Jack, S., & Dobbins, M. (2010). Transformative learning utilization in nursing practice: A missing link. *Worldview on Evidence Based Practice, 7*, 25–35.

McAlister, M., Tower, M., & Walker, R. (2007). Gentle interruption transformative approaches to clinical teaching. *Journal of Nursing Education, 46*, 304.

McGonigal, K. (2007). Teaching for transformation from learning theory to teaching strategies. *Speaking of Teaching, 14*(2), 1–5.

Mezirow, J. (1997). Transformative learning theory to practice. *New Directions for Adult & Continuing Education*. Retrieved from http://dx.doi.org/10.1002/ace.7401

Parker, B., & Myrick, F. (2010). Transitional learning as a context for human patient simulation. *Journal of Nursing Education, 49*(6), 326. Retrieved from http://dx.doi.org/10.3928101484834–20100224-02

Therese Hulme

TRANSITION INTO PRACTICE

DEFINITION

Transition into practice is the progression of a new graduate nurse as he or she advances from the role of a student nurse to a competent professional registered nurse and a leader at the bedside (Manzano, Rivera, & Sullivan, 2013).

APPLICATION

As the nursing shortage and the complexity of patient care continue to increase, it is imperative that the new graduate is integrated into practice autonomously and successfully. Evidence from the National Council of State Boards of Nursing demonstrates that there is a gap between nursing education and the application of knowledge to practice. Employers stated that new graduate nurses were not adequately prepared to provide safe care (Spector & Li, 2007).

A successful strategy and a best practice in improving the transition to practice for new graduate nurses is a formalized Nurse Residency Program (NRP; Little, Ditmer, & Bashaw, 2013). The Institute of Medicine (IOM, 2011) strongly recommends the development and implementation of NRPs to improve retention of nurses and expand existing competencies, in order to foster improved patient outcomes and quality of care (Little et al., 2013).

SYNOPSIS

The aim of an NRP is to "improve a new graduate's organizational ability and technical skills; encourage the use of outcome data to promote patient safety; strengthening commitment to lifelong learning; and enhance the commitment to nursing as profession" (Manzano et al., 2013, p. 371).

A white paper published by The Joint Commission (2005) states that the University Health System Consortium/American Association of Colleges of Nursing (UHC/AACN) NRP "could serve as a critical model for more broadly based nursing residency programs" (Goode, Lynn, McElroy, Bednash, & Murray, 2013). The UHC/AACN NRP is an evidence-based program consisting of a series of learning seminars and work experiences with a focused curriculum developed in collaboration with the Chief Nursing Officers Council of the UHC and deans from baccalaureate schools of nursing from the AACN (2009) (Goode et al., 2013). The program emphasizes three principal content areas: "leadership, with a focus on managing resources for patient care and collaborating with interprofessional teams; patient safety and outcomes, which enhances knowledge of quality, safety and nurse-sensitive outcomes; and professional role, which includes professional practice issues, managing changing patient conditions, ethics and end-of-life care" (Goode et al., 2013, p. 74).

Measuring the success of an NRP can be performed using metrics such as a favorable return on investment (ROI) rate and a decreased turnover rate for new graduate nurses in the first year of employment (Anderson, Hair, & Todero, 2012; Pine & Tart, 2007). Many studies have shown a positive ROI and decreased turnover after implementation of an NRP (Casey, Fink, Krugman, & Propst, 2004; Williams, Goode, Krsek, Bednash, & Lynn, 2007). In addition, the Casey–Fink Graduate Nurse Experience instrument is widely used to measure the success of the new graduate's transition. The new graduate completes the online survey at the time of hire, after 6 months, and after 1 year of employment. Progression is measured in five main areas: stress, support, organization and prioritizing, communication with leadership, and professional satisfaction (Goode et al., 2013). Data consistently show that all domains of the Casey–Fink demonstrate favorable outcomes after a new graduate nurse completes an NRP (Goode et al., 2013).

RECOMMENDATIONS

Structured NRPs have been effective in assisting the new graduate nurse with the transition into practice (Little et al., 2013). After reviewing the literature, the following recommendations can be made: all new graduate nurses should complete a transition into practice program, such as an NRP that is 1 year in length (Goode et al., 2013; Krugman et al., 2006; Rush, Adamack, Gordon, Lilly, & Janke, 2013; Williams et al., 2007). Second, the NRP's structure should align with the organization's mission, vision, values, and care model to further support the assimilation into the organization's culture (Little et al., 2013). Third, there should be metrics to measure the effectiveness of the program, such as a favorable ROI (Pine & Tart, 2007). Finally, an advisory board should be established to include interprofessional health team members and an academic partner to foster the collaboration between academia and practice to increase organizational buy-in and ensure continued evolution of the NRP to meet the needs of the new graduate nurses.

American Association of Colleges of Nursing (AACN). (2009). *Post baccalaureate nursing residency program: Executive summary.* University Health System Consortium. Retrieved from http://www.aacn.nche .edu/Education/nurseresidency.htm

Anderson, G., Hair, C., & Todero, C. (2012). Nurse residency programs: An evidence-based review of theory, process, and outcomes. *Journal of Professional Nursing, 28*(4), 203–212.

Casey, K., Fink, R., Krugman, M., & Propst, J. (2004). The graduate nurse experience. *The Journal of Nursing Administration, 34*(6), 303–311.

Goode, C. J., Lynn, M. R., McElroy, D., Bednash, G. D., & Murray, B. (2013). Lessons learned from 10 years of research on a post-baccalaureate nurse residency program. *The Journal of Nursing Administration, 43*(2), 73–79.

Institute of Medicine (IOM). (2011). *The future of nursing: Leading change, advancing health.* Washington, DC: The National Academies Press.

Krugman, M., Bretschneider, J., Horn, P. B., Krsek, C. A., Moutafis, R. A., & Smith, M. O. (2006). The national post-baccalaureate graduate nurse residency program: A model for excellence in transition to practice. *Journal for Nurses in Staff Development, 22*(4), 196–205.

Little, J. P., Ditmer, D., & Bashaw, M. A. (2013). New graduate nurse residency: A network approach. *The Journal of Nursing Administration, 43*(6), 361–366.

Manzano, W., Rivera, R. R., & Sullivan, R. (2013). What we have learned from a model nurse residency program: Ideas for linking service and education. *Nursing Education Perspectives, 34*(6), 371.

Pine, R., & Tart, K. (2007). Return on investment: Benefits and challenges of baccalaureate nurse residency program. *Nursing Economics, 25*(1), 13–18, 39, 3; quiz 19.

Rush, K. L., Adamack, M., Gordon, J., Lilly, M., & Janke, R. (2013). Best practices of formal new graduate nurse transition programs: An integrative review.

International Journal of Nursing Studies, 50(3), 345–356.

Spector, N., & Li, S. (2007). A regulatory model on transitioning nurses from education to practice. *JONA'S Healthcare Law, Ethics and Regulation, 9*(1), 19–22.

The Joint Commission. (2005). *Heath care at the crossroads: Strategies for addressing the evolving nursing crisis.* Retrieved from http://www.jointcommission.org/Strategies_for_Addressing_the_Evolving_Nursing_Crisis_/

Williams, C. A., Goode, C. J., Krsek, C., Bednash, G. D., & Lynn, M. R. (2007). Postbaccalaureate nurse residency 1-year outcomes. *The Journal of Nursing Administration, 37*(7–8), 357–365.

Kelly A. Gallagher
Reynaldo R. Rivera

U

UNIVERSITY PARTNERSHIP

DEFINITION

University partnerships are formed among colleges, universities, and their local communities (Office of University Partnerships, 2014). These partnerships can assist communities in addressing local problems and providing students with learning opportunities and a mechanism for development of community awareness. There are seven categories of university partnerships: service learning, service provision, faculty involvement, student volunteerism, community in the classroom, applied research, and major institutional change (Martin & Smith, 2005).

APPLICATION

Each of the categories has distinct applications in nursing education. Service learning involves students in activities in the community as part of their regular coursework. At Auburn University, the School of Nursing partnered with the Early Head Start Program as part of the pre-licensure (bachelor of science in nursing [BSN]) nursing students' childbearing course to provide services to teenage mothers and to develop community service knowledge of nursing of vulnerable populations (Bentley & Ellison, 2005).

Service provisions are long-term coordinated projects involving a specific component of the community (Martin & Smith, 2005). The University of Akron School of Nursing opened its Nursing Center for Community Health in 1982. This center provides nonemergency, episodic, primary care service to the university community as well as the underserved and vulnerable populations in the local community. It provides clinical education for undergraduate and graduate nursing students, medical students, residents, and other health professionals; it also helps generate and share clinical research (The University of Akron School of Nursing, 2014).

Faculty involvement initiatives are projects in which a faculty member is the driving force behind a community activity or initiative (Martin & Smith, 2005). An example of a faculty involvement project is that of a monthly BP clinic at an outreach center for the community supported by the college. The faculty worked with the city health department to determine the high-risk population in the area and invited students to participate in the faculty-managed screening clinic.

Student volunteerism includes voluntary activities that students participate in who are not in any course of instruction (Martin & Smith, 2005). A program at the Massachusetts College of Pharmacy and Health Sciences provides physician assistants and pharmacy and nursing students the opportunity to volunteer at a Head Start Preschool in southern New Hampshire (Gallagher, Cooper, & Durand, 2010).

Community in the classroom is an activity to enhance community growth and education (Martin & Smith, 2005). At the East Tennessee State University School, students developed and delivered a community-based employee wellness program for a rural county school district as one of the course requirements (Florence & Behringer, 2011).

Applied research involves students and faculty in data collection and analysis *u*

(Martin & Smith, 2005). At the Harris College of Nursing of Texas Christian University, undergraduate nursing students who were bilingual and bicultural served as data collectors with Spanish-speaking cancer caregivers in a research project investigating cultural beliefs that influenced caregiving behaviors (Wells & Cagle, 2009).

Major organizational change is needed in order to foster more community and university engagement (Martin & Smith, 2005). Strategic planning at Lorain County Community College (LCCC) involves a 100-member team comprised of external community and regional stakeholders, faculty staff, and students (Mission, Vision, and Values, 2014). The resulting strategic planning process formed the University Center, which provides 40 bachelor and master degree academic partnership programs based on the needs of the local community. One of these was for a registered nurse (RN)–BSN completion program. The University of Akron provides this program on-site as a 3 + 1 program with the associate degree nursing (ADN) program of LCCC, providing more than $40,000 in tuition savings compared to the traditional pre-licensure BSN program by offering all general education courses for the ADN and BSN through LCCC at the community college tuition rate (The University Partnership, 2014).

SYNOPSIS

There are seven types of university partnerships (Martin & Smith, 2005). Service learning engages students in activities in the community as part of a specific course. Service provision is a continuous project involving a specific component of the community, which provides learning experiences for students. Faculty involvement is an initiative in which a faculty member is participating and invites students to participate. Student volunteerism is an activity in which students participate that is not part of any course or requirement. Community in the classroom is a project developed to better the community as part of a specific course

requirement. Applied research utilizes faculty and students in data collection and analysis in community-related research. Major institutional change is accomplished for the purpose of bettering the community the college or university is serving. Furthermore, students were found to have increased community awareness based on the partnership experience (Gallagher et al., 2010).

RECOMMENDATIONS

Nursing education programs have had close working partnerships with local communities in the form of clinical affiliations; however, nursing educators need to expand the partnerships within the framework of university partnership models. Numerous research studies have been carried out to validate the benefits of these university partnership activities for students including personal outcomes, such as personal efficacy, spiritual growth, moral development, and leadership and communication skills; social outcomes, such as cultural sensitivity, social responsibility, citizenship, commitment to service, and volunteerism; learning outcomes, such as academic learning, application to practice, and critical thinking; career development; and a stronger relationship with faculty (Eyler, Giles, Stenson, & Gray, 2001).

Bentley, R., & Ellison, K. J. (2005). Impact of a service-learning project on nursing students. *Nursing Education Perspectives, 26*(5), 287–290.

Eyler, J., Giles, D. E., Jr., Stenson, C. M., & Gray, C. J. (2001). *At a glance: What we know about the effects of service-learning on college students, faculty, institutions and communities, 1993–2000* (3rd ed.). Nashville, TN: Vanderbilt University.

Florence, J., & Behringer, B. (2011). Community as classroom: Teaching and learning public health in rural Appalachia. *Journal of Public Health Management and Practice, 17*(4), 316–323.

Gallagher, H., Cooper, M., & Durand, C. (2010). Effects of an interdisciplinary volunteer experience on students' knowledge of and attitudes toward the health care team. *The Journal of Physician Assistant Education, 21*(3), 27–30.

Martin, L. L., & Smith, H. (2005). Bridging town & gown through innovative university community partnerships. *The Innovation Journal: The Public Sector Innovation Journal, 10*(2), 20th ser. Retrieved from http://www.innovation .cc/peer-reviewed/martin_Bridging%20 town_partnerdships_final4v10i2a3 .pdf

Mission, Vision, and Values. (2014). *Vision 2.0 strategic plan. Building on our past. Designing for our future.* Retrieved from http://www .lorainccc.edu/About+Us/About+LCCC/ Mission_Vision_and_Values.htm

Office of University Partnerships. (2014). Retrieved from http://www.huduser.org/ portal/oup/home.html

The University of Akron School of Nursing. (2014). *The nursing center for community health.* Retrieved from http://www .uakron.edu/nursing/community-engagement/nursing-center-for-community-health.dot

The University Partnership. (2014). *Experience Ohio's best value in higher education.* Retrieved from http://www.lorainccc .edu/UP

Wells, J. N., & Cagle, C. S. (2009). Preparation and participation of undergraduate students to inform culturally sensitive research. *Nurse Education Today, 29,* 505–509.

Hope M. Moon
Mary T. Quinn Griffin

UNSAFE STUDENT

DEFINITION

A student labeled as unsafe, due to the presence of internal and/or external conditions, is unable to uphold patient safety consistent with educational expectations and professional standards. The presence of a singular or combination of compromised physical, affective, cognitive, behavioral, social, and ethical characteristics render students vulnerable to unsafe practice. External conditions, whether associated with academic or health care contexts, may exacerbate the risk for unsafe practice by individual students. Students unable to self-assess and communicate with competent educators struggle in consolidating a professional identity composed of cognitive and performance dimensions.

APPLICATION

Safety is a shared responsibility among educators, students, and clinicians. Despite the best efforts of these individuals, the sanctity of safety is continually threatened (Attree, Cooke, & Wakefield, 2008). Nurse educators, therefore, must be mindful in the selection and provision of appropriate classroom, laboratory, and clinical learning opportunities to facilitate student development commensurate with safeguarding the public. In addition, educators are obligated to enact evidence-informed educational strategies; be vigilant for risks; detect unsafe students and unsafe circumstances; accommodate and remediate, if appropriate; and remove unsafe students from practice.

As students advance through programs of study, the breadth and depth of the responsibility for patient safety increases. Therefore, it is imperative that leveled cognitive, affective, and practice expectations are explicitly detailed and consistently upheld to avoid the progression of unsafe students. Purposeful dialogue among educators, students, and clinicians about patient safety is a precursor to safe practice. A learning partnership, characterized by mutuality, trust, and open communication (Gillespie, 2005), allows students to integrate formative constructive feedback to support safety in practice. Despite appropriately guided learning and timely evaluative appraisal, unsafe students are unable to achieve minimal expectations for safe practice.

U

SYNOPSIS

The presence of unsafe practitioners involved in the care of individuals, families, and communities is a global concern. As novices, students are susceptible to compromising safety at many points during their learning processes. The etiology of unsafe practice is a complex interplay of individual student factors and system circumstances. In response, educational programs have been developed with an overt focus on safety competencies (National Patient Safety Foundation, 2014; Quality and Safety Education for Nurses Institute, 2014; World Health Organization, 2011). Shared foci across such programs include evidence-informed knowledge; patient-centeredness; roles and responsibilities; clinical reasoning; health informatics; and theories of communication, systems, and risk management. Emergent programs, primarily created to generate safe practitioners, emphasize the need for comprehensive safety curricula (Brady, 2011).

From the perspective of senior nursing students, the profile of an unsafe student includes compromised professional accountability, uncritical knowledge transfer, non-patient-centeredness, impaired interactions, unsatisfactory clinical performance, and unsubstantiated clinical progression (Killam et al., 2012). Educators are held accountable for their role in upholding the safety mandate and protecting the public (American Association of Colleges of Nursing [AACN], 2013; Canadian Nurses Association, 2014). The evidence to date does not specify a definitive educational approach to mitigate the presence of unsafe students in their learning. However, much of the available research has used nonexperimental designs to investigate teaching and learning strategies to facilitate student safety. Problem-based learning, for example, has been identified as a promising strategy to bridge the gap between theory and practice, ultimately promoting safety (Khan, Ali, Vazir, Barolia, & Rehan, 2012; Larue, 2008). Similarly, simulation assists educators to evaluate application of safety competencies

with the advantage of providing immediate performance feedback both during and following the learning activity. This offers students the opportunity to reflect upon, refine, and correct their performance prior to direct patient contact (Shearer, 2013).

There is much evidence addressing medication errors, which may or may not lead to adverse patient events or the designation of an individual student as unsafe. Such errors are attributable to an interaction of individual, clinical, and programmatic variables (Sulosaari, Kajander, Hupli, Huupponen, & Leino-Kilpi, 2012). For the development of medication competency, Ramjan (2011) emphasized the need to integrate "real" world clinical situations across written, visual, and hands-on learning experiences. Such activities must be designed to mitigate knowledge deficits, address systems issues, and promote adherence to appropriate procedural practices (Reid-Searl, Moxham, & Happell, 2010).

RECOMMENDATIONS

All nursing programs must purposefully integrate opportunities for students to develop and refine safety competencies as they progress toward graduation. Adequate human, physical, and financial resources must be allocated to plan, deliver, and evaluate safety curricula. Regardless of curricula structure, educators are charged with the formidable responsibility of supporting the development of safe students. In doing so, they must continuously deliberate students' right to learn against patients' right to safety. Deliberations must be guided by clear organizational policies and practices that uphold safety. Ultimately, educators must be prepared to identify, intervene, and remove unsafe students from practice.

Given that purposeful dialogue about patient safety is identified as a precursor to safe practice, communication among students, educators, and clinicians is essential. The development of formal collaborative partnerships between academic and practice organizations may provide the structure to allow for regular and recorded communication. Communication about patient safety that meets learning needs, identifies risks for unsafe practice, evaluates learning outcomes, and complies with professional and practice setting policies will mitigate the presence of unsafe students in practice.

American Association of Colleges of Nursing (AACN). (2013). *Fact sheet: Creating a more highly qualified nursing workforce.* Retrieved from http://www.aacn.nche.edu/media-relations/NursingWorkforce.pdf

Attree, M., Cooke, H., & Wakefield, A. (2008). Patient safety in an English pre-registration nursing curriculum. *Nurse Education in Practice, 8*(4), 239–248.

Brady, D. S. (2011). Using quality and safety education for nursing (QSEN) as a pedagogical structure for course redesign and content. *International Journal of Nursing Education Scholarship, 8*(1), Article 5.

Canadian Nurses Association. (2014). *Competencies for entry-level registered nurse practice.* Retrieved from http://www.cno.org/Global/docs/reg/41037_EntryToPracitic_final.pdf

Gillespie, M. (2005). Student-teacher connection: A place of possibility. *Journal of Advanced Nursing, 52*(2), 211–219.

Khan, B. A., Ali, F., Vazir, N., Barolia, R., & Rehan, S. (2012). Students' perceptions of clinical teaching and learning strategies: A Pakistani perspective. *Nurse Education Today, 32*(1), 85–90.

Killam, L. A., Montgomery, P., Raymond, J. M., Mossey, S., Timmermans, K. E., & Binette, J. (2012). Unsafe clinical practices as perceived by final year baccalaureate nursing students: Q methodology. *BMC Nursing, 11*, 26.

Larue, C (2008). Group learning strategies for nursing students: Reflections on the tutor role. *International Journal of Nursing Education Scholarship, 5*(1), Article 30.

National Patient Safety Foundation. (2014). *Patient safety curriculum.* Retrieved from http://www.npsf.org/online-learning-center/patient-safety-curriculum-2/

Quality and Safety Education for Nurses Institute. (2014). *Project overview: The evolution of the quality and safety education for nurses (QSEN) initiative.* Retrieved from qsen.org/about-qsen/project-overview/

Ramjan, L. M. (2011). Contextualism adds realism: Nursing students' perceptions of and performance in numeracy skills tests. *Nurse Education Today, 31*(8), e16–e21.

Reid-Searl, K., Moxham, L., & Happell, B. (2010). Enhancing patient safety: The importance of direct supervision for avoiding medication errors and near misses by undergraduate nursing students. *International Journal of Nursing Practice, 16*(3), 225–232.

Shearer, J. E. (2013). High-fidelity simulation and safety: An integrative review. *Journal of Nursing Education, 52*(1), 39–45.

Sulosaari, V., Kajander, S., Hupli, M., Huupponen, R., & Leino-Kilpi, H. (2012). Nurse students' medication competence—an integrative review of the associated factors. *Nurse Education Today, 32*(4), 399–405.

World Health Organization. (2011). *Patient safety curriculum guide: Multi-professional education.* Malta, Greece: WHO.

Phyllis Montgomery
Sharolyn Mossey
Laura Killam

U

V

VIRTUAL LEARNING

DEFINITION

Virtual learning (VL) is an online educational process that allows students to access, communicate, share, and/or acquire knowledge with the teachers and fellow students. Using software applications and computer systems available on the Internet, VL can take place regardless of geographic and time zones. The VL environment (VLE) supports activities mediated by information and communication technology (ICT) such as real-time video or web conference. VLE mimics what traditional classrooms provide by posting predefined course requirements through bulletin boards, e-mail notification, and forums/blogs through asynchronous communication, or conducting real-time classroom lectures or question-and-answer sessions via chat rooms or instant messaging through asynchronous communication. VL is interchangeably identified as similar to other educational technologies such as distance learning, e-learning, or online learning due to the use of ICT.

APPLICATION

Franceschi, Lee, Zanakis, and Hinds (2009) described virtual worlds as online sites with virtual landscapes, buildings, and artifacts, where multiple users adopt fantasy identities, role-play, and interact simultaneously through the use of avatars (a virtual person that represents the computer user) in a three-dimensional (3D) simulated environment. The most common and distinguishing characteristics of virtual worlds include the support of multiple players, a persistent 3D environment, social-networking capabilities, and visual similarity to the real world. Second Life (Skiba, 2007), Mirror Lake (Curran, Elfrink, & Mays, 2009), Stillwell, and The Neighborhood (Giddens, Shuster, & Roehrig, 2010) are examples of virtual communities that use innovative approaches to frame scenarios in an authentic, relevant, and safe environment. The application of these virtual worlds in nursing education is intended to augment student learning, as well as provide problem-based experience, social and group interaction, and patient engagement. Key standards of nursing care that could be taught in the virtual community are composed of characters with various demographic backgrounds and health care agencies. Medical records, photos, and videos enhance the VLE. Learning contents incorporated in VL can run over several academic terms including clinical reasoning on patient health risk factors, relationship-based care across care settings, clinical indicators of chronic disease processes, social consequences of disease, and influence of environmental factors.

Grady (2011) applied techniques from telehealth to implement a virtual clinical practicum in a Pennsylvania nursing program to address barriers related to distance, time, and specialty faculty expertise using video teleconferencing. The virtual clinical practicum focused on a complex case and progression of care for a patient who had suffered burn injuries in a remote war-torn area. This type of specialized clinical experience would not have been available to these students without the innovative VLE.

SYNOPSIS

The VL strategies and ICT provide methods to enhance the traditional nursing education, balance the challenges with nursing faculty shortage, and accommodate limited classroom and clinical space (Murray, 2013). An integrative review of literature on the use of virtual worlds in nursing and health care education identified three top design considerations in VL. These are clinical reasoning skills, student-centered learning, and instructional format (De Gagne, Oh, Kang, Vorderstrasse, & Johnson, 2013). The virtual clinical practicum allowed an opportunity for dialogue with the instructor, critical reflection, and synthesis of events via technology.

RECOMMENDATIONS

Nursing faculty must engage with students, strive to facilitate a sense of belonging, and ensure a safe learning environment to fully realize the benefits of VL techniques in nursing education (De Gagne et al., 2013; Grady, 2011). Providing orientation sessions on the use of VL is an important aspect to consider in minimizing students' frustration due to technical issues. Availability of technical resources for the course can enhance positive and effective learning experiences (De Gagne et al., 2013). The success of implementing a sound web-based instruction program using virtual worlds requires thoughtful planning, committed faculty, and administrators who are willing to invest in technical support and equipment. Further studies will support and expand the evidence base of VL strategies to justify a return on investment in meeting current and future demands of nursing education.

Curran, C. R., Elfrink, V., & Mays, B. (2009). Building a virtual community for nursing education: The town of mirror lake. *Journal of Nursing Education, 48*(1), 30–35.

De Gagne, J. C., Oh, J., Kang, J., Vorderstrasse, A. A., & Johnson, C. M. (2013). Virtual worlds in nursing education: A synthesis of the literature. *Journal of Nursing Education, 52*(7), 391–396. doi: 10.3928/01484834–20130610-03.

Franceschi, K., Lee, R. M., Zanakis, S. H., & Hinds, D. (2009). Engaging group e-learning in virtual worlds. *Journal of Management Information Systems, 26*(1), 73–100. doi:10.2753/MIS0742–1222260104.

Giddens, J. F., Shuster, G., & Roehrig, N. (2010). Early student outcomes associated with a virtual community for learning. *Journal of Nursing Education, 49*(6), 355–358. doi: 10.3928/01484834–20100217-03

Grady, J. L. (2011). The virtual clinical practicum: An innovative telehealth model for clinical nursing education. *Nursing Education Perspectives, 32*(3), 189–194.

Murray, T. A. (2013). Innovations in nursing education: The state of the art. *Journal of Nursing Regulation, 3*(4), 25–31.

Skiba, D. J. (2007). Nursing education 2.0: Second Life. *Nursing Education Perspectives, 28*, 156–157.

Mary Joy Garcia-Dia
Amy Reiterman

VIRTUAL LEARNING ENVIRONMENTS: SECOND LIFE

DEFINITION

A virtual learning environment (VLE) is an interconnected set of tools and resources used to manage, deliver, and assess online learning. One example of a VLE is Second Life (SL). SL is a virtual, three-dimensional application that is fully interactive and mimics the real world. Individuals are represented graphically in SL by avatars that allow them to engage with the environment and other avatars (people). As a VLE, SL is an engaging and collaborative learning experience.

APPLICATION

Nurse educators and administrators are finding that SL is a potent learning space for nursing education. This graphically robust virtual world can address diverse learning styles while providing a variety of learning experiences. SL can be used to provide passive learning methods, such as lectures, posters, or exhibits. However, an advantage of teaching in virtual environments is that engaging learning strategies can be offered to students. Through the social interactivity in SL, there is a sense of presence that improves learning outcomes through the following learning activities: immersion, collaboration, building, and communication.

SL provides many opportunities for students to immerse in the virtual environment and to try on professional roles in a safe, supportive environment. Students engage in scenarios, simulations, and gaming to learn concepts and develop their future roles. For example, a scenario in which students role-play with other avatars in a culturally diverse virtual working environment can provide a safe space to simulate the challenges experienced in the real world. Using programmed clinical simulations, students can also learn to prioritize actions to take when practicing procedures, such as medication and blood administration, and to practice the critical thinking needed to provide professional care.

Students can collaborate, practice critical thinking skills, and problem-solve with each other in virtual meetings, explorations, treasure hunts, and building projects. Virtual hospitals, clinics, and colleges serve as clinical sites where students can work through a clinical case study and plan care based on research evidence.

SL provides both geographical spaces and opportunities to develop projects related to learning outcomes. For example, students can build and set up equipment and supplies for virtual hospitals and clinics, colleges, and even entire communities. They can also write business plans; develop curriculum plans; and apply evidence to real clinical, educational, and administrative issues.

Students can practice interprofessional communication skills in SL in addition to interacting with patient avatars in clinical encounters, counseling sessions, or support groups. SL's virtual space can be used by organizations to offer continuing professional development sessions and professional meetings that do not require travel, thus reaching out to practitioners in rural, underserved areas or other far-off places.

SYNOPSIS

Newer generations of college students are accustomed to technological teaching methods, authentic assignments, gaming, simulation, and interaction with other learners. Thus, they are open to exploring and learning in virtual environments (Veltman, Connor, Honey, Diener, & Bodily, 2012). The advantage of teaching and learning in SL is that students build on previous learning in a socially interactive environment, resulting in deeper learning. Realistic physical spaces, such as hospitals or clinics, can be designed for students to practice clinical skills. Students and faculty can access these spaces across the world (Veltman et al., 2012). In terms of student engagement, working with avatar-based case studies is well received by students (Anderson, Page, & Wendorf, 2013; Foronda, Liu, & Bauman, 2013).

Research on using virtual environments helps students meet learning outcomes, enhances student satisfaction and confidence, promotes collaboration and communication, and helps students meet clinical competencies (Aebersold, Tschannen, Stephens, Anderson, & Xuefeng, 2012; Anderson et al., 2013; Foronda et al., 2013; Miller & Jensen, 2014). SL is an effective environment for learning how to work with culturally diverse patients (Games & Bauman, 2011). Additionally, participating in simulations in a VLE promotes communication skills and professional behavior (Veltman et al., 2012) as well as interviewing skills (Sweigart & Hodson-Carlton, 2013).

SL is a learner-centered methodology where power is shared by faculty and students, content is background to developing skills, teachers facilitate learning, student autonomy is encouraged, and assessment of learning is multifactorial with the goal of improving learning (Foronda et al., 2013; Miller & Jensen,

V

V

2014). Students enjoy defining their own characteristics in SL by turning their avatars into representatives of their own racial–ethnic identities (Lee & Park, 2011). Although student satisfaction with learning in SL is high (Anderson et al., 2013; Bai, Lavin, & Duncan, 2012), further research is needed on how learning in VLEs affects learning outcomes (Foronda et al., 2013; Miller & Jensen, 2014).

RECOMMENDATIONS

Faculty members should first decide why they want to use SL and how it can be used to meet learning needs. Faculty also need to be committed to the virtual environment. Anyone can enter a public island in SL, so purchasing an island that allows for secure access is recommended. The charge for educational institutions to purchase islands has historically been less expensive than for individuals. Unless the organization has the appropriate personnel on staff, consultants are available for planning and building physical environments in the organization's islands as well as for developing scenarios and simulations. Personnel who are working in SL will need training and practice time, so building an adequate timeline is important. Support is also needed to handle any technical issues.

Policies on correct dress and behavior of students while they are in SL mimics comparable policies in real settings. Be aware, though, that students are likely to want to alter their avatars with respect to race and culture. Students will need orientation and training in order to learn the motor skills featured in SL. Walking, running, flying, opening doors, and other activities in SL need to be practiced. Providing Second Life URLS (SLURLS) is useful to help students find where they need to go in SL to participate in educational activities.

Integrating SL into courses and curricula begins with learning about using VLEs and exploring SL to make informed decisions about how to integrate SL into the curriculum. Scrutinizing the literature to discover SL's advantages and disadvantages is important so the advantages can be leveraged and the disadvantages minimized. Multiple ways

of using SL should be explored to determine the best approach for the learners to be able to meet the learning episode outcomes. With a focus on learner-centered educational activities, SL can be a rich resource that provides opportunities for learning to transcend the real world in a safe environment.

Aebersold, M., Tschannen, D., Stephens, M., Anderson, P., & Xuefeng, M. (2012). Second Life in education nursing students. *Clinical Simulation in Nursing, 2012*(8), 469–475.

Anderson, J. K., Page, A. M., & Wendorf, D. M. (2013). Avatar-assisted case studies. *Nurse Educator, 38*(3), 106–109.

Bai, X., Lavin, J., & Duncan, R. O. (2012). Are we there yet? Lessons learned through promoting 3D learning in higher education. *The International Journal of Learning, 18*(6), 1–14.

Foronda, C., Liu, S., & Bauman, E. B. (2013). Evaluation of simulation in undergraduate nurse education: An integrative review. *Clinical Simulation in Nursing, 9*(10), e409–e416. doi:10.1016/j.ecns.2012.11.003

Games, I., & Bauman, E. (2011) Virtual worlds: An environment for cultural sensitivity education in the health sciences. *International Journal of Web Based Communities, 7*(2), 189–205. doi:10.1504/IJWBC.2011.039510

Lee, J. E., & Park, S. G. (2011). "Whose second life is this?" How avatar-based racial cues shape ethno-racial minorities' perception of virtual worlds. *Cyberpsychology, Behavior and Social Networking, 14*(11), 637–642.

Miller, M., & Jensen, R. (2014). Avatars in nursing: An integrative review. *Nurse Educator, 39*(1), 38–41.

Sweigart, L., & Hodson-Carlton, K. (2013). Improving student interview skills: The virtual avatar as client. *Nurse Educator, 38*(1), 11–15.

Veltman, M., Connor, K., Honey, M., Diener, S., & Bodily, D. (2012). Collaborative practice through simulations in a multiuser virtual environment. *Computers, Informatics, Nursing, 30*(2), 63–67.

Rebecca J. Sisk
Dee McGonigle

W

WIKI TECHNOLOGY

DEFINITION

Developed in 1994, *wiki*, the Hawaiian word meaning quick or fast, refers to technology that enables collective authorship of associated web pages (Martin, 2012). Wikis have been used in higher education since the late 1990s and allow students to read, edit, exchange ideas, reorganize, add content, and peer review documents. The history function of wiki tools tracks edits and contributions of visitors, allowing page edits to be saved or reversed to an earlier version. Tracking the edits demonstrates the accumulation of knowledge over time. Considerations on security, cost, ease of use, and accessibility when selecting wiki tools are important decision choices (Beyer, 2012). The most recognizable wiki is Wikipedia, an online encyclopedia.

APPLICATION

One of the greatest advantages of wikis is the ability to facilitate group work or projects in nursing education. Ciesielka (2008) used a wiki with graduate-level nursing students in a community health course. Martin (2012) conducted a mixed-methods study of both qualitative and quantitative data to improve graduate-level nursing education students' writing skills through the use of a wiki and then evaluated their satisfaction with the assignment and technology. Beyer (2012) used group wiki in conjunction with simulation as a debriefing tool for students to share immediate feedback about their experience. The use of wiki in these various learning processes enables students to collaborate online, and share information, resources, and experiences with peers as well as the course instructor (Kardong-Edgren et al., 2009). Through discussion boards, creation of wiki pages, and question-and-answer postings, students are able to analyze data, identify problems, and develop action plans, thus facilitating cooperative learning and interactive communication with peers (Ciesielka, 2008). Stutsky and Doak (2013) used a wiki as the platform for the creation of a collaborative online textbook in a baccalaureate program for nurses. The collaborative design lends to peer feedback for review of content, improvement of writing skills, and potential opportunity to self-publish (Kardong-Edgren et al., 2009). The wiki can also be used in any nursing course for written assignments such as care plans, concept maps, clinical worksheets, research papers, literature reviews, annotated bibliographies, and book writing. In addition, a wiki is a useful administrative tool for faculty and committees (Kardong-Edgren et al., 2009), allowing participants to communicate with each other, brainstorm, postminutes, share documents for review, and save resources. Wiki technology is also useful in simplifying preparation of collaborative reports and other documents that require information from multiple sources. A wiki can be used for clinical preceptor development by including course outlines, resources, clinical requirements, student goals, and a discussion board to explore strategies for working with students in the clinical setting. Faculty members can use a wiki for developing course documents, instructional materials, and for sharing teaching strategies with colleagues (Kardong-Edgren et al., 2009). The wiki writing assignment introduces

W

students, faculty, and the community to student projects while exposing students to new technology. The wiki assignment encourages active engagement and deeper learning.

SYNOPSIS

Wikis are effective in teaching subject matter that benefits from collaborative efforts, knowledge development, and content-building experience (Billings, 2009).

The ease of use and simple design of wiki technology allow both students and educators to use the tool, offering opportunities for continued learning (Martin, 2012). Applying wiki in nursing education and clinical settings can promote interprofessional collaboration, simplify project development, provide peer support, and link users to information provided by national health care organizations.

RECOMMENDATIONS

Wikis are effective innovative tools to promote active student engagement and deeper learning, allowing a collaborative approach for any type of nursing project (Martin, 2012; Stutsky & Doak, 2013). Providing a nurturing and supportive environment for students is important to allow students to understand wiki capabilities and limitations. Demonstrating how to create a basic wiki page using design aesthetics by bringing experts and allowing students plenty of practice time can minimize frustration. Additional research is needed with larger sample sizes to increase the generalizability of the results and to test the efficacy and effectiveness of

wikis as a pedagogical method in nursing education. Further studies are needed to support and expand on the initial evidence base of innovative technology tools to assist educators to meet the current and future demands of nursing education.

Beyer, D. A. (2012). Enhancing critical reflection on simulation through wikis. *Clinical Simulation in Nursing, 8*(2), e67–e70. doi: 10.1016/j.ecns.2010.12.003

Billings, D. M. (2009). Wikis and blogs: Consider the possibilities for continuing nursing education. *The Journal of Continuing Education in Nursing, 40*(12), 534–535.

Ciesielka, D. (2008). Using a wiki to meet graduate nursing education competencies in collaboration and community health. *Journal of Nursing Education, 47*(10), 473–476.

Kardong-Edgren, S. E., Oermann, M. H., Ha, Y., Tennant, M. N., Snelson, C., Hallmark, E.,... Hurd, D. (2009). Using a wiki in nursing education and research. *International Journal of Nursing Education Scholarship, 6*(1), doi:10.2202/1548–923X.1787

Martin, C. T. (2012). Promoting pedagocial experimentation: Using a wiki in graduate level education. *Computers, Informatics, Nursing, 30*(12), 655–660.

Stutsky, B. J., & Doak, K. (2013). Engaging students in the creation of a collaborative wiki textbook. *Computers, Informatics, Nursing, 31*(7), 299–304. doi:10.1097/NXN.0b013e3182a06e99

Amy Reiterman
Mary Joy Garcia-Dia

INDEX